Fitness and Well-Being for Life

Second Edition

Carol K. Armbruster, PhD

Indiana University Bloomington, Professor Emeritus

Ellen M. Evans, PhD

Indiana University Bloomington

Catherine M. Laughlin, HSD, MPH

Indiana University Bloomington

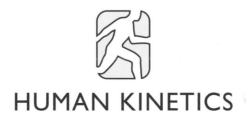

HUMAN KINETICS

Library of Congress Cataloging-in-Publication Data

Library of Congress Cataloging-in-Publication Data
Names: Armbruster, Carol Kennedy, 1958- author. | Evans, Ellen M., 1965-
author. | Laughlin, Catherine M. 1965- author.
Title: Fitness and well-being for life / Carol K. Armbruster, PhD., Indiana
University Bloomington, Professor Emeritus, Ellen M. Evans, PhD.,
Catherine M. Laughlin, HSD, MPH, Indiana University Bloomington.
Other titles: Fitness and wellness
Description: Second edition. | Champaign, IL, USA : Human Kinetics, [2025]
| Originally published: Fitness and wellness.1st edition, 2019. |
Includes bibliographical references and index.
Identifiers: LCCN 2023039517 (print) | LCCN 2023039518 (ebook) | ISBN
9781718213463 (paperback) | ISBN 9781718213470 (epub) | ISBN
9781718213487 (pdf) | ISBN 9781718221055 (loose-leaf)
Subjects: LCSH: Physical fitness--Study and teaching (Higher)--Canada. |
Exercise--Study and teaching (Higher)--Canada. | Health--Study and
teaching (Higher)--Canada.
Classification: LCC RA781 .K446 2025 (print) | LCC RA781 (ebook) | DDC
613.7071/171--dc23/eng/20231018
LC record available at https://lccn.loc.gov/2023039517
LC ebook record available at https://lccn.loc.gov/2023039518

ISBN: 978-1-7182-1346-3 (paperback)

ISBN: 978-1-7182-2105-5 (loose-leaf)

Senior Acquisitions Editor: Amy N. Tocco; **Senior Developmental Editor:** Christine M. Drews; **Managing Editor:** Melissa J. Zavala; **Copyeditor:** Heather Gauen Hutches; **Proofreader:** Joyce H.-S.Li; **Indexer:** Rebecca L. McCorkle; **Permissions Manager:** Laurel Mitchell; **Senior Graphic Designer:** Sean Roosevelt; **Cover Designer:** Keri Evans; **Cover Design Specialist:** Susan Rothermel Allen; **Photograph (cover):** © Tashi-Delek/E+/Getty Images; **Photographs (interior):** © Human Kinetics, unless otherwise noted on the Photo Credits pages; **Photo Asset Manager:** Laura Fitch; **Photo Production Manager:** Jason Allen; **Senior Art Manager:** Kelly Hendren; **Art Style Development:** Joanne Brummett; **Illustrations:** © Human Kinetics, unless otherwise noted; **Printer:** Walsworth

Printed in the United States of America   10 9 8 7 6 5 4 3 2 1

The paper in this book was manufactured using responsible forestry methods.

Human Kinetics
1607 N. Market Street
Champaign, IL 61820
USA

United States and International
Website: **US.HumanKinetics.com**
Email: info@hkusa.com
Phone: 1-800-747-4457

Canada
Website: **Canada.HumanKinetics.com**
Email: info@hkcanada.com

E8634 (paperback) / E9072 (loose-leaf)

CONTENTS

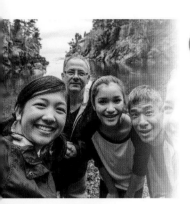
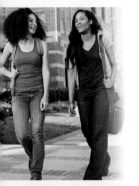
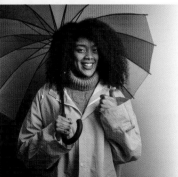
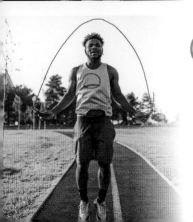

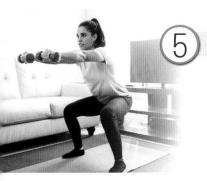

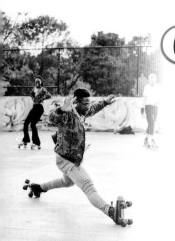

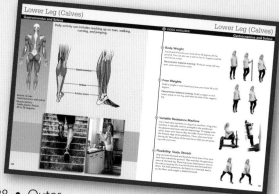

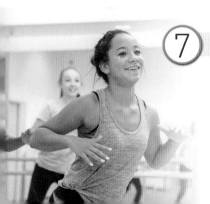

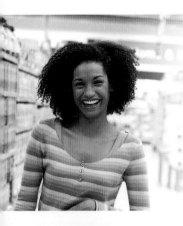

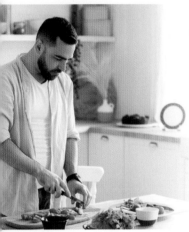

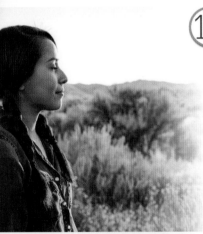

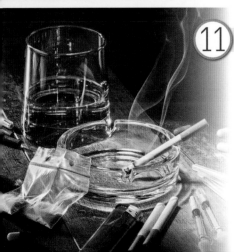

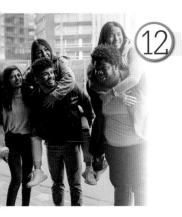
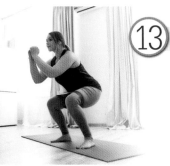
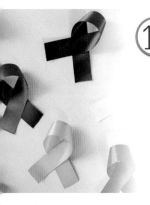
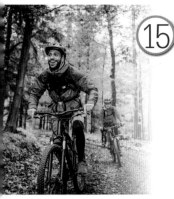

PREFACE

Welcome to *Fitness and Well-Being for Life, Second Edition*. We are glad you are joining us for this exciting journey. The behaviors you start now will become your daily habits that determine your lifestyle. If these behaviors, healthy or less healthy, continue after your college years, your lifestyle will have major consequences for your functional fitness. We hope you invest in your health and incorporate the healthy choices described in this book now and for the rest of your life. Our intent is to help you improve your quality of life by intentionally applying evidence-based concepts of health and well-being to your daily living practices. Our overall philosophy is that a healthy body is the key to a healthy mind and a life well lived.

This book is a labor of love by three professionals, academics, and mothers who have over 80 years of combined experience in the health and well-being profession. We watched our children grow up in the Internet age and saw outdoor play be replaced by organized activities and screen time. We also experienced face-to-face conversations being replaced by email, text messages, tweets, and more. In response to these lifestyle changes in today's society, we developed this book with you and our children in mind. We want to give you the tools you need to successfully manage your life and your health behaviors so you can live your life to the fullest.

Concepts in this book involve the following:

- Focusing on your personal behavior choices rather than following a prescription for health and well-being
- Appreciating the complexity of health behavior change and learning how to tackle your less healthy habits through goal setting and the application of behavior change concepts
- Applying evidence-based research and government guidelines regarding physical activity, exercise, and sedentary behavior to your daily movement habits
- Incorporating evidence-based recommendations regarding dietary intake and sleep into your daily routines to obtain quality fueling and optimal restoration

- Dealing with sensitive health issues related to sexuality, stress management, and mental health (such as anxiety and depression) that may influence your lives and those of the people you love
- Understanding that your health behavior choices greatly influence your functional fitness now and as you progress through your ages and stages of life.

Functional Fitness and Well-Being Integrated

We regularly hear from our students that they do not have enough time to take care of themselves. Our students also frequently complain about being stressed out and tired. One of the major goals of this book is therefore to educate you about what to do (i.e., recommendations by experts) and then give you tools to help you manage your health behaviors. We all recognize that our modern environment does not help us make the healthy choice the easy choice. It is our hope that you will gain some realistic behavioral strategies and motivational muscles to help you make healthier choices most of your days.

As you invest time and effort into your daily health behaviors and practices, you will improve your functional fitness and your general well-being. This means you will both feel better and function better. For example, you will find that your sleep quality will improve, and your anxiety will likely be reduced. You might also have less neck and back pain from the required computer screen time for your academics. Your concentration will likely improve, and your academic work will be less stressful. In sum, you will have more energy to do all the tasks and activities you *have* to do, with energy left to do all the things you also *want* to do. It is likely that the concepts covered in this textbook will greatly change your way of thinking about your behaviors and your health and well-being. A key concept is to design your life to make the healthy choice the easy choice. For example, instead of, or in addition to, paying for a fitness facility membership and making time for an intentional exercise routine, you can focus on moving more throughout the day. With this approach, your physical and social environment become "fitness facilities." Try taking the stairs instead of the escalator, or go to class with a walking partner or biking buddy instead of taking the bus. Or plan a hike in nature with your friends to stay socially connected. Perhaps you can organize a group exercise gathering in your residence hall or your apartment complex using high-intensity interval training techniques, and everyone can bring a different piece of equipment. Similar ideas can be used for healthy eating, with your friends gathering for a group study session and bringing their favorite dish to share—a strategy that also saves money.

Our Functional Fitness Training section after chapter 6 shows you the purpose for strengthening specific muscles and includes exercises that you can perform both inside and outside of a fitness facility. Most of these exercises have a corresponding video on HK*Propel*, where you'll also find workouts with video samples to help you maintain your routine and reach your fitness goals. We hope that this book will help you rethink what it means to take care of yourself so that you can do so more simply, making the healthier choice the easier choice.

How This Book Is Organized

Fitness and Well-Being for Life, Second Edition, has 15 chapters. We realize that many people begin their journey toward healthy practices with physical movement; therefore, chapters 1 to 6 focus on the guidelines for exercise, physical activity, and sedentary behavior, as well as the importance of functional fitness choices. The beginning of the book helps you evaluate your physical health behaviors for moving and choosing not to move. Thinking about being more physically active and being aware of the consequences of too much sitting time can motivate you to incorporate movement into your day. Habitual movement can help us feel better, work better, and sleep better so that we can live our best lives.

Chapters 7 to 9 tackle healthy body composition, eating practices, and weight management, which are often difficult to achieve with the college lifestyle and even more so as you leave college and life typically gets more complicated. We provide you with the tools you need to manage your health behaviors even as your environment changes. Chapters 10 to 15 help you round out your awareness and practice of wellness with information on stress, sleep, addictions, healthy sexuality, and reducing risks for metabolic syndrome and cancer.

Special Features of This Book

This book will help you reach your goals. Each chapter has key terms to help you focus your study efforts and Behavior Check sidebars with specific ideas for integrating health concepts into your daily practices. These sidebars encourage small steps, which are helpful for removing barriers to change. Also included in each chapter are Now and Later sidebars, which help you realize how the positive choices you make today will lead to a healthier tomorrow. Immunity Booster sidebars are especially important, given the recent COVID-19 pandemic. The focus on immune function is an important but often underappreciated aspect of functional fitness.

Throughout the book, you will find infographics, figures, and evidence-based tables to reinforce the information you are learning in an easy-to-understand way. We make an extensive effort to connect research to practice and emphasize that making the healthy choice the easy choice is often about simple daily decisions that make a huge difference in your health, today and in the future.

Instructor Resources

Fitness and Well-Being for Life, Second Edition, is supported by a complete set of ancillaries: presentation package, image bank, instructor guide, test package, and chapter quizzes.

- The instructor guide contains semester- and quarter-based syllabuses; chapter overviews, objectives, and outlines; class activities to engage discussion and promote self-reflection among students; and answers to the in-text chapter review questions.

- The presentation package provides more than 600 PowerPoint slides with selected illustrations and tables from the text.
- The image bank contains most of the figures, tables, and content photos. You can use these images to supplement lecture slides, create handouts, or develop your own presentations and teaching materials.
- The test package contains over 450 questions in a mix of true-false, multiple-choice, fill-in-the-blank, and essay formats.

- The ready-made chapter quizzes allow you to check students' understanding of the most important chapter concepts. Both the test package and chapter quizzes are available in a variety of formats and can be imported into most learning management systems.

All these instructor ancillaries are provided to adopting instructors via the instructor pack on HK*Propel*.

Behavior Check sidebars help you integrate health concepts into your daily practices

Now and Later sidebars encourage you to consider how your actions now will affect you in the future

Immunity Booster sidebars provide tips on improving immunity

Labs found in HK*Propel*

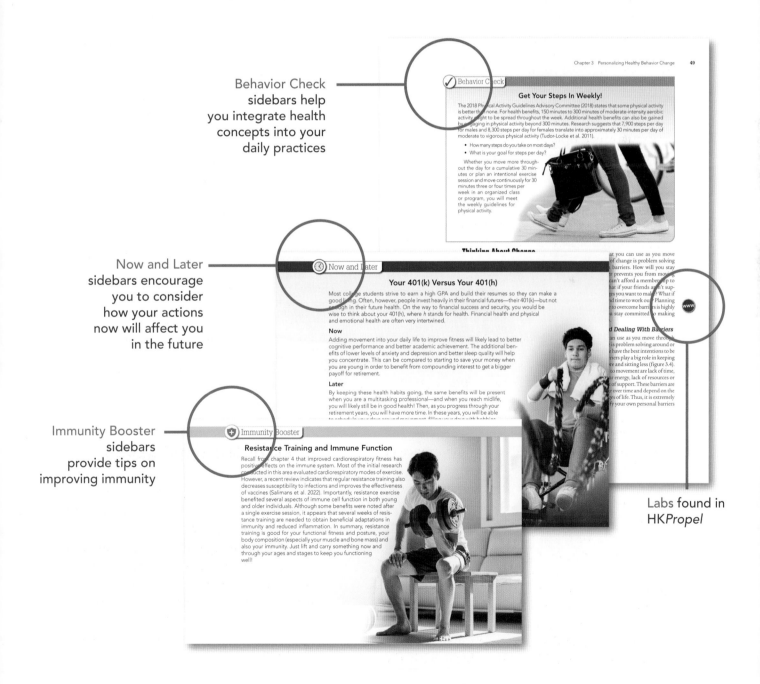

Functional Fitness Training **exercises, with**
video available in HK*Propel*

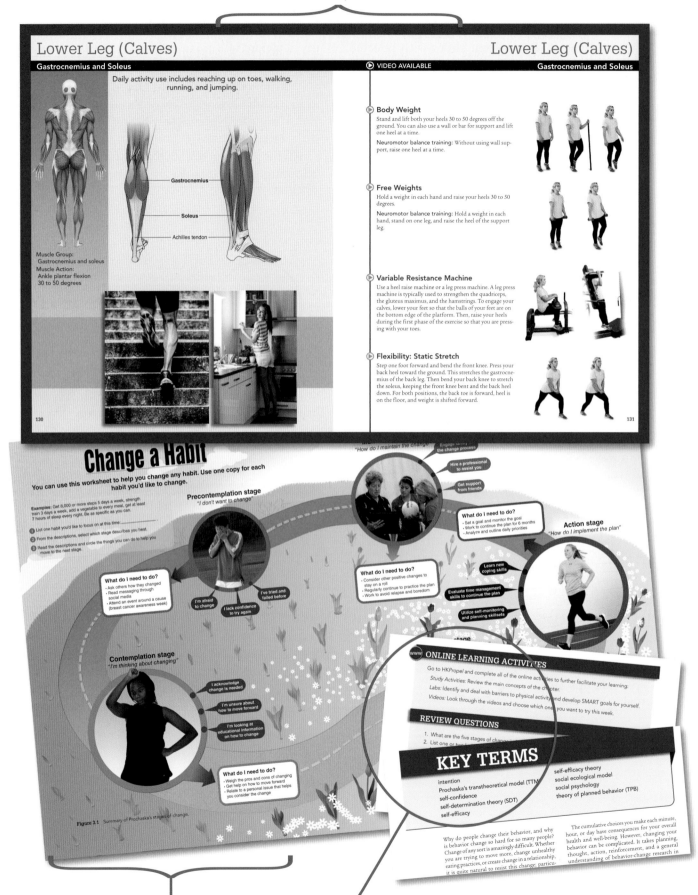

Infographics, **evidence-based**
tables, and figures

Key terms **and**
Review questions

Student Resources

The online learning activities are a powerful resource for students. All online content is provided in HK*Propel*. Interactive study activities will strengthen your understanding of key chapter concepts. Lab activities are provided for every chapter; these can be downloaded, completed, and then submitted to your instructor through a learning management system. The labs include video instructions and demonstrations that involve assessment of fitness components. These assessments focus on your individual scores and provide an opportunity for personal goal setting over the course of a quarter, a semester, or an entire year, even after you have finished the course. HK*Propel* also includes a Functional Fitness Training section, which provides instructions, photos, and videos demonstrating exercise techniques for all major muscle groups. Finally, sample workouts are provided in video format, or you can create your own workouts using any of the exercises demonstrated.

Not only will these online learning activities help you develop a full understanding of course content, but they will also help you evaluate your own fitness and well-being behaviors. Through the lab activities, you will establish goals in the areas of physical activity, exercise, minimizing sedentary behavior, and other key aspects of health—including nutrition, sleep, and stress—and you will be encouraged to make plans that will keep you healthy and well for life!

See the Online Learning Activities section on the next pages for more information.

Final Thoughts

The primary goal of this book is to provide a personal, evidence-based interactive tool to help you lead a healthier, happier, and more productive life. Learning how to take care of yourself so you can take care of others is the first step in making a difference in the world. Although we are rarely encouraged to practice prevention early in our lifetime, we need to take responsibility for charting our own paths to a state of well-being. Taking charge of your health, rather than waiting for medicine to cure you after you've gotten sick, is an enlightening concept—one that we hope energizes you to be proactive.

Taking care of yourself will help you have the energy you need to be successful in college and beyond. People who love life and have a positive attitude are often those who are the healthiest and happiest—physically, mentally, and emotionally. We are excited to give you the tools you need to embrace healthy behavior changes in your life. Kudos to you for taking this class and being open to the possibilities of what healthy living can do for you, now and in your future. Let's do this!

ONLINE LEARNING ACTIVITIES

HK*Propel* is your source for learning activities that will equip you to make lifestyle changes that matter. You'll find study activities, labs, and videos to support your learning. Your instructor might also assign chapter quizzes and tests through HK*Propel*.

The interactive study activities are designed to help you deepen your understanding of key chapter concepts by interacting with the content in unique ways. Activities include evaluating how virtual characters engage with various components of wellness; analyzing goals and making decisions for virtual characters in preparation for setting your own goals; and thinking more deeply about stress, addiction, and other health and well-being issues.

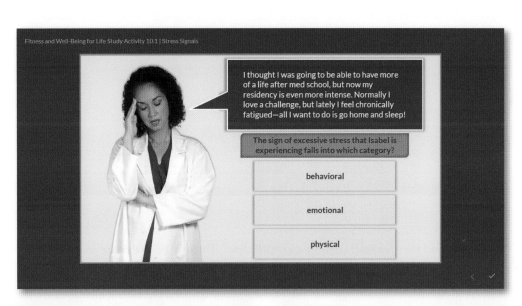

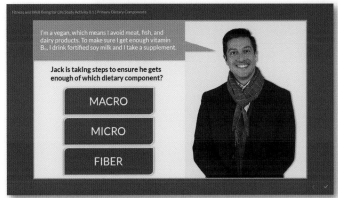

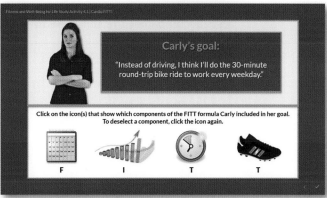

The Functional Fitness Training section, a resource filled with instructions, photos, and videos, can become your personal guide to selecting movement activities that work with your lifestyle and preferences. For every muscle group, we have included several videos demonstrating exercise techniques. We have also included two work-out videos to help you reach your personalized goals.

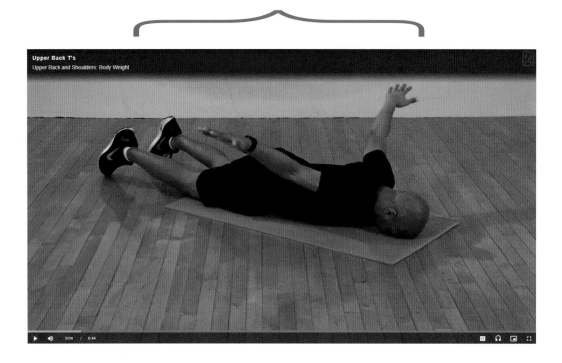

You'll also find labs for each chapter in HK*Propel*. These labs will help you personalize the content as you do such activities as create a family wellness history, consider pros and cons of changing habits, assess your fitness components and set individualized goals, consider aspects related to nutrition, and tackle tough subjects such as body image, addiction, sexual assault, and cancer. A video demonstrating fitness tests accompanies the self-assessment labs.

PHOTO CREDITS

Table of content photos in chronological order: PamelaJoeMcFarlane/E+/Getty Images; Blend Images - Peathegee Inc/Brand X Pictures/Getty Images; AaronAmat/iStock/Getty Images; Supersizer/E+/Getty Images; Antonia Diaz/iStock/Getty Images; Thomas Barwick/DigitalVision/Getty Images; FatCamera/E+/Getty Images; HBSS/Corbis/Getty Images; Fizkes/iStock/Getty Images; Tony Anderson/DigitalVision/Getty Images; Monticello/iStock/Getty Images; Thanit Weerawan/Moment/Getty Images; Lanastock/iStock/Getty Images; John Kevin/iStock/Getty Images; Vm/E+/Getty Images

Page 1: PamelaJoeMcFarlane/E+/Getty Images

Page 2: Biggunsband/iStock/Getty Images

Page 7: South Agency/E+/Getty Images

Page 12: Westend61/Getty Images

Page 13 (from left to right): Maskot/Getty Images; Andresr/E+/Getty Images

Page 14 (from top to bottom): Caiaimage/Sam Edwards/OJO+/Getty Images; Damircudic/E+/Getty Images

Page 15 (from left to right): Tom Merton/Caiaimage/Getty Images; Nathaphat/iStock/Getty Images

Page 16: Yan Lu/iSTock/Getty Images

Page 17: Jordan Siemens/DigitalVision/Getty Images

Page 20: Kali9/E+/Getty Images

Page 21: Tetra Images/Getty Images

Page 22: Tetra Images/Getty Images

Page 23 (clockwise from top): skynesher/E+/Getty Images; Tetra Images/Getty Images; BryanRupp/iStock/Getty Images; Monkeybusinessimages/iStock/Getty Images; Inti St Clair/Blend Images/Getty Images

Page 25: Blend Images - Peathegee Inc/Brand X Pictures/Getty Images

Page 27\: Adam Glanzman/Getty Images

Page 28: Artur Debat/Moment/Getty Images

Page 29: Sadeugra/iStock/ Getty Images

Page 31 (from left to right): Martin Novak/Moment/Getty Images; Wavebreakmedia/iStock /Getty Images Plus

Page 33: Stockbyte/Stockbyte/Getty Images

Page 35: Symphonie/The Image Bank/Getty Images

Page 39: Juanmonino/E+/Getty Images

Page 43: AaronAmat/iStock/Getty Images

Page 44: Hero Images/Getty Images

Page 49: olaser/E+/Getty Images

Page 50: Plume Creative/DigitalVision/Getty Images

Page 54: Westend61/Getty Images

Page 56: Mike Kemp/Tetra Images/Getty Images

Page 59: Westend61/Getty Images

Page 61: Supersizer/E+/Getty Images

Page 62: Martin-Dm/E+/Getty Images

Page 65: Innocenti/Cultura/Getty Images

Page 66: PeopleImages/iStock/Getty Images Plus

Page 69 (from left to right): Mike Kemp/Blend Images/Getty Images; Wavebreakmedia/iStock/Getty Images Plus; Peathegee Inc/Blend Images/Getty Images

Page 69 (bottom): Oliver Eltinger/Corbis/Getty Images

Page 71: Hero Images/Getty Images

Pages 72-73 (from left to right): The Good Brigade/DigitalVision/Getty Images; Image Source/DigitalVision/Getty Images; Jordan Siemens/Getty Images

Page 75: Hero Images/Getty Images

Page 76: technotr/E+/Getty Images

Page 78: Jasmin Merdan/Moment/Getty Images

Page 80: Sturti/E+/Getty Images

Page 81: Westend61/Getty Images

Page 83: Dirima/iStock /Getty Images Plus

Page 84: Idea Images/DigitalVision/Getty Images

Page 85: D Keine/E+/Getty Images

Page 87: Antonia Diaz/iStock/Getty Images

Page 88: Gahsoon/E+/Getty Images

Page 90: David Larson/iStock/Getty Images Plus

Page 91: Laurence Mouton/PhotoAlto Agency RF Collections/Getty Images

Page 93: PeopleImages/iStock/Getty Images

Page 94 (clockwise from left to right): gpointstudio/iStock/Getty Images Plus; diego_cervo/iStock/Getty Images Plus; Antonio_Diaz/iStock/ Getty Images Plus; Tom Merton/Caiaimage/Getty Images; patrickheagney/iStock/Getty Images Plus; skynesher/E+/Getty Images;

Page 96 (from top to bottom): SolStock/E+/Getty Images; Hero Images/Getty Images; Tony Ding/Icon SMI/Corbis/Icon Sportswire via Getty Images; Hill Street Studios/Blend Images/Getty Images

Page 97 (clockwise from top left): PeopleImages/DigitalVision/Getty Images; Dimitri Otis/DigitalVision/Getty Images; Copyright Christopher Peddecord 2009/Moment/Getty Images; Mihailomilovanovic/E+/Getty Images

Page 98: JLPH/Image Source/Getty Images

Page 102: JackF/iStock/Getty Images

Page 105: GoodLifeStudio/E+/Getty Images

Page 107: SolStock/E+/Getty Images

Page 109: Thomas Barwick/DigitalVision/Getty Images

Page 112 (from clockwise from left): AndreyPopov/iStock/Getty Images; Julio Ricco/iStock/Getty Images; Paul Bradbury/Caiaimage/Getty Images; Sam-Stock/iStock/Getty Images; Santa1604/iStock/Getty Images Plus

Page 114 (from left to right): Laurence Mouton/PhotoAlto Agency RF Collections/Getty Images; Luminola/iStock/Getty Images; AndreyPopov/iStock/Getty Images

Page 115: Phynart Studio/E+/Getty Images

Page 116: PeopleImages/DigitalVision/Getty Images

Page 118 Edwin Tan /E+/Getty Images

Page 119 (from left to right): Sam Edwards/OJO Images/Getty Images; Joos Mind/DigitalVision/Getty Images

Page 122: PeopleImages/E+/Getty Images

Page 124: Kali9/E+/Getty Images

Page 129 : Jupiterimages/Goodshoot/Getty Images Plus

Page 130 (from left to right): DaveLongMedia/E+/Getty Images; Philipp Nemenz/Cultura/Getty Images

Page 132 (from left to right): Trinette Reed/Blend Images/Getty Images; Peathegee Inc/Blend Images/Getty Images

Page 134 (from left to right): Klaus Vedfelt/DigitalVision/Getty Images; DK IMAGES / Science Source

Page 136 (from left to right): GROGL/iStock/Getty Images; Maskot/Getty Images

Page 138 (from left to right): Dave and Les Jacobs/Blend Images/Getty Images; Westend61/Getty Images

Page 140 (from left to right): stevecoleimages/E+/Getty Images; BERKO85/iStock/Getty Images

Page 142 (from left to right): laindiapiaroa/Blend Images/Getty Images; Sam Edwards/Caiaimage/Getty Images

Page 144 (left): BJI/Blue Jean Images/Getty Images

Page 146 (from left to right): Bambu Productions/DigitalVision/Getty Images; Westend61/Brand X Pictures/Getty Images

Page 148 (from left to right): Peathegee Inc/Blend Images/Getty Images; technotr/Vetta/Getty Images

Page 150 (from left to right): Tanya Constantine/Blend Images/Getty Images; Malorny/Moment/Getty Images

Page 152 (from left to right): iprogressman/iStock/Getty Images Plus; Sam Edwards/Caiaimage/Getty Images

Page 155: FatCamera/E+/Getty Images

Page 158: Ming H2 Wu/Blend Images/Getty Images

Page 160 (bottom): BSIP/UIG Via Getty Images

Page 161 (top to bottom): © Ellen Evans; BSIP/Universal Images Group/Getty Images; © Ellen Evans; © Ellen Evans

Page 162: Microgen/iStock/Getty Images

Page 163 (top): CHRISTOPHE VANDEREECKEN/REPORTERSf/SCIENCE SOURCE

Page 164: laflor/E+/Getty Images

Page 167: © Ellen Evans

Page 168: Mikolette/E+/Getty Images

Page 169: © Ellen Evans

Page 170: Westend61/Getty Images

Page 171: Meg Haywood-Sullivan/Getty Images

Page 173: Plan Shooting 2/Imazins/Getty Images

Page 175: HBSS/Corbis/Getty Images

Page 177 (from left to right): Jared C. Tilton/Getty Images; Xavierarnau/E+/Getty Images

Page 181: Maskot/Getty Images

Page 183: Anthony Lee/Caiaimage/Getty Images

Page 185: FG Trade Latin/E+/Getty Images

Page 186: Anthony Lee/Caiaimage/Getty Images

Page 189: Maskot/DigitalVision/Getty Images

Page 190: PeopleImages/DigitalVision/Getty Images

Page 192: Anouchka/E+/Getty Images

Page 196: Bjorn Holland/Image Source/Getty Images

Page 197: Maridav/iStock/Getty Images

Page 198: Steve Debenport/E+/Getty Images

Page 199: Jay_Zynism/iStock/Getty Images Plus

Page 203: Fizkes/iStock/Getty Images

Page 205: SolStock/E+/Getty Images

Page 208: Milena Magazin/iStock/Getty Images

Page 212: David Lees/ DigitalVision/Getty Images

Page 216: Eternity In An Instant/DigitalVision/Getty Images

Page 217: Jose Luis Pelaez Inc/DigitalVision/Getty Images

Page 222: Donald Iain Smith/Blend Images/Getty Images

Page 223: monkeybusinessimages/iStock/Getty Images

Page 225: Tony Anderson/DigitalVision/Getty Images

Page 227: Jacob Ammentorp Lund/iStock/Getty Images

Page 231: Jacob Ammentorp Lund/iStock/Getty Images

Page 233: Trokantor/E+/Getty Images

Page 234 (clockwise from top left): National Archives; National Archives; Pete Souza/National Archives; Xinhua/Yin Bogu via Getty Images; Ken Cedeno-Pool/Getty Images; TIM SLOAN/AFP/Getty Images

Page 236: Carol Yepes/Moment/Getty Images

Page 237: Daisy-Daisy/iStock/Getty Images

Page 238: EMS-Forster-Productions/DigitalVision/Getty Images

Page 239: Westend61/Getty Images

Page 242: Svetkid/E+/Getty Images

Page 244: Paolo Cordoni/iStock/Getty Images

Page 245: Monkeybusiness/iStock/Getty Images

Page 247 Monticello/iStock/Getty Images

Page 248: zodebala/Vetta/Getty Images

Page 252: Frankreporter/iStock/Getty Images

Page 254: sturti/E+/Getty Images

Page 256: Elva Etienne/Moment/Getty Images

Page 258: Skodonnell/E+/Getty Images

Page 259 (from top to bottom): Heath Korvola/Digital Vision/Getty Images; FotoMaximum/iStockphoto/Getty Images

Page 260 (from top to bottom): Artem_Furman/iStock/Getty Images; Johner Images/Getty Images

Page 261 (from top to bottom): mikroman6/Moment RF/Getty Images; Daniel Kaesler / EyeEm/EyeEm/Getty Images

Page 262: Spencer Platt/Getty Images

Page 264: BackyardProduction/iStockphoto/Getty Images

Page 267: PeopleImages/E+/Getty Images

Page 271: Joe Raedle/Getty Images

Page 273: Joe Raedle/Getty Images

Page 274: InkkStudios/iStockphoto/Getty Images

Page 279: Sabrina Bracher/iStock/Getty Images

Page 281: Beavera/iStock/Getty Images

Page 290: Science Photo Library/Getty Images

Page 294 (from top to bottom): BSIP/UIG Via Getty Images; Getty Images; BSIP/UIG Via Getty Images

Page 296: Blair_witch/iStock/Getty Images

Page 302: CDC / Science Source

Page 303: lolostock/iStock/Getty Images

Page 306: Courtney Hale/E+/Getty Images

Page 307: THOM LEACH / Science Source

Page 308: BSIP/UIG Via Getty Images

Page 311: BSIP/UIG Via Getty Images

Page 310: Portra/DigitalVision/Getty Images

Page 311: PeopleImages/iStock/Getty Images

Page 313: JackF/iStock/Getty Images

Page 317: Lanastock/iStock/Getty Images

Page 319: Peathegee Inc/Blend Images/Getty Images

Page 325: Vanessa Nunes/iStock/Getty Images

Page 330: Luke Chan/E+/Getty Images

Page 331: PeopleImages/iStock/Getty Images

Page 333: Ivan Pantic/E+/Getty Images

Page 336: monkeybusinessimages/iStockphoto/Getty Images

Page 337: John Kevin/iStock/Getty Images

Page 338: FatCamera/E+/Getty Images

Page 343: Kupicoo/E+/Getty Images

Page 346: FatCamera/E+/Getty Images

Page 348: monkeybusinessimages/iStock/Getty Images

Page 354 (from top to bottom): Caiaimage/Sam Edwards/iStock/Getty Images; Monkeybusinessimages/iStock/Getty Images

Page 356: Pixelimage/iStock/Getty Images

Page 359: Manuel Arias Duran/Moment/Getty Images

Page 362: Adamkaz/E+/Getty Images

Page 365: Vm/E+/Getty Images

Page 366: Thomas Barwick/DigitalVision/Getty Images

Page 367 (from left to right): diego_cervo/iStock/Getty Images; B2M Productions/DigitalVision/Getty Images

Page 369: Blend Images - KidStock/Brand X Pictures/Getty Images

Page 371: Moyo Studio/E+/Getty Images

Page 372: ArtistGNDphotography/E+/Getty Images

Page 375: Urbazon/E+/Getty Images

Page 376: Stnazkul/iStock/Getty Images

Page 377: Javi-indy/iStock/Getty Images

Page 378: Monkeybusinessimages/iStock/Getty Images

Staying Healthy and Well Throughout Life

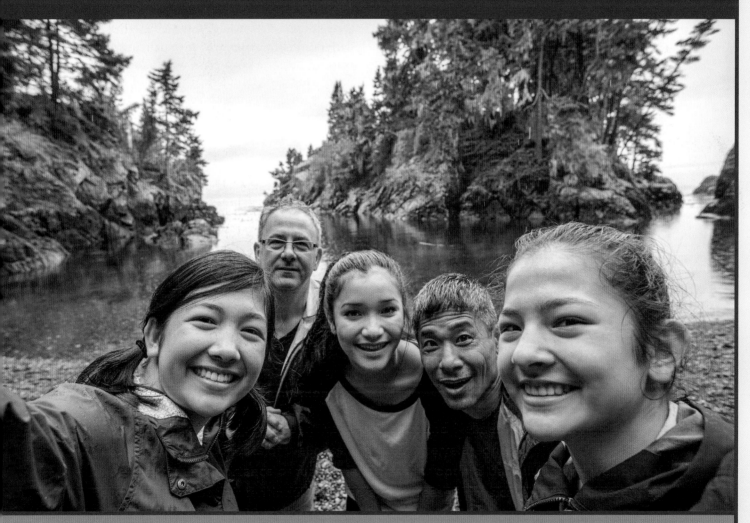

OBJECTIVES

- Explain the relationship between life expectancy and wellness practices.
- Describe the components of wellness and their interrelatedness.
- Understand the importance of functional fitness for optimal daily living and well-being.
- Recognize that both intentional exercise and increased physical activity are essential for functional fitness and well-being.
- Create a personal wellness profile.

KEY TERMS

Wellness, well-being, health, and *fitness* are similar terms that can be defined differently depending on your life circumstances. This book will help you understand what it means to be well—not only to be "not sick" but also improve your day-to-day living so you can enjoy a full and productive life. This textbook will not offer prescriptions or scare you about what will happen if you don't practice healthy behaviors. Instead, it will emphasize how *you* can create healthy lifestyle habits. After all, a lifestyle is the summary of your habits over a long-term period. The **medical model**, used by trained medical experts, focuses on prescribing drugs and procedures to combat illness. The **well-being model** empowers you to use self-management skills to create and maintain healthy habits to help prevent disease and disability over the long-term while also enhancing your functional fitness now. Our overall vision for *Fitness and Well-Being for Life* is to empower, educate, and encourage you to make productive and healthy lifestyle choices.

When you think of people who are healthy and well, what comes to mind? Getting eight hours of sleep a night? Not smoking? Eating broccoli and fresh fruits? Do you think of people accomplishing incredible physical feats or just being generally active most of the time? You may picture hiking with friends, or maybe you're visualizing someone coming out of a yoga class with a deep sense of peace. Do the people you've thought of smile more or seem more positive to you than other people? Or is there something even deeper that marks a person as healthy and well?

Staying Healthy Through the Life Span

A life well lived starts with an understanding of productive health and **well-being** practices. This includes feeling good enough about your body to live well—to eat well, move more, and attend to all aspects of health, including mental and emotional health. The Gallup

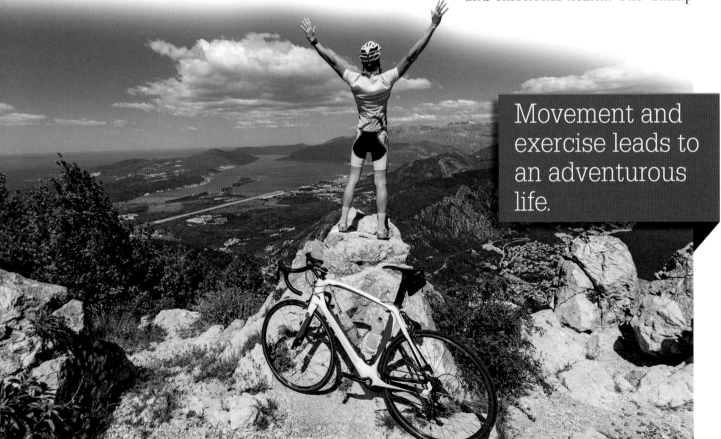

Movement and exercise leads to an adventurous life.

> Be your best you! You are limited less by chance and nature than by your vision of yourself.

World Happiness report (2023), published annually, recognizes the importance of happiness and associated well-being as a key metric of a country's success. Recent books and articles represent a new focus on well-being practices, and people are more aware than ever that health can come in many body sizes. With this awareness, many people are losing interest in fad diets and intense exercise programs. When people love their bodies, regardless of their size, they are more likely to care for themselves and make healthy choices.

The notion of exercise prescription, explained in greater detail in chapter 2, comes out of a medical framework, which does not necessarily align with behavioral science theories of motivation and the reality of how we fit movement into our daily lives (Segar et al. 2020). Interestingly, the most recent World Health Organization global guidelines on physical activity and sedentary behavior have removed the previous recommendation for aerobic activity to occur in bouts of at least 10 minutes duration—a change that may support the perception that increasing one's physical activity is both feasible and relevant (Segar et al. 2020). In fact, lasting behavior change can be achieved by making joyful and meaningful decisions in the moment (Segar 2022).

The **COVID-19** pandemic, as well as the related death, disability, and collective grief worldwide, have changed many of our feelings about and practices around wellness. Kaur et al.'s (2020) qualitative study on the impact of COVID-19 on the practices of fitness enthusiasts found that, after an initial drop in psychological and physical wellness, participants reported a return of positive self-perception and motivation to continue fitness programs at home. As further explored in forthcoming chapters, a recent literature review reported regular and appropriate intensity exercise enhances immune function, which helps prevent being afflicted with the COVID-19 virus (da Silveira et al. 2021). These findings offer us hope that together we can create the change we want to see to improve health and wellness throughout the world.

What's New in Well-Being Trends?

In an article predicting the future of well-being in the workplace, Muldoon (2021) suggests a decreased focus on measuring specific behavior change and an increased focus on whether we feel we are thriving. But what is thriving, especially in the workplace? There is no one accepted definition for workplace well-being, but Muldoon suggests that metrics of importance include (1) a positive work culture and climate, (2) inclusivity, connectedness, and belonging, (3) social support for the moments that matter, (4) decreased worries about health, and (5) more control and flexibility about when, where, and how much we work. As you progress through your college years and start to build your life, think about how your workplace will help or hinder your well-being.

Life Expectancy and Well-Being

Although **life expectancy** in the United States increased from 1980 to 2019, the Centers for Disease Control and Prevention (CDC) revealed that life expectancy at birth in the United States decreased to 77 years in 2020—a decline from 78.9 in 2019, in part a result of COVID-19 (Rakshit et al. 2021). The list of top 10 leading causes of death in the United States has also recently changed. As of 2020, COVID-19 was the third highest cause of death in the United States (Centers for Disease Control and Prevention 2020), after heart disease and cancer (figure 1.1).

Contrast the decrease in U.S. life expectancy (despite the billions of dollars spent on health care in the United States) with the increase in world life expectancy. Why are Americans not living as long as or longer than people in other countries around the world? Could this recent decrease in longevity, independent of the COVID-19 pandemic, also be attributed to our sedentary behaviors and other poor lifestyle choices? Is it because we sit too much and do most daily tasks with a press of a button? Modern medicine has enhanced overall longevity, yet sedentary living and poor dietary choices may be balancing out the influence of modern medicine in terms of overall life expectancy.

The true meaning of being well therefore has less to do with medical interventions and more to do with how we choose to spend our days and live life. This book will help you learn how to make decisions that will empower a healthy way of thinking and living and ultimately enhance the chance of a long, productive, and energetic life.

Is a longer life a better life? **Life span**, or the number of years you live, can be divided into healthy years and unhealthy years. **Health span** describes how *well* those later years of life are lived. Most people want to live many years but also want to have as many healthy years as possible, with unhealthy years limited to the very end of life. Taking care of your body, mind, and soul is critical for adding more years to both your life span and your health span. What you put into your body and how you take care of it now will increase the number of healthy years and reduce the number of unhealthy years. Consider your older relatives and friends. Are they leading functionally fit years

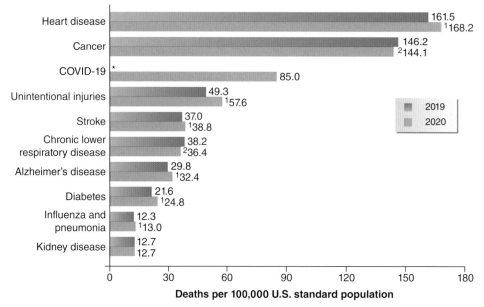

Figure 1.1   Age-adjusted death rates for the 10 leading causes of death in 2020: United States, 2019 and 2020.

[1]Statistically significant increase in age-adjusted death rate from 2019 to 2020 (p < .05).

[2]Statistically significant decrease in age-adjusted death rate from 2019-2020 (p < .05).

Notes: A total of 3,383,729 resident deaths were registered in the United States in 2020. The 10 leading causes accounted for 74.1 percent of all deaths in the United States in 2020. Causes of death are ranked according to number of deaths. Access data table for figure 1.1 at https://www.cdc.gov/nchs/images/databriefs/401-450/db427-fig4.png SOURCE: NCHS, National Vital Statistics System, Mortality.

Data from National Center for Health Statistics, National Vital Statistics System, Mortality, www.cdc.gov/nchs/images/databriefs/401-450/db427-fig4.png.

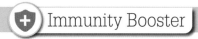 Immunity Booster

Blue Zones and Longevity

Best-selling author Dan Buettner (2020) takes a unique approach to understanding the many factors that affect longevity. He studied places in the world whose populations had the longest life expectancy (which he calls *blue zones*) and discovered that within these areas, people generally had healthy diets and moved more (figure 1.2). He now has a website featuring these thriving communities, with research updates, insights on why certain populations are living longer, and tips for moving more throughout the day (see www.bluezones.com).

What's the Difference Between Life Span and Health Span?

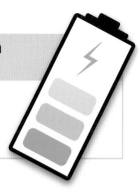

- Life span: The number of years we live from birth to death
- Health span: The number of functional and disease-free years we live from birth to death (i.e., the period of life that does not include unhealthy years)

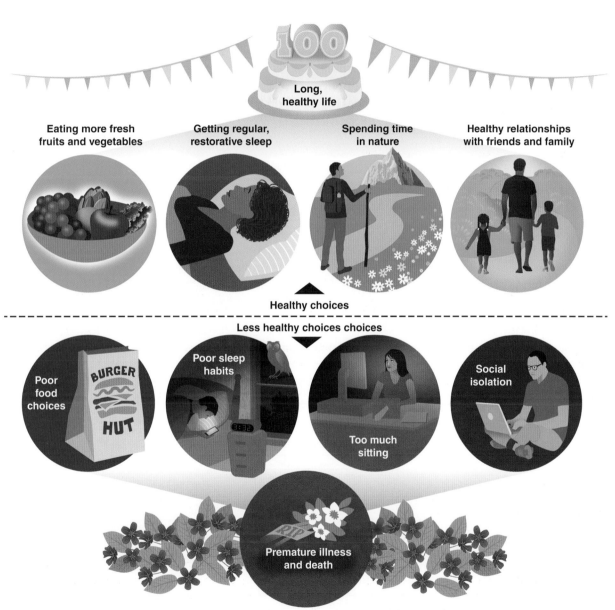

Figure 1.2   Life expectancy is influenced by many factors, including making healthy choices.

as they age? What do you anticipate would be the life span and health span of your closest relatives?

Most medical research is targeted at a single disease in isolation. However, evidence is mounting that physiological changes due to aging interact with lifestyle choices made much earlier in life, subsequently resulting in chronic diseases—many of which are leading causes of death. Just as you need to financially plan for retirement, you need to invest in your well-being so that you can enjoy your later years.

National Health and Wellness Goals

Healthy People 2030 (Office of Disease Prevention and Health Promotion 2022) is a government initiative that sets goals for improving health and wellness in the United States. This initiative provides data-driven decisions on improving quality of life and reducing preventable diseases and premature death. The Healthy People 2030 report provides science-based objectives for improving health and wellness on an individual and national basis. The major goals of Healthy People 2030 are to (1) empower people to make informed health decisions, (2) measure the effect of prevention activities provided by community and government resources, and (3) improve the health of people in the United States. This book will address many of the leading health indicators identified in Healthy People 2030.

Choosing where to live is an important part of well-being. A private digital health company called Sharecare (2022) has a well-being index that includes not only the major components of wellness but also social, community, physical, and

---

✓ Behavior Check

What's Your Family Health Span?

Now that you understand the difference between life span and health span, think about your parents and grandparents or other older people in your life. Would you say they are living well as middle-aged or older adults? If yes, why do you think this? If no, why not? What health habits do you possess that they too have? How are your health habits different (for better or worse)? How do you envision your health span unfolding throughout your life span after watching your own relatives move through theirs?

Figure 1.3 shows life span extension from ages 60 through 90. Note that living with disease and disability from the age of 60 to 90 is not a quality health span. In contrast, a period with disease and disability that is compressed to a few years in your 80s *does* indicate a high-quality health span. Your health habits today heavily influence the life and health paths you will go down later in life.

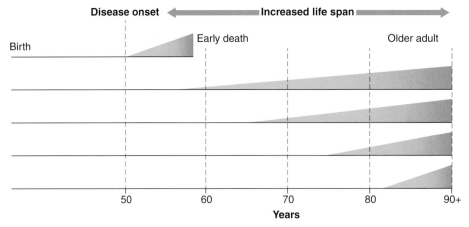

Figure 1.3   By delaying the onset of chronic conditions and diseases, you can increase your life span and your quality of life in later years.

financial indicators. Each year Sharecare's surveys provide enlightening perspectives on community well-being.

Companies have used the Sharecare survey information, along with other factors such as crime rate, commute time, unemployment, and cost of living, to determine where to place their businesses. According to Sharecare (2020), Massachusetts had the highest community well-being index ranking, and Mississippi had the lowest ranking. Notably, analyses indicates that states in the top quintile (top 10 highest well-being scores) achieved better COVID-19 measures compared to the bottom quintile (bottom 10 lowest well-being scores), with more than 20 percent lower incidence rates on average. Figure 1.4 outlines the community well-being index rankings by state.

New Perspectives on Well-Being

Past generations often defined the state of health as the absence of disease, but contemporary thinkers know the limitations of this definition. Arloski (2021), a pioneering architect in the field of health and wellness coaching, depicts wellness coaching as a process to facilitate making choices for a more successful existence. His five keys of coaching for a lifetime of wellness are as follows:

1. Build self-efficacy
2. Nurture visionary and intrinsic motivation
3. Focus on the maintenance stage of the transtheoretical model (discussed in chapter 3)
4. Co-create relapse prevention strategies
5. Coach for connectedness

✓ Behavior Check

How Does Your Location Rank?

Think about where you live. When you compare it to figure 1.4, where does it rank in terms of well-being?

Now think about where you might like to live. Would this place help you move more, sit less, and live well? Does it have good walkability? Will the air that you breathe be of good quality? Give your current living area the walkability test (www.walkscore.com). Consider the following questions and compare it to where you grew up and where you might like to live in the future:

- Can you walk to get to restaurants and stores, or do you need a car?
- How many parks are nearby?
- Can you get to places by bus, by bike, or on foot?
- What is the crime level? Is it safe to walk at all hours of the day or night?
- What is the air quality, and does it allow you to be healthy inside and outside of your home?

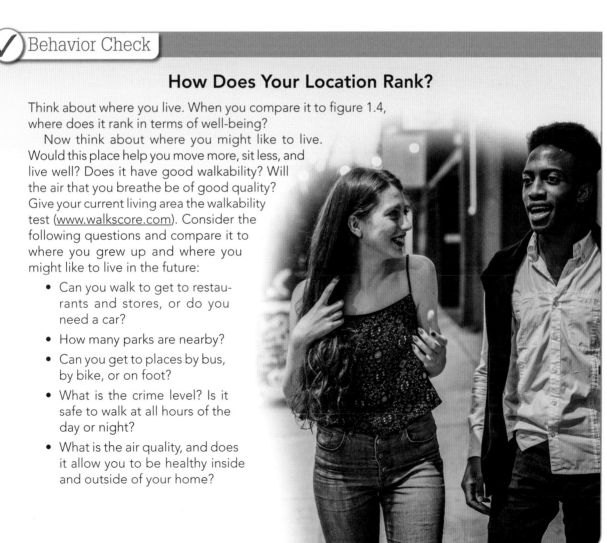

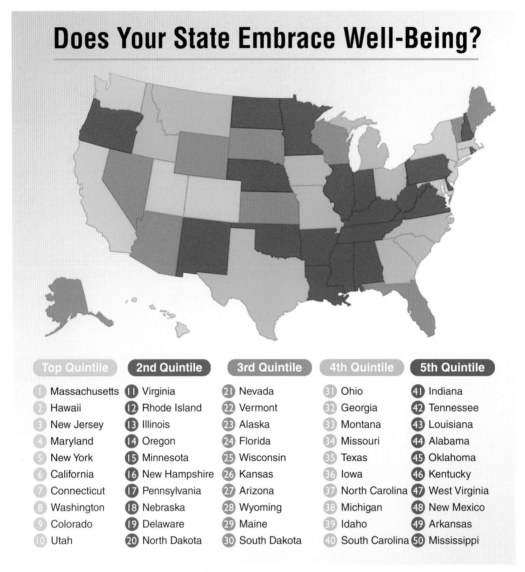

Figure 1.4   Community well-being index rank by states.
Data from Sharecare (2020).

You will see many of these steps reinforced in this book as we help you guide yourself through your own well-being journey. Simply, by learning and applying concepts in this book, you will become your own wellness coach. You will learn tools to improve your situational self-confidence (self-efficacy) to consistently make the healthier choice the easier choice. As will also be reinforced, your habits are highly influenced by the company you keep.

Dr. Jack Travis, an MD who created one of the first wellness inventory surveys nearly 50 years ago, had a mission to shift the focus of the medical culture from authoritarianism and domination to partnership and cooperation. His vision was ahead of its time and in line with current wellness and well-being perspectives. Travis's illness–wellness model (Well People 2011; see figure 1.5) depicts a paradigm where the neutral point is neither illness nor wellness. We move either right or left on this wellness continuum based on personal choices. To the right, high levels of wellness and enhanced health and well-being are realized. To the left are symptoms of physical and mental disability and disease, which can negatively impact our well-being and cause premature death. Dr. Travis was a pioneer in shifting our mindset beyond traditional medical practices into acting as our own well-being coaches. His vision of well-being also aligns with contemporary research on aging, which is shifting away from a primary focus on disease and

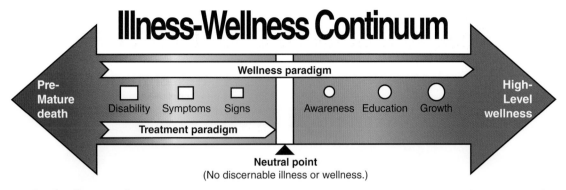

Figure 1.5 The illness–wellness continuum.

Illness-Wellness Continuum © 1972, 1981, 1988, 2004 by John W. Travis, MD. Reproduced with permission, from *Wellness Workbook: How to Achieve Enduring Health and Vitality*, 3rd edition, by John W. Travis and Regina Sara Ryan, Celestial Arts, 2004. www.wellnessworkbook.com.

related pathologies to be more inclusive of other well-being indices.

Dr. Travis also created the iceberg model of wellness, which places one's current state of health at the tip of the iceberg (Well People 2011). The next level of the iceberg is the lifestyle or behavioral level. It includes what to eat, how to move, letting go of stress, and preventing accidents. If you deepen further to the psychological or motivational level, then finally to the spiritual and meaning level, you may improve your health status and longevity. For true well-being, it is important to delve into the connections between all the dimensions of health and wellness over the life span. To maintain a lifestyle change, we must understand why we are making the change. This requires research into the cultural, psychological, motivational, and even spiritual levels of well-being. Overall, changing any behavior is complex. You will need concerted effort, focus, and balance to create a sustained healthy lifestyle.

In addition to Dr. Travis's iceberg model, there are many other ways to break down wellness into workable pieces. See figure 1.6 for a progression of wellness models, culminating in our well-being continuum. This model gets more detailed throughout the life span, with choices that ebb and flow depending on stages of life.

In previous decades, wellness was commonly described as distinct pieces of a pie. However, this model is limiting because the pieces fit perfectly together and do not overlap or mix. The reality is that life is not this perfect. Habits (positive or negative) that form from one aspect of wellness often roll over into others. We may also be working more on one aspect of well-being than another at any given time—for example, a college student's

well-being focus would likely be more on intellectual and social wellness, whereas occupational wellness may take a back seat until graduation. In our 30s or 40s, our focus may be on emotional and occupational well-being (marriage or partnership, children, pets, and work). In our 50s and 60s, there is typically great investment into financial wellness (pun intended!) to prepare for retirement. Finally, in our 70s and 80s, the social and physical aspects of wellness are often a priority for optimal aging. The focus on any one dimension may be impacted by life stage but also by personal interests and challenges. Unfortunately, an investment in one aspect of wellness often compromises others. For example, working very long hours at a stressful job might enhance financial wellness but reduce physical, emotional, and social wellness. Balance is important but can be challenging at all life stages.

Lifestyle changes occur during the transition of working on one or more well-being areas. Well-being is not a single pie piece but rather a holistic summary of collective behaviors (i.e., the whole pie!). Your own well-being model is closely aligned with your reality, where the significance of different areas ebbs and flows throughout life depending on what you value and the choices you make. Well-being is how you juggle all these choices to live a fulfilling and healthy life. Many young adults fail to realize that your 20s is when you may make many life choices that will affect your future, including what college to attend, what career to pursue, or who to marry or partner with and build a life. Meg Jay, a psychologist who wrote a book called *The Defining Decade: Why Your Twenties Matter and How to Make the Most of Them Now* (2012), calls this accumulation of personal assets *identity capital*, with which you "purchase" jobs and relationships.

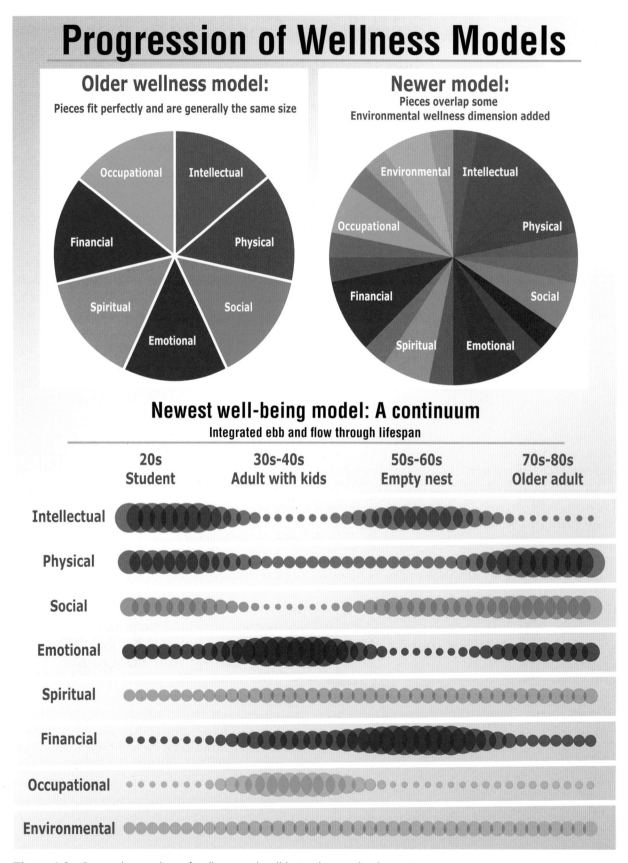

Figure 1.6   Our understanding of wellness and well-being has evolved over time.

⏱ Now and Later

Well-Being Priorities

Throughout this book we will present Now and Later boxes to remind you of the big picture of *why* a focus on your health in your earlier years will pay off in all dimensions in your later years.

Now

What are the top three well-being areas you are working on right now as a college student? See the elements under the "20s Student" in figure 1.6. How do your priorities align with those of your friends? We have illustrated the four areas of intellectual, physical, social, and emotional wellness as typical priorities for college students in figure 1.7. Does this match your experience? Why or why not? How would you illustrate the balance of these four elements of well-being?

Later

Think about your family members at older life stages, including your parents, grandparents, siblings, aunts, and uncles. Using their example as a guide, guess what your well-being focus will be as you age. Draw your well-being journey throughout your life span as depicted in the wellness continuum in figure 1.6.

Take Home

Well-being and life values go hand in hand. List the main well-being components that you want to focus on throughout your life span and explain why these are important to you.

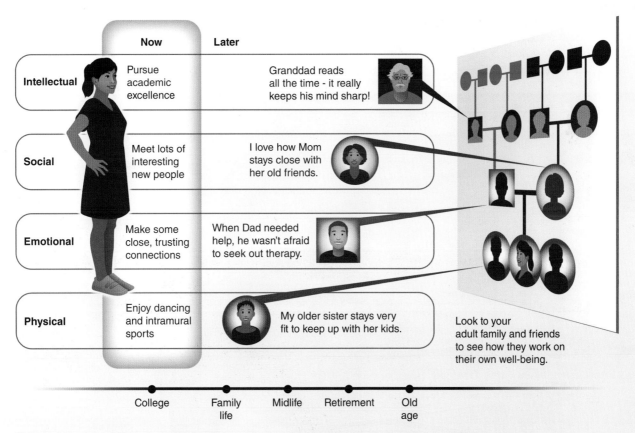

Figure 1.7 What does the balance of these four elements look like in your life as a college student?

Classic Components
of Wellness

The classic components of wellness from the older wellness models—in which the pieces fit together perfectly and are generally the same size—include seven major areas: intellectual, physical, social, emotional, spiritual, financial, and occupational. An eighth dimension, environmental wellness, is also now well accepted. As you read about the eight major areas of wellness in the next section, we will compare and contrast the traditional pie chart models with the newer well-being continuum. We urge you to pay close attention to this analysis, and as you do, write down a few ideas you might want to focus on to improve your well-being across all dimensions. The chapter 1 labs in HK*Propel* will provide you with opportunities to utilize knowledge of the traditional wellness components to help you construct a personal plan to enhance your well-being.

Intellectual Wellness

People who possess good intellectual wellness are lifelong learners. Enjoying intellectual wellness involves constantly being challenged mentally, thinking logically, and solving problems to meet life's challenges with creative ideas. It is being open to learning new ways of thinking and working. Intellectual well-being also involves being curious and motivated to master new skills and become a critical thinker who possesses the courage to question the status quo. Being motivated to learn and adapt to change will be a critical skill in the modern workplace. Think of the last time you got a new cell phone and had to learn how to use it efficiently: That involved intellectual challenge.

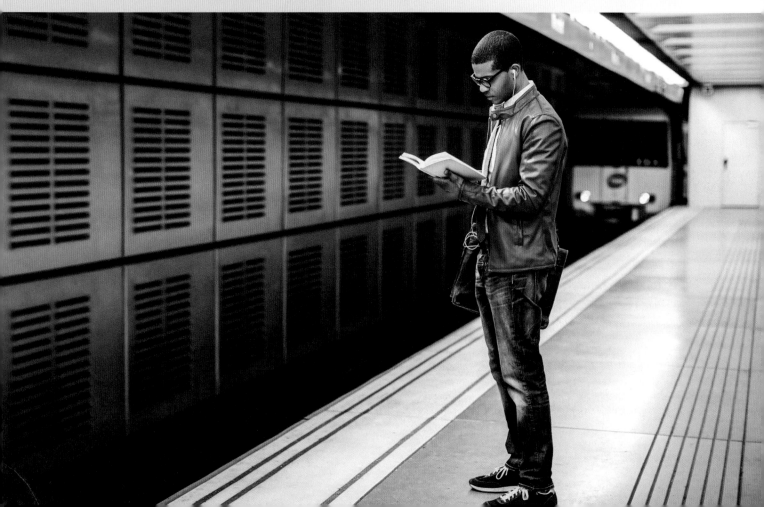

Physical Wellness

Physical wellness is much more than exercising to become physically fit and look good (although these goals are important too!). Although definitions can vary, physical wellness generally starts with adequate physical activity, healthy foods, and optimal sleep. It is also concerned with preventing illness and injury and managing chronic conditions. Having physical wellness also means having enough physical health to perform activities of daily living with vitality throughout the day.

To have a state of physical wellness, you will need to make informed health decisions and manage your personal health behaviors. Beyond being physically active and eating healthy, it also includes getting quality sleep, using alcohol and drugs responsibly, not texting while driving, and using sunscreen, as a few examples. Finally, it can also include practicing good self-care by making intentional and responsible sexual choices and managing injuries, illnesses, and pandemics effectively. A large portion of this book is dedicated to the physical aspect of wellness and well-being. Often, having adequate physical wellness influences other aspects of well-being, as will be discussed in the following chapters.

Social Wellness

Social wellness can be thought of as having a sense of connection and belonging, the ability to interact with others in meaningful ways, and a well-developed social support system. Human beings are social animals. We strive to maintain positive and satisfying interpersonal relationships, which requires effective communication skills. A person with a strong level of social well-being is generally engaged in life rather than lonely. They also have a capacity for intimacy. The most critical skills for social well-being are engaging in social relationships, giving support, being assertive, practicing self-disclosure and emotional expression, and managing conflict. Finally, engaging in community activities, helping others, and listening are important for building positive social skills.

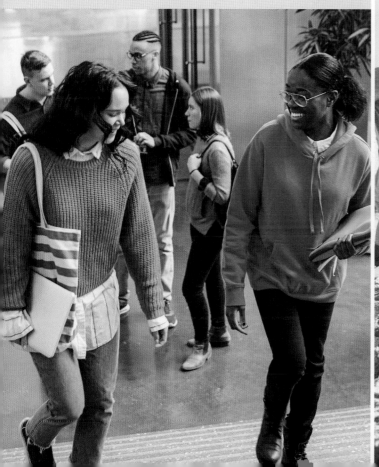

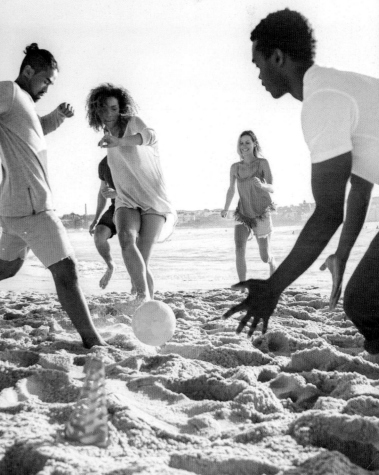

Emotional Wellness

Emotional wellness is your ability to carry out day-to-day activities with self-confidence and optimism. It means having the ability to understand and accept your feelings. It is also about being free from emotional and mental illnesses such as anxiety and major depression. Sharing feelings with others and going through life more often happy than depressed are important for having a fulfilling life. The well-being model for emotional wellness includes possessing a positive outlook on life and being stable, dependable, positive, and persistent. It also includes living and working independently as well as reaching out to others or finding professional help when needed.

Spiritual Wellness

Spiritual wellness is related to having a sense of purpose and meaning in life, as well as possessing values and beliefs to live by. A spiritually well person knows how to make the best of a bad situation, recover from loss, and forgive and forget with gratitude. Organized religion often helps with the development of spirituality, but it is not the only source of spiritual strength. Meditation, a walk in the forest with a friend, drawing, listening to music, or yoga can all help you gain spiritual well-being.

> You cannot teach people anything; you can only teach them to find it within themselves.

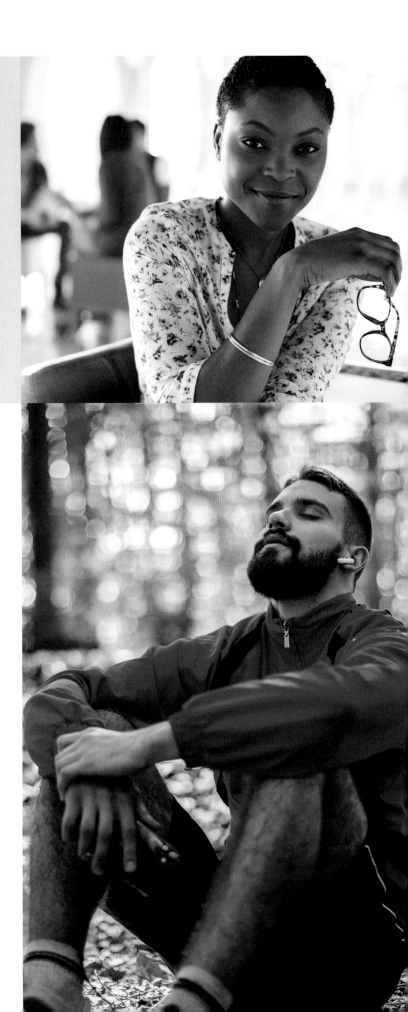

Financial Wellness

Managing your finances is often a task that requires critical thinking, self-discipline, and financial planning. Having financial wellness involves living within your means, working to stay out of debt, and being realistic about your spending habits. Keeping emotions in check related to your financial well-being is also important. Using multiple credit cards, letting friends make financial decisions for you, gambling, or having unrealistic expectations can cause emotional stress. Having a budget can help set realistic expectations and keep spending under control. Just as tracking your movements can help you know how many steps you take in a day, so too will tracking your expenditures give you an idea of where your money goes. We often think that making more money will help us feel happier. Many researchers have reported, and many people you know would agree, that a larger paycheck *does* buy happiness, but only up to the point that your needs are met and you do not have money worries. Of course, the dollar number that enables you to feel like you have enough money and don't have to worry will differ for everyone and their specific situation. The point is that earning an ever-larger paycheck and having an ever-larger financial portfolio does not guarantee happiness. The research suggests a few key principles to bring you the most happiness for your money, including (1) spending your money on experiences instead of things, (2) helping others instead of yourself, and (3) buying many small pleasures instead of a few big ones (Baer 2014).

Occupational Wellness

Occupational wellness refers to the level of happiness and satisfaction you gain from your work. Considering the many days you will spend at work over the course of your lifetime, your choice of job is essential to health and wellness. Your well-being is connected to having a job that is meaningful and fulfilling, provides personal satisfaction, and allows you to use your skills to contribute to society. Having good occupational wellness is more than being paid well. If you don't value your work or gain personal satisfaction from it, it often will not matter how well you are paid. In an ideal job, your supervisors recognize your work, you generally enjoy your coworkers, and the work is satisfying. Finding fulfilling work upon college graduation is often challenging. However, if you are seeking an occupation that enhances your well-being, you are heading in the right direction for a job *and* career you might enjoy for years to come.

> The only way to do great work is to love what you do. Look for a job but seriously hunt for a career.

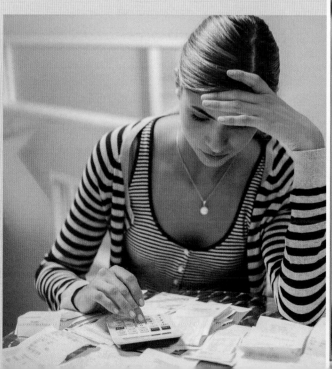

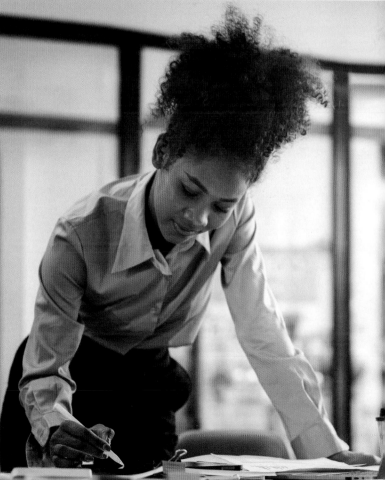

Environmental Wellness

A relatively new component of well-being is environmental wellness, which can be thought of as occupying pleasant and stimulating environments. For example, when you moved into your college space, did you bring some items that made you feel more at home? If you did, you were creating your own sense of place so you could feel comfortable in a new environment. This work of settling in is important no matter where you live or work. This concept has a lot to do with your environmental wellness on a day-to-day basis.

Having a strong sense of place will help you carefully select where to live, which will influence your environmental well-being. Remember the states where people had the highest level of well-being? Sense of place also relates to deeply feeling an emotion or sense of identity when you go to a particular place. Sociologists and urban planners study why certain places hold special meaning to people, a process called *place mapping*. Buettner's blue zones (2020) are an example of place mapping.

Think about how it feels to go home from college. All your things are in place where you put them, the family dog comes to greet you, and you feel comfortable, safe, and relaxed in this space. It even smells like home! Now, think about where you will live when you leave college. Is there a history of violence where you choose to live? Is your environment walkable? Can you take steps to make sure your lifestyle is respectful of the environment and contributes to sustainability (human and ecological)? Are recycling programs and gardening spaces available? Essentially, what is the livability of your surroundings, and do they meet your expectations for a happy and healthy environment? If not, then how can you make sure you live in an environment that meets your expectations? What is your plan to make this happen?

Many college alumni revisit their alma maters. As they explore campus again, they relive both positive and negative experiences. Thus, college campuses are a common site for the place-mapping process.

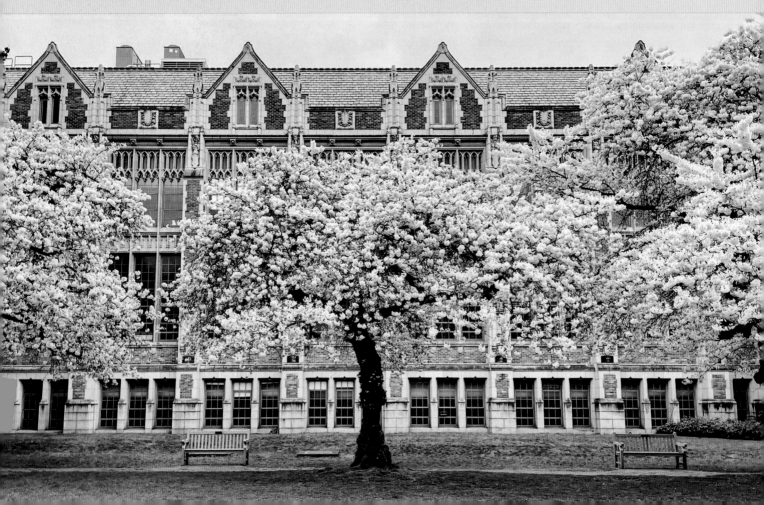

Summing Up the Dimensions of Wellness

Making healthy choices in your 20s can have major impacts on your life trajectory. For example, you might find a life partner at the recreational center and make well-being a core part of your partnership and future family. Alternatively, you might find your partner at the local bar and overindulgence on alcohol may be a primary activity in your relationship. You might learn the important skill of living within your means by carefully budgeting and managing your spending habits, or you might manage your funds so poorly that you have extensive credit card debt upon graduation, which will impact your next steps in life. Learning and practicing good habits in this defining decade can have a profound impact on the remaining decades of your life.

The Functional Fitness and Well-Being Connection

Investing time and effort to optimize all dimensions of wellness summarized in figure 1.6 will greatly enhance your overall well-being now as well as increase your chances for a long life span and health span later. Although there is much more to well-being than moving more, we will focus here on physical activity as a key behavior related to physical well-being—it requires you to make daily choices in environments where the healthy choice is often not the easy choice, and it is related to weight management and a healthy body composition, a primary topic of interest to many college students.

 Now and Later

Your Daily Choices Matter!

Now

In terms of staying healthy through the life span, the choices made in your 20s matter.

Later

Imagine this eulogy: "She passed away peacefully in her sleep at the age of 100, after her final one-mile walk with her dog."

Take Home

Now that's a lifetime of living well! Living well requires honest reflection about your behaviors, the perseverance to make healthy choices most of the time, and a joy for taking care of yourself so you can also take care of others. Going beyond physical aesthetics to empower an internal sense of well-being will have big implications for an enjoyable life.

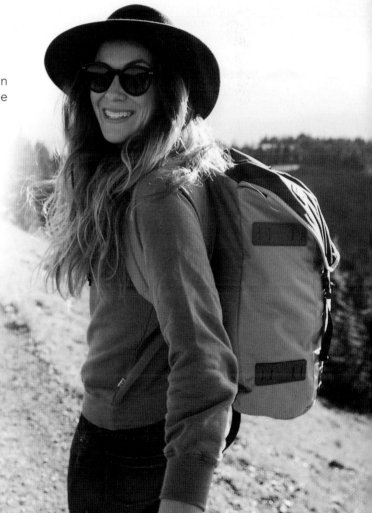

Åstrand coined the term *functional training* in a landmark article titled "Why Exercise?" He stated, "If animals are built reasonably, they should build and maintain just enough, but not more structure than they need to meet functional requirements" (1992, 153). Dr. Åstrand was ahead of his time with the belief that physical movement should be performed to positively influence function rather than aesthetics. For the purposes of this book, we will define **functional fitness** as possessing the necessary fitness to perform daily functional movements, especially physical activities, throughout your life. Thus, functional fitness is your ability to reach up and pull down your suitcase from the overhead bin of an airplane. It is your ability to rush up a flight of stairs as you are running late to class. It is your ability to pick up a large box of books and move them to another room in your apartment. Because our contemporary lives involve countless minimal detectable movements that involve many postural muscles, functional fitness is also your ability to stand or sit in front of a computer screen without back or neck pain.

This important concept of functional fitness for your well-being will appear again and again throughout this textbook. Although most of this book will center on physical function and how to move to improve your physical functional fitness, a second important concept is that your physical functional fitness can greatly influence other dimensions of wellness, including your emotional and social well-being, your cognitive health, and even your financial wellness. In this way, better health habits, especially physical movement habits, can have major implications for your overall daily function in many dimensions (e.g., attention, memory, mood, motivation).

In order to improve your functional fitness so you can meet the demands of your lifestyle, it is important to incorporate **functional fitness training**, which is deliberate and intentional training to improve functional fitness, usually using resistance training and stretching and often simulating functional movements. This book includes a special Functional Fitness Training section after chapter 6 to help you better understand how to perform functional fitness training to meet your daily lifestyle needs. In that section, you'll find distinct exercise and movement patterns that you can do anytime and anywhere, focusing on free weight or resistance band exercises, body weight movements, variable resistance machine exercises, and stretches. You can also find videos demonstrating these movements on HK*Propel*.

In addition to benefiting from the Functional Fitness Training section, you can also improve your functional fitness by choosing to incorporate more functional movements throughout the day. A few examples of easy ways to incorporate movement into your daily life include walking to class rather than getting dropped off by a friend, taking the stairs instead of the elevator, and wearing your backpack over both shoulders to strengthen your core muscles as you walk to class. Making active choices on a daily basis in addition to planning and engaging in intentional exercise sessions will positively impact your functional fitness and increase your ability to maintain your physical well-being now and in the future. The next chapter will more fully discuss the difference between exercise, which is planned and intentional, and physical activity, which can include recreational activities, transportation, domestic chores, or movement related to your occupation. Many college students previously played a sport but may not be training during their college years—therefore, engaging in intentional exercise training, increasing daily physical activity, and reducing sedentary behaviors is typically a new but essential transition in thinking. A key theme of this textbook is that to attain and keep your functional fitness now and later, you will have to make the choice to move every day, even when the environment makes unhealthy choices seem easier. Over time, your choices will become habits, and your habits will become your lifestyle.

All Your World Is a Fitness Facility

Having been professors in the exercise field for a long while, the authors of this textbook have managed many fitness programs and facilities over the decades. We have nothing against fitness facilities, fitness programs, and gym memberships. If a person uses these movement options on a regular basis, benefits to physical fitness and wellness will occur. However, the data clearly indicate that most people do not purchase fitness memberships, and if they do, they do not use them regularly. Even more important is the emerging science, explained more fully in forthcoming chapters, that indicates a single intense workout won't offset the sedentary aspects of our contemporary lifestyle. Thus, when evaluating your daily and weekly patterns of movement, you will need to plan to incorporate various types of exercise and physical activity throughout your day to gain optimal functional fitness. In addition, you will also need to strategize to reduce your sitting behaviors or break up your sitting time in an intentional way.

Let's look at an example of walking movements of varying intensity over a workday for three individuals at a typical workplace, shown in figure 1.8. We have selected walking because walking is central to our quality of life and is considered a fundamental aspect of functional fitness by many people, especially beyond middle age. Sedentary Sam (orange line) sits at his desk all day and gets very little movement throughout his day. He even takes a short afternoon nap at his desk because he is tired. Is that mental fatigue or physical fatigue? Could a short walk instead of a nap help him have more energy to do his work? On the other hand, Moving Mary (blue line) parks farther away from her building, having purchased the economy parking pass (also helps financial wellness!) and walks to her office. She takes the stairs at work, walks to lunch and back, and takes frequent movement breaks throughout the day by delivering messages in person and scheduling walking meetings. Finally, Moving Mary takes her dog on a long after-dinner walk while she talks to her parents or best friend in another state on her phone. Moving Mary expends much more energy in her daily activities than Sedentary Sam; however, note that she does not have a planned exercise routine. Then there is Exercising Eric (green line). His workday is much like that of Sedentary Sam, but he takes a break at lunch to drive to the local fitness facility and walks at a moderately high intensity (speed and grade) on a treadmill, then goes back to work and continues to sit at his desk all day.

Although we used the example of walking, a cardiorespiratory activity (discussed in chapter 4), these patterns could also be compared using the example of functional resistance training—for example, contrasting the use of a facility weight room (Exercising Eric) with the use of resistance-based functional movements throughout the day using body weight, bands, and other options (Moving Mary). This creative idea will be explained more fully in chapters 5 and 6.

Ideally, a combination of the routines of Exercising Eric and Moving Mary represents healthy movement patterns. If you do not prefer to spend

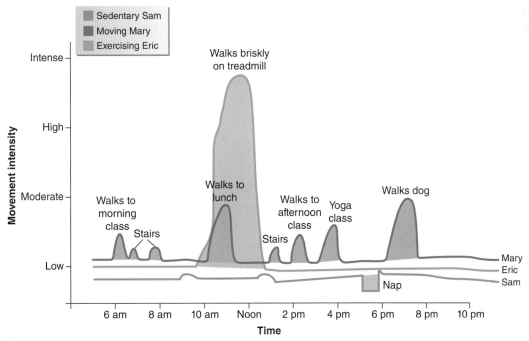

Figure 1.8 Example daily patterns of walking: lifestyle physical activity (blue line), intentional exercise (green line), and sedentary living (orange line).

Based on Blair, Kohl, III, and Gordon (1992).

the time and money on a fitness membership or you do not like to engage in intentional exercise, then be like Moving Mary and incorporate physical movement into your lifestyle on most days of the week. If you know you will have to sit in a chair most of the day in class, then Exercising Eric's day might work for you. Ideally, though, you are encouraged to blend the two approaches—intentional exercise and a lifestyle of increased physical activity. Exercising Eric could certainly benefit from more movement throughout his day, especially to break up the sitting time. Moving Mary could benefit from more intense exercise training sessions, at least a few times per week. The message here is that going to a fitness facility or intentionally planning a walking workout is not the only way to get movement into your day, and other options count. You have many ways to acquire functional fitness. All movement (whether in a fitness facility or throughout the day) is *good* movement and improves your health and well-being.

This brings us to the concept of sedentary behavior, another aspect of a healthy lifestyle to consider. Emerging research suggests that even people who visit fitness facilities or have planned exercise bouts throughout the week may still engage in sedentary behaviors to the point of adversely affecting their health. The World Health Organization (Bull et al. 2020) suggests that a single activity break each day is likely not enough movement to offset the

harmful physiological and psychological effects of sitting so much. The specific recommendations regarding sedentary behaviors (e.g., minutes) are evolving; however, most experts agree that reducing sedentary behaviors is recommended across all age groups and abilities. In essence, performing a daily exercise bout to offset sedentary behavior may no longer be enough to maintain physical health. Engaging in movement opportunities throughout the day, often described as part of one's lifestyle, is also essential. You will read more about these concepts in chapter 2.

The increasing popularity of the standing desk is a social testimony that we are trying to maintain screen productivity but also reduce our sitting time. In a study comparing sitting, standing, or regular breaks within a desk job, Peddie et al. (2021) noted that although the use of a standing desk had positive effects on health, frequent movement breaks rather than replacing sitting with standing mattered the most to overall health improvement. To keep up with the current literature on sitting time, check out the website www.JustStand.org, which contains evidence-based studies on sitting time that are updated regularly. Debate about sitting time and the health risks of being sedentary for long periods of time will continue, and we will likely see workplaces and classrooms change dramatically in the future to reduce our sitting time.

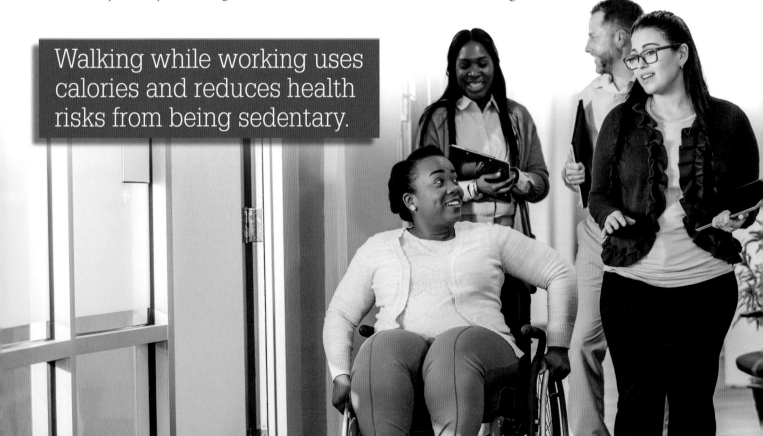

Walking while working uses calories and reduces health risks from being sedentary.

✔ Behavior Check

Daily Movement Choices: Expending Energy and Gaining Energy

Let's make it simple: All movement matters for your health, whether it occurs inside or outside a fitness facility. For example, table 1.1 provides the calorie expenditure for a 150-pound (68 kg) person doing basic life tasks such as cleaning and yard work. These small tasks can be planned throughout the day to break up sitting time while studying. Importantly, because sitting can be mentally draining, taking movement breaks also helps you gain energy to tackle the brain work. For example, while writing this textbook, your author set a timer to complete one chore after each hour of sitting. A sequence looked something like this: write, do dishes, write, vacuum, write, wash a load of laundry, write, dry a load of laundry, and so on. At the end of the day lots of writing and chores were completed! As you will realize, movement takes planning and can be woven into your daily life. Think of your environment, wherever you are, as a fitness facility! Be creative.

Table 1.1 Calories Utilized by a 150-Pound Person During Daily Activities

Activity	Calories per hour
Raking leaves	147
Gardening or weeding	153
Moving (packing and unpacking)	191
Vacuuming	119
Cleaning the house	102
Playing with the kids (moderate activity level)	136
Mowing the lawn	205
Strolling	103
Sitting and watching TV	40
Biking to work (on a flat surface)	220

Based on McCoy (2009).

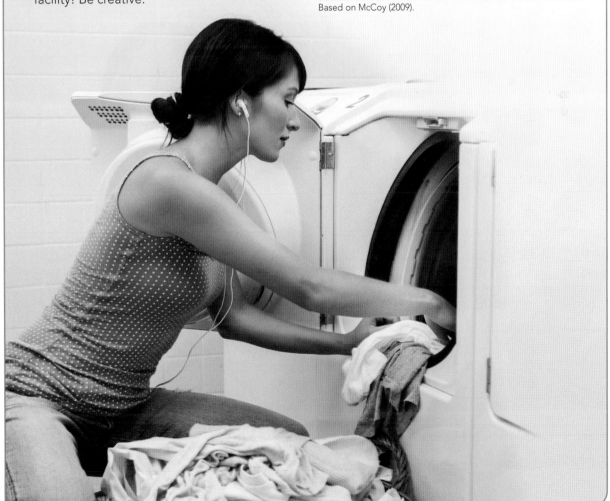

Eating and Sleeping Habits: Keys to Functional Fitness and Well-Being

Although most of this textbook will center on human movement, particularly on exercise, physical activity, and sedentary behavior, your nutritional habits and sleeping routines are two other health behaviors that have major implications for your functional fitness. Beyond weight management, how and when you fuel your body—your engine—has major implications for how fast and far you can go as you tackle your daily to-do list. Chapters 7 to 9 will provide information about body composition, healthy eating practices, and weight management, as well as behavioral strategies to stick to your new healthier routines to create habits that will become your lifestyle. We all recognize that you must drink and eat to live, and you need to make numerous decisions all through your waking hours about what, when, and how much to eat. In our environment of "good and plenty," it takes lots of willpower to make the healthy choice most of the time.

Sleep habits are another factor that greatly influences your functional fitness. Going through your days exhausted greatly compromises how you feel and how you function—physically, cognitively, emotionally, and socially. In our collective experience as college professors, the two main complaints of students are feeling tired and stressed. This less-than-optimal state indicates compromised functional fitness and well-being during the college years for many students. Chapter 10 will discuss strategies to better manage sleep and stress.

Learning the basics and developing tools to manage healthy eating and sleeping behaviors, when combined with healthy moving habits, will dramatically improve how you feel and function during your college days. And importantly, these behavioral tools will help expand your life and health span later.

It is the little things that matter the most over time when it comes to evaluating a lifestyle. Think of life as a game and then ask yourself how you want to play it over the long term. A life well lived is one in which you come sliding into home plate at the end with a lot of energy.

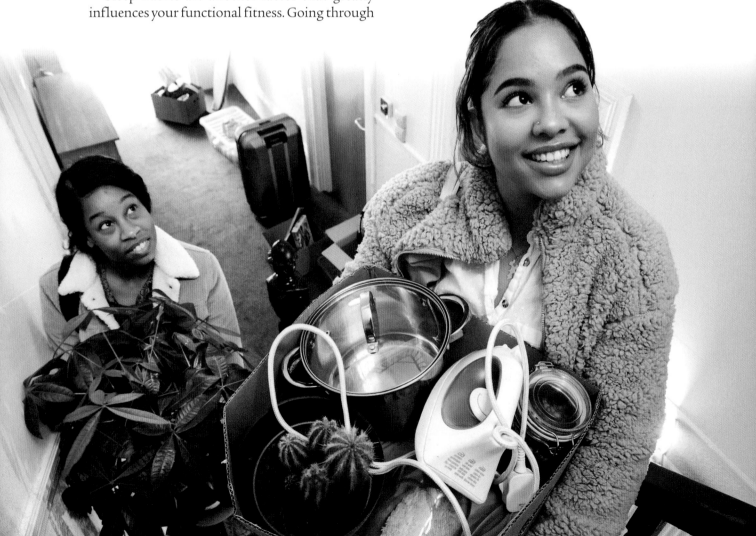

Lifestyle Choices of Real People

What gets in your way when it comes to being healthy and well?

Take a moment and make a list of habits you could turn into healthy lifestyle choices. Begin to think about the real choices you make.

1. Take the stairs instead of an elevator.
2. Walk home instead of having a friend pick you up.
3. Go to a local restaurant known for growing their own food instead of an all-you-can-eat local food chain for dinner.
4. Have a dinner party where your closest friends bring healthy choices.
5. Park far away instead of finding the closest parking space when shopping and carry your own bags to the car.
6. Shovel snow or rake leaves instead of using a blower to clean the yard.
7. Instead of sitting to have coffee or tea with friends, walk and talk while enjoying your drinks.
8. Go on a hike with friends instead of going out to dinner together.
9. Walk your dog with a friend and their dog instead of leisurely surfing the Internet.

These are just a few examples of typical movement and eating choices we make every day that can become habits and then contribute to your lifestyle of health and wellness. We often make unhealthy choices when we are hungry, angry, lonely, or tired. This textbook will help you HALT the poor behavioral choices and move forward with healthier habits.

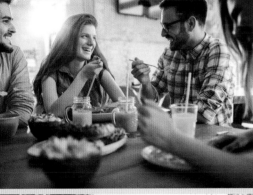
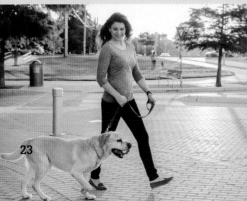
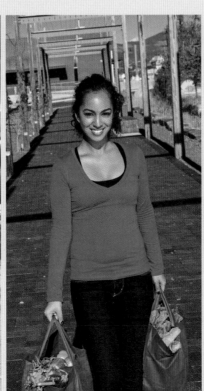
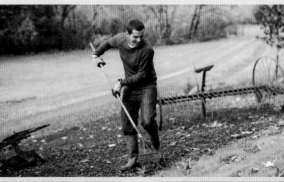
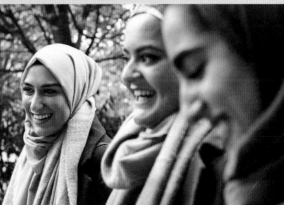

> A great life is not about great huge things—it's about small things that make a big difference.

The book *Making Learning Whole: How Seven Principles of Teaching Can Transform Education* (Perkins 2009) discusses how college classes build on one another to create a learning experience that will one day culminate into workforce readiness, typically in the form of a career. You may wonder why taking chemistry will make you a better doctor or how a psychology class will make you a better accountant. The point is that you will one day put the cumulative effect of your college learning into a career as a productive member of society, and it will all make sense. The same is true with well-being. Learning about the various dimensions of wellness and how and why they impact your functional fitness will become integrated. The little choices you make every single day will become your habits and these habits will become your lifestyle and your wellness life. It might seem like taking the stairs instead of the elevator each time you are greeted with this choice cannot mean much, but over a lifetime, it can make a huge difference for your health.

Summary

This book will help you think about your health habits, especially your daily movement choices, and how they can impact your functional fitness in the short term and your life and health span in the long term. The game of life—your life—is greatly impacted by these choices. The goal of this textbook is to teach you how to be your own coach, to work hard as a team player, and to show up with energy and enthusiasm to play every day. By scoring highly in all of the wellness dimensions, you are setting yourself up for a life well lived.

ⓌⓌⓌ ONLINE LEARNING ACTIVITIES

Go to HK*Propel* and complete all of the online activities to further facilitate your learning:

Study Activities: Review the main concepts of the chapter.

Labs: Complete the labs your instructor assigns.

Videos: Look through the videos and choose which ones you want to try this week.

REVIEW QUESTIONS

1. What is the difference between life span and health span?
2. Name the eight components of wellness. Which three are you doing well in? How do you know you are doing well in these three areas? Make a list that shows your successes in these areas and a list to work on over time.
3. Describe the neutral point of the illness–wellness continuum created by Dr. Jack Travis.
4. Explain functional fitness and how it can go beyond just the physical dimension.
5. List three specific behavioral changes, other than intentionally exercising, you can make to move more and sit less in your daily college routine.
6. Is there a difference in energy expenditure between walking on a treadmill for two miles in a fitness facility and taking a two-mile walk with a friend? Defend your answer in two to three sentences.

Functional Fitness and Movement Choices

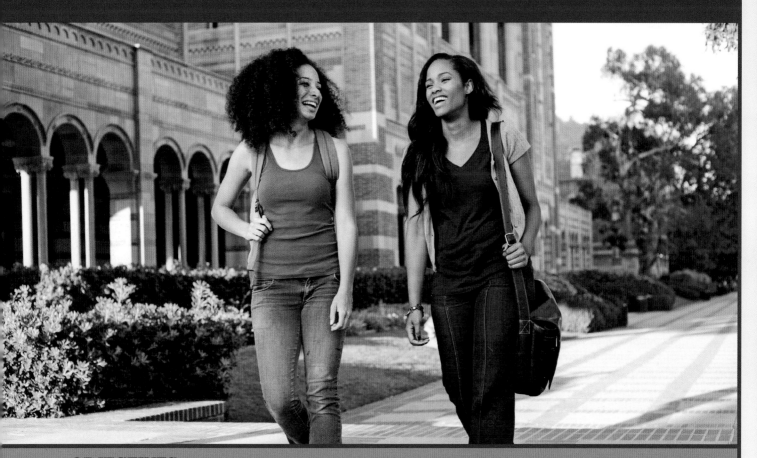

OBJECTIVES

- **Understand the HHS Physical Activity Guidelines (PAG), the ACSM exercise guidelines, and the 24-hour activity cycle (24-HAC) paradigm.**
- **Explain the emerging risk factor of sedentary behavior.**
- **Recognize that intentional exercise, physical activity, and reductions in sedentary behavior should be planned into most days of the week.**
- **Analyze how environmental choices influence movement opportunities, which in turn affect your overall well-being.**
- **Understand how to perform a personal screening and safety inventory analysis prior to creating your movement program.**
- **Practice setting SMART goals.**

KEY TERMS

24-hour activity cycle (24-HAC) paradigm
ACSM exercise guidelines
exercise
functional fitness
functional fitness training
HHS Physical Activity Guidelines (PAG)

PAR-Q+
physical activity
RICE principle
sedentary behavior
SMART goals

This chapter introduces the current guidelines for human movement, including exercise, physical activity, and sedentary behavior. Experts agree that all types of movements matter, and most current, contemporary thinking is concerned with patterns of various intensities of movement (e.g., light or vigorous) and their interaction with sleep behaviors in a 24-hour period—a new paradigm commonly referred to as the 24-hour activity cycle.

There are a few important concepts to keep in mind as you learn about the movement recommendations introduced in this chapter and begin thinking about how to practically apply this information to your own life. Ultimately, the end goal is to design a personal daily movement plan to improve and maintain your functional fitness as you go about your college days and beyond. This can be achieved using many different types of movements and activities and does not require going to a fitness facility or purchasing expensive equipment. Making your movement dependent on space and place is a serious threat to your commitment to a consistent movement program—the best program is the one you will do on a consistent basis. Being a consistent mover in our contemporary world will require strategic thinking, active planning, and a good dose of creativity. Every little bit of movement counts: For example, you could put on your exercise gear, go to the student recreation center, jump on a treadmill, put your earbuds in, and tune out the world for 30 minutes. Or you could plan to meet a classmate near the entrance to your apartment complex and review concepts for the upcoming exam while you walk briskly to campus for 30 minutes. Or you could put on your hiking boots, get out of the city, and walk briskly for 30 minutes while listening to the birds tweeting in the nearby nature preserve. Although you may perceive these three examples very differently, the truth is that they all "count" toward your movement program, and if the intensities are similar, your physiological systems will not know the difference. At the end of this chapter, you will reflect on your current day-to-day movement choices and consider your exercise, physical activity, and sedentary living habits. After doing a quick safety check, you will then create a movement plan using SMART goals for success.

Understanding Movement Recommendations

This chapter will provide an overview of the American College of Sports Medicine (ACSM) exercise guidelines, the U.S. Department of Health and Human Services (HHS) Physical Activity Guidelines (PAG), and the emerging health risks of sedentary behavior, or excessive sitting time (Yang et al. 2019). This three-part human movement focus of **exercise, physical activity**, and **sedentary behavior** is directly linked to health and well-being (figure 2.1). Although the benefits of exercise and physical activity have been known since the 1950s, Americans have not kept up with movement guidelines. Alarmingly, nearly 80 percent of adults fail to meet the Physical Activity Guidelines and a greater percentage fail to meet ACSM guidelines. Additionally, Ussery et al. (2018) studied sitting time of adults and found the greatest proportion of adults reported sitting for six to eight hours per day and being inactive. Clearly, Americans of all ages have a movement problem.

Before we discuss the current movement guidelines to increase exercise and physical activity, it will be useful to explore some history to understand how these guidelines emerged and how intentional exercise and fitness became such a focus in our society over the past several decades.

Live to Move and Move to Live

Functional fitness, introduced in chapter 1, will be a consistent theme in this textbook. However, an important question for you to consider is "Why do you want to be fit?" Often, especially for young adults, the goal is to look good and feel good about how you look. Beyond this, we encourage you to think about how you want to function in your daily life. For example, maybe you want to be able to hike steep hills on the weekend or take an exotic hiking vacation on spring break. Choosing to walk around campus with a loaded backpack as active transportation will prepare you for these experiences. Thus, this functional movement choice—carrying the backpack—works as functional fitness training for hiking. In a similar manner, an older adult might be motivated to walk the neighborhood so that they can take long walks and have some memorable talks with their grandchildren on vacation. This functional training concept is key for physical activity choices. More importantly, these reasons help your motivational muscles by connecting to your "why." Typically the "whys" relate to social connections and pleasurable activities—reasons that are much more important than looking good, especially as you go through life. Move functionally to function well in your life.

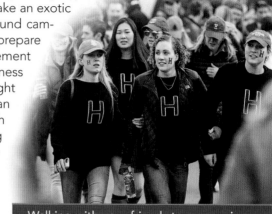

Walking with your friends to a game is a great way to enjoy an active transportation opportunity. The social connections are pure bonus!

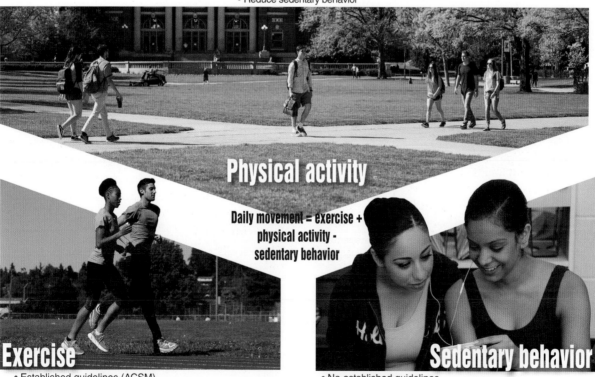

• Established guidelines (PAG) • Moderate-to-vigorous aerobic physical activity • Muscle strengthening activity
• Reduce sedentary behavior

Physical activity

Daily movement = exercise + physical activity - sedentary behavior

Exercise
• Established guidelines (ACSM)
• Cardiovascular (aerobic), resistance training, and flexibility
• Frequency, intensity, time, and type

Sedentary behavior
• No established guidelines
• General recommendation by ACSM and PAG
• Reduce sedentary behavior
• Move more and sit less

Figure 2.1 Healthy daily movement patterns incorporate exercise, physical activity, and minimal sedentary behavior.

A Brief History of Intentional Exercise Practices

The term *prescription* is often defined as a written order by a physician or clinician for the administration of medicine. The definition of a prescription is simple: It is a piece of advice. The expression "exercise prescription" has been a staple of many fitness and medical professionals for decades. In practical terms, a contemporary version of this prescription might read, "Move more, sit less, and rest well."

As we all recognize, the rise of automation and technology has effectively engineered movement out of our lives, and now many of us spend our days sitting. But consistent movers know that once you start to move you too will feel better. Moving is common sense. We were designed to move. In the past, exercise prescriptions often left out the physical activity that we do just for the joy of moving. Our minds are broadening to include movement habits beyond our historical concept of intentional exercise practices—however, change can be hard.

The Early Years

The history of the exercise prescription is best seen through updates from the ACSM, specifically their *Guidelines for Exercise Testing and Prescription*. Often referred to as the best evidence-based source for exercise prescription, the various revisions of the ACSM guidelines provide a chronological record and contextualization for the changes to the specifics of the exercise prescription. The acronym FITT (frequency, intensity, time, and type) was also introduced by ACSM to provide a useful way for remembering a science-based exercise prescription.

Although the details of the past position statements are not of primary interest, several changes in focus are important to note. The first ACSM position statement was published in 1978. As a result of the increase in the number of Americans diagnosed with heart disease in the 1970s, its primary focus was cardiorespiratory (aerobic) training (discussed in detail in chapter 4). This statement also advocated for performing movements that involved large muscle groups

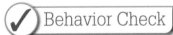 Behavior Check

Stairs Versus the Escalator

Think about the last time you were greeted with a scene like the one in this photo. Would you choose those glorious stairs in the middle to charge up, or would you find your way to the escalator on the side of the stairs? Often, we see crowds of people taking the escalator or waiting in line for an elevator. Perhaps you can be the one who chooses the stairs next time. Remember, small decisions like choosing to take the stairs add up over time and equate to better overall health and functional fitness.

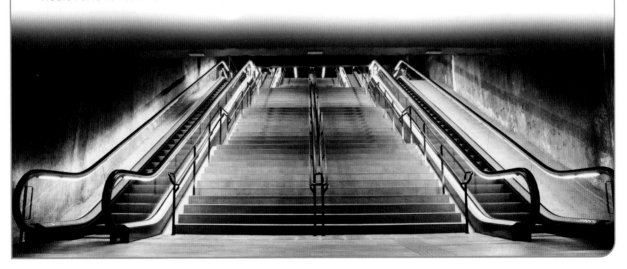

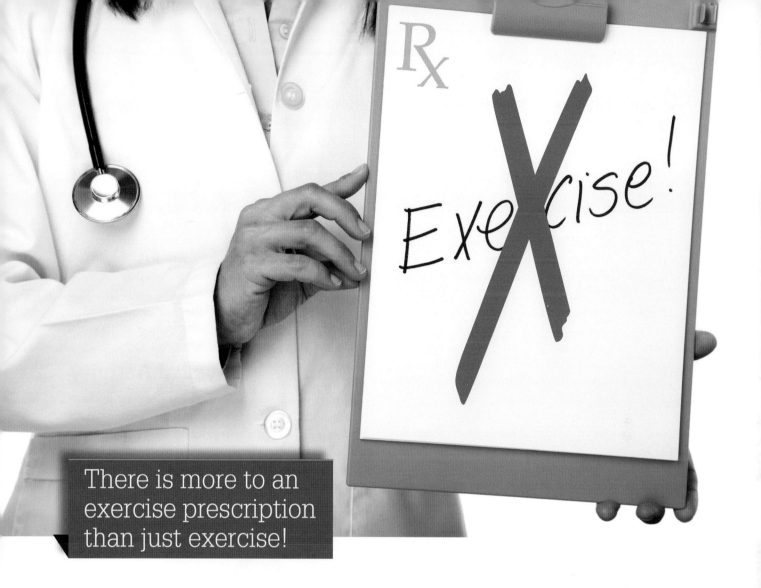

There is more to an exercise prescription than just exercise!

and doing sessions of moderate- to high-intensity activity for 15 to 60 continuous minutes three to five times per week (American College of Sports Medicine 1978).

1990s to Present

In 1990, a major revision occurred to the ACSM position statement with the addition of muscular strength and endurance training twice per week for all major muscle groups (American College of Sports Medicine 1990). More substantial changes were made in 1998: Cardiorespiratory exercise sessions could be either 20 to 60 continuous minutes or more frequent 10-minute bouts that accumulated to 20 to 60 minutes, the muscular strength and endurance training prescription was altered to reflect different intensities for individuals over the age of 50, and flexibility training was added as a new mode of exercise (American College of Sports Medicine 1998). The 2006 ACSM position stand provided more detailed guidance about intensity and duration for the primary modes of cardiorespiratory, resistance, and flexibility training—notably, the initial FITT frame was preserved, with the addition of a musculoskeletal focus (American College of Sports Medicine 2006). Finally, neuromotor practices, to be explained in chapter 6, were included in the 2018 ACSM guidelines (American College of Sports Medicine 2018) but were removed from the 2022 ACSM guidelines for lack of evidence-based information (American College of Sports Medicine 2022). See figure 2.2 for a visual summary of the current ACSM guidelines.

Future of Fitness Across the Life Span

The baby boomers—those born between 1946 and 1964—had the most influence on intentional fitness practices. This generation often used fitness facilities as a social outlet for getting out of the house and for improving how they looked and felt, and they are still active participants in the fitness facility model. They were also the first generation to show us that we needed to modify our intentional movement choices as we age.

In the 1970s, when boomers were in their 20s, they participated in high-impact aerobics and ran 10K races in droves. In the 1980s and 1990s, boomers transitioned to low-impact aerobics, 5Ks, step and slide classes, water exercise, indoor cycling, and yoga. The next two decades, when boomers were in their 50s and 60s, led to exercise with stability balls, core strength, and TRX devices to improve neuromuscular and proprioceptive fitness. As boomers age into their 70s, look for them to be more involved in walking, corrective exercise, and water exercises. Just as baby boomers changed their choices of fitness activities across their life span, so will your generation!

You may be a runner in your 20s, but you might need to move to gentler activities such as cycling or walking later in life. If you are not moving, you may experience musculoskeletal issues later in life. How many of your older relatives have had hip or knee replacements? Your body is the vehicle that drives your health and well-being throughout your life span. If you take care of it, you can get many miles out of it without replacing parts. Listening to your body and changing your activities based on what it is telling you is another important secret to a long, healthy life of functional fitness. To help you reflect on this topic, complete the chapter 2 labs on HK*Propel*, where you will consider your personal movement history, current practices, and projected changes as you progress into your later adult years.

Exercise + Physical Activity

Since the initial 1978 ACSM statement on how much exercise is enough, much more detailed research has been done. The exercise prescription

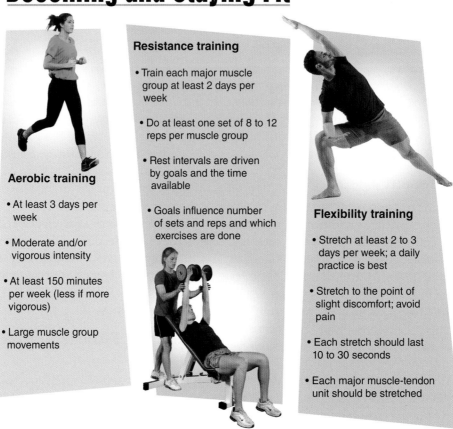

Becoming and Staying Fit

Aerobic training

- At least 3 days per week
- Moderate and/or vigorous intensity
- At least 150 minutes per week (less if more vigorous)
- Large muscle group movements

Resistance training

- Train each major muscle group at least 2 days per week
- Do at least one set of 8 to 12 reps per muscle group
- Rest intervals are driven by goals and the time available
- Goals influence number of sets and reps and which exercises are done

Flexibility training

- Stretch at least 2 to 3 days per week; a daily practice is best
- Stretch to the point of slight discomfort; avoid pain
- Each stretch should last 10 to 30 seconds
- Each major muscle-tendon unit should be stretched

Figure 2.2   American College of Sports Medicine recommendations for physical fitness.

Data from *ACSM's Guidelines for Exercise Testing and Prescription* (2022).

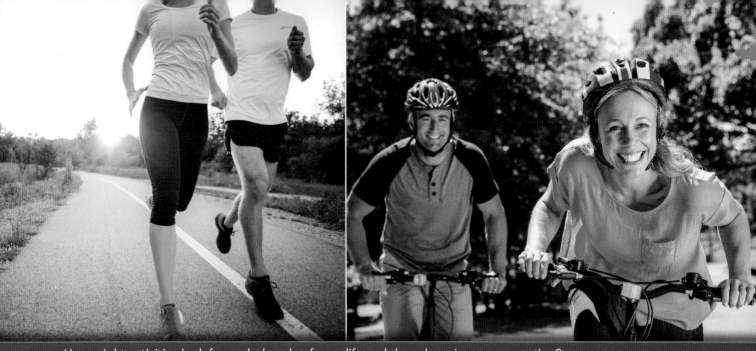

How might activities look for each decade of your life and those born in your generation?

is now so complex it can be overwhelming, even with our simplified version (see figure 2.2). Many exercisers have struggled to determine what to do, how intensely to do it, and how often to do it. Some started running and then learned walking was okay; some ran continuously for 30 minutes and learned that smaller increments of movement accumulated throughout the day were enough. Ultimately, the best exercise is the one you will do! But intentional and planned exercise, although important for health, was only one piece of the movement puzzle. The 1990s also brought the idea of physical activity into the health conversation.

In 1995, Pate and colleagues published a landmark recommendation on behalf of both the U.S. Department of Health and Human Services (HHS) and ACSM advocating that every adult in the United States accumulate at least 30 minutes of moderate-intensity physical activity on most, preferably all, days of the week. The message was intended to increase public awareness of the health-related benefits of moderate-intensity physical activity. The 1996 Surgeon General's report on physical activity and health (U.S. Department of Health and Human Services 1996) aligned with the ACSM statement, emphasizing that health benefits occur at a moderate level of physical activity (moving approximately 150 minutes per week). Hence, the first HHS Physical Activity Guidelines (PAG) included a simple explanation stating that all movement counts, no matter the intensity (U.S. Department of

Health and Human Services 2008). Compared to the exercise-focused ACSM guidelines—which we now know less than 20 percent of the population determined they could fit into their busy lifestyles—the HHS's 2008 PAG emphasized 150 minutes of weekly movement and a lifestyle approach that highlights how active transportation choices, occupational activities, leisure and recreation activities, and domestic chores can be incorporated into a weekly physical activity plan.

More recently, the 2018 Scientific Report, used to inform the most recent PAG, demonstrates that, in addition to disease prevention benefits, regular physical activity provides a variety of benefits that help individuals sleep better, feel better, and perform daily tasks more easily (2018 Physical Activity Guidelines Advisory Committee 2018). The 2018 Physical Activity Guidelines built on the first edition and formed recommendations for federal physical activity and education programs (U.S. Department of Health and Human Services 2018). Importantly, the first edition of the Physical Activity Guidelines for Americans stated that only 10-minute bouts of aerobic physical activity (such as walking) counted toward meeting the guidelines. The second edition removed this requirement to encourage Americans to move more frequently throughout the day as they work toward meeting the guidelines, emphasizing: *Any amount of physical activity has some health benefits*. The latest guidelines also reinforced the importance of muscle strengthening activities (to be explored in chapter 5). Beyond this brief history lesson, the

> Find activities that bring you joy and do those! If you do, you're likely to meet the current guidelines without even thinking about it.

most important point is that you should move—with intentional exercise and different types of physical activity on most days of the week.

We are getting back to finding joy in movement without a detailed prescription so that movement is a regular part of life rather than another thing we must fit into an already busy schedule. Would you stick with an activity that is higher intensity, or is moving more throughout the day a better option for your health? Or would you prefer a mix-and-match approach? Think about it.

Exercise + Physical Activity – Sedentary Behavior

The **ACSM exercise guidelines**, written by scientists and intended for delivery by fitness professionals, are highly detailed and can be hard for a regular person to understand. Alternatively, the **HHS Physical Activity Guidelines (PAG)**, which align closely with the current ACSM guidelines, are much simpler to understand and implement. One important goal of the PAG is to offer an under-standable method for putting physical activity behaviors into daily practice with many options that do not necessarily include intentional structured exercise. The PAG and ACSM guidelines are also well aligned in encouraging the reduction of sedentary behaviors. This brings us to the last but very important topic of movement—reduce your sitting! In our contemporary daily lives, sitting and other very low-intensity activities make up the great majority of our waking time. Current research highlights how too much sitting can harm your health.

Health Effects of Sedentary Behavior

As movement recommendations advanced beyond planned and intentional exercise to include physical activity obtained during occupational requirements, active transportation choices, domestic chores, and leisure pursuits, the effect of too much sedentary behavior was emphasized. Although definitions vary in the literature, a common theme for sedentary behavior is activities that typically occur in a sitting or lying position and do not increase energy expenditure much above resting level (this does not include sleeping). The new focus on avoiding excessive sedentary behavior is in part linked to our culture's increasingly sedentary, screen-based lifestyle. The expression

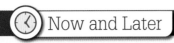

Now and Later

Everybody Walk

Now

Kaiser Permanente, in collaboration with many partners, created a 30-minute documentary called *The Walking Revolution*. It outlines the evidence-based practices of physical activity and why it is important to think about moving differently than we have in the past. Google "The Walking Revolution" and check out either the full 30-minute version or the shorter 8-minute version. Approximately how many minutes do you walk per day?

Later

Now let's analyze how many minutes you think you will be walking per day when you are 60 or 80 years old. What are your parents or other adults in your life currently doing for movement experiences? What about your grandparents? Will you be like these adults, or will you be more or less active?

Take Home

Now that you have watched the video and thought about your family movement history, what are your goals for walking and moving more throughout the day? How will you accomplish this goal? If you own technology that tracks your steps, such as a phone app or an activity tracker, what will your daily step goal be?

"sedentary behavior" has frequently been used as a synonym for not exercising, but the two are not synonymous, and sedentary behavior has serious consequences that are independent from those occurring from lack of exercise. This new way of thinking about movement emphasizes the distinctions between not exercising, physical inactivity, and sedentary behavior (Young et al. 2016):

1. Spending significant time in sedentary behaviors increases disease risk independent of physical activity and exercise; therefore, sedentary behavior has distinctly different negative health effects.

2. Prolonged sitting can further increase disease risk in people who are already insufficiently physically active.

3. The molecular and physiological responses to too much sitting are not simply the opposite of responses that follow a bout of physical activity or exercise.

4. Physical activity and exercise cannot make up for the consequences of too much sitting.

Dr. James Levine's work at Mayo Clinic determined that the negative effects of six hours of sedentary time were similar in magnitude to the benefit of one hour of exercise on fitness levels. His trade book called *Get Up! Why Your Desk Chair Is Killing You and What You Can Do About It* (2014) describes his research to the average population and was one of the first educational pieces to introduce the concept that today's chair-based world has negative consequences for our health.

> Stand up and walk around during TV commercials or breaks in video games, walk around when on the phone, or drop down to do a plank to break up your study session.

Although the 2022 ACSM exercise guidelines and the PAG outline the recommendations for exercise and physical activity, the recommendations regarding sedentary behavior are less detailed due to a lack of comprehensive research. For example, the World Health Organization (2020) recommends the reduction of sedentary behaviors across all ages and abilities, but the evidence is not available to

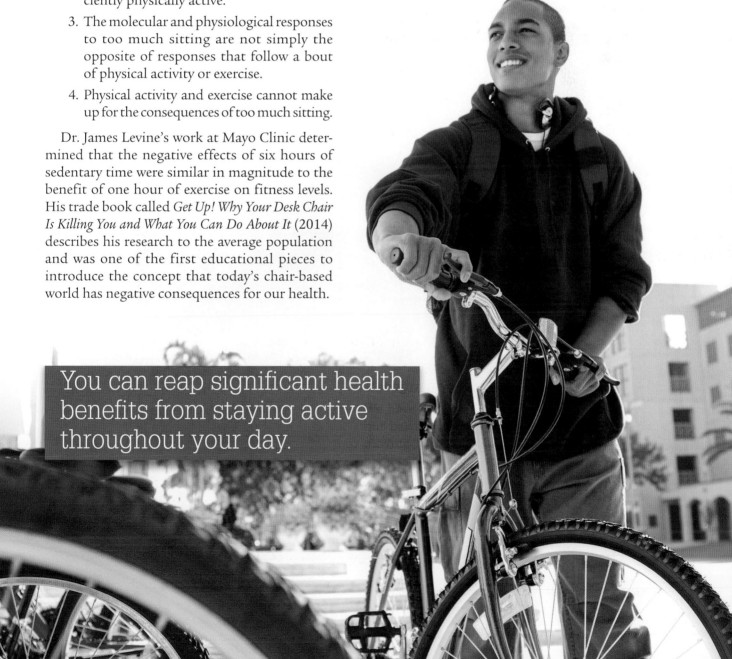

You can reap significant health benefits from staying active throughout your day.

quantify a sedentary behavior threshold. Future research will provide more guidance as to specific recommendations, but the evidence at this time points to sedentary behavior being an important health issue to address independent of physical activity and exercise. In fact, a meta-analysis study on sitting time by Nguyen et al. (2020) indicated that sedentary behavior interventions were better than physical activity interventions or combined physical activity and sedentary behavior interventions in reducing sitting time. Even physically active adults can benefit from reducing the total time they engage in sedentary pursuits by mixing in frequent, short bouts of standing and physical activity between periods of sedentary activity.

A Day in Your Life: The 24-Hour Activity Cycle (24-HAC) Paradigm

Contemporary research is now looking at the interrelatedness of sleep, sedentary behavior, light-intensity physical activity, and moderate-to vigorous-intensity physical activity. In 2019, Rosenburger et al. created the **24-hour activity cycle (24-HAC) paradigm** comprising these four elements to represent a new model for how we think about human movement (figure 2.3). It is likely (though currently not well researched) that time spent in one behavior affects another. For example, improving sleep possibly increases time in moderate or vigorous physical activity. The

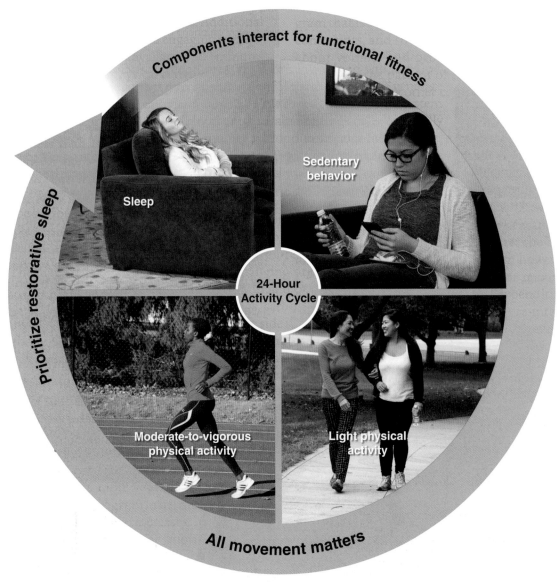

Figure 2.3   The 24-hour activity cycle paradigm.

Adapted from Rosenberger et al, (2019); Figure 1.

reverse is also generally true—that is, high-intensity physical activity often improves sleep.

A recent study of college students concluded there is a need to better identify the relationships within the 24-HAC paradigm to understand the integrated impact of sleep, sedentary behavior, and physical activity (light and moderate to vigorous intensities) on mental and physical energy and fatigue (Frederick et al. 2021). As evidence supporting the interrelatedness of these behaviors and their impacts on health continues to accumulate, it is almost certain that sleep will be a major component. Sleep will be discussed in detail in chapter 10.

Organizations have already begun to incorporate light, moderate and vigorous physical activity, sedentary behavior, and sleep into comprehensive 24-HAC guidelines. For example, the Canadian Society for Exercise Physiology (2020) has developed separate 24-HAC guidelines for

distinct population age groups (ages 0 to 4, 5 to 17, 18 to 64, and 65+). Certainly, as the research advances, more countries will follow along in the same manner. The PAG will likely include more detailed guidelines for sedentary behavior in future revisions as well.

Fitting Movement Into Everyday Life

The ACSM exercise guidelines and PAG both include summaries of extensive research showing the positive physiological and psychological benefits of regular exercise and physical activity across the life span. Many of the benefits will be described in detail in the following chapters. Benefits for young adults tend to be related to decreased stress, anxiety, and depression, as well as improved weight management. But as they move toward middle age, more important benefits include

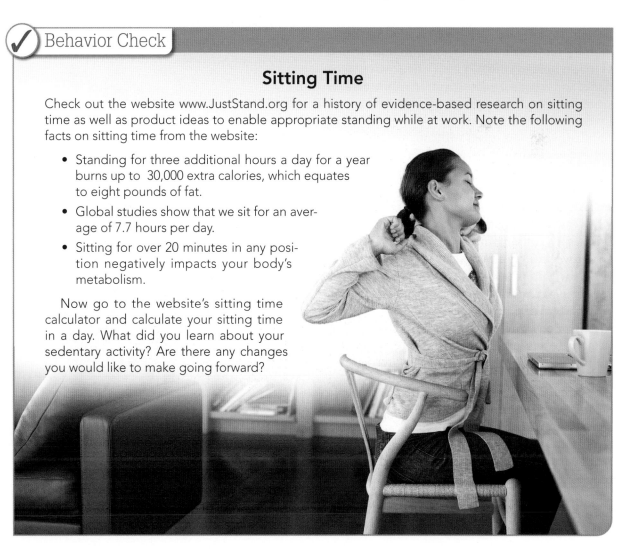

✓ Behavior Check

Sitting Time

Check out the website www.JustStand.org for a history of evidence-based research on sitting time as well as product ideas to enable appropriate standing while at work. Note the following facts on sitting time from the website:

- Standing for three additional hours a day for a year burns up to 30,000 extra calories, which equates to eight pounds of fat.
- Global studies show that we sit for an average of 7.7 hours per day.
- Sitting for over 20 minutes in any position negatively impacts your body's metabolism.

Now go to the website's sitting time calculator and calculate your sitting time in a day. What did you learn about your sedentary activity? Are there any changes you would like to make going forward?

decreased risk of chronic diseases and conditions, as compared to middle-aged and older individuals who do not move daily and who sit a lot. The goal at the end of a long life is to preserve the capability for independent living and lots of social activity. Regular physical movement is necessary not only to look better, but also to enjoy leisure activities well into your 80s and even 90s.

Experts suggest that a better way of increasing physical activity is to look beyond guidelines and recommendations and focus more on creating environments built for easy access to movement experiences. For example, creating walking and biking paths could enhance movement access and opportunity, thus making this healthy choice an easy choice. If we build it, will they use it? Some literature suggests this is true, but a more important question is—will *you* choose to use it? The majority of college campuses in the United States are highly walkable, cycle-friendly, and safe. We encourage you to make the most of this easy access to a safe, walkable environment.

To integrate consistent movement into your daily movement choices, focus on your behaviors as well as how you interact with your environment daily. Start thinking about your environment as your new gym. Your opinion of hills, stairs, and loaded backpacks might start to change. Remember that walking to class will contribute to your collective health outcomes—every movement counts! Take those stairs every chance you get! Your body needs to move, but your mind must make the decision to move more and sit less even when easier choices are available (e.g., the campus bus). Often you will find that when you move consistently throughout your day you will feel more energetic, and your sleep will improve.

As you go through your life stages, you will need to work hard to continue to incorporate movement into your day wherever you are located and with whatever equipment you can locate. For example, milk jugs filled with water or sand make great resistance training equipment for many middle-aged and older adults. And of course, walking is the most accessible activity for most individuals. Figure 2.4 presents very accessible ways you can incorporate physical activity into your busy days on campus. The chapter 2 labs on HK*Propel* will provide an opportunity to reflect on your personal fitness and daily movement history and preferences.

Setting SMART Goals for Movement

Setting **SMART goals** (ones that are specific, measurable, attainable, realistic, and time bound) is an efficient way to begin any new behavior (see figure 2.5). Let's briefly review how to set a SMART goal using physical activity (steps) so you can start to think about the goal-setting process for your health habits. This will be a behavioral warm-up for chapter 3.

Following is an example of how one person set a SMART movement goal based on steps:

Specific. I would like to increase my steps per day so I get a weekly average of 10,000 steps a day by the last week of the semester.

Measurable. I'll use my activity tracker to measure my steps per day and get a weekly average.

Attainable. Currently, I am getting 5,000 steps per day, so I believe that 10,000 steps per day is attainable as a goal.

Realistic. I currently get on the nearest bus to get to campus. I will skip the bus and walk to campus two times a week when I do not have early classes.

Time bound. I'm giving myself the entire semester to work up to my steps goal by increasing an average of 500 steps per day over the remaining 10 weeks in the class. By the last week of the semester, I will get an average of 10,000 daily steps.

The chapter 2 labs on HK*Propel* will help you set SMART goals for physical activity, exercise, and sedentary behavior. Use the same process mentioned in the previous example and make sure your goal meets the SMART criteria.

Once you have created a SMART goal, it's time to break your goal down even further with specific behavioral components (discussed further in chapter 3). Let's take

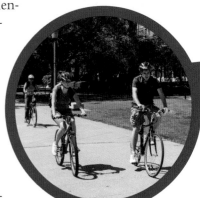

Let's roll!
Biking saves gas, reduces emissions, and keeps you moving!

the example of doing 150 minutes of movement a week. If you said you were going to do 30 minutes of physical activity each day for five days and you planned to do this by walking for 10 minutes three times a day, what behaviors must you change to do this? How would you measure the success of the goal? Do you need to enter the 10-minute breaks on a smartphone app? Will you buy an activity tracker and check out movement distances?

Maybe you need to create a walking route that is 10 minutes long so you can walk it three times daily. Be sure to personalize your plan by choosing options that are going to work for you.

Stand or walk while you work

Use a standing desk, take breaks from your chair and screen, and schedule walking meetings.

Use the stairs

Health permitting, choose the stairs every time. They are also a good option to break up prolonged sitting at your computer.

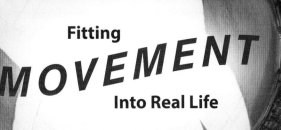

Fitting

MOVEMENT

Into Real Life

Take a walk in nature

Take a "nature bath" while you walk. Appreciate the sights, sounds, and smells. Ask a friend to join you.

Incorrect

Correct

Figure 2.4 Get creative with how to fit movement into your daily life on campus.

Wear backpacks over both shoulders

Wearing a backpack correctly over both shoulders strengthens your postural muscles.

As you progress through the chapter 3 content and lab, you will continue to practice SMART goal setting to set a health goal that is not movement based. You'll also prioritize your goals, choosing which ones to work on first. These might include more sleeping, changing your eating patterns, or drinking more water. Choose a goal that feels important to address now. If you want ideas for health goals outside of the physical activity realm, feel free to look ahead at other chapters in this book for inspiration, which discuss sexuality, stress, and addiction issues. Choose behaviors you'll need to change to meet your health goal. If your health goal is to eat more vegetables, what strategies will help you do that? For example, maybe you'll want to add vegetables you like to eat to your shopping list or change which aisles of the grocery store you choose to walk down.

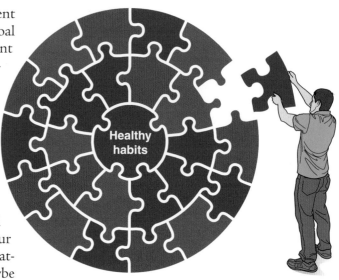

Figure 2.5   Build healthy habits one piece at a time through conscious goal setting.

Safety First: Getting Started With a Personal Movement Program

Before you start a personal movement or exercise program, it is important to plan for safety to prevent injury. Injuries, especially ones that become chronic, can hinder your ability to stick with your daily movement program. Preventing injuries in the short term enables lifelong movement. Strategies for injury prevention start with screening and are enhanced by good planning and practices. It is also important to understand care strategies if you do suffer an acute or chronic injury.

Screening for Major Challenges to Moving Safely

The major challenge to moving safely is related to heart and lung function. Most young adults have healthy cardiorespiratory systems, but some people experience conditions that make it more challenging to move safely, such as a heart murmur or asthma. The chapter 2 labs on HK*Propel* include a preparticipation screening questionnaire that will help you understand whether you need to consult your physician before initiating a movement or exercise program. As part of the chapter 2 lab experiences, you will access http://eparmedx.com and work through the questions on the Physical Activity Readiness Questionnaire for Everyone (**PAR-Q+**) to see if you are healthy enough to participate in exercise or physical activity without consulting a physician. If you have a chronic medical condition or must use certain medications on a regular basis, you should consult your personal physician to talk through the specific details.

You may have musculoskeletal limitations that are not covered as thoroughly in this screening process. If you have pain in your muscles or joints with movement, consult your physician to have a thorough evaluation before engaging in moderate- or vigorous-intensity movement or exercise. The "no pain, no gain" mentality simply does not work. If you experience pain, listen to these signals, and seek professional medical assistance.

Injury-Prevention Strategies

How you create and execute your movement plan can have a major effect on your risk for injuries. Of course, the type of activity you want to do will determine which strategies are most appropriate. An intense weightlifting session requires different strategies than an all-day hike. Figure 2.6 illustrates the keys to moving safely.

Planning for Your Future Moving Self and Health

Now

Let's say you start to move more and sit less now by walking to classes and getting some regular exercise when you can. You are also aware of sitting too much of the time. You might even ask your professors for a break to stand and stretch in the middle of class.

Later

In midlife—your 30s to 50s—you can keep these good habits going. Most college students do not have chronic conditions such cardiovascular disease, type 2 diabetes, or cancer. Indeed, these conditions typically occur in middle age. However, the biological processes underlying these conditions typically start in young adulthood. For example, plaque buildup in the coronary arteries, which causes many heart attacks, typically begins in young adults.

Take Home

Engaging in moderate- and vigorous-intensity physical activity over your life span will make you feel better, perform better, and prevent many chronic diseases. Think of movement as a tool you can start using now to help you function well and enjoy more years with greater health span.

Getting Care for Injuries

If you need to manage a minor exercise injury to a soft tissue such as muscles or tendons, use the **RICE principle**:

- *Rest.* Try to rest the injured body part. Stay off your feet if any part of your leg is injured.
- *Ice.* In the first 24 hours after an injury, apply a cold compress for 20 to 30 minutes and remove it for 20 to 30 minutes. Repeat as needed. Do not apply heat.
- *Compression.* Wrap a sprain or strain in a compression bandage for the first day or two after an injury. Make sure toes or fingers have some blood flow.
- *Elevation.* If possible, try to keep the injured part above the heart.

Other important strategies include seeking professional help when needed and using reputable resources for information such as WebMD (www.webmd.com) or the National Athletic Training Association (www.nata.org). Finally, do not ignore nagging or chronic injuries, which often progress into serious situations that are more challenging to resolve.

Injury-Prevention Strategies

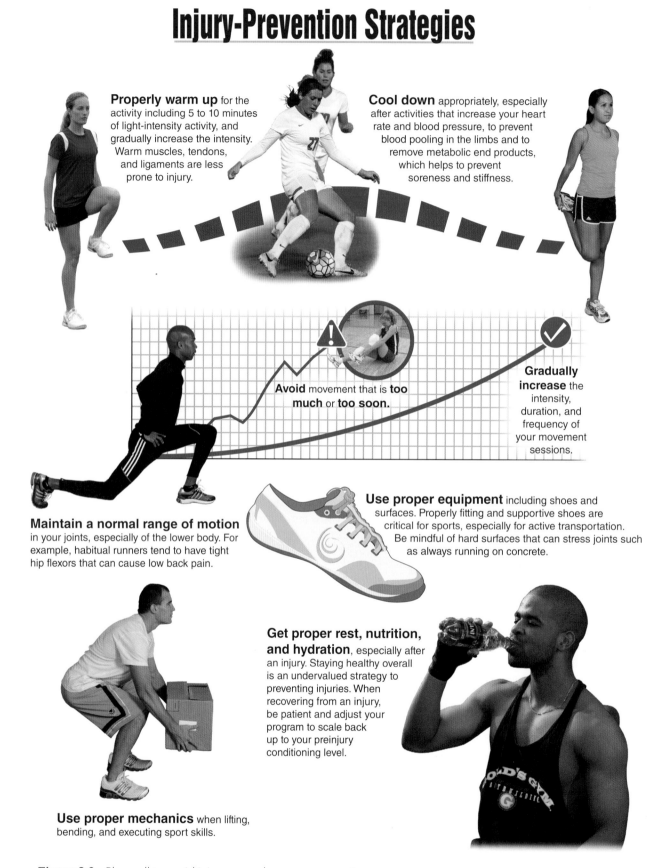

Properly warm up for the activity including 5 to 10 minutes of light-intensity activity, and gradually increase the intensity. Warm muscles, tendons, and ligaments are less prone to injury.

Cool down appropriately, especially after activities that increase your heart rate and blood pressure, to prevent blood pooling in the limbs and to remove metabolic end products, which helps to prevent soreness and stiffness.

Avoid movement that is **too much** or **too soon.**

Gradually increase the intensity, duration, and frequency of your movement sessions.

Maintain a normal range of motion in your joints, especially of the lower body. For example, habitual runners tend to have tight hip flexors that can cause low back pain.

Use proper equipment including shoes and surfaces. Properly fitting and supportive shoes are critical for sports, especially for active transportation. Be mindful of hard surfaces that can stress joints such as always running on concrete.

Get proper rest, nutrition, and hydration, especially after an injury. Staying healthy overall is an undervalued strategy to preventing injuries. When recovering from an injury, be patient and adjust your program to scale back up to your preinjury conditioning level.

Use proper mechanics when lifting, bending, and executing sport skills.

Figure 2.6 Plan well to avoid injury as you become more active.

Summary

Although the evidence is clear that all movement is essential to health, the benefits cannot be realized if you don't choose to move regularly. Both the ACSM and the HHS acknowledge that maintenance of movement behavior is challenging, because society has largely engineered movement out of our daily lives. Over the past few decades, we have gotten better at unlocking the behavioral keys to moving more and sitting less. To get regular physical activity, we must embrace the concept that healthy physical movement does not have to include intentional exercise in a fitness facility. Indeed, as explained in this chapter, physical activity obtained through occupational, domestic, transportation, and leisure choices can add many wonderful opportunities to move throughout the day. The important concept of reducing your time spent in sedentary behavior and breaking up your sitting time was also reinforced. Finally, a new model for considering the interrelated factors of sleep, sedentary behavior, light-intensity physical activity, and moderate- to vigorous-intensity physical activity, known as the 24-hour activity cycle (24-HAC) paradigm, was introduced.

The take-home point is that all movement matters. Every day, wake up and think this mantra: Move more and sit less! However, you will need to strategize, plan, and create ways to make it happen, because our modern world tries to steal your steps and capture your attention with a screen at every opportunity. Chapter 3 will build upon your SMART goal and dive deeper into behavioral concepts that will better enable you to manage your personal movement plan.

www ONLINE LEARNING ACTIVITIES

Go to HK*Propel* and complete the online activities to further facilitate your learning:

Study Activities: Review the main concepts of the chapter.

Labs: Complete the labs your instructor assigns.

Videos: Look through the videos and choose which ones you want to try this week.

REVIEW QUESTIONS

1. What is the main difference between intentional exercise and physical activity? Explain how attaching your daily movement choices to your larger life purposes can help you move to live and live to move. Provide an example from your life.

2. In what main ways are the ACSM exercise guidelines and the HHS Physical Activity Guidelines the same? How do they differ?

3. Intentional exercise practices (such as going to a fitness facility) are one partial solution for getting more movement into your day. Does exercise make up for sitting too much during the day? Why or why not?

4. What are three ways you can incorporate more physical activity into your day?

5. What does the SMART acronym mean, and why do we use it to set goals?

6. Practice writing both a movement and other health (e.g., eating, sleeping) SMART goal.

7. What are five injury-prevention strategies to consider to safely move?

8. What is the RICE principle of first aid?

Personalizing Healthy Behavior Change

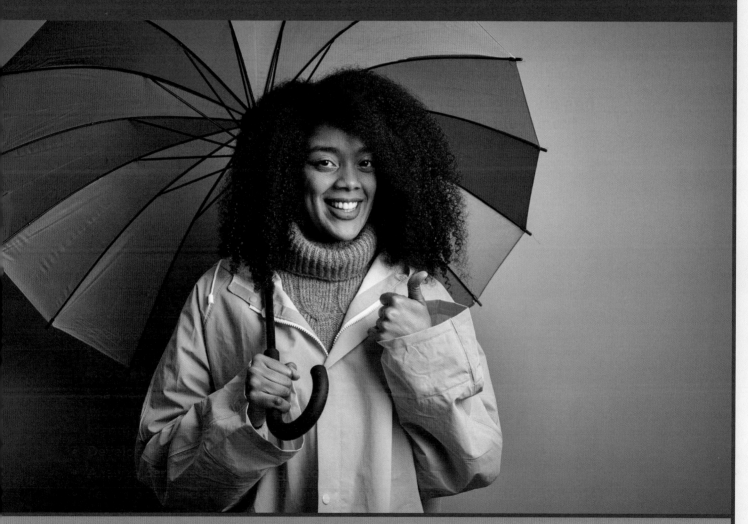

OBJECTIVES

- Identify how behavior influences your health and well-being.
- Develop behavior change strategies.
- Analyze barriers and challenges to behavior change.
- Set up goals and strategies for integrating movement and health behavior change into daily living practices.
- Use movement ideas from chapter 2 and behavioral theories from this chapter to choose and integrate a health-based behavior change process that works for you.

KEY TERMS

intention

Prochaska's transtheoretical model (TTM)

self-confidence

self-determination theory (SDT)

self-efficacy

self-efficacy theory

social ecological model

social psychology

theory of planned behavior (TPB)

Why do people change their behavior, and why is behavior change so hard for so many people? Change of any sort is amazingly difficult. Whether you are trying to move more, change unhealthy eating practices, or create change in a relationship, it is quite natural to resist this change; particularly if you do not see an immediate reward or if you perceive the outcome as negative. Leaving an unhealthy relationship might mean that you do not have anything to do on weekend nights. Maybe you have set a goal to walk to class, but today it is raining outside. Do you get out your rubber boots, look for your umbrella or waterproof jacket, and walk to class, or do you find a ride?

The cumulative choices you make each minute, hour, or day have consequences for your overall health and well-being. However, changing your behavior can be complicated. It takes planning, thought, action, reinforcement, and a general understanding of behavior-change research in order to create sustainable lifetime practices. For example, an article by prominent researchers Gaesser and Angadi (2021) concluded that shifting the focus away from weight loss and instead focusing on increasing physical activity to improve cardiorespiratory fitness may be prudent for treating obesity-related health conditions. This is a much different message than our predominant focus

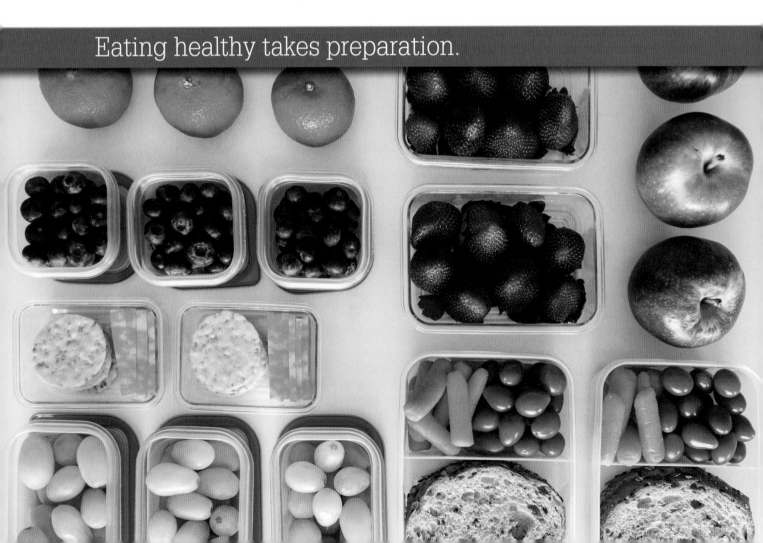

Eating healthy takes preparation.

The key to changing a behavior is understanding how habits work. If you want to sleep more but can't find the time, then focusing on where you use your time, rather than working on sleeping more, may be the start of changing that habit (Duhigg 2014).

on dietary changes or physical activity to lose or manage weight. The key here is to make the focus on daily movement so you gain greater functional fitness so that you can do more in your life now and in your future. While striving to reach one fitness goal, weight management might be an added benefit.

This chapter introduces several theories of behavior change and provides practical examples of how to integrate evidence-based behavioral practices into daily living. At the end of the chapter, you will apply behavioral methods and tools to your fitness and well-being goals to finalize an overall health goal. Our hope is that this chapter will help you have a better understanding about how you can integrate established health behavior theories into personal practice to tackle a specific behavior change and achieve your personalized goals.

Leveraging Models and Theories for Your Positive Behavior Change

It is interesting that the last two editions of the ACSM *Guidelines for Exercise Testing and Prescription* (2018, 2022) have a final chapter on behavioral theories and strategies. Behavior is sometimes considered an afterthought when in fact, it is imperative that one acts on their intentions in order to reap the health benefits of movement. Fortunately, health behaviorists have done research that can help guide the change process and show you how to begin. Several behavioral theories are discussed in this chapter that provide evidence-based insights on the behavior change process, including Prochaska's transtheoretical model, the self-efficacy theory, the self-determination theory, the theory of planned behavior, and the social ecological model. Although many of these models and theories have been used for numerous health behaviors (e.g., eating, smoking),

notably they have all been researched with movement behaviors. As you learn about these models and theories, keep in mind that no one model or theory is the right or perfect one. You likely will benefit from combining multiple approaches as you construct the perfect plan for you, and your plan will need to change throughout your life.

Before we dive into this content, take a moment to reflect on a process for behavior change that has worked for you. Close your eyes and think of a behavior that you wanted to change in the past. Perhaps you wanted to make a habit of flossing your teeth daily or eating the recommended daily servings of vegetables. Whatever the change was, think for a moment: Why were you successful or not successful? What strategies helped facilitate the change process for you? What barriers made the change process difficult? Keep your previous experiences in mind as you review the models and theories that follow and start to formulate a plan to use the next time you are attempting to change a behavior.

Prochaska's Transtheoretical Model (TTM)

Prochaska's transtheoretical model (TTM) of behavior change can help you conceptualize where you are in the change process (Prochaska and DiClemente 1984). The TTM initially came from research centered on smoking cessation, but it has been modified and applied to other behaviors. With our main health behavior focus being movement and functional fitness, we use the TTM as a way to outline beginning a new program.

Figure 3.1 summarizes the TTM. If you are not currently thinking about being physically active or exercising regularly, you are in the precontemplation stage of change, where moving more is not on your immediate radar. If you begin researching ways to move more (i.e., thinking about making a positive change), you are more likely in the contemplation stage. If you determine how you might create this change (for example, thinking, "tomorrow I might go for a short walk"), then you are in the preparation stage. If you start to walk three or four times per week for 30 minutes daily, you are in the action stage of change. If you continue to walk three of four times per week for 30 minutes a day for six months, you are in the maintenance stage of change.

Change a Habit

You can use this worksheet to help you change any habit. Use one copy for each habit you'd like to change.

Examples: Get 8,000 or more steps 5 days a week, strength train 3 days a week, add a vegetable to every meal, get at least 7 hours of sleep every night. Be as specific as you can.

1 List one habit you'd like to focus on at this time: _____ .

2 From the descriptions, select which stage describes you best.

3 Read the descriptions and circle the things you can do to help you move to the next stage.

Precontemplation stage
"I don't want to change"

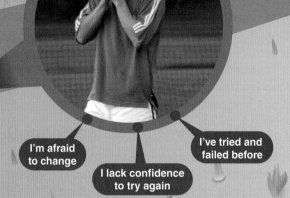

What do I need to do?
- Ask others how they changed
- Read messaging through social media
- Attend an event around a cause (breast cancer awareness week)

I'm afraid to change

I lack confidence to try again

I've tried and failed before

Contemplation stage
"I'm thinking about changing"

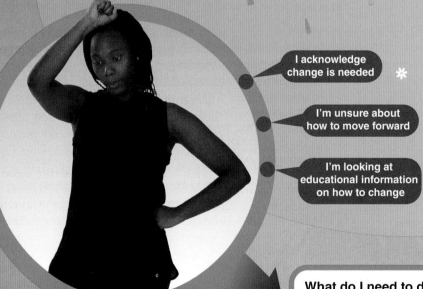

I acknowledge change is needed

I'm unsure about how to move forward

I'm looking at educational information on how to change

What do I need to do?
- Weigh the pros and cons of changing
- Get help on how to move forward
- Relate to a personal issue that helps you consider the change

Figure 3.1 Summary of Prochaska's stages of change.

Maintenance stage
"How do I maintain the change"

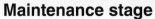

Engage family in the change process

Hire a professional to assist you

Get support from friends

What do I need to do?
• Set a goal and monitor the goal
• Work to continue the plan for 6 months
• Analyze and outline daily priorities

Action stage
"How do I implement the plan"

What do I need to do?
• Consider other positive changes to stay on a roll
• Regularly continue to practice the plan
• Work to avoid relapse and boredom

Learn new coping skills

Evaluate time management skills to continue the plan

Utilize self-monitoring and planning skillsets

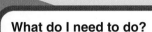

Preparation stage
"How do I move from thinking to doing"

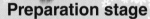

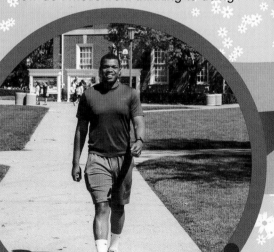

What do I need to do?
• Make a plan to reach your goals
• Evaluate where you are in relation to where you want to be
• Begin to move from thinking about the action to actually doing it

Start planning and getting ready; hire someone to help you

Make a plan and detail it out for a few months

Seek out information and get educated

Note that sometimes things happen that cause you to move from maintenance back to precontemplation. Maybe your running partner transfers to a different school, your favorite fitness facility closes, or you move and need time to learn about your new environment. After a life change, it is easy to move from maintenance all the way back to precontemplation. After moving back to precontemplation, it is quite a process to get back to the maintenance stage of change. Change is never quick or permanent; it is a constant work in progress! You will most likely move back and forth through the stages of change before a behavior becomes a natural practice in your daily life.

Beginning a new behavior starts with increasing your knowledge, caring about the effect of your health on yourself and others, and understanding the benefits gained. Once you begin to prepare for this change, looking for options, finding social support, and using reminders and rewards become important. The TTM guides the change process by helping you consider action items for various stages of change. Figure 3.2 contains a list of common action items that may help with your change process, depending on your stage of change.

Developing Tools for Processes of Change Using the TTM

To help you get started on your own physical activity and health goals, let's integrate the TTM into practice. Bridging the gap between theory and practice is how you take research-based information and apply it to your own life. Let's use Prochaska's TTM to help you understand where you are in the behavior change process.

If you are not thinking about change, you are in the precontemplation stage of change. To encourage yourself to start thinking about change, you might use these processes: Increase your knowledge (for example, learn more about eating healthier or doing more physical activity), think about what kind of role model you want to be to others, examine your attitudes and self-talk, or do some research about the benefits of this change.

> You'll never change your life until you change something you do daily. The secret of your success is found in your daily routine.

To move to the contemplation stage of change, where you are thinking about changing but are not yet acting on it (see figure 3.3), weigh the pros and cons of this behavior change. You might also journal about your behavior, imagine the effects of this change on your life overall, and link the benefits of changing with what you want for yourself long term.

Once you are in the preparation stage of change, sign a contract with yourself, your friends, and your family about your commitment to making a behavior change, and find tools and information that will help you change. For the action and maintenance stages of change, find a partner who will work with you, ask friends and family members to send you reminders, or find a support group.

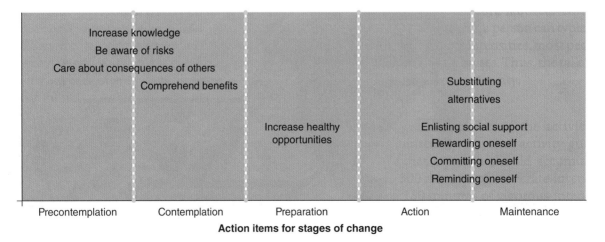

Figure 3.2 Action items for different stages of change.

✓ Behavior Check

Get Your Steps In Weekly!

The 2018 Physical Activity Guidelines Advisory Committee (2018) states that some physical activity is better than none. For health benefits, 150 minutes to 300 minutes of moderate-intensity aerobic activity ought to be spread throughout the week. Additional health benefits can also be gained by engaging in physical activity beyond 300 minutes. Research suggests that 7,900 steps per day for males and 8,300 steps per day for females translate into approximately 30 minutes per day of moderate to vigorous physical activity (Tudor-Locke et al. 2011).

- How many steps do you take on most days?
- What is your goal for steps per day?

Whether you move more throughout the day for a cumulative 30 minutes or plan an intentional exercise session and move continuously for 30 minutes three or four times per week in an organized class or program, you will meet the weekly guidelines for physical activity.

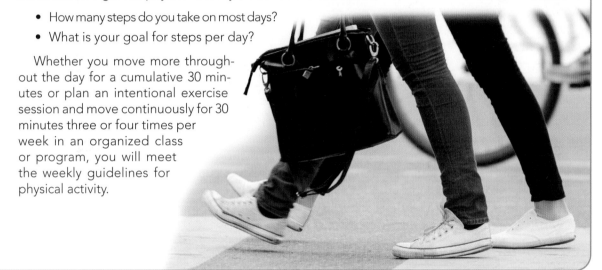

Thinking About Change

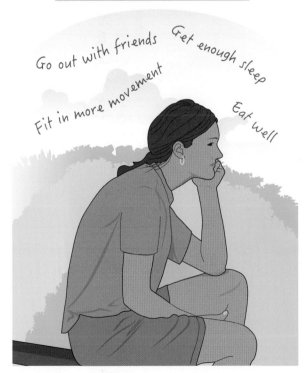

Figure 3.3 Thinking about change is a process.`

Another tool that you can use as you move through the stages of change is problem solving around or through barriers. How will you stay active if the weather prevents you from moving outdoors or if you can't afford a membership to a fitness center? What if your friends aren't supportive of the changes you want to make? What if you can't seem to find time to work out? Planning strategies in advance to overcome barriers is highly effective to help you stay committed to making changes in your life.

Recognizing and Dealing With Barriers

We have the best intentions to be more active, but barriers play a big role in keeping us from moving more and sitting less (figure 3.4). The biggest barriers to movement are lack of time, lack of motivation or energy, lack of resources or equipment, and lack of support. These barriers are real, and they change over time and depend on the obligations and stages of life. Thus, it is extremely important to identify your own personal barriers and develop strategies and solutions to overcome those barriers. Take a moment to consider the

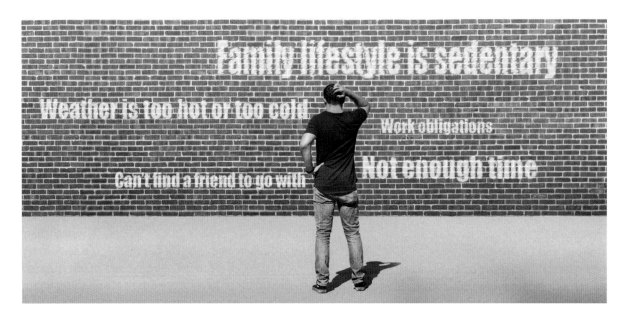

Figure 3.4   What are your barriers to changing your movement behaviors and how will you get around them?

 barriers to physical activity that most commonly affect you, then dive into this a bit further by completing the chapter 3 labs in HK*Propel*.

Self-Efficacy Theory

The **self-efficacy theory** is grounded in **social psychology**. What is self-efficacy? In general, **self-efficacy** is your confidence in your ability to control your motivation, behavior, and social environment. Specific self-efficacy is your belief in your ability to succeed at a designated task, such as walking three days per week to class instead of taking the bus. Self-efficacy theory (Bandura 1977; McAuley 1994) therefore suggests that the higher your self-efficacy (i.e., confidence), the more likely you are to be able to make a change in a habit or behavior (Nigg 2014).

Self-confidence is a common term for self-efficacy; however, the two terms differ slightly in meaning. Self-confidence refers to your belief or trust in your abilities, qualities, and judgment. Self-efficacy is more situational in nature and thus more specific. An important concept is that self-efficacy is both a predictor and an outcome in behavior change such as movement. Thus, the greater you can build your self-efficacy for your movement plan, the more you will move, and the more you adhere to your movement program, the more your self-efficacy to do so increases. In essence, you are building your "motivational fitness."

When you like the activity you've chosen and you feel like you can do it well, you will be more likely to stick with it.

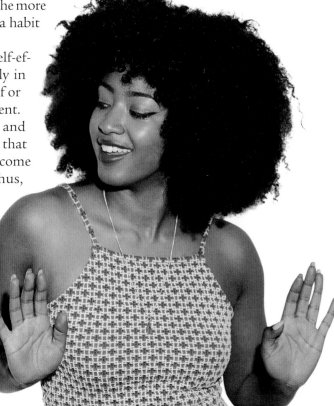

Self-Determination Theory (SDT)

Self-determination theory (SDT), another theory grounded in social psychology, is a theory of human motivation and personality (Deci and Ryan 1985; Fortier et al. 2012; Teixeira et al. 2012). According to SDT, people have three basic psychological needs: autonomy, or self-determination; competence, or mastery; and relatedness, or ability to experience meaningful relationships (American College of Sports Medicine 2022). When these three needs are fulfilled, optimal motivation, performance, and well-being are enhanced.

Autonomy is feeling in control of our own behaviors and goals (e.g., I choose to move). Do you remember a time when someone told you to do something that really irked you and made you *not* want to do whatever they asked? This is an example of someone taking your autonomy away. *Competence* refers to the need to learn and gain mastery of skills (e.g., I am good at exercising regularly). Think about a time you did a challenging exercise that made you feel successful and capable, like jumping rope, sprinting, or mastering a difficult lift in the weight room. The sense of accomplishment you feel is competency. *Relatedness* refers to our need to feel a sense of belonging and connection with others in our environment (e.g., I feel accepted and can relate to the people in my fitness class). Each of us wants to feel understood and cared for by others—including when we're

trying to be physically active. Overall, this theory suggests that you can achieve high self-determination if your needs for competence, relatedness, and autonomy are fulfilled (see figure 3.5).

Theory of Planned Behavior (TPB)

The **theory of planned behavior (TPB)**, which links beliefs and behavior, holds that your attitude, subjective norms, and perceived behavioral control work together to shape your behavioral intentions (Ajzen and Driver 1992). Intentions are a determination to act a certain way. The TPB comes from the theory of reasoned action, which states that intentions often predict actual behavior outcomes. A meta-analysis applying these two theories to exercise (Downs and Hausenblas 2005) suggests that your attitude strongly influences your intention, which is the strongest determinant of your behavior. As mentioned earlier, a recent review of obesity treatment by Gaesser and Angadi (2021) suggests that adherence to physical activity may improve if health care professionals consistently emphasize the benefits of physical activity and cardiorespiratory fitness rather than weight loss. In this way, focusing on moving more and sitting less rather than on losing weight transforms the intention behind the change. Also, the knowledge that your movement program does not have to be hard, continuous, uncomfortable, or formal in order to provide health benefits can

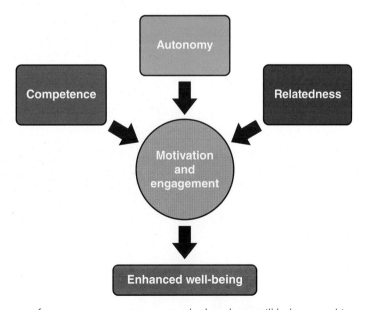

Figure 3.5 Having a sense of competence, autonomy, and relatedness will help you achieve your long-term goals.

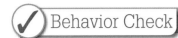
Behavior Check

Using Self-Determination Theory to Help Set Goals

Stop for a minute and take a brief inventory of your psychological needs for a movement goal you might set for this class.

Psychological needs	Your reflections about your movement experience
Competence: A sense of mastery and confidence that we are adequate and effective.	1. Describe a time when you felt competent. 2. Describe a time when you did not feel competent. 3. What can you do to keep feeling competent in the future?
Autonomy: A feeling that we are in control of our lives and make our own choices.	1. Describe a time when you did not feel that you had autonomy. 2. What can you do to keep feeling that you have autonomy in the future?
Relatedness: A sense of belonging and connection with others.	1. Describe a time when you felt connected with others. 2. Describe a time you did not feel connected with others. 3. What can you do to keep feeling connected with others?

1. What is one of your anticipated movement goals? _____

   _____

2. Work through the table for this movement goal by answering the questions asked in each component of the SDT model. As you work toward this goal, consider the following:

   - What can you do to keep feeling competent as you move?

     _____

     _____

   - What can you do to keep feeling that you have autonomy when you move?

     _____

     _____

   - What can you do to feel connected to others when you move?

     _____

     _____

change your attitude about engaging in these important health behaviors. Let us consider some positive attitudes that can influence your intentions now that you are starting to explore the goal-setting process:

1. *Behavioral attitude.* I like to move; it makes me feel better.
2. *Subjective norm.* My friends like to move. I know a few people I can ask to go running or walking with me.
3. *Perceived behavioral control.* I can walk to class on my own, and it counts as a part of my daily movement.

These three constructs help us predict our intentions and are similar to the self-efficacy theory in that they require you to be confident in order to act on a behavior. The TPB can also apply to any other health practice. For example, it's often difficult in college to engage in healthy sleeping patterns. Let's work through an example using sleep as the health behavior you want to improve or change:

1. *Behavioral attitude.* I feel and think better when I get eight hours of sleep.
2. *Subjective norm.* I will let my roommates know sleep is important to me and ask them to enter the room quietly if they see me sleeping.
3. *Perceived behavioral control.* I will wear earplugs to prevent my roommates from distracting or interrupting my sleep on the weekends.

Social Ecological Model

Moving forward to another model that can influence your health behaviors, especially your movement plan, is the **social ecological model** (Sallis et al. 2012). Could the city you live in or the friends around you predispose you to health risks? Think back to the Sharecare survey on state well-being rankings in chapter 1. With states like California and Hawaii ranking among the top 10 in well-being and states like Alabama and Kentucky near the bottom, there are most likely environmental aspects at work. The social ecological model considers five levels of influence on behavior: individual, interpersonal, organizational, community,

and policy systems. A key principle of the social ecological model is that interventions are most effective when they consider the influence of all of these factors on one another.

Figure 3.6 outlines the constructs of the social ecological model. The model begins with the individual but then ripples out into relationships, institutions and organizations, the community, and then into larger policies and systems (Sallis, Owen, and Fisher 2015).

Ecological models consider the social environment when examining what determines behavioral choices. Think about the company you keep, especially close friends and romantic partners. If your best friend leads a sedentary lifestyle, you may be more sedentary as well. Consider a 75-year Harvard study of adult development that followed Harvard graduates with a mean income of $105,000 at age 50 and an inner-city cohort that had a mean income of $35,000 at age 50. The study found that social well-being was more important than financial success for successful aging. Specifically, the quality (not quantity) of close relationships and stable, supportive marriages led to a happy life. If you are interested in the details of the study, search for Robert Waldinger's TED Talk, "What Makes a Good Life? Lessons From the Longest Study on Happiness." The study's initial author, George Vaillant, also wrote a book in 2002 called *Aging Well* that is based on the study's outcomes.

The social ecological model also examines the broader perspective of the physical environment—including where you live and what facilities are available to you (Deci and Ryan 1985)—as well as larger systemic factors. This model suggests that urban planning, including transportation systems, parks, and walking trails, is a key contributor to increasing physical activity (Bauman et al. 2012). Health behavior sustainability is much more widespread if barriers are removed, and convenient choices are available (Sallis et al. 2012). For example, social distancing related to COVID-19 reduced bus and train usage and increased biking and walking outside to prevent disease transmission. A Lime company scooter survey of five major cities found that 68 percent of respondents said they would use share scooters in the future (Yobbi 2020)—a 25 percent increase compared to pre-COVID-19 use. Sallis, Owen, and Fisher (2015) also make the case that activity-friendly

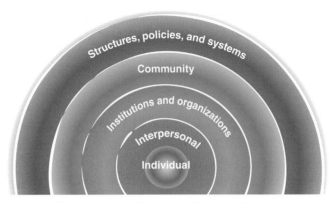

Figure 3.6   Example of the ripple effect of the social ecological model of behavior change.

environmental design shows strong evidence of additional environmental benefits like reduced pollution and carbon emissions. This is a perfect example of the social ecological model in action.

As you determine where you want to live, work, and play, carefully consider the environment around you. Do you avoid riding your bike to school or work because there are no bike lanes where you feel safe? Do you find it difficult to purchase healthy food because many nearby restaurants are fast food establishments? Given the growing epidemic of obesity and sedentary lifestyle practices in the United States and other countries, we need to pay more attention to the features of our communities and neighborhoods that either create or remove barriers to making healthy choices (Sallis and Spoon 2015).

Summary of Behavioral Theories

Prochaska's transtheoretical model, self-efficacy theory, self-determination theory, and the theory of planned behavior are all individually based behavioral theories for making good health behavior choices. The social ecological model has personal choices at its center but reminds us that there is much more to making good lifestyle

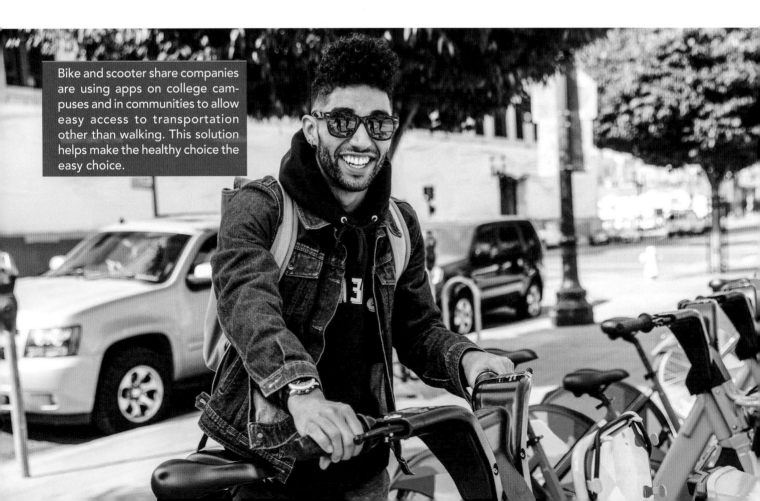

Bike and scooter share companies are using apps on college campuses and in communities to allow easy access to transportation other than walking. This solution helps make the healthy choice the easy choice.

choices than our own motivation and intentions. Where we choose to live, work, and play influences our happiness and contribute to healthy lifestyle practices, as do greater social and political circumstances, for better or worse. These theories also teach us that personal goal setting is a major key to focusing on lifestyle changes regardless of what is happening environmentally.

Personalizing the Behavior Change Process

Before revisiting the SMART goal process to help you manage your own behavior, it is a good idea to remind yourself that changing behavior is a complex interaction of many factors. At any age it can

be challenging, but for college students who are in the stage of life that is inherently full of change, it can be extra challenging (see figure 3.7). Gather your motivation and strategies to make positive health changes, but also be kind to yourself while on the journey to a high level of well-being.

Recall in chapter 2, you were asked to set SMART (specific, measurable, attainable, realistic, time-bound) goals for specific behaviors you wanted to change. To best apply behavior change theory to SMART goals, let's revisit the big picture of how habitual movement and health combine to create a fulfilling life. An article from the Centers for Disease Control and Prevention (2021) on the benefits of physical activity reminds us that engaging in regular physical activity behaviors is one of the most important health choices we can

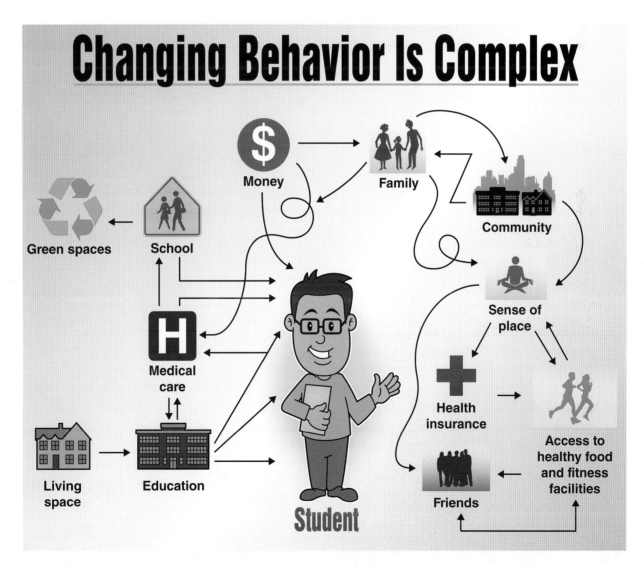

Figure 3.7   There are many factors to consider in the change process.

make. Van Cappellen et al. (2017) also reminds us that moving more and sitting less makes us feel good, thus influencing our decisions to repeat those behaviors. If you enjoy doing something, you will be more likely to do it again. If you do not like running, then consider walking or hiking outdoors. You get the same amount of movement whether you walk two miles (3.2 km) or run that distance; one will just take you longer. Which one will you enjoy more? The behavior you enjoy is the one you will continue to do.

Goal Setting Revisited

Goal setting is a process that is key to changing health behaviors and enhancing your daily lifestyle. Think of setting a goal that is relevant and

meaningful to you as an ongoing self-experiment. Following is a review of some principles of goal setting to ponder that were introduced at the end of chapter 2. Recall that the SMART acronym of goal setting basics included the following: specific, measurable, attainable, realistic and time bound. We will review them again now that you have a better understanding of how behavior theories, grounded in social psychology, can help get you moving and keep you moving.

Former football player and coach Lou Holtz said, "If you are bored with life—you don't get up every morning with a burning desire to do things— you don't have enough goals."

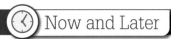

Now and Later

Choose What You Like to Do

Now

The scientific focus on movement and exercise has helped many people, but it has not proven effective for changing population-wide movement trends. As obesity and inactive sedentary behaviors continue to increase in the United States, more work is clearly needed to develop healthy lifestyles that are sustainable and effective. Could a focus on doing what feels good help us enjoy movement more? Could selecting a mode and type of movement that works for you make a difference in adherence to moving more and sitting less? What if everything we do counts? Would you rather run two miles alone or walk two miles while talking to your friends?

Later

Choosing activities that you will continue to enjoy for years to come is essential for long-term health behavior change. And as you leave college and start to build your life, your social and physical environment will undoubtedly change. What will you do to add movement to your lifestyle? Choose an activity that you like to do on a regular basis.

Take Home

If you focus on healthy behaviors that feature things you enjoy or that you find useful in your daily life, you're more likely to stick with them. Self-determination theory teaches us that motivation is a personal choice. Some people find fitness centers useful in prioritizing and sustaining physical activity patterns throughout their lifetime, but if you have found it hard to go to a fitness facility, consider your many other options. This would help it become a part of your lifestyle instead of something you feel obligated to do. Considering the *why* related to movement and behavior change and pairing your why with feel-good movements are essential for long-term adherence. Fitness fads come and go, but enjoyment goes a long way toward a lifelong commitment to being physically active.

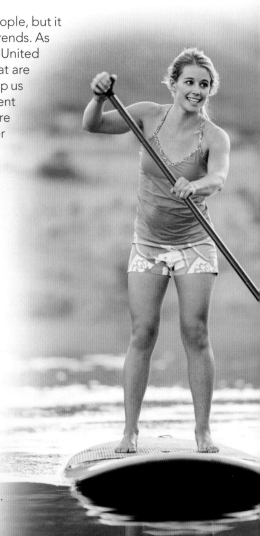

1. ***Set specific and measurable goals.*** Successful goals are specific, measurable, and established in behavioral terms. SMART goals are needed to measure progress, potentially adjust course, and ultimately determine success.

2. ***Set moderately difficult but realistic goals.*** The best goals are difficult enough to challenge you but realistic enough to be achieved. Set short-term goals that are no more than 5 to 15 percent above current performance levels (see figure 3.8). The secret is to balance goal challenge and achievability. Use the chapter 3 labs in HK*Propel* to evaluate the goals you set in the chapter 2 labs.

3. ***Set process, performance, and outcome goals.*** Goal setting works best in a backward design process. Start with your desired outcome, then create process and performance goals on how to acquire your end movement goal. See figure 3.9 for the relationship between different types of goals. The key is knowing when to focus on each type of goal.

Outcome goals are usually long term and focus on the result (i.e., the *what*) you want to achieve rather than how to achieve it. It is best if outcome goals are determined first, then broken down into performance and process goals that will lead to the desired outcome. Examples of outcome goals for the semester might be to lose 10 pounds, improve your 1.5-mile walk/run time by 15 to 20 percent to improve cardiorespiratory fitness, or increase the time you can hold your abdominal plank to 2 minutes for your core muscular fitness.

Performance goals focus on specific standards—for example, comparing your body mass index to health standards or 1.5-mile walk/run time with the norm for

Leo Tolstoy said, "Everyone thinks of changing the world, but no one thinks of changing himself." Be sure to set goals that are uniquely yours.

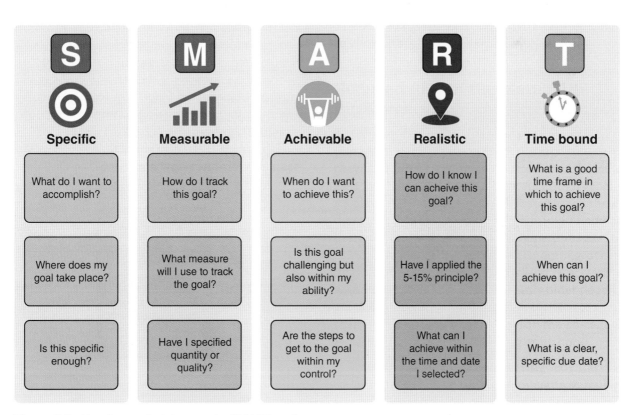

Figure 3.8 Use these principles to write SMART goals.

your age group. Reflect on your previous performance goals and change or modify them accordingly. For this reason, performance goals tend to be more flexible. These goals, although being linked to standards, can also be personal as they move you closer to your outcome goals. Examples of performance goals are losing a pound a week for 15 weeks, walking the 1 mile to campus 30 seconds faster each week, or increasing your core plank time by 10 seconds every week.

Process goals focus on specific strategies or steps (i.e., the *how*) that will help you achieve your performance or outcome goals. They are also very flexible and personal. These goals can be developed by thinking through barriers you are facing and brainstorming solutions for overcoming those barriers. Think of process goals as personal trial-and-error experiments. Examples of process goals may be practicing intermittent fasting (e.g., not eating for 12 hours overnight) for 15 weeks to assist with your performance goal of losing 10 pounds, walking to class every day to support your goal of improving your walking time, or completing your core plank exercise in front of your favorite Netflix show.

4. ***Record and monitor goals.*** Track your progress by posting goals in a place you see them every day to hold you accountable and to keep you motivated.

Develop goal achievement strategies. Setting goals without thinking through how you know you achieved the goal is like going on a road trip without your GPS. You need strategies to support the goals you set. Strategies should be flexible and involve numbers (e.g., how much, how many, and how often). Instead of planning to walk to class on Monday, Wednesday, and Friday, it might be better to focus on walking any three days of the week. You are more likely to achieve a goal by remaining flexible than by forcing yourself to stick to arbitrarily specific parameters that lack flexibility

Identify barriers and action plans. Not every goal set will come without difficulty. If you struggle reaching a goal, spend some time thinking through what is standing in your way. What are some things you know will help you reach your goal? The best way to overcome barriers is to map out a plan or strategy.

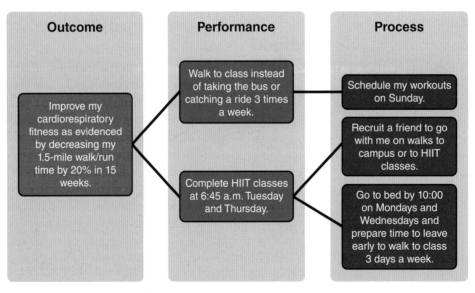

Figure 3.9 Relationship between the different types of goals.

Behavior Check

Goal Importance and Confidence Check-Ins

Use the following two scales to check in with yourself about how you are doing on your goal. Rating your importance and confidence helps you keep track of your progress.

On a scale of 1 to 10, rate how important reaching this goal is to you (select one).

Not important at all in my life   **Most important thing in my life**

1   2   3   4   5   6   7   8   9   10

On a scale of 1 to 10, rate how confident you are in your ability to reach this goal (select one).

Cannot do at all   **Moderately confident**   **Highly certain**

1   2   3   4   5   6   7   8   9   10

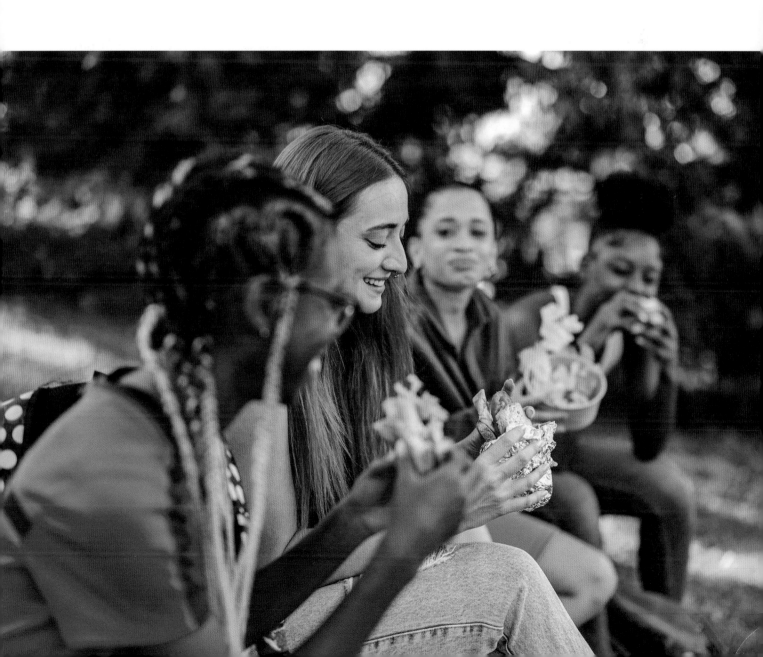

Summary

Incorporating behavior change models and theories into your daily movement planning may require you to dig deeper into why you started and stopped exercise or other movement choices in the past. You have a better chance at lasting success in meeting your movement goals if you also consider research-based implications for behavior as a piece of successful goal-setting practices. Using personal behavior change ideas and integrating them into constructs such as self-efficacy, self-determination, and awareness of where you are in the change process prior to beginning your journey will help overall success. Also, the TPB reminds us that your attitude, the support of friends and family, and perceived control over the change are also essential. Remember that the strategy is to start or continue your movement plan now and also build a personal movement behavior management took kit so you can remodel your program throughout your life.

Research shows the importance of a behavior change being your own idea, not someone else's (Zenko, Ekkekakis, and Kavetsos 2016). A good coach or trainer will work with you by asking what *you* want out of the program. Coaches or trainers who give you their workout are not doing their job of helping you enjoy the experience so you can continue it on your own. The medical profession has taught us to prescribe behavior, but the human aspect of decision making is critical for ongoing behavior change (Segar 2022). If you want to move, make the decision to move, and choose movements that you enjoy, then you will have a much better chance of continuing to move regularly for a lifetime of healthy living.

(www) ONLINE LEARNING ACTIVITIES

Go to HK*Propel* and complete all of the online activities to further facilitate your learning:

Study Activities: Review the main concepts of the chapter.

Labs: Complete the labs your instructor assigns.

Videos: Look through the videos and choose which ones you want to try this week.

REVIEW QUESTIONS

1. What are the five stages of change in Prochaska's transtheoretical model?
2. List one or two behavioral action items for each of the five stages of change in Prochaska's transtheoretical model.
3. How might the behavior of others impact your goals for behavioral change both from a positive and negative perspective?
4. Explain the social ecological model of behavior change and apply it to your personal goal setting for exercise or movement.
5. Why is it important to consider process and performance goals when setting specific SMART outcome goals for exercise or movement?

Cardiorespiratory Fitness

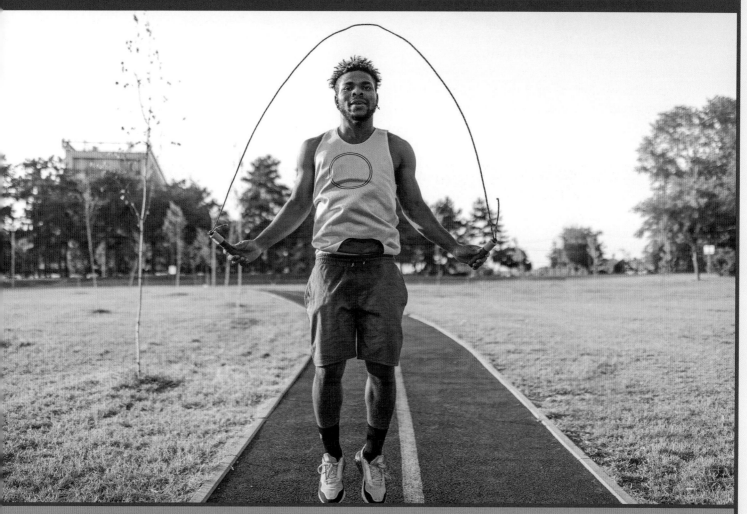

OBJECTIVES

- **Understand how your body obtains and uses energy for physical movement.**
- **Describe methods for assessing your cardiorespiratory fitness.**
- **Appreciate ways in which cardiorespiratory fitness can enhance your health and make you feel better.**
- **Design a personalized plan to improve your cardiorespiratory fitness.**

KEY TERMS

adenosine triphosphate (ATP)

adenosine triphosphate–phosphocreatine (ATP-PC) system

carbohydrates

cardiorespiratory endurance

cardiorespiratory fitness

diastole

dietary fats

dose–response association

glucose

glycogen

heart rate reserve (HRR) method

high-intensity interval training (HIIT)

maximal oxygen consumption ($\dot{V}O_2$max)

metabolic equivalents (METs)

metabolism

nonoxidative (anaerobic) system

oxidative (aerobic) system

protein

rating of perceived exertion (RPE)

specificity of training

systole

talk test

Cardiorespiratory fitness is a key component of health-related fitness. A well-trained and fit cardiorespiratory system helps you enjoy recreational pursuits and complete your daily activities with greater ease. The heart and lungs, the primary components of the cardiovascular and respiratory systems, need to be challenged regularly to effectively deliver oxygen to the working muscles—after all, the heart is also a muscle. Cardiorespiratory fitness also plays an important role in the prevention of chronic diseases.

Your Energy Needs: Supply and Demand

The human body's ability to adapt is amazing. Energy systems provide muscles with the fuel needed to contract and produce movement. The cardiorespiratory system produces most of the energy for general day-to-day movement. This chapter will help you design a safe and effective program to enhance your cardiorespiratory fitness so you can live a life filled with mental and physical energy.

Cardiorespiratory System

The cardiovascular and respiratory systems, commonly referred to together as the *cardiorespiratory system*, are responsible for many critical functions. These functions can be classified into the following four primary categories:

1. Delivery of oxygen, nutrients, and hormones and other chemical messengers

2. Removal of carbon dioxide and waste products

3. Maintenance of body temperature and acid-base balance (pH)

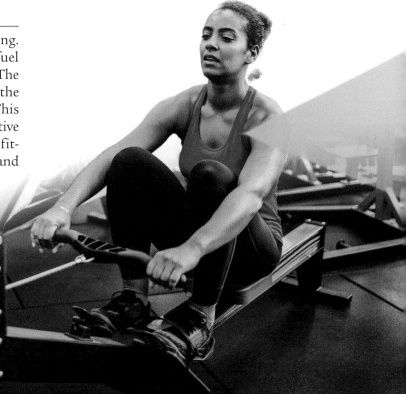

4. Prevention of infection as assisted by the immune system

The cardiorespiratory system is made up of the heart, blood vessels, and lungs. Of course, the blood flowing through the cardiorespiratory system is also of primary importance. As discussed in chapter 13, cardiovascular diseases are the number one cause of death in most countries in the world. A healthy cardiorespiratory system makes you feel good now and helps you live a long life in the years to come.

The Heart as Your Pump

The heart is a large muscle located just behind and slightly to the left of the breastbone. It has four chambers and two circulatory systems that work in nearly perfect harmony (see figure 4.1). The left side, or systemic circulation, distributes oxygenated blood to the rest of the body for use by various organs and tissues, including the muscles. The right side, or pulmonary circulation, accepts deoxygenated blood returning from the body and then delivers it to the lungs for waste removal and reoxygenation.

The heart can be thought of as a powerful muscular pump. As such, with every beat of the heart, a healthy heart performs a perfectly choreographed dance. The cells within the heart muscle undergo electrical depolarization, which causes them to contract. This perfectly synchronized depolarization–contraction sequence sends nearly equal volumes of blood to the lungs and the rest of the body. This contraction phase is termed **systole**. In the relaxation phase, or **diastole**, the chambers fill in preparation for the next heartbeat. Therefore, although the pulmonary and systemic circulations are separate, they must work together for healthy heart function. Each

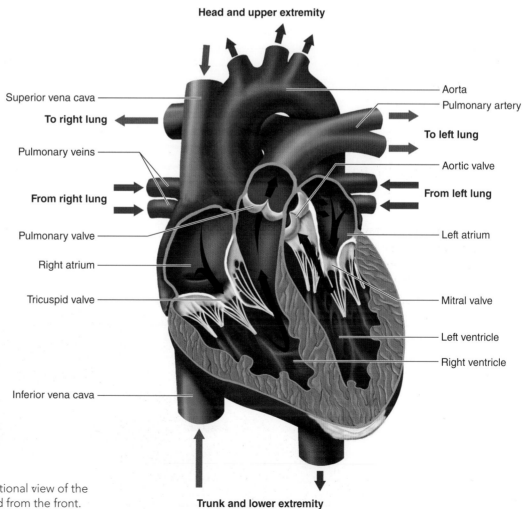

Figure 4.1 Cross-sectional view of the human heart, as viewed from the front.

of the heart chambers has valves that must function well, serving as doors through which the blood moves in and out. The heart muscle must also be strong. Each contraction must generate enough pressure to move the blood volume from the left ventricle and deliver it to the rest of the body. Thus, a healthy left ventricle is especially important during exercise, when the muscles have a greater need for oxygenated blood.

Vessels Provide Blood Transportation

The blood vessel system within the body is an amazing arrangement of paths for blood delivery. Just as a city has a variety of roadways, such as large

interstate highways, state routes, and one-way city streets, the human body has vessels that vary in function and size (figure 4.2). Arteries, which carry oxygenated blood away from the heart and deliver it to the body, are characterized by thick elastic walls that can expand or contract to direct blood to tissues that need it. In this manner, the arterial system acts like a traffic controller for blood delivery within the body. The aorta, which leaves the heart just next to the left ventricle, absorbs the highest pressure within the circulatory system. The aorta branches into smaller and smaller vessels, ultimately ending in capillaries located in all tissues of the body. These tiny capillaries are the

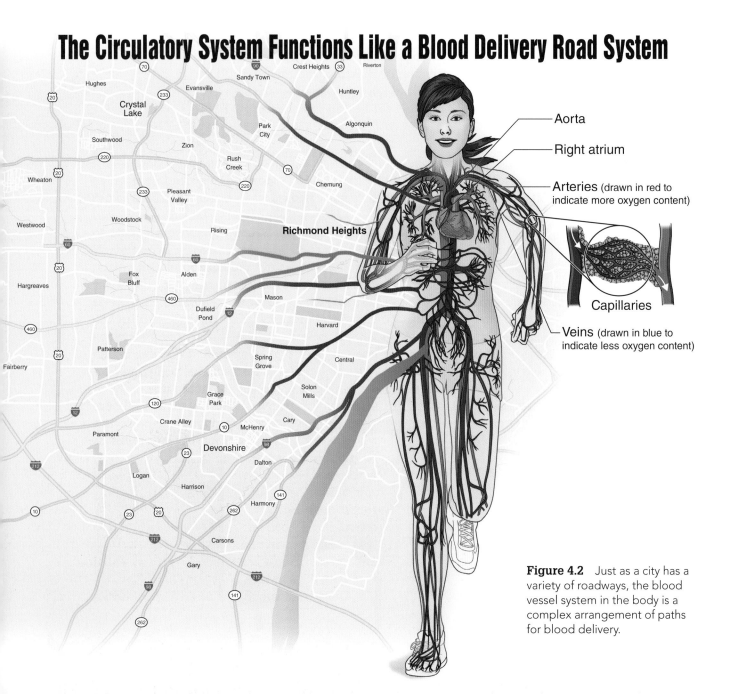

The Circulatory System Functions Like a Blood Delivery Road System

Figure 4.2 Just as a city has a variety of roadways, the blood vessel system in the body is a complex arrangement of paths for blood delivery.

site of oxygen, nutrient, and carbon dioxide waste product exchange within the body.

After this exchange in the individual muscle cell (capillary level), blood travels to small veins called *venules* and then progresses through veins that increase in size until the blood reaches the heart, emptying into the right atrium. There, the cycle begins again. Veins have thin, stretchy walls that allow them to expand and hold larger volumes of blood. When we have blood drawn from our arms in a medical clinic, the thin walls of the veins allow the needle to easily puncture them. Veins also have valves that help keep blood flowing in the right direction back to the heart with minimal pressure in the system. If you have ever stood in a warm environment for a long period of time, you might have noticed that the veins in your legs became larger and visible and sometimes have small bumps due to the values. In this way, the veins and cardiovascular system play a critical role in thermoregulation of the body.

A well-designed and managed road system (i.e., vascular system) is important, but if there is no transportation vehicle, delivery will not occur. Therefore, blood can be thought of as the cars and trucks of the vascular road. An average-sized person has approximately 5 liters of blood that circulate around the body once every minute during rest. Imagine the contents of two and a half 2-liter soda pop bottles of blood circulating through your system every minute. During strenuous exercise such as running, which uses large muscle groups, the body can require as much as 25 liters per minute (see figure 4.3)—that's 12-1/2 2-liter pop bottles of blood per minute!

Blood pressure is defined as the pressure exerted on the arteries. An average blood pressure is 120 over 80 measured in millimeters of mercury (mmHg). The systolic blood pressure (the first number; 120) occurs during the heart's contraction. Diastolic blood pressure (the second number; 80) occurs during its relaxation phase. Pressure is highest when the blood is ejected into the aorta (the main artery of the body) from the left ventricle and decreases as the blood travels throughout the circulatory system.

Blood pressure management is a common health topic due to the negative health consequences of hypertension (high blood pressure), described in chapter 13. However, low blood

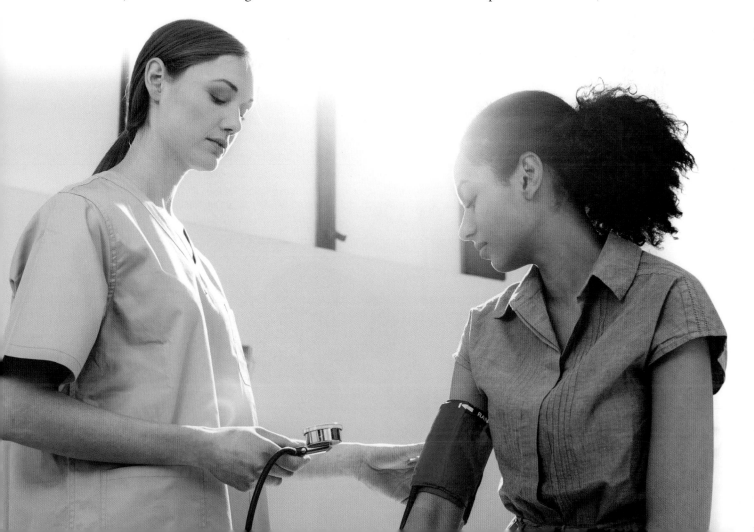

Amount of Blood Circulating per Minute

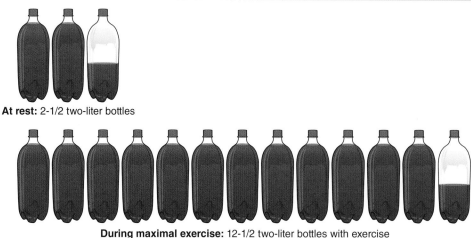

At rest: 2-1/2 two-liter bottles

During maximal exercise: 12-1/2 two-liter bottles with exercise

Figure 4.3   The amount of blood needed to circulate per minute at rest and during maximal exercise.

pressure is also very serious. If blood pressure is too low, blood will not flow appropriately and in the correct direction. A major role of the heart is to generate enough pressure so that the pumped blood will flow through the arterial system and back to the heart. Signs of low blood pressure are fainting spells, especially when standing or working in hot environmental conditions, and feeling light-headed or seeing stars when quickly standing up. Typically, low blood pressure in young healthy individuals is a result of dehydration.

Respiratory System

The respiratory system, including all the passages from the nose and mouth to the lungs, is a critical partner to the heart for delivery of oxygen, removal of carbon dioxide, and maintenance functions of the cardiorespiratory system (figure 4.4). The diaphragm contracts and relaxes, changing pressure within the chest cavity. This pressure change allows air to flow in and out. As blood flows from the right ventricle to the capillaries in the lungs, carbon dioxide and oxygen are exchanged. Oxygen-rich blood flows to the left side of the heart to be pumped to the body. Carbon dioxide passes from the capillaries into the lungs and leaves the body through the nose and mouth during exhalation.

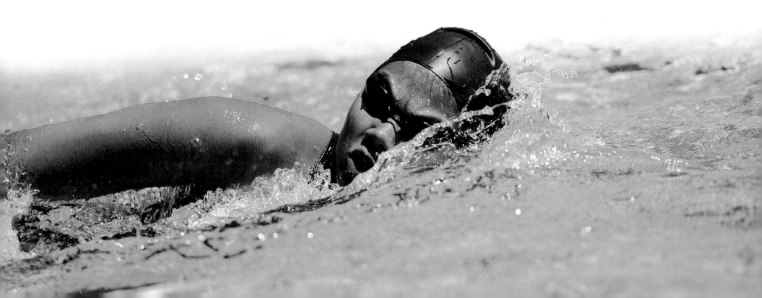

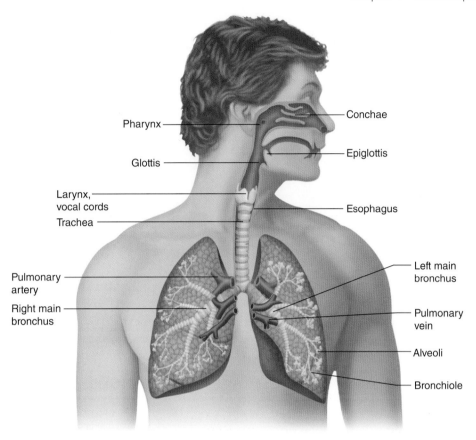

Pharynx

Conchae

Glottis

Epiglottis

Larynx,
vocal cords

Esophagus

Trachea

Pulmonary
artery

Left main
bronchus

Right main
bronchus

Pulmonary
vein

Alveoli

Bronchiole

Figure 4.4 Anatomy of the respiratory system.

Cardiorespiratory Systems Are Challenged by Exercise

When you are at rest or doing light activity, your cardiorespiratory system functions easily. A healthy person has a relatively steady resting heart rate of 60 to 100 beats per minute, breathing rate of 12 to 20 breaths per minute, and blood pressure at or near 120/80 mmHg. However, when you are exercising or engaging in physical activity at a moderate or vigorous intensity, these systems must provide your working muscles with oxygen and fuel to perform the work. This coordinated effort by the nervous and endocrine systems, both of which are controlled by the brain, increases breathing and heart rate and redistributes the blood supply to the working muscles. Figure 4.5 summarizes a few of the many changes that occur when the body changes from rest to maximal exercise.

Energy Production Systems

Metabolism refers to the breakdown and transformation of food into energy through various chemical processes. This available energy fuels muscle contraction and moves the human body during physical activity. People often think about metabolism as it refers to weight management—for example, a person who can consume a large quantity of calories without any weight gain is often said to have a high metabolism.

The unit used to describe the energy available in various foods or expended by the human body is the kilocalorie (kcal). The body's total energy need is a person's metabolic rate and is expressed in kilocalories per day. As described in chapter 9, many factors influence both your energy intake and energy expenditure.

Dietary Intake: The Energy for Life

The food and drink you consume is converted through complex biochemical processes into a substance the body can use to do biological work or store energy for later use. Energy transfer is never completely perfect: A lot of heat is lost during this conversion from chemical energy to biological energy. Also, there are times in the day when we are not eating. If energy were not stored

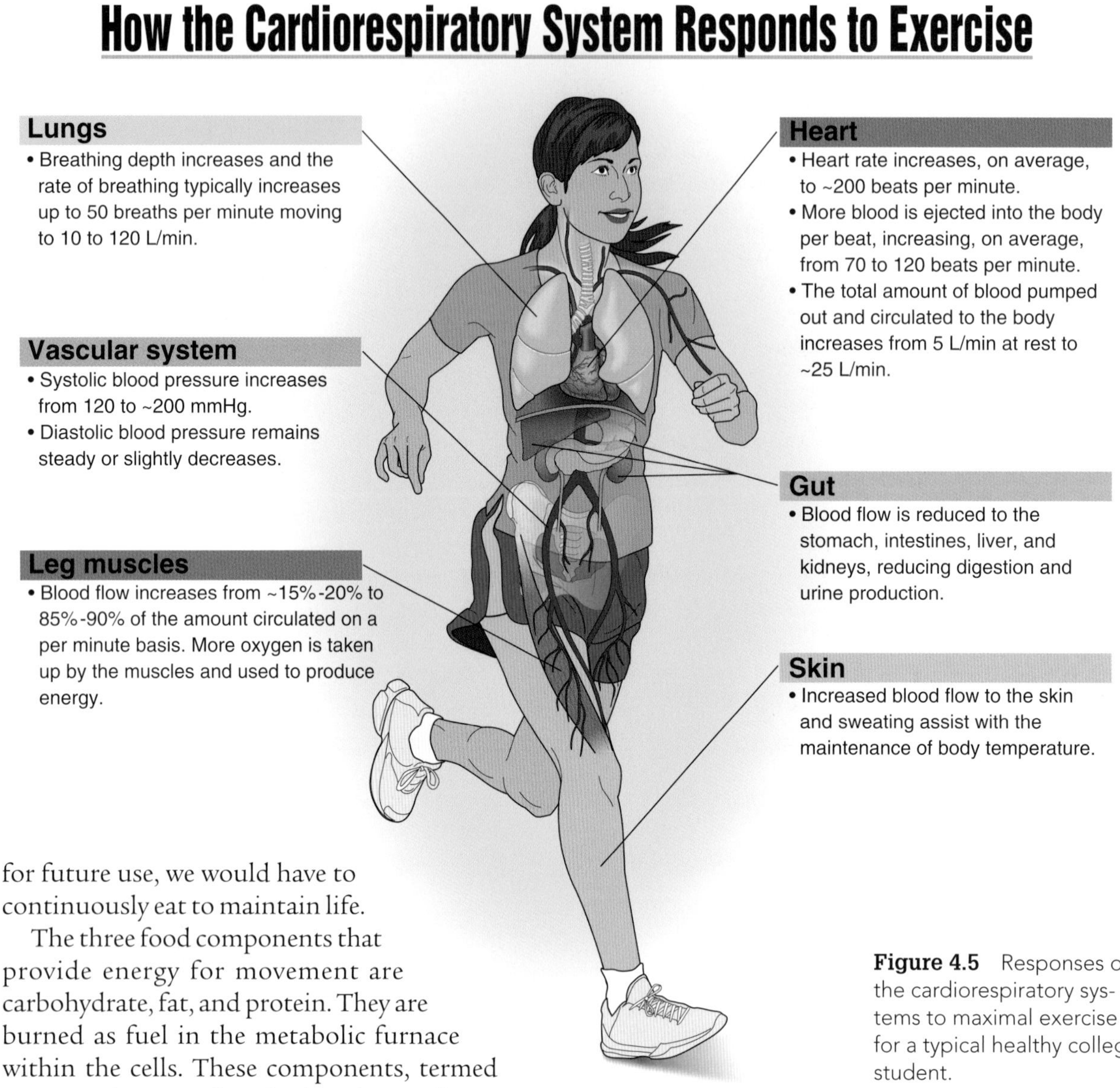

How the Cardiorespiratory System Responds to Exercise

Lungs
- Breathing depth increases and the rate of breathing typically increases up to 50 breaths per minute moving to 10 to 120 L/min.

Vascular system
- Systolic blood pressure increases from 120 to ~200 mmHg.
- Diastolic blood pressure remains steady or slightly decreases.

Leg muscles
- Blood flow increases from ~15%-20% to 85%-90% of the amount circulated on a per minute basis. More oxygen is taken up by the muscles and used to produce energy.

Heart
- Heart rate increases, on average, to ~200 beats per minute.
- More blood is ejected into the body per beat, increasing, on average, from 70 to 120 beats per minute.
- The total amount of blood pumped out and circulated to the body increases from 5 L/min at rest to ~25 L/min.

Gut
- Blood flow is reduced to the stomach, intestines, liver, and kidneys, reducing digestion and urine production.

Skin
- Increased blood flow to the skin and sweating assist with the maintenance of body temperature.

Figure 4.5 Responses of the cardiorespiratory systems to maximal exercise for a typical healthy college student.

for future use, we would have to continuously eat to maintain life.

The three food components that provide energy for movement are carbohydrate, fat, and protein. They are burned as fuel in the metabolic furnace within the cells. These components, termed *macronutrients*, are described in chapter 8.

Think back over your day. What movement activities have you done? For example, you might have sat in your room studying for several hours, slowly walked to lunch, and then jogged to reach your next class, run to catch the bus, or played a sport. Each macronutrient and energy system contributed in specific ways to help you accomplish these tasks. Your body relied primarily on fat for energy when you slowly walked to lunch but used mainly carbohydrate when you ran to catch the bus.

Carbohydrates, either simple or complex, are a ready energy source. They are easily digested, especially simple sugars, and converted to glucose and released into the blood. Glucose can be stored in the form of glycogen within muscles and the liver and then made available later. If immediate needs are met and glycogen storage needs are at maximal capacity, the extra carbohydrate will be stored as body fat.

In today's world, where struggles with weight management are common, **dietary fats** have a bad reputation, but they are a great energy source. Dietary

Although the term *calorie* often has a negative connotation, it is just a unit of energy that allows your body to move!

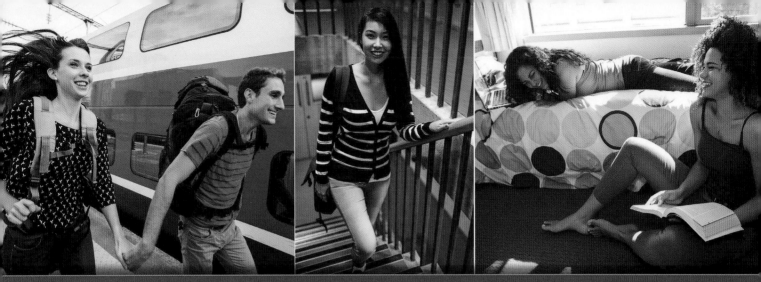

Carbohydrate, fat, and protein contribute in specific ways to help you accomplish a range of physical movement activities.

fats are a great choice when energy is needed for long-duration, lower-intensity movement. For example, trail mixes often contain nuts because they contain lots of energy (due to their fat content) and are easy to carry when hiking for hours. However, like carbohydrates, once immediate energy needs have been met, any extra dietary fat will be stored as body fat.

Protein provides amino acids, which are the building blocks of tissues for new growth and repair. It also can be used for energy production, although this is typically as a last resort when carbohydrate and fat are lacking. As with carbohydrate and fat, any excess protein consumed is stored as body fat.

> If we think of body fat as stored energy, it can have a positive connotation. However, remember that storing too much energy can harm your health.

 Behavior Check

Break a Sweat

In today's showered and groomed world, it is often not acceptable to be sweaty unless exercising or performing physical labor. Because humans are machines that are not very efficient, we give off heat when we move. In fact, we have about a 22 percent efficiency, which is not very good compared to contemporary refrigerators or wood-burning stoves! This means that nearly three-quarters of our energy is given off as heat.

Our bodies have adaptive ways to get rid of this extra heat through sweating. If you try to avoid sweating, you are missing out on chances for movement opportunities. Plan to sweat a little throughout the day. For example, in the morning, put a small toiletry kit and perhaps some extra undergarments into your backpack, or stay cooler while walking across campus by going through air-conditioned buildings. Thinking strategically can allow you to take lots of daily steps.

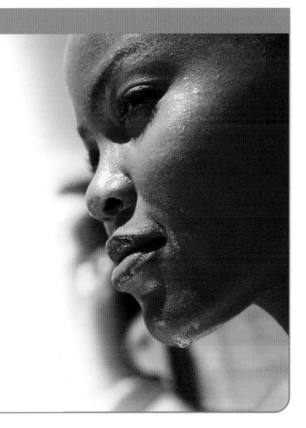

ATP: The Energy Bucks of the Human Body

All cells need energy for biological work, which is gained through the bond breaking of **adenosine triphosphate** (**ATP**). Thus, the body is constantly using ATP for biological functions like muscle contraction and gaining it back through the metabolism of food—carbohydrate, fat, and protein. Therefore, ATP can be thought of as the "energy bucks" of the human body (see figure 4.6). Like your bank account, the ATP dollar is constantly being deposited (generated) in the cells and then withdrawn (used) for energy production.

Three Energy Systems

Muscle cells within the body are fueled by three energy systems that cooperate to provide ATP. These three systems vary in their metabolic machinery, the fuel they use, and the types of physical activities that primarily use them (table 4.1). For example, if you need to walk for two miles due to parking far from campus or sprint to your car when it's raining, the systems in place work well and in collaboration with each other. The energy systems collaborate for many sport activities as well. For example, soccer players conserve their energy when the ball is downfield from them but are ready to sprint into action as needed. Although all three energy systems contribute to almost all activities, typically one or two energy systems are used the most depending on the duration and intensity of the activity. Flexibility in fuel source and the range of energy production options are critical to our daily functioning.

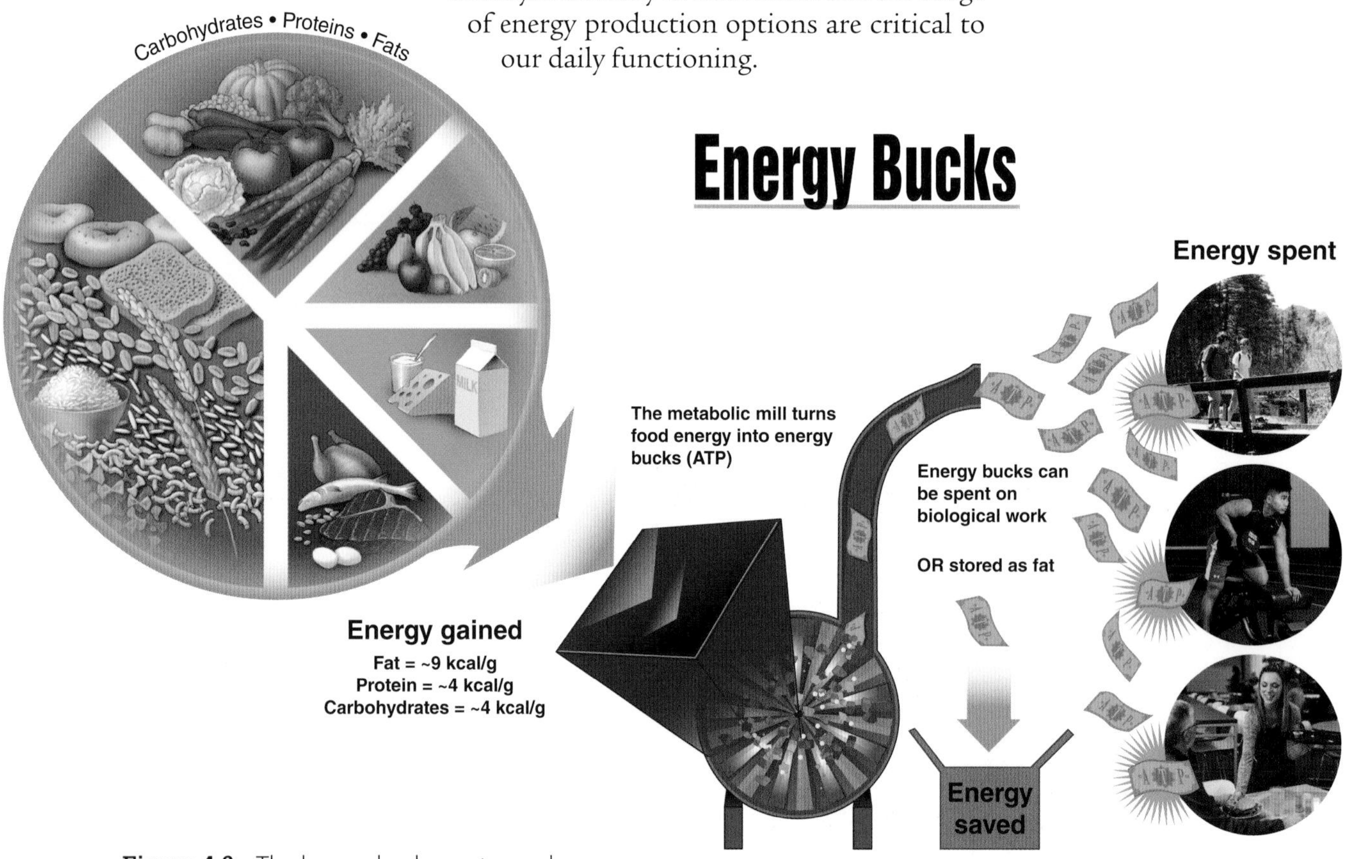

Carbohydrates • Proteins • Fats

Energy Bucks

The metabolic mill turns food energy into energy bucks (ATP)

Energy gained

Fat = ~9 kcal/g
Protein = ~4 kcal/g
Carbohydrates = ~4 kcal/g

Energy bucks can be spent on biological work

OR stored as fat

Energy spent

Energy saved

Figure 4.6   The human body creates and uses energy from ATP stored in cells, much like we earn and spend money from our bank accounts.

Table 4.1   Movement Energy Systems: Summary and Comparison

| | ENERGY SYSTEMS | | |
Characteristic	Immediate (ATP-PC)	Nonoxidative (anaerobic)	Oxidative (aerobic)
Rate of ATP production	Immediate	Rapid	Slow
Duration of activities where system is most used	≤10 seconds	10 seconds to 2 minutes	>2 minutes
Intensity of activities where system is most used	High	High	Low to moderate
Fuel source	ATP and PC	Muscle glucose and glycogen	Liver stores of glycogen (glucose), fat, protein
Example sports	Golf swing Weightlifting	200-meter hurdles 50-meter swim	Running a marathon Distance cycle race
Example leisure activities	Playing catch with a football or baseball	Intense gardening and yard work	Hiking at moderate pace
Example daily activities	Carrying shopping bags	Running through the airport to catch a flight	Walking on campus

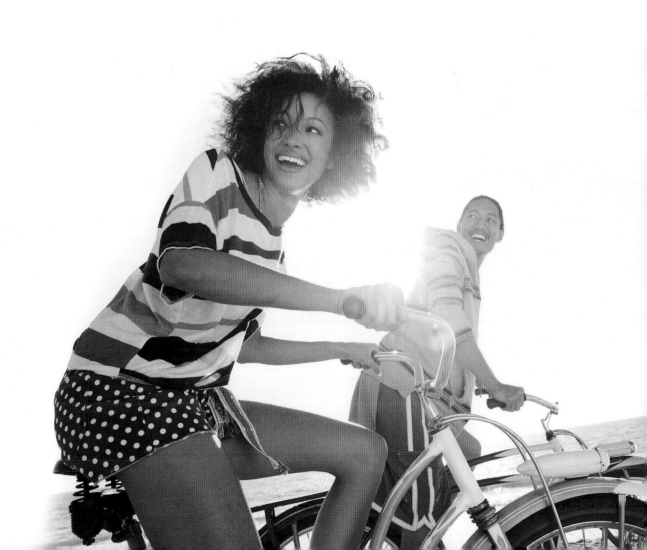

The immediate energy system, or the **adenosine triphosphate–phosphocreatine (ATP-PC) system**, is fueled by a small amount of ATP stored in the cells. The benefit of this system is that it provides energy very quickly. The downside of this system is that it has a very short supply of ATP, so activities that are fueled by this system can last only a few seconds (about 10 seconds maximum). After that, unless other systems provide the energy, muscle fatigue and failure will occur, and movement will stop.

The **nonoxidative (anaerobic) system** is critical at the beginning of activity and for higher-intensity movement lasting approximately 10 seconds to 2 minutes. The fuel source used for this system is carbohydrate—**glucose** or **glycogen**. Because this system does not require oxygen, it is often termed *anaerobic*. (It is also sometimes called the *glycolytic system* because it uses glycogen.) The advantage of this system is that energy is readily available at a relatively high supply. The disadvantages of this system are that (1) the body does not store much glucose or glycogen, so fuel supply is limited, and (2) bioproducts of this pathway result in metabolic acids, such as lactic acid (lactate), that reduce your muscles' ability to contract and contribute to muscle fatigue and discomfort. A real-life example of this physiology in action is high-intensity interval training (HIIT). Although highly effective, HIIT activities are not always very comfortable because the by-product of lactic acid causes discomfort during the exercise bout.

Finally, the system most often used is the **oxidative (aerobic) system**, termed so because it requires oxygen. This system is used during activities that last longer than two minutes and are of low to moderate intensity. This system has many advantages, including the use of numerous fuel sources (carbohydrate, fat, and protein) and the ability to supply a large amount of ATP. Therefore, this system powers most of our activities of daily living, including when muscles are used for posture during sitting and standing. The only major downside to this energy system is that it cannot provide ATP very quickly. It is therefore not used to fuel the first few minutes of movement or any activity of high intensity such as sprinting for the campus bus.

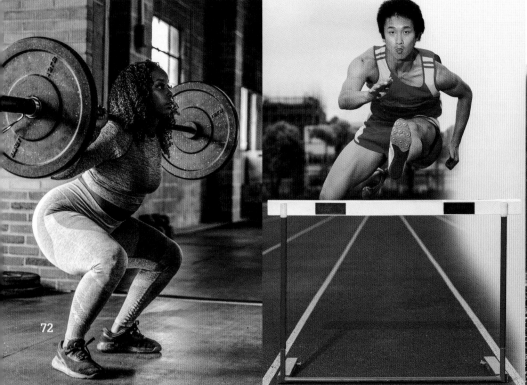

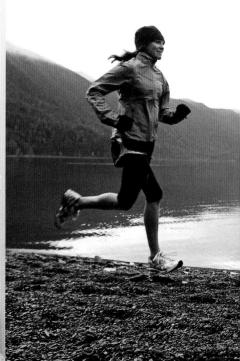

Energy Expenditure for Human Movement: The Continuum

Although the three energy systems appear to have distinct time frames when they contribute to energy production (i.e., less than 10 seconds, 10 seconds to 2 minutes, more than 2 minutes), they do not turn on and off with a timer. These energy systems have great teamwork to provide ATP, the energy bucks needed for movement. We use all three of the energy systems during daily movement, especially when we exercise. Therefore, in determining the energy system being used for a given activity or movement bout, it is useful to think of the *relative contribution of the system*. Very few activities obtain 100 percent of their ATP from a single energy system to generate movement. When considering which energy system is predominately being used for an activity bout, think about both duration and intensity.

If your energy systems are working well, you likely will not worry about them much. However, what if you want to train for a specific activity to improve your performance? A major concept in the field of exercise science is **specificity of training**. Specificity is particularly important for energy systems. If you want to enhance performance in a certain activity, train the energy system that supports the energy production for that activity. However, it is important to note that training one system can reduce the performance of another system. For example, sprinters who add distance running to their training program typically experience reduced sprinting performance. This is because a sprinter relies on a well-conditioned anaer-

obic system, whereas a distance runner uses a trained aerobic system. Training to enhance all your energy systems is important for optimal health, but the relative importance of each will depend on the sport, recreation, and occupational activities in your daily routine. Training the aerobic energy system is often considered the most important because it enhances cardiorespiratory fitness and prevents many chronic diseases.

> If you want to enhance performance in a specific activity, train the muscles and the energy systems that support that activity. For example, if you want to run better, run often!

Cardiorespiratory Fitness Benefits Your Daily Life

Maintaining your cardiorespiratory fitness will not only prevent chronic diseases later in life but will also give you a higher level of functional fitness for daily tasks, including cognitive function and mood regulation. A high level of aerobic fitness adds life to your years and years to your life. The following sections summarize how optimal cardiorespiratory fitness can help you feel better in the short and long term.

Reduced Risk of the Metabolic Big Three

Three major diseases affect most people at some point in life, either personally or through someone they love. These diseases are cardiovascular disease, type 2 diabetes, and cancer. Although genetics play a role, the common risk factor for all three diseases are lifestyle choices. The human body is designed to move. A lack of movement results in unhealthy use of metabolic fuels, among other negative outcomes for various bodily systems. Although it may appear that mainly older people get these diseases, it is critical to appreciate that many of the disease processes for the so-called *metabolic big three* begin in young adulthood.

- *Cardiovascular diseases.* Being sedentary is a major risk factor for many cardiovascular diseases (CVDs), which are the number one cause of death. As described in chapter

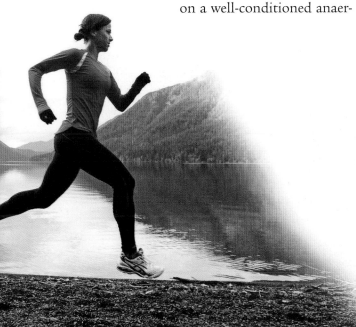

13, regular engagement in cardiovascular endurance activities, especially of moderate to vigorous intensity, can enhance the health of the cardiovascular system, positively affecting the heart, the blood vessels, and the quality of the blood in the circulatory system.

- *Type 2 diabetes.* Because CVD and type 2 diabetes have so many common risk factors, they are often thought of together as *cardiometabolic diseases.* Type 2 diabetes occurs when blood glucose is too high. Because regular muscle contraction causes glucose to move from the blood into the cells more easily, physical activity is a key strategy for both the prevention and management of this disease.

- *Cancer.* It is well accepted that physical activity is very important for the prevention of several cancers, especially cancers of the colon and breast. Chapter 14 provides detailed information on how healthy lifestyle choices can help prevent cancer.

> The disease process for CVDs, type 2 diabetes, and cancer begins in young adulthood. Get moving and act now to prevent these diseases.

Improved Weight Management

Do you equate exercise and physical activity with weight management? Many people do. In fact, a common goal for an exercise program is to manage weight and become or stay lean. As explained in chapter 9, regular movement, especially moderate- to high-intensity exercise, is very important for managing body composition, which is the proportion of fat, muscle, and bone in your body. Energy expenditure through movement allows you to splurge on a few extra calories with your favorite foods and drinks while remaining in energy balance.

Easier Daily Physical Tasks

When you have a high level of cardiorespiratory fitness, the physical tasks you do each day, like walking and going up and down stairs, will be easier. With cardiorespiratory fitness, you will reap the following benefits:

- For any given physical challenge, your heart rate and breathing rate will be lower.

- Your muscles will produce less lactate and lactic acid, which means that physical challenges will feel easier and stress your body less.

- You will need less time to recover from physical tasks. For example, carrying a heavy backpack across campus will not be as tiring.

Enhanced Work, Recreation, or Sport Performance

The better your cardiorespiratory fitness, the less stress your body will experience from physical work, recreation, and sports:

- If you have a service job (e.g., retail or waitstaff) that requires you to be on your feet for many hours, you will experience less physical stress and fatigue by the end of your shift.

- You can enjoy the outdoors during hiking without undue fatigue or performance worry.

- You will enjoy recreational sport activities and group fitness classes more when you can keep up with the team or the class.

Improved Sleep and Psychosocial Well-Being

The many benefits of regular cardiorespiratory exercise include stress management, better sleep, and improved mood, as described in chapter 10. Regular physical movement, especially moderate to vigorous physical activity that results in improvement or maintenance of cardiorespiratory fitness, can improve the following aspects of daily life.

- You will sleep better. Good restorative sleep is critical for many physiological and psychological processes that are important to daily life. Being tired is a primary complaint from students of all ages—better sleep quality will help you feel better.

⊕ Immunity Booster

Cardiorespiratory Fitness and Immune Function?

Regular exercise and physical activity generally have positive effects on the immune system. Those who are physically fit have been shown to get fewer colds and upper respiratory tract infections compared to people who are sedentary (Martin, Pence, and Woods 2009). Emerging evidence also strongly suggests that being physically active, along with the associated benefits of improved fitness, can prevent COVID-19 by enhancing immune function, as well as potentially enhance the effectiveness of the COVID-19 vaccine and recovery from COVID-19 infection (Nieman 2021). In addition to maintaining your physical fitness, protect yourself by tending to other key health behaviors, including healthy dietary choices, optimal sleep, stress management, and good hygiene practices like hand washing. Optimal immune function is important for daily risk exposures as well as longer-term immune challenges such as cancer.

- You will be less affected by daily stressors and have less anxiety.
- You can help avoid depression. This is particularly important because the prevalence of anxiety and depression, unfortunately, is increasing on college campuses.
- You will add vitality and energy to your day. Having enough energy to complete your daily tasks is critical to success as a student.

Better Brain Function and Academic Achievement

Higher levels of physical activity and cardiorespiratory fitness is positively associated with cognition and enhanced brain structure and function, most notably in children, adolescents, and older adults (2018 Physical Activity Guidelines Advisory Committee 2018). In other words, by engaging in moderate- to vigorous-intensity physical activity

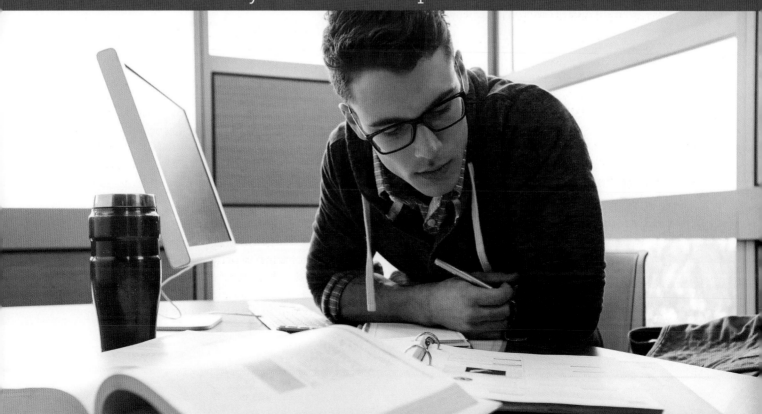

Having cardiorespiratory fitness can help enhance your academic performance!

and having higher cardiorespiratory fitness, the brain works better. However, the aforementioned indirect benefits of being physically active (e.g., stress management, enhanced sleep, and prevention of depression) may also improve academic performance. The college years, by definition, are cognitively challenging—you think hard and study for long hours! For optimal personal performance, regular physical activity, especially at an intensity that improves cardiorespiratory fitness, can greatly enhance your academic life.

In summary, we admire people of all ages who have lots of energy and a high engagement in their lives. By investing in your cardiorespiratory health, you will have more energy to do the things you have to do, plus energy to do all the things you want to do. Physical activity and cardiorespiratory fitness ultimately help you live your best life.

> Having good respiratory fitness not only makes you healthier, but it also helps you feel better!

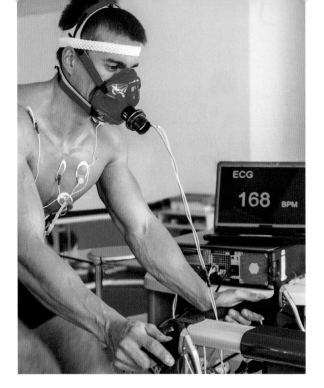

Assessing Your Cardiorespiratory Fitness

Now that you are aware of its many benefits, it will be useful for you to be able to determine your cardiorespiratory fitness. If you are sedentary, you will have low levels of cardiorespiratory fitness, even if you are otherwise healthy. Assessing your cardiorespiratory endurance will establish a baseline, motivate you to improve it, and help you track progress. Embarking on a program to improve your cardiorespiratory fitness brings you closer to a wellness lifestyle that can make you feel better and live longer. But first, let's make sure you understand exactly what the term *cardiorespiratory fitness* means.

Cardiorespiratory Fitness Defined

Cardiorespiratory fitness, also referred to as **cardiorespiratory endurance**, is the ability to provide oxygen to the working muscles in order to perform large muscle movements for a prolonged period. The greater your cardiorespiratory fitness, the longer you can perform an activity at a given intensity without fatigue (American College of

Sports Medicine 2022). In real-life terms, if you are winded after walking up a set of stairs, you need to train your cardiovascular system. Physical exertion takes a coordinated effort between the cardiovascular, respiratory, and muscular systems.

The higher the intensity of your exertion, the more oxygen you will consume until you must stop the activity. The point at which you must stop activity is termed **maximal oxygen consumption ($\dot{V}O_2max$)**. This is the maximum amount of oxygen a person can take in and use to perform dynamic exercise with large muscle groups. Maximal oxygen consumption is considered an objective measure of cardiorespiratory fitness.

Laboratory Methods of Assessment

Maximal oxygen consumption ($\dot{V}O_2max$) is well accepted in the exercise science field as the gold standard measure of cardiorespiratory fitness. The most common laboratory method uses a system, typically called a *metabolic cart*, that measures the amount of air a person inhales, the oxygen that is used from that air, and how much carbon dioxide is then exhaled during an exercise bout. Essentially, a person performs exercise at an increasing intensity (e.g., treadmill or cycle test) with a goal to reach exhaustion in approximately 10 minutes. Metabolic carts are costly, and tests need to be conducted by professionals trained in exercise science, especially if the person being tested has chronic health conditions. Because of these challenges, numerous simpler assessment methods have been developed that rely on the relationship between oxygen consumption and heart rate.

Field Methods of Assessment

The relationship between exercise intensity and heart rate is like the one between exercise intensity (or relative work capacity) and oxygen uptake—both are linear (see figure 4.7). This allows us to use the measurement of heart rate as a field method of cardiorespiratory fitness assessment to make good estimates about a person's oxygen consumption and overall cardiorespiratory fitness (American College of Sports Medicine 2022).

Field methods do not require a laboratory and special equipment. They can be performed at home, in a fitness facility, or on an outdoor track. There are two main types of field methods for estimating cardiorespiratory fitness (American College of Sports Medicine 2022):

- *Run/walk tests.* To complete a run/walk test, you complete either the farthest distance possible in a defined time limit (e.g., 12 minutes) or a defined distance (e.g., 1.5 miles) in the shortest time possible. You

then use an equation to estimate $\dot{V}O_2$max from either time or distance.

- *Step tests.* In these tests, you step at a fixed rate, at a fixed height, or both. The lower your HR response during or after exercise, the greater your cardiorespiratory fitness.

The chapter 4 labs in HK*Propel* provide detailed directions on how to conduct a personal assessment of your own cardiorespiratory fitness.

Designing Your Plan to Improve Cardiorespiratory Fitness

Now that you know how your cardiorespiratory system and muscles collaborate to power muscle movement and you understand the benefits of improving your cardiorespiratory fitness, the next step is to formulate a personal plan so that you can develop and maintain cardiorespiratory fitness throughout your life.

The Plan Depends on the Goal

Your plan to develop cardiorespiratory fitness is highly dependent on your goal. Your personal goals may be influenced by your recreational interests. For example, maybe you want to enjoy some rigorous hiking in the nearby mountains, you want to participate in a fun run with your friends, or perhaps you play on a recreational basketball league and your performance would benefit from a good conditioning base. Alternatively, you may want to manage your weight so that you look good and feel good. Maybe you want your cardiorespiratory program to reduce your anxiety about your academic performance and help you sleep better. Your goals may cross several domains of sport performance, health, body image, and academic performance.

Regardless of your goals, at a minimum, strive to meet the HHS Physical Activity Guidelines (U.S. Department of Health and Human Services 2018) and the ACSM exercise guidelines (American College of Sports Medicine 2022) discussed in chapter 2. If you want to reach other goals, such as for sports performance or weight management, you will need to use slightly different strategies.

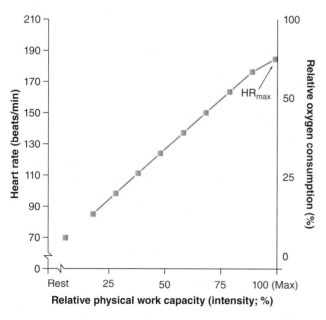

Figure 4.7 The relationship of physical work capacity or exercise intensity to oxygen consumption and heart rate.

Adapted by permission from W.L. Kenney, J.H. Wilmore, and D.L. Costill, *Physiology of Sport and Exercise*, 6th ed. (Champaign, IL: Human Kinetics, 2015), 197.

FITT Approach for Cardiorespiratory Fitness

The fundamental frame to organize your program will follow the FITT principles of frequency, intensity, time, and type (figure 4.8). These components interact with each other in terms of their benefits. Remember that the best program for you depends on your goals and interests. Selecting activities that you enjoy is very important, because if you don't stay with your program, you won't be able to both achieve and maintain your cardiorespiratory fitness.

Frequency

The U.S. Department of Health and Human Services (2018) and the American College of Sports Medicine (2022) agree that most people need to engage in moderate- to vigorous-intensity aerobic activities throughout the week. The American College of Sports Medicine (2022) indicates that a minimum of three days per week and spreading the exercise sessions across the three to five days per week is likely the best strategy to meet the goal. Specific frequency is influenced by intensity level. For example, performing moderate-intensity activity five times per week and vigorous-intensity activity three times per week may provide similar cardiorespiratory fitness benefits. Even performing aerobic exercise only once or twice per week can bring about health benefits if the intensity is high enough. Thus, consider mixing and matching your frequency (sessions per week) with your exercise intensity. More than five bouts of exercise per week may increase risk for musculoskeletal

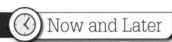

Now and Later

Your 401(k) Versus Your 401(h)

Most college students strive to earn a high GPA and build their résumés so they can make a good living. Often, however, people invest heavily in their financial futures—their 401(k)—but not enough in their future health. On the way to financial success and security, you would be wise to think about your 401(h), where h stands for health. Financial health and physical and emotional health are often very intertwined.

Now

Adding movement into your daily life to improve fitness will likely lead to better cognitive performance and better academic achievement. The additional benefits of lower levels of anxiety and depression and better sleep quality will help you concentrate. This can be compared to starting to save your money when you are young in order to benefit from compounding interest to get a bigger payoff for retirement.

Later

By keeping these health habits going, the same benefits will be present when you are a multitasking professional—and when you reach midlife, you will likely still be in good health! Then, as you progress through your retirement years, you will have more time. In these years, you will be able to schedule your days around movement, filling your days with hobbies and travel and enjoying family and friends. You will have the energy and health to do this because of your lifelong investment in physical activity, exercise, and other health behaviors.

Take Home

Engaging in moderate- and vigorous-intensity physical activity over your life span will help you feel better, perform better physically and cognitively, and prevent many chronic diseases. Your movement habits and resulting fitness just might help you have a great 401(h) and 401(k)!

injury in some individuals, especially if the activity stresses the same joints repeatedly. Cross-training, which involves using different modes of exercise (e.g., three days of running and two days of cycling), may help reduce risk of injury and prevent boredom.

Intensity

Intensity of aerobic exercise is a major factor influencing cardiorespiratory fitness. The cardiorespiratory system, muscles, and energy systems adapt in response to a repeated stress. Thus, the greater the intensity of training, the greater the benefit. However, risk of injury also increases, especially in people with unhealthy cardiorespiratory or musculoskeletal systems. The actual intensity needed for improving cardiorespiratory fitness is influenced by age, health status, recreational activity, and other factors. Heart rate (HR) can be used to estimate exercise intensity and is often prescribed using a target HR zone. Adjust intensity in response to environmental stress (e.g., hot and humid conditions) or when recovering from an illness or injury. You can use several methods of varying complexity to monitor endurance exercise intensity. You might want to consider mixing and matching them depending on your physical activity choice and how you feel.

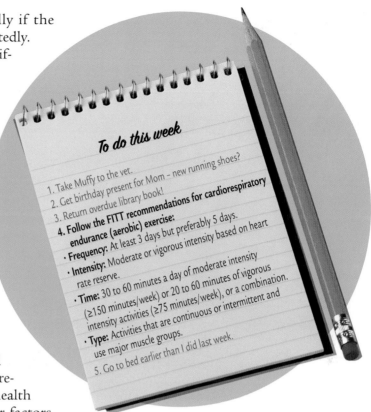

Figure 4.8   Make a weekly to-do list that includes the FITT recommendations to enhance cardiorespiratory fitness.

One method for monitoring intensity is called the **heart rate reserve (HRR) method**, calculated as the difference between resting heart rate (RHR) and maximal heart rate (MHR). According to the American College of Sports Medicine (2022), moderate-intensity exercise is 40 to 59 percent of HRR, and vigorous exercise is 60 to 89 percent of HRR. Maximal heart rate is calculated by subtracting age from the number 220. For example, for a typical 20-year-old, MHR is approximately 200 beats per minute (bpm), RHR is approximately 70 bpm, and HRR is 140 bpm. A target HR zone for moderate-intensity endurance exercise (40 to 59 percent) would be estimated as follows:

$$(140 \text{ bpm} \times 40 \text{ percent}) + 70 \text{ bpm} = 126 \text{ bpm}$$

$$(140 \text{ bpm} \times 59 \text{ percent}) + 70 \text{ bpm} = 153 \text{ bpm}$$

So, the target heart rate zone for this 20-year-old individual would be 126 to 153 bpm.

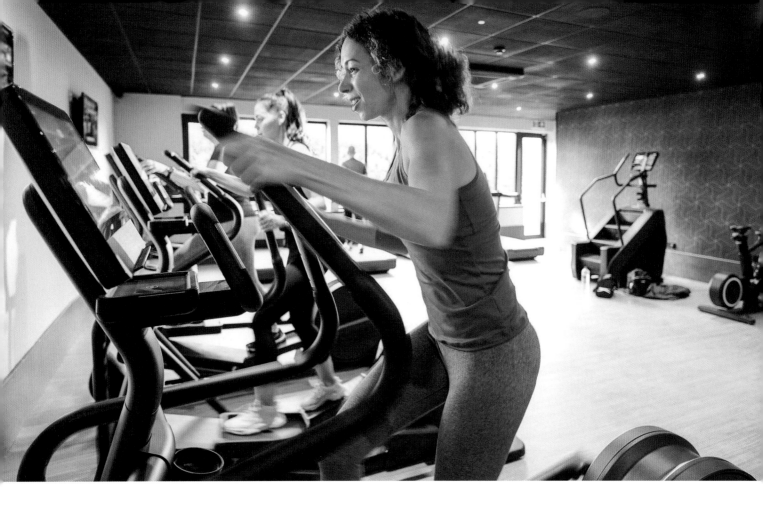

A second way to measure exercise intensity is using **metabolic equivalents (METs)**, which can be used to express the rate of energy expenditure during an activity in comparison to the rate of energy expended at rest, defined as 1 MET. Therefore, an activity that is 2 METs is twice the resting metabolic rate. For typical young adults specifically, activities in the range of 3 to 6 METs are considered moderate intensity, and activities of 7 to 10 METs are considered vigorous. Aerobic activities greater than 10 METs are considered near-maximal or maximal intensity (American College of Sports Medicine 2022).

When you become accustomed to exercising, especially when you regularly perform the same activity such as jogging or cycling, you will begin to feel how hard you are working subjectively. Using the **rating of perceived exertion (RPE)** scale in combination with other methods (e.g., HR) can provide another measure of intensity. The American College of Sports Medicine (2022)

> An easy fitness test is to walk quickly up a hill on campus with a full backpack and see how out of breath you get!

endorses a scale that ranges from 6 (near rest) to 20 (maximal effort), with moderate intensity being 12 to 13 and vigorous intensity 14 to 17. To learn this technique, start to associate an RPE rating with exercise in your target heart rate zone. Over time, this can be an easy way to monitor intensity.

Finally, the easiest method of all for estimating exercise intensity is a validated method called the **talk test**. Because higher levels of exertion require greater oxygen demand, respiration rate increases as intensity increases. At higher intensities, your breathing rate becomes more labored. During moderate-intensity exertion, a person can typically talk; however, at vigorous intensities, most people can speak only in small phrases. Thus, the talk test can help you gauge your intensity.

Time

The recommended duration of the activity is influenced by intensity. Physical activity guidelines indicate that a person should accumulate *at least* 150 to 300 minutes of moderate-intensity activity, 75 to 150 minutes of vigorous-intensity activity, or an equivalent combination of moderate- and vigorous-intensity aerobic activity per week, preferably spread throughout the week (U.S.

✓ Behavior Check

Integrating Aerobic Physical Activities Into Your Life

Not all your aerobic physical activity will be obtained with intentional exercise (e.g., going out for a run or going to the recreation center to use a machine), especially as you graduate and start your career. It is useful to think of physical activity in the four categories of occupation, domestic chores, transportation, and leisure. Examples of activities aligning with the four categories may include the following:

- Occupation: Scheduling a walking meeting with a colleague
- Domestic: Mowing the lawn with a push mower
- Transportation: Parking at a remote lot and walking to the office every day
- Leisure: Weekend hiking with partner, children, or dogs

Which of these ideas for incorporating aerobic movement into your daily life appeals to you? On a college campus, most students engage in moderate to vigorous physical activity primarily through transportation and leisure categories:

- If you live off campus, walk or bike instead of driving to campus. You might also take the bus or ride with a friend to campus and plan to briskly walk home at the end of the day.
- Use active transportation (e.g., walk or bike) while on campus by not taking the bus or an Uber on campus. Choose walking or biking routes that have the most hills to build some intensity into your movement.
- Supplement your active transportation with a few sessions of planned vigorous activity, such as a group exercise class, running, cycling, or swimming.
- Join a campus recreation club sport or intramural team that includes a lot of aerobic activity, such as rowing, cycling, Ultimate Frisbee, or soccer.

The best program for developing cardiorespiratory fitness will be the one that allows you to meet physical activity recommendations and reach your personal goals within the constraints of your weekly schedule, as well as offers you the enjoyment and motivation to keep moving and elevating your heart rate for a lifetime!

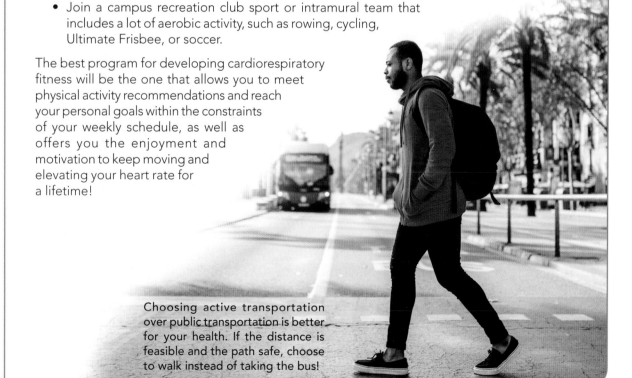

Choosing active transportation over public transportation is better for your health. If the distance is feasible and the path safe, choose to walk instead of taking the bus!

> There are many ways to move to gain cardiorespiratory fitness—the key is to move at least at a moderate intensity on a nearly daily basis!

Department of Health and Human Services 2018). The American College of Sports Medicine (2022) has similar weekly recommendations but also recommends that most adults should strive to get 30 to 60 minutes per day of moderate-intensity activity (≥150 minutes per week), 20 to 60 minutes per day of vigorous-intensity activity (≥75 minutes per week), or a combination of daily moderate and vigorous activity to obtain the recommended volume of exercise. A general guideline is that 2 minutes of moderate-intensity aerobic exercise is equivalent to 1 minute of vigorous-intensity aerobic exercise. Additional health benefits are gained from engaging in physical activity beyond the equivalent of 300 minutes of moderate-intensity physical activity per week.

However, and very importantly, moving from being physically inactive to any amount of physical activity can enhance health, with short bouts of less than 10 minutes showing benefits, especially for the sedentary or minimally active individual. Pattern of time within the activity can also vary. For example, an endurance activity could be performed in a continuous session or in multiple sessions of 10 minutes or more to reach the desired duration or volume for a given day (American College of Sports Medicine 2022). As explained in chapter 9, longer durations may be needed for weight management, especially if the rest of your day is spent sitting.

Type

You can use many modes of activities to enhance cardiorespiratory fitness. Rhythmic aerobic exercise that requires little skill and involves large muscle groups, especially the legs (as physical capabilities allow), is recommended for all adults for health. Sports that require a higher level of skill or fitness are options for people who have the training and conditioning base to safely engage in these activities (American College of Sports

Medicine 2022). The most popular activity is walking, because it is easily accessible to nearly everyone and requires only a good pair of shoes. Other common choices are running, cycling, swimming, and the use of exercise equipment. Doing cross-training and finding many ways to move will add variety and keep you interested and motivated. Figure 4.9 provides examples of common cardiorespiratory endurance activities that vary in skill and fitness requirements.

Volume, Progression, and Pattern

The FITT framework provides a great approach to developing a cardiorespiratory fitness program. Frequency, intensity, and time can interact when you organize your weekly movement plan around a variety of activities. After determining the program that is right for you, your interests, schedule constraints, and so on, your next step is to think about volume and progression. As mentioned previously, the pattern of how you exercise may also influence the other components.

Volume

Exercise volume is the product of frequency, intensity, and time. For example, if you exercise vigorously, you can move for less time and get health benefits like those of a longer program at moderate intensity. This concept is known as a **dose–response association**. The greater amounts of physical activity you do, the greater the health and fitness benefits you will obtain; however, it is less clear if there is a minimum or maximum amount. A total amount of energy expenditure of about 1,000 kcal per week of moderate-intensity physical activity is associated with the prevention of cardiovascular disease and thus is a reasonable target for most adults for heart health. This level of energy expenditure is approximately equal to 150 minutes per week of moderate-intensity activity (American College of Sports Medicine 2022).

Activity trackers and pedometers can be useful for estimating physical movement volume in steps per day. Contemporary wearable technologies can also provide an easy way to track intensity, with a walking pattern or cadence of at least 100 steps

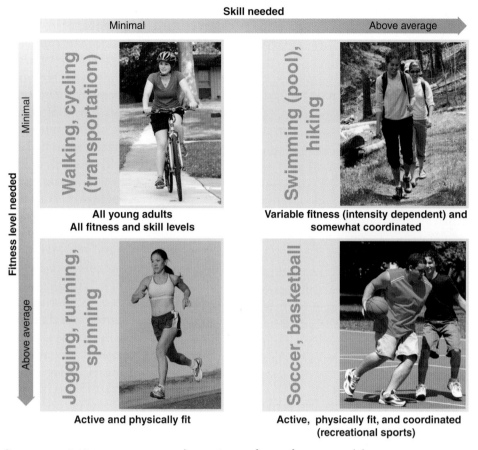

Skill needed

Minimal → Above average

Fitness level needed

Minimal → Above average

Walking, cycling (transportation)
All young adults
All fitness and skill levels

Swimming (pool), hiking
Variable fitness (intensity dependent) and
somewhat coordinated

Jogging, running, spinning
Active and physically fit

Soccer, basketball
Active, physically fit, and coordinated
(recreational sports)

Figure 4.9   Common activities to promote cardiorespiratory fitness for young adults.

per minute meeting the minimum pace for moderate-intensity physical activity. Although 10,000 steps per day is often cited as a health goal, a daily step count of 7,000 to 8,000 steps per day, with at least 3,000 steps being taken at a brisk pace, is a reasonable minimal daily target for health benefits. It is best to use a combination of step counts and frequency, intensity, and time components when designing your aerobic exercise or physical activity program.

You can estimate your exercise intensity by monitoring your heart rate.

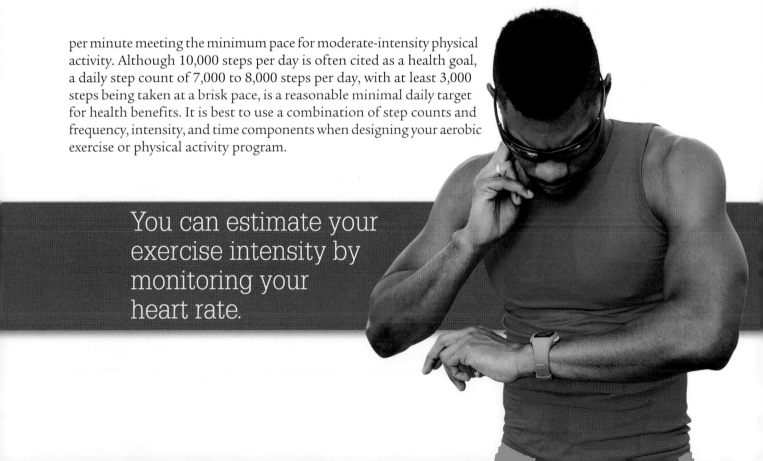

Progression

Progression of the cardiorespiratory endurance program is highly dependent on a person's health status, current fitness level, and exercise program goals. You can accomplish progression by advancing any of the FITT components. Generally, increasing time first is often the best option: An increase of approximately 5 to 10 minutes per session every few weeks is recommended. You can then gradually advance other components over four to eight months (American College of Sports Medicine 2022). Most importantly, progression should be slow and planned to avoid muscular soreness, injury, and undue fatigue. The risk of going too hard, too fast, too long, and too soon is not just related to physiological outcomes. If you experience a lot of muscle soreness and fatigue, you will not feel motivated to adhere to your fitness program. Therefore, progress slowly, listen to your body, and think of this adventure as something you will maintain throughout your life with modifications as needed.

Pattern

Although it is not a formal component of the guidelines and recommendations outlined previously, pattern of movement can be altered by the week, day, or even the workout session. Recall that the guidelines target weekly amounts (e.g., five hours per week) spread out over most days of the week. The daily accumulation of time spent in moderate-intensity activity aligns well with the typical life of a college student, in which demands of life often change day to day. For example, some days will allow for a longer, more intense exercise session, whereas other days will accommodate only intermittent bouts of moderate walking for transportation on campus. Thus, small bouts of movement can be accumulated throughout a given day to provide big benefits to you and your overall health.

With respect to the pattern of training within a given exercise session, a popular choice is interval training, which is broadly defined as periods of more intense exercise or physical activity interspersed with periods of rest or recovery. More specifically, **high-intensity interval training (HIIT)** is a hot topic among avid exercisers (American College of Sports Medicine 2022; U.S. Department of Health and Human Services 2018). Essentially,

short, high-intensity bursts of activity are interspersed with longer bouts of low-intensity activity or rest periods. It does not matter what type of activity you use for this type of aerobic training, but the most common types are running, cycling, rowing, and swimming. Large muscle group calisthenic exercises, such as jumping jacks, squats, or stair sprints, are also gaining popularity, but remain to be adequately researched. Research studies document the effectiveness of HIIT that used protocols of 30 seconds of near-maximal exercise followed by a rest period of three to five minutes of lower-intensity activity. Typical protocols consist of vigorous- to maximal-intensity exercise (20 to 240 seconds) followed by equal or longer bouts of light- to moderate-intensity exercise (60 to 360 seconds). For example, a runner might sprint very vigorously for 30 seconds, then walk fast or jog for four minutes to recover, and then repeat the cycle four to seven times in each workout.

Research in healthy young adults specifically suggests that using HIIT for longer than two weeks can improve cardiorespiratory fitness better than a conventional endurance training protocol (Milanovic, Sporis, and Weston 2015). Thus, HIIT workouts are a very time-efficient way to enhance cardiorespiratory fitness. They can also be quite useful for adding variety to an exercise routine.

The potential drawback of HIIT is the risk of injury. It can be dangerous for people with health

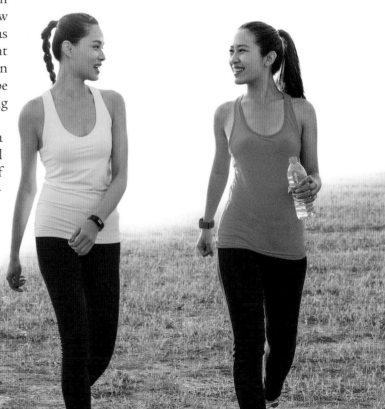

conditions involving the cardiorespiratory system to train this intensely. Even healthy people might trigger abnormal heart rhythms with intense exercise of this nature. Intense exercise can also greatly strain the joints, tendons, and muscles and therefore poses a high risk for musculoskeletal injuries. Finally, HIIT can be extremely fatiguing. Therefore, this type of training is best for people who already have a very good conditioning base. If you do decide to try HIIT, start slowly, build slowly, and listen to your body and adjust accordingly.

Your Plan + Modern Life = Creativity Required

The cardiorespiratory training recommendations outlined in this chapter provide a great framework for designing an individual program. The components of frequency, intensity, time, type, volume, progression, and pattern can be mixed and matched to produce a movement program that is both effective and enjoyable. Find activities that motivate you to keep moving, elevating your heart rate, and working hard to obtain and maintain your cardiorespiratory fitness level. If you can figure out how to incorporate these behaviors into your days, you will experience the fitness benefits. In today's highly sedentary world, you will need to be creative to obtain the volume of activity needed to improve and maintain cardiorespiratory fitness and positively influence your health. The chapter 4 labs in HK*Propel* will help you design your own program for developing cardiorespiratory fitness.

Safety First: Getting Started With Cardiorespiratory Fitness

Recall from chapter 2 the topics of safe movement and the importance of screening before beginning your program. In addition to doing an adequate prescreening with the PAR-Q+, other primary keys

---

✓ Behavior Check

HIIT: Just Do It Anywhere

Common excuses for not exercising include not having enough time to get to the gym. However, if you have the conditioning base and your primary joints are healthy, most college students have awesome opportunities right out their door to engage in HIIT. All you need is a safe place to obtain the high-intensity part of the training. This could be a running track or a trail on campus, a street with a good incline, a steep driveway, or even a set of indoor or outdoor stairs to increase intensity of the activity. Your routine might also incorporate jumping jacks, burpees, or other calisthenics to increase the intensity, or perhaps these exercises could be mixed and matched with sprints. The only factors to keep track of are the duration of the high-intensity and recovery components and the total number of intervals. Using convenient activities will enhance the chance that you will be stronger than your excuses. Plan a HIIT date with friends and turn the workout into a social fitness event with the bonus of accountability for adherence.

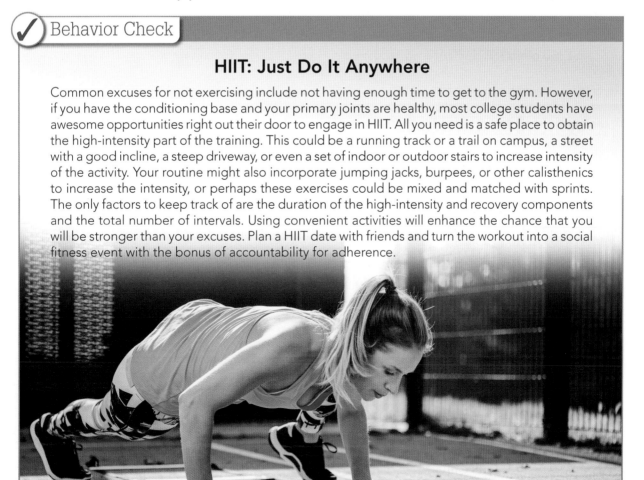

for moving safely include a proper warm-up and cool-down. When heart rate, blood pressure, and breathing rate are elevated during moderate or vigorous activity, keep a few other considerations in mind.

- *Air quality.* Depending on where you live, watch your air quality. Poor-quality air can hinder your performance and enjoyment of aerobic activities. This is especially true if you have a chronic lung condition such as asthma. On poor air days, you may need to exercise indoors.
- *Hot weather.* Because the body is an inefficient machine, you give off heat when you move. This causes your blood to move toward the surface of your body and produces sweating. If you perform intense or longer-term exercise in the heat, you could be at risk of a hyperthermic event such as heat cramps, heat exhaustion, or heat stroke. Proper hydration and clothing are keys to prevention.
- *Cold weather.* Hypothermia and frostbite are two common challenges when exercising outside in cold environments. Proper clothing is essential. Avoid wearing wet clothing in a cold environment for long periods of time and wear layers that do not hold moisture.

Summary

Cardiorespiratory endurance is a key component of health-related fitness. Your body's energy systems work with your cardiorespiratory system to supply energy for muscle contractions of all types. When you challenge these systems, they adapt, allowing you to meet physical challenges with less stress. Cardiorespiratory fitness is important not only for sport performance but also for activities of daily living. A regular movement program that you enjoy and are motivated to do on a weekly basis will help you feel great, perform your academic work better, and avoid illness now. Cardiorespiratory fitness also plays a key role in the prevention of several important chronic diseases and increases your chances for a long, healthy life.

ONLINE LEARNING ACTIVITIES

Go to HK*Propel* and complete all of the online activities to further facilitate your learning:

Study Activities: Review the main concepts of the chapter.

Labs: Complete the labs your instructor assigns.

Videos: Look through the videos and choose which ones you want to try this week.

REVIEW QUESTIONS

1. List and describe the four critical functions that the cardiorespiratory systems perform in the human body.
2. Compare and contrast the three movement energy systems in terms of (a) rate of ATP production, (b) duration and intensity of activities where the system dominates, and (c) sample sport, leisure, and activities of daily living that primarily rely on the system.
3. Explain the physiological basis of why the step test can be used as a measure of cardiorespiratory fitness.
4. Name the so-called "metabolic big three" diseases and describe the primary way that cardiorespiratory fitness prevents them.
5. Name three primary ways that cardiorespiratory fitness benefits the typical college student.
6. Describe the benefits and risks of HIIT and how a student could use HIIT to meet the ACSM exercise recommendations for cardiorespiratory exercise.

5

Muscular Fitness

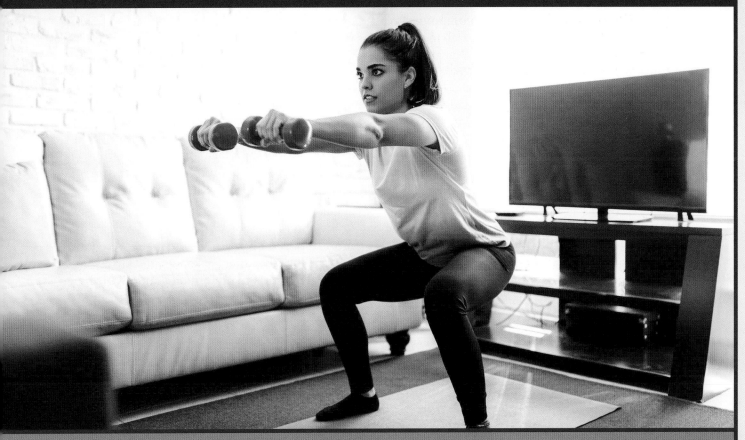

OBJECTIVES

- Understand how muscles work so the body can move.
- Identify the major muscle groups and their primary actions.
- Appreciate that muscular fitness has several components important for health- and skill-related physical fitness, including muscular strength, endurance, power, and hypertrophy.
- Recognize the importance of muscular fitness for looking good, feeling great, and functioning well today and in the future.
- Design a personalized plan to improve muscular fitness based on your health and fitness goals.

87

KEY TERMS

anabolic-androgenic steroids (AAS)
ergogenic
fast-twitch fiber
isometric
isotonic concentric
isotonic eccentric
muscle fiber

muscular endurance
muscular fitness
muscular hypertrophy
muscular power
muscular strength
slow-twitch fiber

Muscular fitness is an essential component of physical fitness. Traditionally, the elements of muscular strength and muscular endurance were considered important for health-related physical fitness, whereas muscular power was deemed important for skill- or performance-related fitness. However, the American College of Sports Medicine (ACSM) now recognizes that health and performance are an integrated part of overall fitness. And because muscle mass is also important for muscular fitness, ACSM defines muscular hypertrophy as a fourth component of muscular fitness (American College of Sports Medicine 2022). This chapter therefore focuses on these four aspects of muscular fitness, which are important for sport performance, functional fitness for your lifestyle, and living well for a lifetime.

These muscular fitness components are also important for living free of pain and injury. Joint and muscle pain may be the furthest thing from your mind right now; however, with our increasingly sedentary lifestyles, painful and stiff joints are getting more common even in younger individuals. Adequate muscular fitness is important for your activities of daily living, such as walking long distances while carrying a heavy load of books, working a shift on your feet as waitstaff, or playing recreational sports. As you reach middle age and beyond, muscular fitness, along with flexibility and neuromotor fitness, will become even more important for joint health, pain prevention (especially of the lower back, hips, and knees), and physical function to prevent falls and to continue living independently.

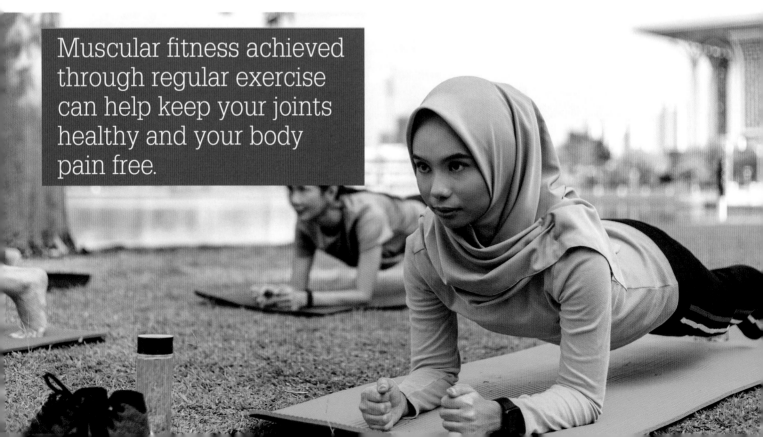

Muscular fitness achieved through regular exercise can help keep your joints healthy and your body pain free.

Your Body Was Designed to Move

We certainly move less for survival than our ancestors did, but we still need to move for our health and quality of life. The muscles, bones, and joints provide us with an amazing ability to move in big and small ways and in lots of directions. For example, walking is a large motor movement with little skill required, whereas eye tracking requires small fine motor movements. The purpose of this chapter is to help you understand basic muscle physiology so you can design a personal muscular fitness program.

Muscle Anatomy and Contraction Physiology

Although the body is complex, the fundamentals of movement are quite simple. Muscles are attached to bones by tendons. When a muscle contracts and produces force on the tendon connected to a bone, this causes movement. Muscles can only pull; they cannot push. Thus, muscles are typically arranged in pairs to allow movements in both directions. Muscles differ in their force production abilities, which is the rate at which they can produce force and how long they can produce force based on their physiology.

Muscle Fibers

Individual muscle cells are the building blocks of all muscles. These cells are called **muscle fibers** and are clustered into bundles called *fascicles* (figure 5.1). A muscle, no matter how small or large, is made up of many bundles of muscle fibers that are combined into a unit called a *myofibril*. Finally, myofibrils are arranged into *sarcomeres*, which are made up mostly of actin and myosin. When actin attaches to the myosin molecules, the muscle contracts and pulls on the tendons, and muscle shortening occurs. This muscle shortening comes from a coordinated effort by many muscle cells arranged in work teams.

Recent estimates indicate that approximately 80 percent of adults do not meet the HHS Physical Activity Guidelines, especially the muscle-strengthening activities (U.S. Department of Health and Human Services 2018). Beyond looking good, muscular fitness is important to function well now and in your future!

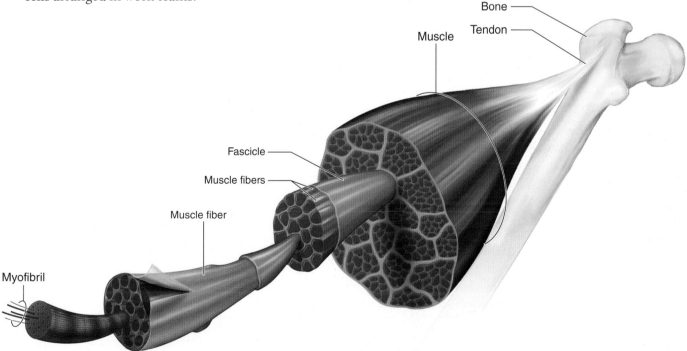

Figure 5.1   The basic structure of muscle.

Not all muscle fibers are created equal. They are often broadly categorized as **slow-twitch** or **fast-twitch fibers** based on their speed of contraction, force output, and the primary energy source used to fuel the contraction. Slow-twitch fibers contract more slowly and resist fatigue better. They also primarily use the oxidative (aerobic) system to gain their ATP, or energy bucks. Recall that the oxidative system can provide a lot of energy bucks but at a slower rate. Slow-twitch fibers are often reddish (darker) in color as a result of the myoglobin stored in the muscle fibers, which provide a quick source of oxygen. In contrast, fast-twitch fibers contract more forcefully and rapidly but fatigue more quickly than slow-twitch fibers. The primary fuel system for these fibers is the nonoxidative (anaerobic) energy system. Fast-twitch fibers are often whitish in color. Each fiber type has a preferred work output in terms of magnitude and rate of force production that is often matched to the movement requirements. The turkey and duck provide a relative comparison when we consider their different distributions of dark and white meat (figure 5.2).

Nearly all muscles contain a mixture of both slow-twitch and fast-twitch fibers, with the relative balance varying by the muscle and the individual as well as the person's requirements for daily movement. Fiber-type distribution is largely fixed at birth, but changes can occur with shifts in exercise or physical activity as well as through the aging process. Essentially, when given muscle fibers and their related energy system are overloaded, they will adapt to meet the demands placed on them. This is often referred to as the *specificity of training principle* (discussed in chapter 4).

The different functional abilities of the fiber types allow us greater flexibility to meet our constantly changing movement demands. To use an analogy, think of the slow-twitch fibers as a car like a Toyota Prius, which gets great gas mileage but does not accelerate very fast. In contrast, fast-twitch fibers could be represented by a Lamborghini, which accelerates very quickly but gets very poor gas mileage. Most cars blend these factors so that they get good gas mileage but can accelerate rapidly enough for safety (for example, when pulling out into traffic). In a typical day on campus, you might need your slow-twitch fibers to walk across campus and maintain your sitting and standing postures. You might also need to dash to catch the campus bus; this primarily taxes your fast-twitch fibers.

Motor Units

For a muscle to contract, it must be stimulated by the nervous system. This communication is accomplished by the motor unit, which is a nerve connected to several muscle fibers. Motor units can range from very small, with a ratio of one motor nerve to two muscle fibers, to very large, with a ratio of one motor nerve to several hundred fibers. Slow-twitch fibers are generally smaller motor units, whereas fast-twitch fibers are generally larger motor units. All motor units, regardless of size, abide by the all-or-none principle. This means that if they receive an adequate stimulus from the nervous system, all muscle fibers associated with that motor nerve and unit contract. In this way, the magnitude of force produced is determined by the number and type of motor units recruited. For example, you use smaller and fewer motor units when picking up a pencil compared to a large box of books. Keep in mind when we talk about neuromotor movement

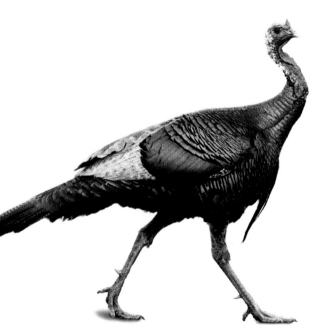

Figure 5.2 Turkeys walk and do not fly much, heavily using slow-twitch fibers in their legs. For this reason, turkeys have dark meat in their legs and white meat in their breasts. In contrast, ducks fly and do not walk much; therefore, they have dark meat in their breasts and white meat in their legs.

in the following chapters that the nervous system controls if, when, and how we move.

Muscular Fitness Defined

Muscular fitness is the ability of your muscles to perform different types of movements at different speeds and levels of force. It is comprised of **muscular strength**, **muscular endurance**, and **muscular power**. Because muscle size often relates to strength, endurance, and power, **muscular hypertrophy** (i.e., muscle mass or size) is also considered a primary component of muscular fitness.

Compared to cardiorespiratory fitness (explored in the previous chapter), muscular fitness is a multifaceted concept. You might be asking yourself, which muscular component is important for functional well-being? The answer is all of them—but which component is the *most* important may differ based on your personal demographics (e.g., age, biological sex), health status, activities of daily living, and health and fitness goals. And importantly, as your life changes, especially from stage to stage and decade to decade, your muscular fitness priorities will undoubtedly change as well.

Physiological Adaptations to Muscular Overload

Per the specificity of training principle, physiological systems adapt in response to the physical load placed on them. In addition to other systems in the body, this has direct implications for the cardiorespiratory system, energy production (metabolic) system, and certainly the musculoskeletal system. If you begin to challenge your muscles, they will adapt to these new stresses, ultimately making the challenge less challenging.

How exactly do muscles gain fitness? How do they get stronger, increase their endurance, or develop the ability to generate more power? Generally, in response to resistance training, there is

an interplay between neuromotor adaptations and changes in muscle size. In the early period of resistance training (first few months), neural factors explain most of the muscular fitness adaptation, whereas muscle fiber hypertrophy increasingly influences strength after longer periods of resistance training. Importantly, neural adaptations always accompany strength gains. Primary neural changes include an increased frequency and improved ability to recruit motor units as well as more synchronized motor unit firing to cause muscle contraction. Primary muscle fiber changes for most health and recreational resistance trainers (i.e., not elite bodybuilders) include increased cross-sectional area of the individual muscle fibers (i.e., larger actin and myosin filaments) and potentially increased number of muscle fibers. The nonoxidative (anaerobic) energy system, introduced in

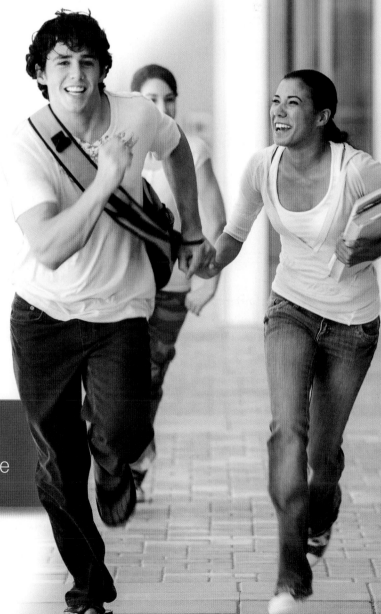

You use slow-twitch fibers when you are walking at a leisurely pace and fast-twitch fibers when you are running to catch a bus.

Components of Muscular Fitness

Muscular fitness is generally categorized with the following characteristics (American College of Sports Medicine 2022):

- **Strength.** The maximal amount of force that can be produced for a specific movement at a given speed by a muscle.
- **Endurance.** The ability of a muscle to hold or repeat a contraction without fatigue.
- **Power.** The rate at which work can be produced by the muscle or the product of force (strength) and velocity.
- **Hypertrophy.** An increase in the size of the muscle, sometimes referred to as the maintenance of muscle mass.

chapter 4, also increases in response to resistance training (figure 5.3).

How the muscles adapt will depend on how they are challenged (how much, how often, how fast) and other key factors such as your genetics, health status, hormones, and dietary intake. Your muscle adaptation is also influenced by your baseline levels of muscular fitness. For example, are you very sedentary and just starting a new resistance training program? Or perhaps you are starting a resistance training program in the student recreation center, but you are already very physically active working on the family farm. Finally, muscle adaptations may be influenced by other types of physical activity in your movement routine, especially cardiorespiratory activities.

As discussed at the end of this chapter, your goals will influence the design of your muscular fitness program. In addition to keeping the key principle of specificity of training in mind, a few other factors are important.

- **Hypertrophy and atrophy.** Remember that adaptations go in both directions. All the adaptations just described are reversed when you decrease or stop challenging your muscles with resistance training activities. Extensive research has documented the muscle physiology and performance changes in response to bed rest or cast immobilization, with strength being reduced more than muscle mass due to reductions in neural changes

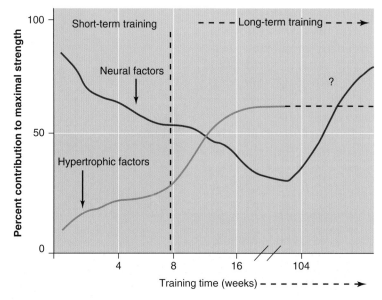

Figure 5.3   Resistance training results in movement tension, metabolic stress, and muscle damage that causes adaptations at the muscle cell level and subsequently increased muscle capacity (e.g., strength).

Adapted by permission from S.J. Fleck and W.J. Kraemer, *Designing Resistance Training Programs*, 4th ed. (Champaign, IL: Human Kinetics, 2014), 108.

(Clark 2009). Certainly, other factors described previously also influence the loss of muscular fitness (age, health status, hormones, other physical activity, etc.). When it comes to muscular fitness, use it (resist it) or lose it!

• *Sex and gender disparities in behavior and equality in adaptation.* From high school to older adults, males have greater participation rates in muscle-strengthening activities, likely as a result of higher sport participation and other social and cultural factors (U.S. Department of Health and Human Services 2018). As most people recognize, biological males, on average, have larger muscle mass and greater muscular strength and power compared to biological females. However, strength and hypertrophy gains are similar between the sexes in response to the same resistance training protocol if starting from the same baseline (Roberts, Nuckols, and Krieger 2020). Although some females still avoid resistance training due to fear of "getting bulky muscles," this concern is not warranted, especially when the muscular fitness program is designed more for strength or endurance. Resistance training is for everybody!

• *Overload is overload.* The principles of an exercise prescription to develop muscular fitness components will be described in detail later. However, here it should be reinforced that your muscles adapt when a force is repeatedly developed against a resistance. Muscle cells do not know or care if the resistance is a perfectly matched set of bars and weights or a bale of hay or a bag of dog food. Anything can be used to provide overload, including many items in your home—be creative! Just lift and carry something!

All pumped up! Temporary hypertrophy, or the increase in muscle size during and immediately after an exercise bout, mainly results from fluid accumulation in the extracellular fluid spaces and between the muscle cells.

Key Definitions

Designing an effective program for muscular fitness involves a thorough understanding of muscular fitness terms. It's important to understand these terms and examples of the movements connected with them so you have the tools to build your personal muscular fitness plan.

Muscle Contractions Defined

The three main types of muscle contractions differ by length of the muscle and movement of the joint: **isometric**, **isotonic concentric**, and **isotonic eccentric**.

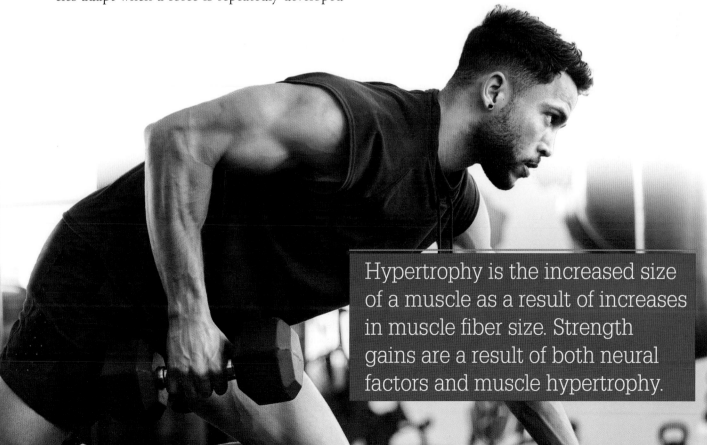

Hypertrophy is the increased size of a muscle as a result of increases in muscle fiber size. Strength gains are a result of both neural factors and muscle hypertrophy.

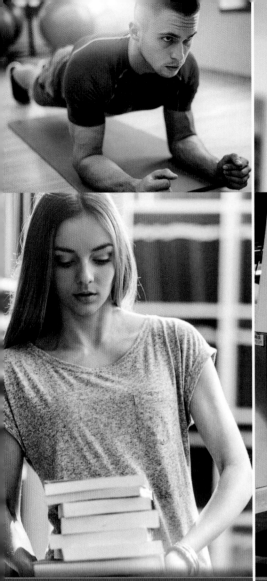

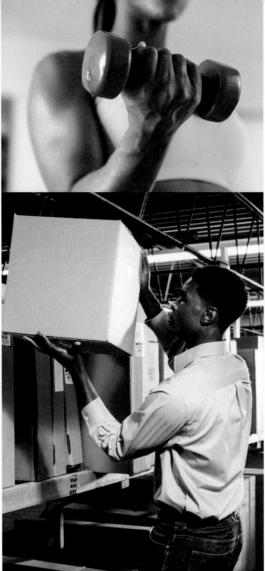

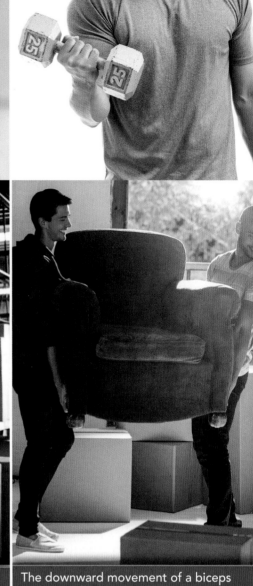

Holding a plank and carrying a pile of books in a fixed position are examples of an isometric muscle contraction.

The up phase of a biceps curl and lifting a box to a shelf are examples of an isotonic concentric muscle action.

The downward movement of a biceps curl and setting down furniture when moving are examples of activities that use an isotonic eccentric muscle action.

- *Isometric.* A static muscle contraction where the muscle length or the joint angle does not change. This type of contraction is important for core muscle development. The core muscles involve the torso and hip muscles, which provide important stabilization functions for daily movements.

- *Isotonic concentric.* During this type of muscle contraction, the tension remains the same while the muscle length changes. The most common type of muscle action use is for nonpostural muscles. The up phase of a basic biceps curl and the functional movement of putting a box up on a shelf both use an isotonic concentric muscle action. In both examples, when the muscle contracts, it shortens and the joint angle decreases.

- *Isotonic eccentric.* This type of muscle contraction is the opposite action of an isotonic concentric contraction. As the muscle contracts, it lengthens and the joint angle increases. This type of contraction is often called a negative in the strength and conditioning room. Most resistance training programs have an eccentric component when the weight is lowered to the ground in a controlled manner. Intense eccentric training can cause rapid strength gains but can also cause much muscle soreness if it is not done properly.

Muscular Fitness Benefits Your Daily Life

Most of us are not competitive athletes. We do not need to have high muscular fitness to perform well academically, make a living, or function independently in our homes and communities. Indeed, in our knowledge-based and technologically advanced society, working on a keyboard in front of a screen does not require much muscular fitness except perhaps that required for good sitting or standing posture. However, like cardiorespiratory fitness, muscular fitness provides more benefits to your daily life than you may realize. For example, if you are a restaurant server and regularly carry large trays of food, you need adequate muscular strength and endurance in your arms, upper body, and core to perform your duties well and prevent joint and muscle pain. If you are interested in having a well-toned physique on the beach for spring break, you might be concerned with hypertrophy and design a program that develops muscular strength, endurance, and even power. If you are a recreational athlete, your sport will dictate your approach to muscular fitness to enhance your performance and prevent injury. Importantly, physical activity and exercise approaches to muscular fitness influence body composition and health (discussed in chapters 7 and 9). Starting and maintaining a physical activity and exercise program to maintain muscular fitness will enhance your performance of activities of daily living, prevent injuries and falls, and prevent chronic conditions such as low back pain. Importantly, you will have less fatigue from the activities you *have* to do with energy left over to do the things you *want* to do.

Assessing Your Muscular Fitness

Like assessing cardiorespiratory fitness, the various components of muscular fitness can be assessed using both laboratory equipment and less complicated field tests. However, instead of whole-body measures, assessments of muscular fitness are typically completed for one movement pattern (e.g., a squat) or joint action (e.g., knee extension), which may not be representative of other muscle groups. In a clinical setting, advanced dynamometers are used to assess all aspects of muscle performance, especially muscular strength and endurance. These assessments inform training regimens and rehabilitation programs for people of all ages and fitness levels. Field tests for each component of muscular fitness might help you inform your personal muscular fitness program.

Muscular Strength

Strength is assessed by measuring the maximal amount of weight a person can lift or move in a single effort, commonly called a *one-repetition maximum* (1RM). You could assess the 1RM for all muscle groups using free weights or machines. However, the 1RM can be intense for your muscles, tendons, and joints and is not without risk. Thus, an alternative strength test is a submaximal effort using repetitions that can help predict your strength.

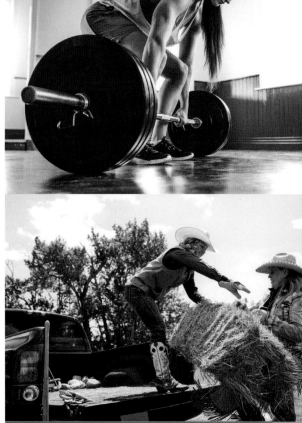

Both performing a deadlift in a strength and conditioning room and lifting a bale of hay require muscular strength.

Muscular Endurance

Muscular endurance is the ability to hold a muscle action or to repeat contractions that are not maximal. This component of muscle capacity is assessed by either the maximum number of repetitions that can be performed (e.g., push-ups) or the length of time a position can be held (e.g., planks). Like muscular strength, good muscular endurance is important for both sport performance and daily living, especially carrying heavy backpacks on campus. Muscular endurance is also important for good posture. The chapter 5 labs in HK*Propel* provide different options you can use to assess your muscular endurance.

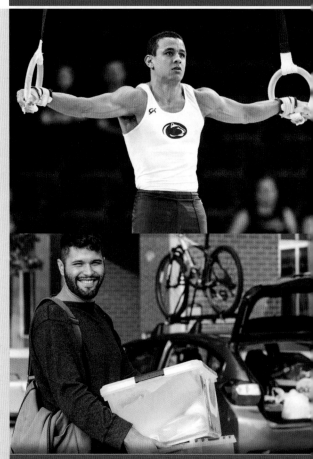

Both holding an iron cross position during gymnastics and carrying boxes while moving involve muscular endurance.

Muscular Power

Muscular power is the ability of a muscle or muscle group to produce a force quickly. The definition of muscular power is force multiplied by distance divided by time. Muscular power is not assessed as often as muscular strength and endurance for health and fitness; however, it deserves mention for its role in daily functional movement. Although its contribution to optimal function is less critical for young adults, the role muscular power plays in daily function for older adults is very important. Muscle power can be assessed with field tests by using a broad jump test or measuring how quickly an older adult gets out of a chair.

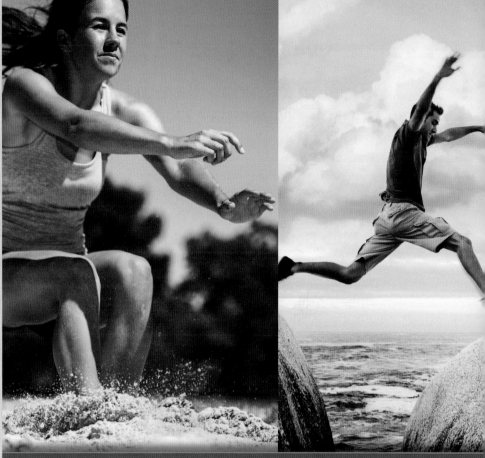

Performing a broad jump and jumping from one rock to another are both examples of a muscular power movement.

Muscular Hypertrophy and Tone

Many people are interested in resistance training for aesthetic or physique reasons. Some people want to have large muscles, be lean, or tone their muscles. A regular program of resistance training can enhance muscle size and definition and help you look and feel better. Although having muscle tone and looking lean are qualitative assessments, muscle and fat mass can be quantitatively measured in the research laboratory or clinic, as described in chapter 7.

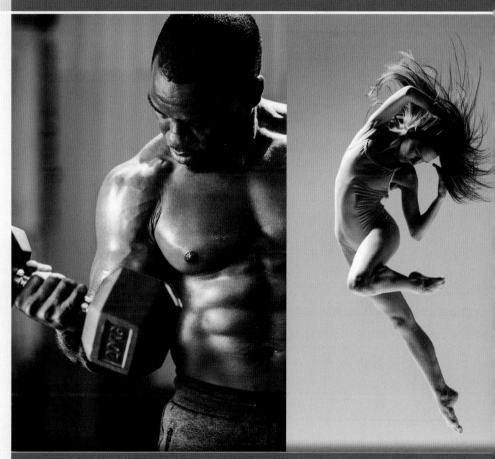

Bodybuilders work on muscle size and tone through resistance training, whereas dancers acquire muscle size and tone by lifting their body weight repeatedly through dance training.

Designing Your Plan to Improve Muscular Fitness

Now that you know how muscles work and how they adapt to overload, you are ready to reflect on your own resistance training program. Formulating a plan to help you realize the benefits of muscular fitness is next.

The Plan Depends on the Goal

Like cardiorespiratory fitness, your personal plan depends on your goal. For example, your muscular fitness might be primarily targeting aesthetic values—you want larger muscles or muscle tone to look good. Or perhaps you need a regular pro-gram to help your posture so that you don't have back and neck pain from lots of computer screen time. Or maybe your sport performance would benefit from a targeted program. You might want to be able to carry a large, heavy backpack while hiking on the weekends. To enhance your health and well-being over time, work on meeting the HHS Physical Activity Guidelines (PAG) (U.S. Department of Health and Human Services 2018) and American College of Sports Medicine (ACSM) exercise guidelines (American College of Sports Medicine 2022), discussed in chapter 2. Please note that content in this section is not targeted to strength training programs for the athlete, specific performance goals, or advanced strength training

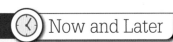

Now and Later

Benefits of Resistance Training

Now

In addition to the many benefits already described, a regular program of resistance training can help you lose inches off your body and greatly enhance your muscle tone. Combined with the benefits for posture and self-confidence, resistance training is a key behavior to looking good and feeling good!

Later

Having muscular fitness is one of the primary keys to aging well, especially in your 60s and beyond. Starting a regular program for your muscular fitness early in life can enhance your bone health and physical functional capacity as you age. It is never too late to start a program and realize the benefits.

Take Home

Older adults need to maintain a regular resistance training program to preserve muscle mass and strength. Importantly, older females are at higher risk of physical disability and females are generally less physically active across the life span compared to their male counterparts. Help the older adults in your life find the motivation to engage in resistance training. Gone are the days of "Let me do that for you." Instead, say, "Grandma (or Grandpa), can you lift that safely? I want you to be independent as long as you can. I know you love living in your own home, so think of it as a fitness center. What can you safely lift every day?" Consider gifting the older adults in your life a set of resistance bands, design a program with them, and text them weekly to see if they have completed their exercises!

techniques such as periodization. If you are interested in moving beyond the general guidelines, we encourage you to consult a personal strength and conditioning coach who has specific expertise for your goal.

Overloading Options

Increasing muscular fitness requires you to overload the muscles in a progressive manner. You can overload a muscle in many ways—muscles respond to the overload, regardless of what is providing the stimulus. The most popular exercise equipment options are resistance machines, free weights, resistance bands or tubes, and body weight; however, you can mix and match these options to design creative workouts. Table 5.1 lists the primary pros and cons for each of these choices. Note that you can improve your muscular fitness without ever going to a strength and conditioning facility.

FITT Approach for Muscular Fitness

The fundamental frame for your muscular fitness program should follow the FITT acronym,

which is an easy way to organize your overload to gain and keep muscular fitness. As we learned in chapter 4, FITT stands for frequency, intensity, time, and type. Figure 5.4 shows how you can fit the PAG and ACSM exercise guidelines into your weekly schedule.

If you are new to resistance training, there a few terms to understand. Commonly, resistance training routines are framed in the following manner:

- *Specific exercises.* Which muscles are overloaded?
- *Load.* How much weight with respect to a 1RM will be lifted?
- *Repetitions (reps).* How many times will the resistance weight be lifted before fatigue or failure occurs?
- *Sets.* How many times will the exercise be repeated in your exercise session?

The ACSM and U.S. Department of Health and Human Services have provided detailed recommendations, with the most important ones described in the following sections. Remember that the best program for you depends on your goals and interests. Unless you enjoy using a strength and conditioning

Table 5.1 Primary Overloading Options and Considerations

Overload option	Positives	Negatives	Considerations
Resistance or stacking weight machines	• Safe • Require no spotter • Easy to understand and use • Easy to target isolated muscle groups • Contain instructional placards on machines • Require little experience	• Expensive • Typically require membership at a fitness facility • Isolate muscle groups, which is not as applicable to real-life functional movement	• Train muscle groups, not movement • Typically work only one or two muscle groups per machine • Require most movements to be performed in a seated position • Require maintenance
Free weights	• Movements are adaptable to real life • Can be used for many different exercises	• Potential for injury is greater • Relatively expensive to purchase for home • May require a spotter for some movements	• Easy to personalize a program • Home use is convenient but requires space
Resistance bands and body weight	• Inexpensive • Easily portable and always available	• Overload for strength may be limited depending on goals and baseline levels	• Inexpensive or free and travel well

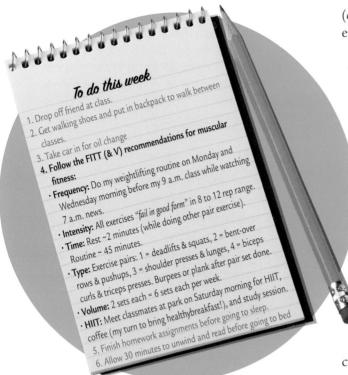

Figure 5.4 Make a weekly to-do list that includes the recommended levels of muscular fitness training.

room or attending a group exercise class, try not to become dependent on a facility or instructor, which can hinder your adherence, particularly over your life span. You may hire a personal trainer or coach to help you design your own program or find a friend who is experienced with resistance training to help you get started. Again, just remember, the best program is the one you will do, so select activities that you enjoy!

Frequency

The HHS Physical Activity Guidelines indicate that adults should engage in resistance training activities of moderate or greater intensity that involve all major muscle groups on two or more days a week (U.S. Department of Health and Human Services 2018). Recommendations by ACSM differ based on experience (American College of Sports Medicine 2022). Novices to resistance training should follow similar advice, overloading each major muscle group at least two days per week. However, for experienced exercisers, frequency is less important than training volume

(discussed later); therefore, the weekly routine for each muscle group may vary.

Most resistance trainers try to give themselves 48 hours between training sessions to allow adaptation and recovery—for example, if you train your quadriceps on Monday, you wouldn't do so again until at least Wednesday. Depending on your schedule and preference, you could train all the major muscle groups in a single session or separate them by splitting the body into regions and alternating your training. For example, a common efficient routine is to alternate working the upper body and the lower body for a total of four days of training a week (e.g., lower body trained on Mondays and Thursdays, upper body trained on Tuesdays and Fridays). Whole-body or split-body routines are equally effective if each muscle group experiences the same volume of overload. You can also choose more functional movements that require balance, stability, strength, and endurance. These types of workouts do not require splitting the body; rather, you would perform total-body functional movements that work several muscle groups simultaneously. Again, once you gain some experience and a conditioning base, there are many effective routines to meet your training volume needs that are dependent on your muscular fitness goals, schedule, and preferences.

Intensity

Your goal will influence the intensity of resistance training. Like other bodily systems, the greater the intensity (i.e., overload or resistance lifted) during training, the greater the benefit; however, there is also a greater risk of injury. For novice trainers, 60 to 70 percent 1RM performed for 8 to 12 repetitions is recommended for improving overall muscular fitness (American College of Sports Medicine 2022). For experienced resistance trainers, a wide range of intensities and repetitions are effective depending on the goal of improving the various muscular fitness components. As you gain a conditioning base, continual improvements will require additional overload with 80 percent or more of 1RM and heavier loads (1 to 6 repetitions) suggested. These intensity recommendations by ACSM align with the PAG suggestions of moderate or greater intensity.

Per ACSM, power gains are best achieved with 1 to 3 sets per exercise performed at maximal velocity with overload differing by muscle groups (30 to 60 percent 1RM for upper-body exercises; 0 to 60 percent 1RM for lower-body exercises). Although research continues to evolve, gains in hypertrophy appear to require performing sets to volitional fatigue. This is often termed "failing in good form." This hypertrophic response can be gained using light to heavy loads, with 6 to 20 repetitions to fatigue being recommended as practical choices.

Optimal endurance routines may vary; low, moderate, and heavy loads have all been shown to be effective to build muscular endurance. Traditionally, lighter loads have been partnered with higher repetitions (15 to 25 or more). Heavier loads with short rest periods could also be used, such as during a circuit routine, interval training protocol, or perhaps a high-intensity functional training session (American College of Sports Medicine 2022). Notably, the popular HIIT format (see chapter 4) can also be incorporated into a muscular fitness routine, although this should be used only by experienced individuals due to risk of injury. The rise in popularity of CrossFit, a branded fitness regimen that involves constantly varied functional movements performed at a high intensity, is a testimony to the interest in fitness activities that are also considered social opportunities.

Time

Unlike cardiorespiratory fitness, time is not a major factor in designing your muscular fitness program. Rather, the time needed for each session will depend on your goals, which influence your exercise choices, repetitions, and sets. How you spread your routine over the days of the week will also impact the time per exercise session. The rest interval between sets can also be altered. Shorter rest intervals (1 to 2 minutes) are more time efficient, whereas longer rest intervals (>2 minutes) between sets may provide greater recovery and thereby allow more total work to be completed in a session. A range of rest intervals have been reported as acceptable to realize muscular fitness gains (American College of Sports Medicine 2022). A common technique to save time during an exercise session is to use a superset, which means to pair two exercises that work opposing muscle groups and alternate them. By exercising one muscle group while the other rests (e.g., biceps

and triceps), rest is built into your routine (see figure 5.5).

Type

As a friendly reminder, lots of options—many in your own home—can effectively provide an overload to your muscles. Beyond recommendations to train the major muscle groups, it makes sense to pick movements that align with your muscular fitness goals to improve your functional fitness and activities of daily living, whether improving your posture after long hours at a computer screen or balancing heavy platters at your weekend server job. More information about program design for functional fitness for your lifestyle is contained in the Functional Fitness Training section, which includes example exercises for the primary muscle groups using free weights or resistance bands, body weight, and variable resistance machines, along with an effective flexibility (stretching) exercise.

Additional recommendations for types of resistance training exercises from ACSM include the following (American College of Sports Medicine 2022):

- Multijoint or compound exercises that affect more than one muscle group (e.g., squats, chest press, bent-over rows)
- Single-joint exercises that target major muscle groups (e.g., leg curl, bicep curl)
- Core exercises that challenge the muscles of the trunk (e.g., planks and curl-ups)
- Exercises that challenge muscles in all actions, including isometric, concentric, and eccentric Exercises that balance opposing muscle groups in a weekly routine (e.g., if you work the biceps, also work the triceps; see figure 5.5)

Notably, this last recommendation is very important to correct imbalances that commonly develop due to our lifestyles. For example, those who perform constant keyboard work sitting in a chair often have tight muscles that cross joints that are in a closed joint position (e.g., pectoralis major, hip flexors, hamstrings), which need flexibility work (see chapter 6). This is often coupled with weak muscles that are not activated or are in a compromised joint position as a result of poor posture (e.g., posterior deltoids, abdominals), which consequently need strengthening. The

✓ Behavior Check

Are You Stronger Than Your Excuses?

Adults meet the HHS Physical Activity Guidelines for muscle-strengthening activities much less often than those for aerobic (cardiorespiratory) activities. Older adults (compared to younger) and females of all ages (compared to males) have the lowest participation rates in resistance training. Why the lack of interest and motivation by so many people? In our research, teaching, and fitness programming experience, we believe it centers on the following three "lacks":

1. Lack of knowledge about personal benefits
2. Lack of how to (safely)
3. Lack of motivation

In our experience, number 3 is the hardest to overcome. We get it! We all need to get personally motivated and help each other engage in resistance training activities to maintain our muscular fitness.

Managing behavior is challenging when we live in a society that encourages us to sit all day long (typically in front of a screen or device). But remember that small choices accumulate toward meeting the PAG over time. For cardiorespiratory fitness, we explored how small steps can add up over the day and week. For muscular fitness, this same notion applies—small lifts also add up. As you go around your living space, on campus, and in your community, think about everything in your environment as a potential resistance training device to improve your functional fitness.

We challenge you to identify 10 unconventional resistance training devices (no bars, plates, or bands!) that currently exist in your environment that you could use to provide overload. Here's an example list of ideas used by one of the authors:

1. Military backpack (great find at a yard sale; handles a large load!)
2. Stairs (take two at a time with the loaded backpack or use for triceps presses)
3. Bag of horse feed or a bale of hay (~50 lb)
4. Full manure cart (~75 lb, uphill to compost pile—a real glute burner!)
5. Bag of dog food or a box of cat litter (40 lb)
6. Dog (~45 lb; helps get steps too!)
7. Firewood and logs (highly variable)
8. 5-gallon buckets of water (great for a farmer carry or suitcase carry)
9. Flooring (for new flooring project; 45 lb per box)
10. Laundry basket (fill it with whatever you want and carry it—it's that simple)

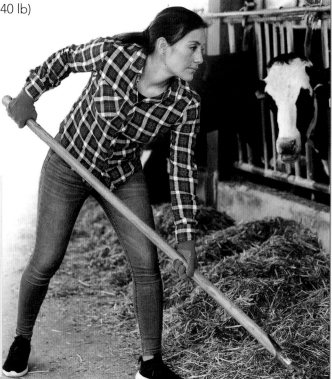

This author says, "My muscular fitness will help me be physically functional so that I can play with and tend to my horses and dogs, engage in do-it-yourself projects, and take care of my homestead." Think creatively and let your own *why* for being strong influence your motivational muscles. You got this—you can be stronger than your excuses!

muscles of the lower back are particularly compromised because they tend to be both weak and tight, a key cause of low back pain. Explore table 5.2 closely and think about your sitting behaviors and your daily movement patterns.

When incorporating a combination of exercises into your routine, be mindful of the order and purpose of the exercises. In general, plan to perform exercises for large muscle groups or multijoint exercises before doing smaller muscle or single-joint exercises. Fatiguing the small muscle groups first limits your ability to overload the larger muscle groups or complete compound exercises. Thus, for example, you should first perform sets for squats, then leg extensions (compound versus single-joint exercise), followed by calf raises (larger versus smaller muscle groups). See table 5.2 for common muscle imbalances.

Volume, Progression, and Pattern

The FITT approach provides a framework for your weekly routine to achieve muscular fitness, but volume, progression, and pattern also influence your planning, regardless of your fitness goals.

Volume

Contemporary recommendations indicate that the volume of a resistance training program is

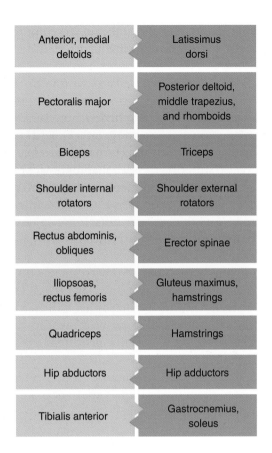

Figure 5.5   Common Muscle Imbalances
Reprinted by permission from C. Kennedy-Armbruster and M.M. Yoke, *Methods of Group Exercise Instruction*, 3rd ed. (Champaign, IL: Human Kinetics, 2014), 44.

Table 5.2   Common Muscle Imbalances

Muscle	Problem	Typical cause	Correction
Pectoralis major	Tight	Poor posture when sitting and standing	Stretch
Posterior deltoids, middle trapezius, rhomboids	Weak, overstretched	Poor posture when sitting and standing	Strengthen
Shoulder internal rotators	Tight	Poor posture, carrying and holding objects close to body	Stretch
Shoulder external rotators	Weak	Poor posture	Strengthen
Abdominals	Weak	Poor posture, obesity	Strengthen
Erector spinae	Tight (and often weak)	Poor posture, obesity	Stretch (and strengthen)
Hip flexors	Tight	Poor posture, sedentary lifestyle	Stretch
Hamstrings	Tight	Sedentary lifestyle	Stretch
Calves	Tight	Wearing high heels	Stretch
Shins	Weak	Not enough use in daily activities	Strengthen

Reprinted by permission from M.M. Yoke and C. Kennedy-Armbruster, *Methods of Group Exercise Instruction*, 4th ed. (Champaign, IL: Human Kinetics, 2020), 28.

determined by the total number of sets completed of a given exercise or movement pattern in a week (American College of Sports Medicine 2022). The PAG indicates that adults who perform a minimum of 1 set per session realize important improvements in muscular fitness; however, 2 to 3 sets per session may provide greater benefits (U.S. Department of Health and Human Services 2018). ACSM also supports the idea that for novice resistance trainers, 1 set per session is adequate to gain benefits. Thus, low-volume protocols (defined as less than 4 weekly sets per muscle group) are an acceptable option for untrained individuals or those with limited time.

Individuals beyond the novice stage who are seeking greater gains in muscular fitness, especially strength and hypertrophy, will need to embrace the dose–response relationship—that is, greater exercise volume produces greater improvements. Moderate-volume protocols are defined as 5 to 9 sets per muscle group per week, whereas high-volume routines are 10 or more sets per muscle group per week. It is important to recognize that for individuals who have progressed beyond the novice stage, volume of training per week is more important than frequency for gains in muscular strength or hypertrophy. Notably, volume goals can be met by mixing and matching exercises for a specific muscle group. For example, 9 quadriceps sets could be accumulated over a week, with a combination of squats, leg presses, and leg extensions (e.g., 9 sets of squats; 5 sets of squats, 2 sets of leg presses, and 2 sets of leg extensions; or 3 sets of each exercise).

> By manipulating reps, sets, and rest intervals between sets, you can target muscular strength, endurance, power, or hypertrophy. Make your program work for your goals and your adherence needs!

Progression

If you establish a good weekly resistance training program and you are interested in increasing your muscular fitness, you will need to progressively overload your muscles. There are many options to accomplish this progression, and the best choice will likely depend most on your schedule constraints and preferences. Remember that it is important to progress slowly and pay attention to your body to avoid injury and excessive daily fatigue and to preserve your motivation. Following are examples of effective methods for incorporating progression into your resistance training routine (American College of Sports Medicine 2022):

- *Increase weight.* Reach 10 repetitions for the deadlift using a 100-pound weight for several sessions over a week. The following week, increase the weight lifted by 10 percent and continue the pattern.
- *Increase reps.* Strive to complete 12 reps until you fatigue with the original 100-pound weight.
- *Increase volume per session.* After completing 2 sets of deadlifts in 2 sessions per week, add an additional set per session, increasing exercise volume by 50 percent.
- *Increase volume per week.* After completing 2 sets of deadlifts in 2 sessions per week, add an additional session per week, increasing exercise volume by 50 percent.

However motivated you might be, you will not be able to progress endlessly. As you move closer to your genetic ceiling you will experience the principle of diminishing returns. This means you will have to work harder to get smaller gains in muscular fitness. Or perhaps you have met your muscular fitness goals, you are feeling good, and now want to think about maintenance. The good news is that research shows that one session per week can maintain a healthy muscular fitness level if the intensity and overload is held constant (American College of Sports Medicine 2022). This is important for very busy times of life too. On those weeks that are extra busy, you will be able to maintain your muscular fitness if you can get just one great resistance training session into your schedule.

Pattern

Pattern is not a formal component of the recommendations by ACSM. However, it is an important consideration for your muscular fitness program during your college years and as you progress through life. Your muscular fitness plan, like your cardiorespiratory fitness plan, can be altered by the week, day, or even the workout session.

Because time and other demands of life often change day to day, and because you will want to build rest days into your routine, plan your activity to fit within a week. For example, some days will allow for an intense full-body resistance training session in the student recreation center (complete with a fully resourced weight room!). Other days, you might need to design a routine with resistance bands and body weight to be completed in your living room. Or you might be short on time and motivation and decide to break up your routine by working your core in the morning to help your posture and then complete the other muscle groups that evening in front of your laptop and

---

✓ Behavior Check

Incorporating Muscular Fitness Movements Into Daily Life

In addition to designing a weekly resistance training exercise program to improve and maintain muscular fitness, use these ideas to add muscular strength and endurance movements to your daily life:

- Choose a large backpack, load it down, and carry it (on both shoulders!) when you use active transportation.
- When carrying groceries and supplies into your room or apartment, try to lift as many bags as you can to transport your goods in as few trips as possible.
- Try to find a part-time job that works your muscles, such as with a lawn care service, a moving or cleaning company, or a farm.
- Break up your computer screen time with sets of planks or push-ups in your room.
- Take the stairs instead of the elevator whenever you can and take two steps at a time (joint health permitting).

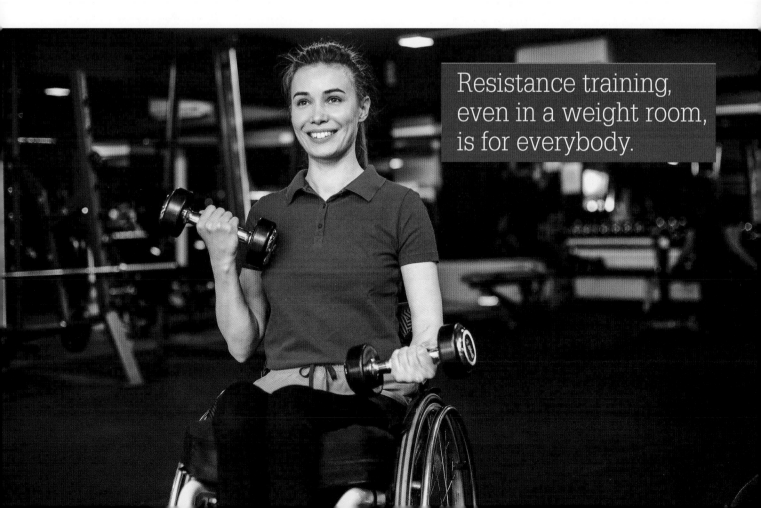

Resistance training, even in a weight room, is for everybody.

your favorite Netflix series. The weekend might bring some needed social time—consider planning a HIIT party in your apartment complex parking lot with your roommates and neighbors. To start designing options, search for "HIIT weight training" (as of this writing, 29.6 million hits came up!).

In closing, when planning your week, think about how you can design your pattern of resistance training to fit within your busy life. Be creative! Be social! And at the end of the week, you will have moved yourself closer to meeting your goals and will be feeling great. Plus, you will have easily met the recommendations for muscular fitness, providing yourself important health benefits.

Analyzing Your Fitness Choices

Although extensive literature exists about exercise adherence, it is a simple fact that if you don't enjoy your movement choices or they are not connected to something you value, you will not continue your program. Try to keep the enjoyment in fitness and make it enhance your daily function. Like cardiorespiratory exercise, there are lots of options to choose from to design your personal program. Think about what activities in your daily life you would like to have more muscular fitness to do and identify which muscle group you want to improve. Do your quads hurt after climbing several flights of stairs to get to a class? Then you will want to strengthen your quadriceps. Do you have difficulty carrying heavy groceries or a pile of books? Strengthening your biceps and deltoids will help with that. Do you want to be able to tuck in your shirt and have good posture and be satisfied that you look and feel good? Working on your core might be your priority. In other words, have a purpose for what you are doing outside of just "working out."

Beginning resistance trainers can find the FITT framework and relatedly, the volume, progression, and pattern components of muscular fitness complicated. Let's make sense out of how you might think about resistance training before you design your own program. Understanding your choices will help you adhere to your program and gradually work up to the recommended guidelines. In the Functional Fitness Training insert (located after chapter 6) you will find a practical method for choosing which exercises to include in your program. You'll start by thinking about which

muscles you use more in daily living. Then you'll use a progression model—moving from functional movement to resistance exercise choices to a relevant flexibility exercise (stretch)—that will be especially helpful if you are new to resistance training.

The muscle groups included in the Functional Fitness Training insert are the muscles of the calves, quadriceps (quads), hamstrings and gluteal muscles (glutes), abdominals, lower back, hip abductors, hip adductors, chest and front of shoulder, upper back and shoulders, latissimus dorsi (lats) and middle back, biceps, and triceps. It is useful to think of your major muscle groups as those that occur in pairs with nearly equal and opposite actions. For example, the chest muscles push away from the body, whereas the upper back muscles pull toward the body. Similarly, the quadriceps of the legs extend the knee joint, and the hamstrings flex the knee joint. Nearly all muscle actions use a combination of the major muscle groups. The Functional Fitness Training insert will help you put this concept into perspective as you perform daily living activities and incorporate practical suggestions for muscular fitness. Flexibility and neuromotor training information, discussed in the next chapter, are also included in this section.

Safety First: Getting Started With Resistance Training

Resistance training can provide many functional fitness and health benefits. However, you must exercise safely to avoid injury and adverse consequences. In this section, we will review safety precautions to take while performing resistance training, followed by a brief discussion of supplements and drugs.

> A good rule for safe resistance training using plates and bars or free weights: If you cannot control it, don't lift it!

Safety While You Train

Follow these special considerations for strength training to avoid injury:

- **Don't skip the warm-up.** Cold muscles and tendons do not respond well to stress. Warming up may reduce the risk of injury, and you will feel better during the session!

- *Mind the joints.* Proper form and technique are very important for injury prevention. For example, spines typically cannot safely twist while bending.

- *Range of motion.* Unless you are performing a static exercise (e.g., plank), complete all exercises through the full range of motion for a given joint.

- *Don't forget to breathe.* Holding your breath can elevate your blood pressure and make you light-headed. Exhale when you are in the concentric or up phase (lifting) and inhale during the eccentric or down phase (lowering).

- *Eccentric training.* Avoid high-intensity eccentric training unless you have a very solid conditioning base; it poses a significant risk for muscle soreness, joint injury, and muscle damage.

- *Use spotters and collars.* When using free weights, always use appropriate collars and spotters to prevent injury to yourself and your fellow exercisers.

- *Progress slowly.* Training too hard and too often is a primary cause of injuries. Start slow and progress appropriately so you can keep up your muscular fitness for a lifetime.

Caution: Supplements and Drugs

Although supplements will be more fully discussed in chapter 8, it is appropriate to provide a brief mention here. Resorting to extreme tactics with little regard for the potential health risks can be dangerous. Although some substances improve performance, the great majority are not regulated by the U.S. Food and Drug Administration (FDA). They may be ineffective, illegal, and in some cases dangerous.

Of special importance is the use and abuse of **anabolic-androgenic steroids (AAS)**, which are **ergogenic** but can be extremely dangerous and have long-lasting health effects. They are rarely prescribed for healthy young people and are not regulated by the FDA. These drugs, marketed as designer steroids, are considered recreational (i.e., illegal). Obtaining a prescription from a physician but using the drugs incorrectly is also illegal. The National Athletic Training Association provides a detailed scientific position statement regarding AAS (Kersey et al. 2012). Another great resource is WebMD (search "anabolic steroids"), which provides an extensive overview of anabolic steroids and the health risks associated with their use and abuse.

Just like you wouldn't want friends to hurt themselves with other types of drug use, watch for

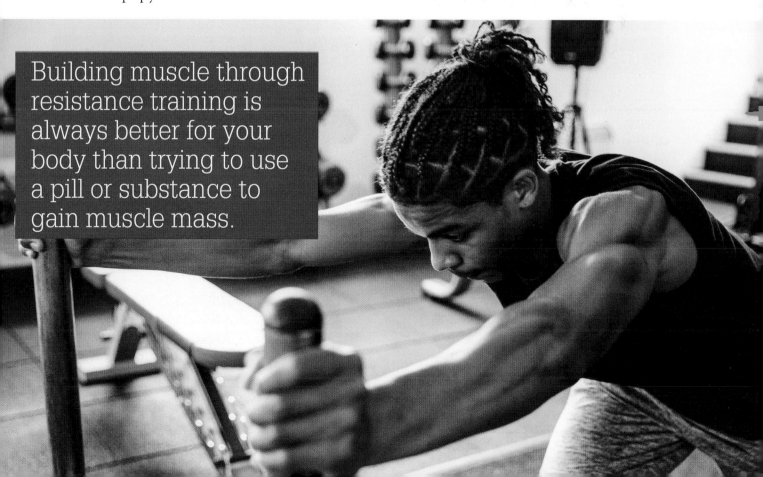

Building muscle through resistance training is always better for your body than trying to use a pill or substance to gain muscle mass.

> Friends don't let friends use steroids! If you suspect use and abuse, be a true friend—confront the situation and assist your friend in getting professional help.

signs and symptoms of steroid use, which include mood swings, secretive actions, and rapid increases in muscular size and fitness. In addition to a regular well-designed resistance program, good health behaviors, including adequate nutrition, hydration, and sleep, are the key strategies to enjoying muscular fitness for a lifetime.

systems provide ATP to your contracting muscles, which pull on your bones to cause movement. When you challenge the muscles with progressive overload using machines, weights, resistance bands, or your body weight, muscles gain fitness due to both neural and muscle fiber adaptations.

Muscular fitness is very important for many sport and recreational activities, as well as activities of daily life. Good muscular fitness is also important for preventing injuries of your muscles and joints during work and play activities. Use the Functional Fitness Training insert, found after chapter 6, to help you design a regular muscular fitness program that you will be motivated to stay with for life. This will help you feel better, look better, reduce your risk of injury and pain, and increase your chance of living a long, independent life. The chapter 5 labs in HK*Propel* provide options for assessing your muscular strength.

Summary

Muscular fitness, which includes muscular strength, endurance, power, and hypertrophy, is a key component of functional fitness. Your body's energy

REVIEW QUESTIONS

1. Muscles contain different types of muscle fibers that allow for different types of movement. What type of muscle fiber helps us run long distances without being tired? What type of muscle fiber allows us to run sprints? For a typical day on campus, which fibers do you use the most and for what activities?

2. List and briefly define the four components of muscular fitness. Which of the components is most important to you as you design your muscular fitness program? Why?

3. List two advantages and two disadvantages each for using (1) resistance machines, (2) free weights, and (3) resistance bands or body weight for resistance training.

4. Understanding muscle imbalances from daily living helps you choose a resistance training routine that will enhance your daily life. What are the opposing muscle groups to the following muscle groups: calves, quadriceps, abdominals, biceps, latissimus dorsi, and rhomboids (see figure 5.5)?

5. Outline a resistance training plan for a typical week using the campus recreational facilities. Calculate your total volume of resistance training based on the weekly sets of exercises. How might you use this volume to help you progress?

6. List five ways you can incorporate muscular strength and endurance training into your daily life using various items available in your environment.

7. Outline three or four safety issues that are important to consider when engaging in resistance training.

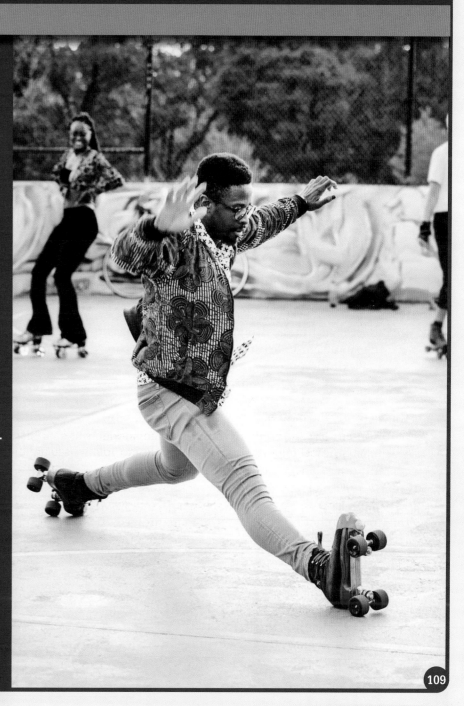

6

Flexibility, Neuromuscular Fitness, and Posture

OBJECTIVES

- Understand the health benefits of flexibility and neuromuscular fitness to enhance your functional fitness.

- Learn the evidence-based guidelines for flexibility.

- Appreciate the multifaceted role that neuromuscular fitness plays in functional fitness and injury prevention.

- Understand how to prevent low back pain with exercise and proper posture.

- Develop a safe exercise plan for enhancing your flexibility and neuromuscular fitness to meet your needs.

- Incorporate strategies into your daily movement routine to enhance flexibility and neuromuscular fitness, including posture.

KEY TERMS

With a solid understanding of cardiorespiratory and muscular fitness, we will now explore the important concepts of flexibility, neuromuscular fitness, and posture, which play key roles in functional fitness. In our experience, most adults neglect their flexibility and neuromuscular training even more so than the muscle fitness guidelines discussed in chapter 5. This is especially true for younger adults, who do not yet recognize or perhaps value the benefits of flexibility and neuromuscular fitness. Both the HHS Physical Activity Guidelines (U.S. Department of Health and Human Services 2018) and the ACSM's *Guidelines for Exercise Testing and Prescription* (American College of Sports Medicine 2022) endorse targeted exercise to enhance flexibility. Although not as well defined with FITT recommendations, neuromuscular training, sometimes referred to as neuromotor training, is also important, especially for core musculature. Together, being flexible and having adequate neuromuscular fitness can assist your functional fitness, including posture to prevent injury and chronic pain, especially low back pain.

Flexibility and neuromuscular training are important for sport-specific performance. For example, a gymnast has very different flexibility and neuromuscular needs than a distance runner or a tennis player. However, beyond sport, recreational or otherwise, you are encouraged to consider the importance of flexibility and neuromuscular fitness to prevent the compromised functional fitness that occurs as a result of our sedentary lifestyles. In this way, think about your flexibility and neuromuscular practices as a primary strategy to prevent injury, thereby making you feel good, so you can keep moving and maintain your functional fitness.

> Consistently engaging in cardiorespiratory and muscular fitness activities but not taking the time for flexibility training is like filling the gas tank but neglecting to change the oil in your car. In the short term it won't be a problem, but in the longer term, like your car's function, your functional fitness will be compromised.

All About Flexibility

Flexibility is the amount of movement that can be accomplished at a joint and is often described as the range of motion (ROM) of a joint or set of joints. Because flexibility is harder to quantify, not as much evidence-based research exists for flexibility compared to cardiorespiratory and muscular fitness. However, less research does not mean it lacks in importance. Let's explore the basics of the physiological determinants of flexibility so that you are well positioned to maintain your flexibility to enhance your daily functional fitness.

What Determines Flexibility?

Have you ever noticed that some people can bend themselves into a pretzel, whereas others can barely get out of a chair after sitting for a while? Flexibility, sometimes referred to as *limberness*, is about how freely your joints move, including the lengthening ability of the muscles that cross a given joint. Several factors can affect your flexibility:

- *Joint structure.* There are many different types of joints in the body, and this affects joint ROM. For example, the ball-and-socket joint in the shoulder has the greatest range of motion of all the joints, whereas the hinge joint of the elbow has much more limited movement.

- *Age and sex.* Flexibility is reduced with age, in part because of changes in the muscle fibers themselves. Females are also more flexible than males throughout the life span as a result of different bone structure and hormones.

- *Connective tissue.* The deep **connective tissues** of the body, including the fascia and tendons, can affect ROM. Fascia is a band of connective tissue below the skin that attaches, stabilizes, and separates muscles and other internal organs. Tendons attach muscle to bone. Ligaments, which attach bones to one another, are not elastic but do respond to regular stretching. Age affects all these connective tissues, making them thicker and less flexible.
- *Muscle size.* When muscles get bigger, ROM may be reduced, particularly in males. For example, having large chest muscles can limit how far you can lift your arms overhead.
- *Proprioceptors.* These tiny sensors are located inside muscle fibers and provide information about joint angle, muscle length, and muscle tension. They can cause reflexes that prevent ROM. The stretch reflex (described later in the chapter) is an example of **proprioceptors** working in the body.
- *Joint injury or repair.* Major injuries to joints that cause scar tissue often reduce ROM. Similarly, joint replacement can make a person less flexible. This typically occurs with knee replacements.

Recall from the previous chapter that muscles often work in pairs. This means that many different muscle groups can influence the ROM of a joint. See, for example, the stretch shown in figure 6.1: The joint being stretched is the shoulder, a ball-and-socket joint that is stabilized by several muscles. Although this stretch is being completed primarily as a triceps stretch, it also involves the posterior deltoid, rotator cuff muscles (teres minor and major), and the latissimus dorsi.

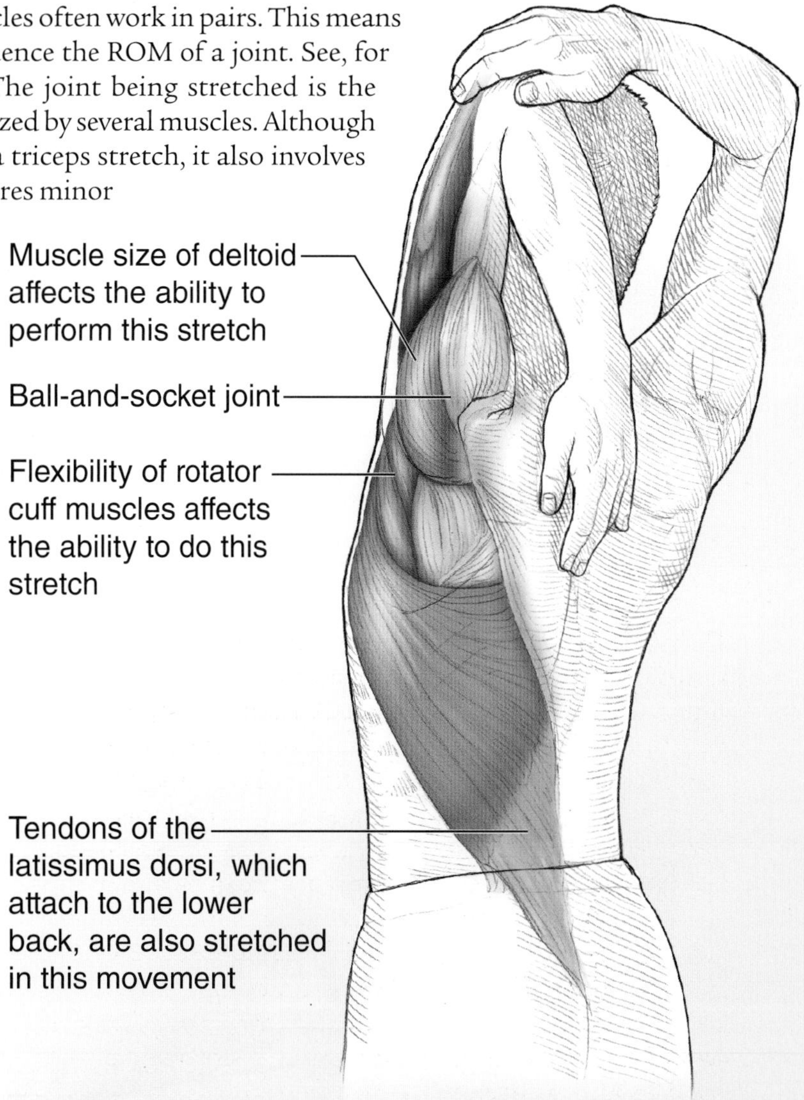

Muscle size of deltoid affects the ability to perform this stretch

Ball-and-socket joint

Flexibility of rotator cuff muscles affects the ability to do this stretch

Tendons of the latissimus dorsi, which attach to the lower back, are also stretched in this movement

Figure 6.1 Notice all the muscles that are involved in the triceps stretch.

✓ Behavior Check

Stretching: Just Do It!

People who adhere to regular flexibility routines often incorporate stretching into daily living activities much like animals do—because it feels good to stretch. The next time your muscles feel tight or you have a tension headache, take a break and try a few stretches. Although flexibility training can be very complicated and include a dedicated regimen such as yoga, this is not required. Many flexibility routines involve no equipment, minimal space, and no special clothing—not even shoes, in many cases! When it comes to flexibility training, keep it simple. Some people find that stretching in the morning starts the day off right, decreasing morning stiffness and increasing blood flow. Or perhaps you can establish a comprehensive flexibility routine that you can do while watching an episode of your favorite Netflix series or while talking to someone special on a video chat. Keep in mind that flexibility training, in comparison to cardiorespiratory or muscular fitness training, requires the least amount of physical effort. Given these important points, the barriers to getting your flexibility exercise are few and the benefits to your life are many. Commit to a flexibility and mobility routine today, and your body will thank you in the future!

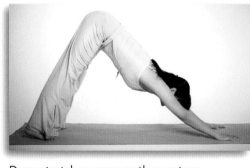

Stretch the front of the shoulder and chest to offset keyboard work, stretch your neck while sitting at your desk, or stretch the glutes and hamstrings at your desk or while standing.

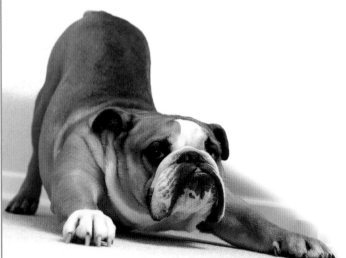

Dogs stretch as soon as they get up; humans should think about doing the same thing!

Strength and Flexibility Can Interact!

A relative balance exists between the strength of a particular muscle group and the flexibility of both the muscle and the joint it crosses. If you already have a great deal of flexibility in a specific muscle group, you may need to emphasize strength movements rather than stretching to avoid injury to joint structures and ligaments. On the other hand, if you are very strong but lack flexibility, then stretching is important. For example, gymnasts are often very flexible and can overstretch the spinal ligaments with their training, causing back pain and hyperflexible joint structures. Thus, to prevent joint pain, many gymnasts also focus on core strengthening to counteract their flexibility. Most of us do not have issues with being too flexible; we are usually too tight in our muscles and joints from lack of movement and sitting. We also generally work in a forward-flexed position in front of a screen. As discussed in chapter 5, balance of opposing muscle groups across the joints is also very important for posture and for pain and injury prevention. To find that healthy balance between being flexible and strong, you will need to understand the evidence-based guidelines of FITT for flexibility exercise training.

FITT Approach for Flexibility

The ACSM has provided recommendations for designing a flexibility exercise program (American College of Sports Medicine 2022) with major factors discussed in the following sections. As you might recognize from the previous chapters, the FITT approach will also work as a frame for your flexibility plan. And certainly, the best flexibility plan for you depends on your goals and interests. Choosing activities that you enjoy and that have minimum resource needs will help you stretch regularly. Figure 6.2 shows how you can fit the guidelines for flexibility training into your weekly schedule. You also might think about incorporating stretching into daily living. Much like the stretches featured in the previous Behavior Check sidebar, think about incorporating stretching movements that feel good throughout the day.

The Functional Fitness Training insert that appears after this chapter outlines ideas for stretching specific muscle groups. Excellent ideas for stretching exercises are also readily available from an Internet search. Think about incorporating stretching into your daily activities as well. For example, when sitting on a bench or couch, turn and put one leg up to stretch your hamstrings, which can get tight from long periods of sitting, especially with your knees bent. When you get up from working at a computer, raise your hands above your head and take a moment to stretch the joints in your lower and upper back and shoulders. Sit back in your chair with arms extended to stretch your neck and upper back muscles. When traveling, find a corner and stretch before boarding,

Figure 6.2 Make a weekly to-do list that includes the recommendations for flexibility training.

To do this week

1. Wear backpack over both shoulders to strengthen lower back.
2. Establish weekend plans with friends.
3. Walk to class and don't forget umbrella and comfortable walking shoes.
4. Follow the FITT (& V) recommendations for flexibility:
   - **Frequency:** Do stretch routine on Tuesday and Thursday during Netflix series after bath. Saturday: video call with Mom after walk.
   - **Intensity:** Hold all stretches to point of discomfort but no pain.
   - **Time:** Hold each exercise for 30 seconds. Routine—15 minutes.
   - **Type:** All major muscle groups—see saved web link.
   - **Volume:** 30 sec/rep x 3 reps/session x 3 (Tues/Thurs/Sat) = for 180 secs weekly total per major muscle-tendon group.
   - **Yoga:** Meet study partner for yoga on Sunday afternoon then study for exam at coffee shop.
5. Watch one episode of my favorite Netflix series after dinner for a break.
6. Do homework 2 hours every evening Monday to Thursday.
7. Go to bed by 10:30 pm.

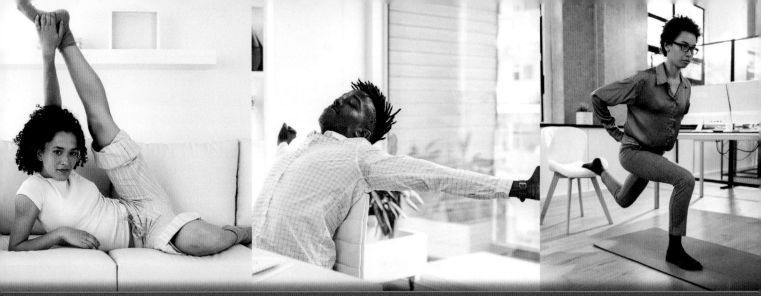

Try stretching your hamstrings while relaxing on the sofa or stretching your chest and shoulders while you are in your chair. You might also stand and stretch your hip flexors while you work.

especially those muscles that will be compromised when buckled into your seat (e.g., hip flexors). These small stretches add up and fit easily into daily living practices, allowing you to meet the guidelines for stretching with minimal time and effort.

Frequency

Everyone, regardless of age, can improve joint ROM. It is never too late to become more flexible. The other great news is that the ROM of a joint is improved immediately after performing targeted exercises, giving instant gratification. You can gain more permanent improvements in flexibility after three to four weeks of a regular stretching program performed two to three times per week. Importantly, although the recommendation is at least two to three times per week, daily flexibility training is the most effective.

Intensity

Determining intensity for flexibility training is less complicated than that required for cardiorespiratory or muscular fitness training. Stretch to the point of feeling tightness or slight discomfort but never pain. If you feel your muscles shaking, then reduce the range of motion slightly. Relaxing the muscle is important when thinking of intensity. Getting the mind and body to work together helps you gain positive outcomes in response to your flexibility practice.

Time

Although several types of flexibility exercises exist, the most common type for nonathletes is static stretching. The time recommendation is to hold each position for 10 to 30 seconds. Another time consideration is when to incorporate stretching into your day and with respect to your other physical activities. Some research suggests that holding a static stretch for more than 60 seconds can negatively affect exercise performance (e.g., sprinting, muscular strength and power, or sport performance). Thus, you may want to avoid stretching before these types of activities. Given that joint-specific exercises to gain flexibility are more effective when the body is warm, it makes sense to stretch after cardiorespiratory or muscular fitness training. Passive warming can also be effective—consider stretching after a hot bath. However, dynamic stretches, especially ones that mimic the upcoming muscle actions are encouraged prior to any exercise or sport activity.

Type

Exercises that improve flexibility target the muscle-tendon units linked to major muscle groups. It is suggested that you perform, at a minimum, flexibility exercises for all major muscle groups in your stretching practices. See the Functional Fitness Training insert for the roster of major muscle groups. You may need to pay more attention to joints that are out of alignment due to daily tasks, particularly muscles on the front side of the body that are in shortened positions due to sitting and keyboard work. The chapter 6 labs in HK*Propel* will help you measure your flexibility to inform your personal flexibility program. The primary types of stretching exercises include the following:

- *Static.* This is what most people think of when they picture stretching. **Static stretching** involves slowly moving into a position and holding it for 10 to 30 seconds. Passive static stretching involves holding the limb or body part, with or without the assistance of a prop (e.g., bar, band, or partner). Active static stretching requires the muscle to be stretched to contract while the opposite muscle group is relaxed and stretched, which often occurs when performing yoga.

- *Slow dynamic.* This method involves a slow transition from one position to another with a progressive increase in the reach or ROM as the movement is repeated. Examples of **dynamic stretching** are lifting the knees high or stretching the inner and outer thigh muscles by slowly lunging side to side to dynamically increase the ROM.

- *Ballistic or bouncing.* Ballistic stretching is not recommended for the average person because the stretch reflex (discussed later) is often initiated, which can lead to injury. With ballistic stretching, momentum produces the stretch and may cause the muscle to contract. If you continue to try to stretch the contracted muscle, you may cause a muscle cramp and possibly injury.

- *Proprioceptive neuromotor facilitation (PNF).* Although many different variations of the PNF method exist, it typically involves an isometric contraction (no joint movement and 3 to 6 seconds of a light to moderate intensity) of a selected muscle–tendon group followed by static stretching (10 to 30 seconds) of the same group. This is often termed *contract–relax stretching.*

The primary types of flexibility exercises can all improve ROM. The best choice depends on your personal goals. For example, if your physical activities require you to perform ballistic movements, such as basketball or dance,

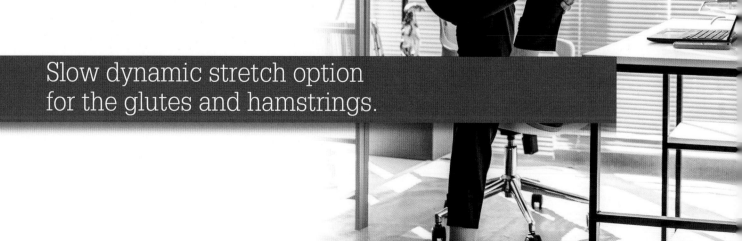

Slow dynamic stretch option
for the glutes and hamstrings.

Benefits of Being Flexible

The return on investment for the time you dedicate to your flexibility routine is not well recognized and is often underappreciated. A consistent stretching practice will give you physical and psychological benefits, positively influencing your well-being.

- Improved physical performance of daily activities
- Increased muscle relaxation
- Enhanced mind–body connection
- Improved posture
- Decreased muscle tension (often linked to neck and back pain and headaches)
- Lowered risk of low back and hip pain
- Lowered risk of muscle or joint injury

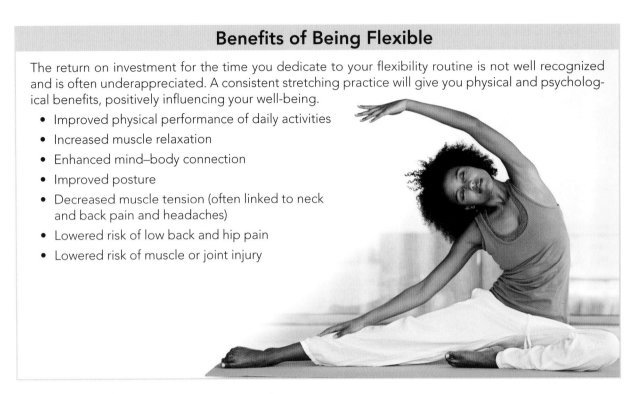

ballistic stretching might be a good choice—but only after you have warmed up your muscles! If you find the complexities of PNF overwhelming, that technique is not a good choice for you. In general, static stretching is the safest and easiest to perform, particularly when muscles are warmed up. As discussed for cardiorespiratory and muscular fitness, mix and match your exercises, and choose options that you will actually do on a consistent basis to obtain and maintain fitness.

Volume, Progression, and Pattern

As with other components of fitness, volume, progression, and pattern are probably important in flexibility training, but little research has been done in these areas. Volume for flexibility training can be considered an interaction of time, repetitions, and frequency (sessions per week). Although the optimal progression is not known, a good target is to perform two to four repetitions of each exercise, which results in about 90 seconds of total stretching time for each flexibility exercise. To increase volume of flexibility training you could do more repetitions of the same stretch in a session (e.g., hold hamstring stretch for 30 seconds and repeat two times; advance to three times the next week) or you could add another session to the weekly routine. As with other fitness components, if you don't use it, you will lose it! And

like cardiorespiratory and muscular fitness, it is much easier to maintain your flexibility than gain it. However, the most optimal program depends on your goals and interests.

Mind the Stretch Reflex!

The body has amazing protective capabilities, and the muscle system is no exception. A basic understanding of the myotatic stretch reflex, commonly called the **stretch reflex**, will help you design a safe and effective flexibility program.

Physiology

Reflexes do not involve the brain but rather operate directly through spinal cord control. This means that a reflex process is quick and cannot be mentally overridden. You might be familiar with reflexes from the knee-jerk test, in which a doctor taps your patellar tendon with a small hammer. This stretches the tendon and quadriceps muscle and immediately results in a spontaneous muscle contraction, causing your foot to move. The stretch reflex is the most important reflex related to muscle movement. Essentially, a stretch reflex is your body's preprogrammed protection mechanism that autoregulates muscle length to prevent muscle tearing. Whenever a muscle experiences a sudden or excessive stretch, special receptors called *Golgi tendon organs* and *muscle spindles* detect the action and immediately send an impulse for two simultaneous muscle actions:

- *Golgi tendon organs.* These contract the muscle, protecting it from being pulled too hard or beyond a normal range. Synergistic muscles are innervated so that they strengthen the contraction and help prevent injury.
- *Muscle spindles.* These relax the antagonist muscles (the opposite muscle groups). Without this inhibitory action, as soon as the stretched muscle began to contract, the antagonist muscle would be stretched, causing a stretch reflex. Both muscles would contract together if it were not for the stretch reflex process.

What Does the Stretch Reflex Mean for You?

The stretch reflex needs to be respected to both prevent injury and maximize your flexibility training. To receive the full benefit when stretching muscles to enhance flexibility and ROM, focus on static stretching and stretching to the point of tension, not pain. If you overstretch or bounce and stretch too vigorously, then the muscle shortens to protect itself. When stretching, remember to relax and be patient. Use gentle, smooth, and pain-free movements to maximize benefits! See figure 6.3 for an illustration of the stretch reflex process.

Neuromuscular Fitness

Defining **neuromuscular fitness** is more challenging than defining the other fitness components of cardiorespiratory fitness, muscular fitness, and flexibility. The American College of Sports Medicine (2022) labels this component neuromotor fitness and addresses it from a balance and fall-prevention perspective, mainly targeting the unique exercise needs of older adults. However, individuals of all ages can benefit from neuromuscular training, which incorporates motor skills such as dynamic balance, coordination, gait and agility, and proprioceptive training.

Neuromuscular training is not new and has been applied to sport performance for many decades. What is relatively contemporary is the application of neuromuscular training to enhance the performance of activities of daily living for younger individuals. At its core (pun intended!) neuromuscular training overloads muscles in complicated and dynamic ways to stress multiple systems at once. Typically, these exercises integrate muscular fitness principles of overload with dynamic balance challenges (i.e., in a destabilized position). Importantly, if programmed correctly, the adaptations in the systems in response to this type of exercise training are highly translatable to movements in our daily lives. Recall the concept of **functional fitness** discussed in chapter 2. The following discussion of neuromuscular training highlights the ways in which it is integrated with functional fitness for daily living. Importantly,

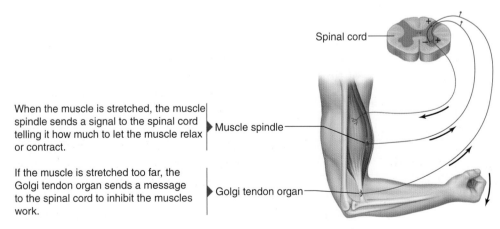

When the muscle is stretched, the muscle spindle sends a signal to the spinal cord telling it how much to let the muscle relax or contract. ▶ Muscle spindle

If the muscle is stretched too far, the Golgi tendon organ sends a message to the spinal cord to inhibit the muscles work. ▶ Golgi tendon organ

Spinal cord

Figure 6.3 The myotatic stretch reflex. Special receptors (Golgi tendon organs and muscle spindles) are active during a strong contraction or stretch. They inhibit or facilitate muscle contraction to protect the muscle. These receptors are connected to the spinal cord, not the brain.

you will quickly appreciate that functional fitness training, to prepare you for moving well for your life choices, is important for individuals of all ages and stages, and not just athletes and older adults. For example, in your daily campus life you use your functional fitness for your lifestyle movements such as when you're carrying your laundry up or down a flight of stairs or when you jump over a puddle and land on one foot while carrying a backpack filled with books.

All exercises benefit daily physical function—some more than others, depending on your health status. However, not all exercises *directly* benefit functional fitness. For example, a bench press is not considered a functional fitness exercise unless you regularly push something heavy off your chest to earn a living or for your recreational fun. Alternatively, the best functional strength training exercise commonly seen in the weight room might be a simple squat. Squats are undoubtedly popular, especially among younger individuals, because they enhance the aesthetics of the gluteal muscle groups (i.e., they "tone the booty"). They also work primary core muscles: The squat action directly translates to sitting and getting up from a chair or bed or a toilet, walking up a hill, climbing steps, and other common activities of daily life.

Beyond individual exercise routines or functional fitness classes, popular exercise formats that are highly functional include yoga and tai chi. The popular program CrossFit also focuses almost exclusively on functional fitness exercises.

Benefits of Functional Fitness

The benefits of functional fitness are well established for older adults—namely, enhanced performance of daily tasks and reduced risk of falling. Many sports training regimens also involve various forms of balance and agility training to enhance performance. The science regarding the importance of functional fitness for activities of daily living in young adults is not well established. However, increasing your functional fitness will provide these primary benefits:

- *Functional strength.* You are only as strong as your core and your base stability. The more stable your foundation, the stronger you will be in your everyday physical movements. For example, shoveling snow is a complex activity that involves many muscle groups and a strong core to prevent

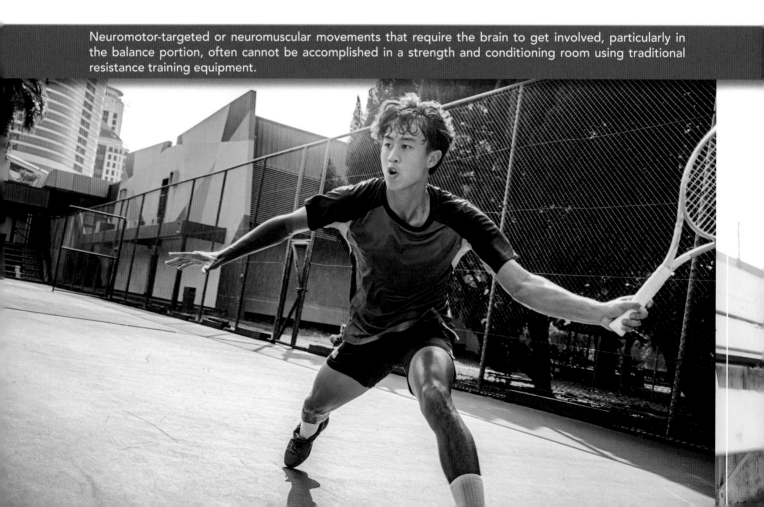

Neuromotor-targeted or neuromuscular movements that require the brain to get involved, particularly in the balance portion, often cannot be accomplished in a strength and conditioning room using traditional resistance training equipment.

back injury. If you are shoveling many heavy loads, you will also be taxing both muscular strength and endurance. Functional training greatly enhances your foundation and often spans many components of muscular fitness (strength, endurance, and power). Although isolation resistance training (exercise targeting a single muscle group) is often quite good for building muscle and definition, it is not as optimal for translation into daily life.

- *Balance and stability.* Although you are likely not worried about falling given your age, you should be aware that falling is more common than you realize. Even if you don't fall all the way to the floor, you may injure a joint or muscle when you catch yourself. The ability to safely regain your balance can be enhanced with training.

- *Reduced risk of injury.* Most physical therapists would attest that back injuries most commonly occur not in the weight room while performing a deadlift or squat but rather during a similar action in daily life executed in a destabilized and often awkward position (e.g., picking up small children, carrying a large load of laundry up the stairs). Lifting and twisting movements are especially problematic. These daily challenges can injure smaller muscles in the back, neck, or shoulder when you least expect it—perhaps as you lift the heavy loaded backpack and swing it onto your back. Functional fitness training will enhance your ability to perform movements in a destabilized position, practicing what you will encounter in real-world settings. Functional fitness training exercises challenge you to manage and balance your own weight plus additional weight, often in a destabilized position. Thus, there is direct application to everyday activities.

Functional Fitness Training

The best way to enhance neuromuscular and functional fitness is not well established from a scientific perspective, and HHS Physical Activity Guidelines and ACSM exercise guidelines do not currently exist for these modalities. However, any activities that translate to your activities of daily

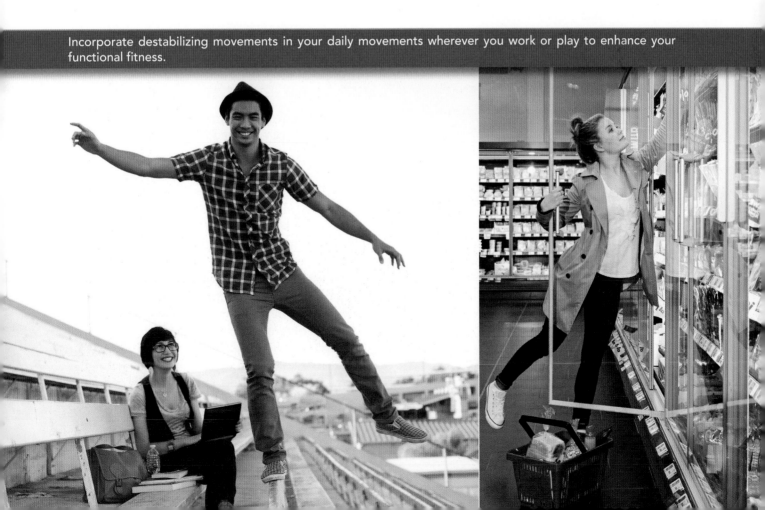

Incorporate destabilizing movements in your daily movements wherever you work or play to enhance your functional fitness.

living and challenge multiple systems (motor, cognitive, vestibular, etc.) will improve your functional fitness. The scientific literature exploring neuromotor, and closely aligned neuromuscular, exercises to improve balance and lower-extremity physical function in older adults typically focuses on the following factors:

1. Base of support (larger versus smaller)
2. Vision (eyes open versus closed)
3. Center of gravity (close to the body versus away from center)
4. Surface (smooth versus rough)

We have a lot to learn about how functional fitness training can improve daily physical and cognitive function for individuals of all ages, not just older adults. Expect more scientific information to emerge about this contemporary form of training. In the meantime, when designing functional fitness aspects of your exercise program, consider the following core elements:

- Choose movements that require core and foundation stability
- Incorporate multiple joints (often from the upper and lower body)
- Overload multiple muscle groups (upper and lower body; crossing multiple joints)
- Use multiplanar movement patterns (performed moving forward, sideways, and with rotation)
- Perform movements in a functional position (mimic activities of daily living)
- Challenge static and dynamic balance (base of support, vision, center of gravity, surface)

Core Stabilization and Progressive Destabilization

To improve functional fitness, you will need to challenge multiple systems in an integrated manner. By mastering complex movements involving the elements described previously and further challenging the systems with destabilization, especially movement with direction changes, you will make the most functional fitness gains. For example, reducing the base of support by standing on one foot will make an exercise harder. If you then shift the center of gravity by moving a handheld weight from your side to straight out in front of your body, it will destabilize the system further. The same exercise performed on a balance disk will be even harder, especially with your eyes closed. Mixing and matching these factors alone can progress the difficulty and neuromuscular overload of the functional exercise.

Progression to gain functional fitness can appear overwhelming to the novice. Whereas muscular fitness can be improved with increases in volume, functional fitness must progress through stages that are less intuitive, at least at first. The following progression system breaks down these stages to help you design your own program (Yoke and Kennedy 2004). Note that there are many effective progressions for functional training, and this is just one example—others may be more effective for your personal program.

In this program, there are typically three main phases: (1) individual muscle groups are isolated for resistance overload to gain a base level of strength; (2) core training is added with the isolation exercise; and (3) the core is overloaded and destabilized with more complex compound movements. Table 6.1 shows an example progression of the reverse fly exercise to work the upper back and shoulders (rhomboids and posterior deltoids). This is a great exercise to offset the effects of long hours spent sitting at a keyboard. A common visualization is to picture a pencil along your spine and try to squeeze it tightly (search your favorite browser for "reverse fly" for more in-depth tips).

Functional Fitness as a Part of Your Movement Plan

Functional fitness training is definitely a whole-body experience! Beyond the complex movements of multiple muscle groups, the higher-level motor control needed for this type of training also tasks cognition, especially as it relates to proprioception. There are many exercise devices on the market to set up a home-based program; however, you can design a high-quality program with minimal cost if you are creative. Just remember to progress slowly and be careful. Functional training, by definition, requires minimal isolated muscle actions—a good thing for functional fitness gains but also an increased risk for injury, especially at the higher levels of destabilization. However, many of our life actions will require these movements. By training in

Table 6.1 Example Progression for the Reverse Fly Through Three Stages: Isolation, Core, and Destabilization

Level	Primary progression task	Exercise and major progression factors
1A	**Isolate** and educate	Prone short-lever reverse fly • Facedown on the floor (no stabilizers needed) • No equipment (body weight only)
1B	**Isolate** and add external resistance	Reverse fly in seated position • Seated position engages core minimally • Use band or tube for resistance (low row position) or resistance machine if available
2A	**Core** training positions	Standing retraction with band or tube • Standing position fully activates core • Use band or tube for resistance with upper arms parallel to the ground (high row position)
2B	**Core** training positions adding increased resistance	Prone reverse fly on stability ball with weights • Facedown on stability ball in plank position • Use free weights and lift arms perpendicular to torso
3A	**Destabilize** using multiple muscle groups, increased resistance, and core challenge	Four-count bilateral bent-over row with external rotation • Feet parallel and shoulder-width apart, abdominals contracted, hinge at the hips • Use free weights to row by (1) bringing elbows up, (2) externally rotating shoulders (palms facing floor), (3) bringing shoulders back to row position, and (4) returning to start
3B	**Destabilize** further by adding balance, speed, and rotational movements	Bent-over unilateral high row on one foot • Repeat level 5 exercise standing on one foot • Alternate one arm at a time; maintain core stability

a controlled manner, unexpected daily challenges should be less likely to cause injuries.

Preventing Low Back Pain

A conversation about flexibility and functional fitness would not be complete without a discussion about **low back pain (LBP)**. Most back pain is acute, lasts a few days to a few weeks, resolves with minimal treatment, and does not involve ongoing loss of function. Chronic back pain is defined as pain that continues beyond 12 weeks even after the underlying cause of acute pain has been resolved. Often chronic LBP is said to be idiopathic, meaning that there is no known cause or event that triggered it. Unfortunately, LBP is a very common health challenge, causing more global disability than any other condition: According to

the National Institute of Neurological Disorders and Stroke (2020), an estimated 80 percent of people will suffer from LBP in their lifetime (see figure 6.4). Unfortunately, older adults are not the only ones impacted, with approximately 25 percent of adults aged 18 to 44 in the United States reporting LBP in the past three months, with females being more afflicted than males (Centers for Disease Control and Prevention 2020a). Like most chronic conditions, preventing LBP with good health and functional habits is important. It is especially important to recognize that once LBP becomes chronic, it is challenging to stop the discomfort and loss of function.

Causes of Low Back Pain

The lower back includes five vertebrae and a complicated composition of muscle, intervertebral discs, and nerves. Because it supports nearly all the weight of the upper body, it is vulnerable to injury—any disruption in the collaboration of these components typically results in pain. Most causes of acute LBP are mechanical in nature. Among young adults, common low back injuries include sprains (ligament related), strains (tendon related) or spasms (muscle related). Certainly, traumatic injuries from sports, car accidents, or falls can also result in low back pain. However, there are many causes of LBP, including congenital (e.g., spina bifida), degenerative (e.g., arthritis), nerve or spinal cord related (e.g., ruptured discs or sciatica), or nonspinal (e.g., pregnancy). Finally, chronic LBP can also result from poor posture and chronic muscle imbalances caused by too much sitting. Importantly, LBP is *variable*. It can range from mild to extreme. It can arrive relatively quickly or be a constant companion. When it arrives and does not go away, it can drastically reduce your quality of life (National Institutes of Neurological Disorders and Stroke 2020).

Although anyone can have LBP, especially as a result of injury, there are many factors that increase your chances of chronic LBP (National Institute of Neurological Disorders and Stroke 2020). Explore this list and consider whether you are at increased risk. Note that the first two factors are out of your control, but the rest can be influenced by your behavioral choices.

- *Age.* The first notable experience of LBP often occurs between the ages of 30 and 50 and becomes more common with increased age. Advanced age typically brings spine issues such as osteoporosis or stenosis (narrowing of the spaces in the spine, putting pressure on spinal nerves). Muscles also begin to get less elastic (especially when not used!), and intervertebral discs lose fluid and flexibility, reducing the ability to cushion impacts.

- *Genetics.* Your family tree can influence your chances of LBP. For example, some forms of arthritis have a genetic component. In comparison to other factors, however, genetic influences will be of relatively small importance.

- *Weight status.* Being overweight or obese or quickly gaining significant amounts of weight can put stress on the back and increase risk for LBP.

- *Physical fitness.* Lower levels of fitness are linked to LBP, likely as a result of low mus-

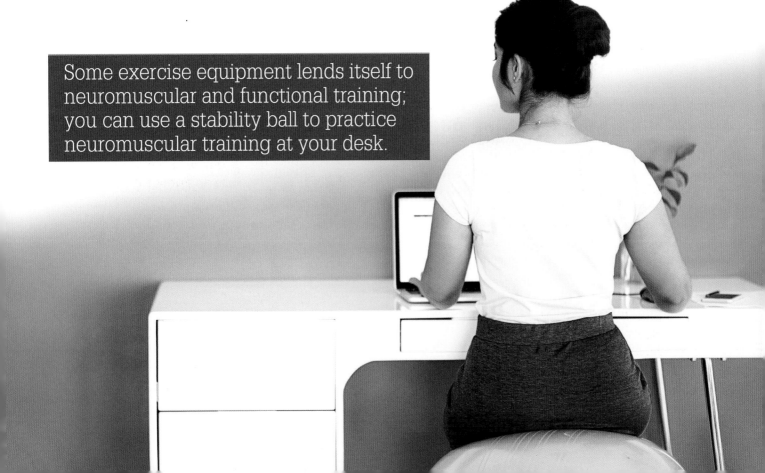

Some exercise equipment lends itself to neuromuscular and functional training; you can use a stability ball to practice neuromuscular training at your desk.

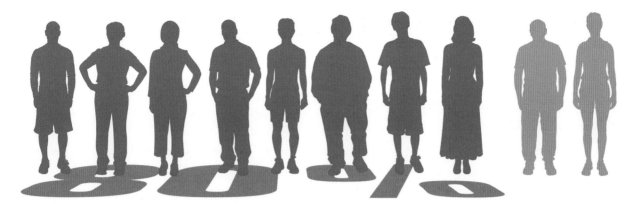

Figure 6.4 Eighty percent of adults will experience back pain at some point in their lifetimes.

cular fitness of the back and abdominal muscles that support the spine. Individuals who are sporadically active are also more likely to get LBP. For example, the person who has a desk job all week and then exercises intensely on the weekend (aka "weekend warrior") often injures the back. Some types of exercise, running being a good example, can also cause LBP due to the repeated impact on the spine or by creating muscle imbalances. In running, muscle imbalances are common due to the repeated motion that causes tight hip flexors that misalign the low back in a hyperextended position. Hip-opening flexibility exercises are important to prevent LBP in most runners.

- *Job-related factors.* Jobs that require regular heavy lifting and carrying often lead to back injuries, especially if the movements twist the spine (e.g., moving furniture). Working in a sitting position all day, particularly with poor posture or in a chair with poor support, can also contribute to LBP. Importantly, too much sitting combined with poor abdominal muscle endurance can cause misalignment of the spine.

- *Psychosocial and mental health.* Stress and anxiety can increase muscle tension, which can lead to LBP. Conversely, having LBP can also cause anxiety, stress, and depression. Reduced psychological well-being, especially depression, can also increase the perception of pain.

- *Backpack behaviors.* Carrying a heavy backpack can cause fatigue and LBP. Incorrect posture while carrying a backpack, especially carrying the bag over one shoulder, can lead to strains, injury, and chronic LBP.

- *Smoking.* Smoking has been linked to LBP because it affects oxygenation of tissues, including spinal discs, which may cause greater degeneration or hinder healing from an acute LBP situation. Yet another reason to quit smoking—or never start!

If you suffer from chronic LBP, visit your personal physician to rule out any major health issues before making lifestyle changes. If you are fortunate enough not to suffer from LBP, reduce your future chances of LBP by reducing these risk factors.

Stand Up Straight

How many times did a parent or grandparent tell you to stand up straight? Having good sitting and standing **posture** is critical to prevent back, shoulder, and neck pain. Good posture is also an important social signal that indicates engagement, energy, self-confidence, and self-respect. One key reason that it is so challenging to keep good posture is that it is not healthy to sit for as many hours as we currently do. Many of us have muscle imbalances caused by regular movement patterns that reinforce bad posture. How can you work on your posture to prevent back pain issues? A well-designed muscular, flexibility, and

> Good posture = more job opportunities? Many employers use posture as an easy way to evaluate confidence and maturity in an applicant. Stand up straight and make a good first impression!

Can Back Pain Be Prevented?

Most of the time, with good behavioral choices, back pain can be prevented, especially in young adults. Your daily choices matter! Check the following 10 behavioral recommendations and see how many you adhere to daily. Do you do the following to reduce your risk for LBP?

- Regularly exercise to obtain neuromuscular fitness and flexibility, especially of core muscles.
- Eat a healthy diet, especially for bone health (see chapter 8).
- Maintain a healthy weight (see chapter 9).
- Manage your stress in healthy ways and prevent or treat depression (see chapter 10).
- Design your workspace to be ergonomically smart including using a quality chair with a lumbar support, setting your computer monitor at the appropriate height, and having good posture.
- Break up sitting time often and change position if possible.
- Wear comfortable, low-heeled shoes with good support.
- Select sleeping positions on firm sleeping surfaces that can open the spine (e.g., fetal position) and rotate your movements to open your hips
- Make smart choices when lifting including lifting with your legs and not your back, being mindful of contracting your abdominals to support your spine, and not lifting objects that are too heavy.
- Don't start smoking, and if you currently smoke, plan to quit today.

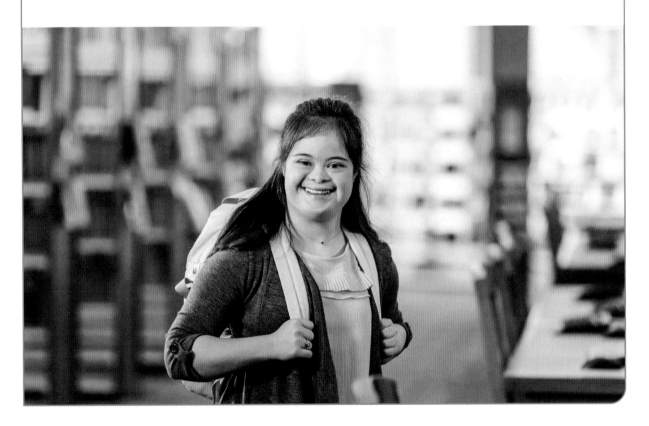

functional fitness program can greatly enhance posture by improving muscular endurance of postural muscles and correcting body mechanics and muscle imbalances caused by too much sitting. Search your favorite Internet browser for "posture correction exercises" to find lots of ideas, many of which require minimal equipment. Other examples are included in the Functional Fitness Training insert.

Good Muscle Balance + Daily Functional Movement = Low Back Pain Prevention

It's important to connect the exercises you do to increase functional fitness with your daily physical tasks so you can appreciate how your efforts help you function in your life. For example, if you wear your backpack over both shoulders as you walk to class, you are essentially strengthening your core

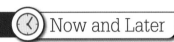

Now and Later

Invest in Your Functional Health

Now

Many young adults take their physical capabilities for granted. Physical function—being able to do whatever you want to—is very important to most people's quality of life. And you typically don't realize how important it is until you lose your function or your activities cause pain. Beyond the good health habits described in this chapter to have good functional fitness and prevent LBP in your college years, there are other considerations to maintain your physical function.

First, prevent injuries by being smart and not taking chances. For example, wear a helmet when cycling (motorized or not): The effects of concussion are underappreciated by most people, and traumatic brain injuries—even mild ones—can have major long-term effects on your cognitive function and brain health.

Second, make functional fitness and injury prevention a priority and establish your health behavior habits during your college years so you are well positioned to maintain them as you start the next stage of your life.

Later

Reductions in functional fitness are very common as people progress through middle age and their older years. Current statistics indicate that one in four adults in the United States have some type of disability, with mobility (e.g., serious difficulty walking or climbing stairs) being the most common type at approximately 14 percent and cognitive (e.g., serious difficulty concentrating, remembering, or making decisions) the second most common at approximately 11 percent (Centers for Disease Control and Prevention 2020b). Adults living with disabilities are more likely to be obese, smoke, or have heart disease or diabetes compared to those who do not have a disability. Maintaining a healthy weight and engaging in adequate daily physical activity and minimal sitting time can do much to ensure optimal physical function later in life.

Take Home

Good health habits, especially eating well and maintaining muscular and functional fitness, will go a long way toward preventing chronic disease and keeping you free from disability. Invest in your functional self now and as you go through life. The return on your behavioral investment will be a major factor in your quality of life!

muscles. As your muscles become fit, you will have less fatigue from a given physical challenge, even if the challenge is transporting your heavy backpack all around campus or on your favorite hiking trail. The ability to complete essential daily tasks will take on new meaning as you age. Muscular and functional fitness, or lack thereof, is a key risk factor for physical disability and falling.

Summary

Flexibility is a key component of health-related fitness. Neuromotor exercises integrate skill-related physical fitness components, including agility, coordination, balance, and reaction time and when done regularly improve your neuromuscular fitness. Collectively, flexibility and neuromuscular fitness determine your functional fitness. Functional fitness is very important for many sport and recreational activities, but it will also enhance your daily life, especially while toting a large backpack and sitting up tall and confident. Like designing a personal program to improve and maintain cardiorespiratory fitness and muscular fitness, you will want to design a regular neuromuscular and flexibility training program that you can adapt throughout your life. Doing so will help you feel better, look better, reduce your risk for injury and pain (especially LBP!), and increase your chance of living a long, independent life.

ONLINE LEARNING ACTIVITIES

Go to HKPropel and complete all of the online activities to further facilitate your learning:

Study Activities: Review the main concepts of the chapter.

Labs: Complete the labs your instructor assigns.

Videos: Look through the videos and choose which ones you want to try this week.

REVIEW QUESTIONS

1. What are some primary factors that determine a person's flexibility?
2. Outline the FITT guidelines to improve and maintain flexibility.
3. List four benefits of being flexible.
4. Explain why the stretch reflex is an important concept to understand to enhance your flexibility training.
5. Define functional fitness training and how it connects to your chosen lifestyle and movement activities. List three elements of functional fitness training and give two examples of exercises or movements you might incorporate into your functional fitness training plan.
6. Define chronic low back pain and describe three modifiable risk factors for it.
7. Explain how neuromuscular fitness and flexibility, and relatedly your functional fitness, can prevent low back pain, especially with respect to sitting behaviors.

Functional Fitness Training

This special section on functional fitness training contains over 60 exercises with photos. A narrated video of most of the exercises is available on HK*Propel*. Use the exercises in this section to help you design a program that fits your goals and interests. Keep in mind that these are just suggestions for exercises to help your functional fitness. As you gain more knowledge and confidence, you will be able to search online to find many different yet effective exercise choices. Thus, if you are a relatively novice exerciser (especially with muscular fitness training exercises), you might start with these options, but you will soon start to think of your exercise routine as a mix-and-match endeavor. And as your day-to-day life changes in terms of available time, motivation and energy, and perhaps equipment and space, you will need to adapt your routine to your changing needs.

The exercises included here provide overload for muscular fitness and flexibility training for 12 primary muscle groups. For each muscle group, you'll find (1) an anatomical illustration showing the location of the muscle group within the body and (2) activities in your daily life that involve the muscle group. Next are instructions for the safe execution of exercises, which include options that use body weight, free weights or bands, or variable resistance machines. Following each body weight, free weight, or band example exercise is a description of a modification to the exercise to further challenge neuromotor systems and balance. Finally, a correct stretch position and related cues for each muscle group are described.

Reminder: Functional Fitness Training Is About Your Why

This section suggests exercise choices for muscular fitness and flexibility exercises for the primary muscle groups to help you look good, feel great, and function well. As discussed in earlier chapters, the selected exercises connect to activities you do every day on campus or during your transportation, occupational, and leisure activities. As described in chapter 6, functional fitness training

often starts with muscle isolation movements that strengthen specific muscle groups. Variable resistance machines, which offer excellent isolation, are often used by many beginning exercisers because they allow the weight being lifted to be controlled, enhancing safety. Also, the movements involved when using the machines are relatively easy to understand for someone who is learning the basics. However, these isolation muscular fitness exercises do not translate very well into movements of daily life and do not challenge balance, and the routine often becomes a bit boring. And because you will likely need a fitness facility membership to use the machines, this limited availability can compromise your adherence to your program. On a positive note, after establishing a conditioning base using variable resistance machines, many beginning exercisers progress to free weight and body weight exercises that train multiple muscle groups. Additionally, many exercisers combine isolation and functional movements for their routines. Finally, different stages of life will present different goals and safety challenges. For example, older adults must be more aware of the risk of falling, and machines can provide overload to the muscles in a safe controlled manner. Thus, there are many good choices for your preferred routine. But we highly recommend a total-body functional regimen, complete with neuromotor challenges to enhance your balance and core stability abilities, and thus enhance your functional fitness so you can function at your best.

This book emphasizes the importance of connecting your fitness training choices with your why: Why do you want to train this way? What is the end game? One reason could be career related; energetic people with good posture fare better when interviewing for jobs. Another reason might be financial; fitness, health, and well-being affect your health care costs. What is your why?

Because your why will change throughout your life, this section presents different options for functional fitness training using various types of simple equipment as well as body weight. If you want to focus on posture and lean abdominal muscles, planks and body weight curl-ups might work best. Alternatively, walking lunges with handheld weights allow you to save time by working on balance and stability along with core training as you address your lower-body muscle groups. If you want to get big biceps, you might use a variable resistance biceps machine for isolation training. This insert will focus on convenient and easily accessible movements that matter for improving overall health and well-being, with a focus on your functional fitness.

There are so many ways to improve the look, feel, and function of your body. Design a program that works best for you and your goals. Find what you like and what matters to you. The best fitness training choices for muscular fitness and flexibility training are the ones you will perform regularly and that are convenient and easy to access.

Safety Reminders

Although much of the following content was addressed in previous chapters, it bears repeating in the context of functional fitness training. Remember that the best fitness program is one that you will do on a regular basis and one that you can do safely.

- Cold muscles are at risk of injury. Always remember to warm up thoroughly before performing muscular fitness and flexibility training exercises. Break a light sweat before you start. You might walk, jog, do some easy bicycling, perform your first set of strengthening exercises with a light weight, or mix aerobic and muscular fitness movements.

- Goals determine exercise sets, repetitions, and volume. Chapter 5 provided detailed guidance about muscular fitness training recommendations from experts. The loads for strength training are determined by your goals and experience with training and overloading. Don't be afraid to experiment to find what works for you and fits your goals. Recall that muscles adapt best through progressive, incremental overload. Although there are a few choices that are not advisable according to scientific evidence, there are many right choices.

Your why matters.

- Progress to neuromotor balance challenges with caution. As discussed extensively in chapter 6, neuromotor challenges often referred to as neuromuscular training, generally integrate balance and stability training into strength and conditioning movements. The unbalanced state that is integral to neuromotor training increases the risk of injuries and falls. You will quickly recognize that you will not be able to lift as much in these unbalanced and unstable conditions. Reduce the weight, perform the exercise, and progress slowly to prevent injury. If you cannot control the weight, don't lift it. Don't overlook flexibility training. Chapter 6 provided extensive information to help you design an effective and safe flexibility training routine. From static stretching routines to more complicated ballistic approaches, the best program is one that aligns with your goals. The body, regardless of age, feels great after a stretching routine. Ironically, the part of the exercise routine that requires the least amount of equipment, space, and effort is often the most neglected part of a person's program. Invest in your future mobility by stretching daily.

Putting It All Together

On the pages that follow, you will find movements and exercises that can help you train the primary muscle groups of the body. Use what you have learned up to this point to design a routine that matches your fitness and well-being goals and that fits into your life.

Establishing a Baseline

If you feel like you need a little more help in putting everything together, you may want to start by establishing a baseline for yourself. Through HK*Propel*, we have included a video that discusses fitness tests that will assess each of the main components of functional fitness training: aerobic, muscular, flexibility, and neuromotor balance. By taking these tests, you can see where you initially are in your fitness journey. You can then use those test results to set SMART (specific, measurable, attainable, realistic, and time bound) goals to help you reach your desired outcomes.

Learning by Example

If you need a little more inspiration, we have put together instructions and some sample workouts for you that use destabilizing techniques and address total body movements and resistance bands. The workouts in these short videos don't require a lot of equipment, so they can be used at home or when traveling to help you with your fitness goals. These videos can be found on HK*Propel*.

Now that you have a better understanding of how to structure your workouts, let's dive into the selected muscle groups.

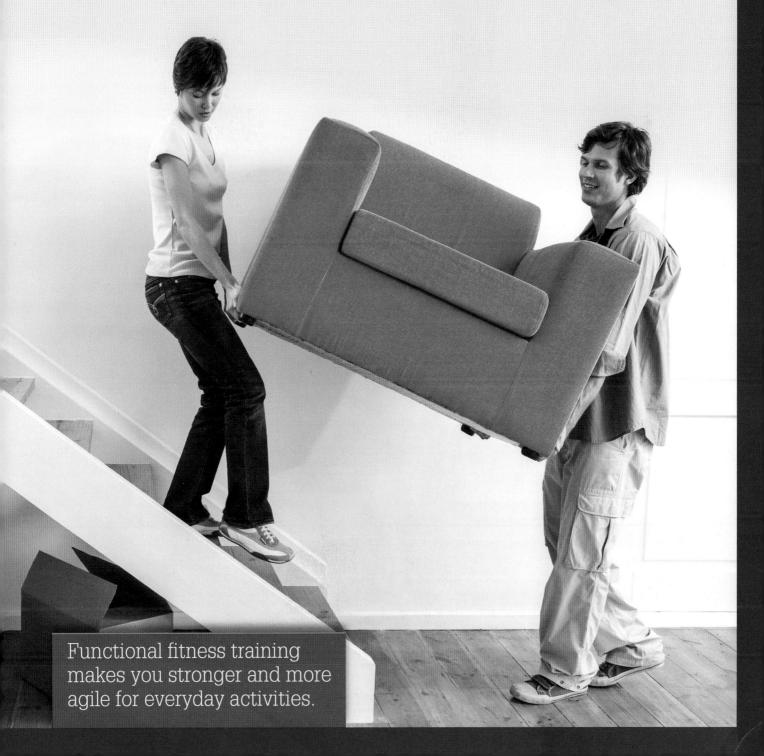

Functional fitness training makes you stronger and more agile for everyday activities.

Lower Leg (Calves)

Gastrocnemius and Soleus

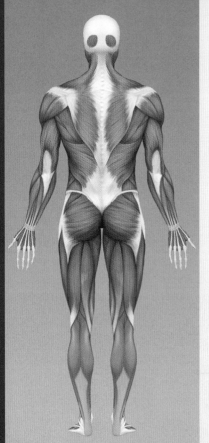

Daily activity use includes reaching up on toes, walking, running, and jumping.

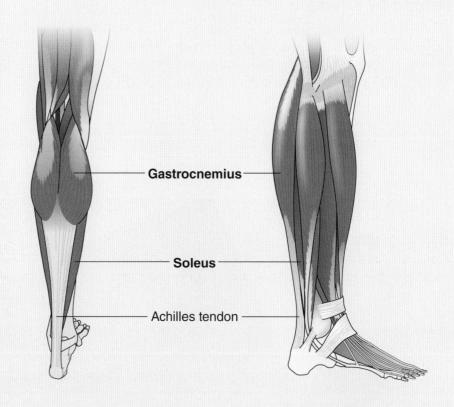

Gastrocnemius

Soleus

Achilles tendon

Muscle Group:
 Gastrocnemius and soleus

Muscle Action:
 Ankle plantar flexion
 30 to 50 degrees

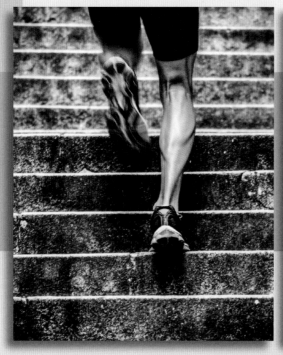

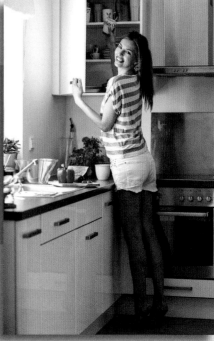

Lower Leg (Calves)

Gastrocnemius and Soleus

▶ Body Weight

Stand and lift both your heels 30 to 50 degrees off the ground. You can also use a wall or bar for support and lift one heel at a time.

Neuromotor balance training: Without using wall support, raise one heel at a time.

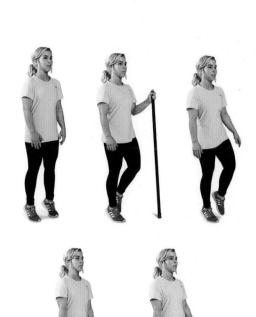

▶ Free Weights

Hold a weight in each hand and raise your heels 30 to 50 degrees.

Neuromotor balance training: Hold a weight in each hand, stand on one leg, and raise the heel of the support leg.

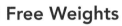

▶ Variable Resistance Machine

Use a heel raise machine or a leg press machine. A leg press machine is typically used to strengthen the quadriceps, the gluteus maximus, and the hamstrings. To engage your calves, lower your feet so that the balls of your feet are on the bottom edge of the platform. Then, raise your heels during the first phase of the exercise so that you are pressing with your toes.

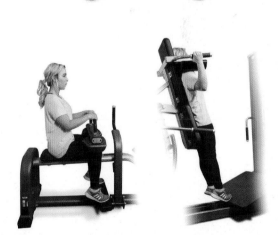

▶ Flexibility: Static Stretch

Step one foot forward and bend the front knee. Press your back heel toward the ground. This stretches the gastrocnemius of the back leg. Then bend your back knee to stretch the soleus, keeping the front knee bent and the back heel down. For both positions, the back toe is forward, heel is on the floor, and weight is shifted forward.

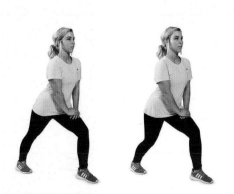

Front of Upper Leg (Quads)

Quadriceps

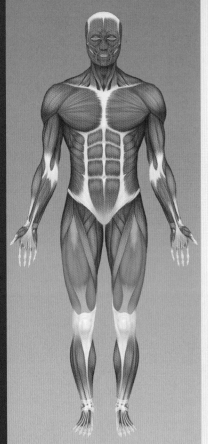

Daily activity use includes getting out of chairs, jumping, walking, and running.

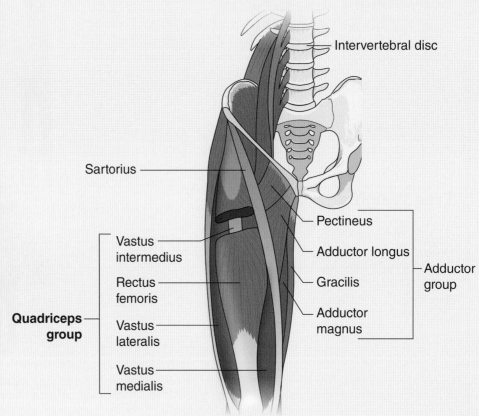

- Intervertebral disc
- Sartorius
- Pectineus
- Adductor longus
- Gracilis
- Adductor magnus

Adductor group

Quadriceps group
- Vastus intermedius
- Rectus femoris
- Vastus lateralis
- Vastus medialis

Muscle Group:
 Quadriceps (rectus femoris, vastus intermedius, vastus lateralis, vastus medialis)

Muscle Action:
 Hip flexion 90 to 135 degrees and knee extension 5 to 10 degrees

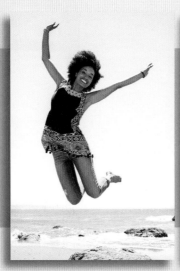

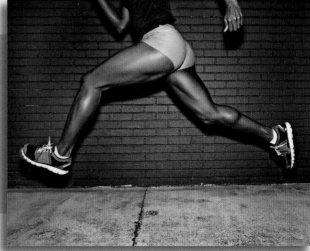

Front of Upper Leg (Quads)

▶ Body Weight

Lower the hips as if to sit and lift the chest; extend your arms in front for balance; flex at the hips 45 degrees; keep your heels on the ground. Return to a standing position.

Neuromotor balance training: Raise one knee up, keeping the shoulders over the hips and balancing on one leg. Simultaneously, raise the arm on the same side of the standing leg straight up by your ear and maintain good posture. To increase the challenge, lower hips and perform a squat but keep your weight on one leg.

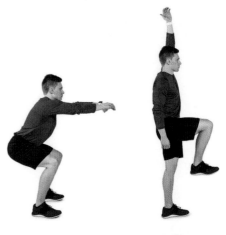

▶ Free Weights

Squat with free weights in hands. Keep your head up and make sure your knees do not go over your toes.

Neuromotor balance training: Do alternating lunges, holding a free weight in each hand.

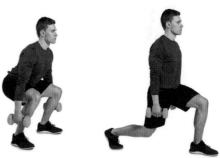

▶ Variable Resistance Machine

To strengthen your quadriceps, you can use a leg press or leg extension machine. Regardless of which machine you choose, be sure that you do not go below a 90-degree angle with your legs to protect your knees and to complete the exercise safely.

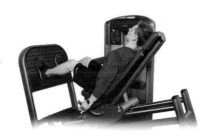
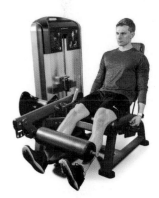

▶ Flexibility: Static Stretch

Lie on your side. Keeping the hips aligned, flex one knee and hold the top of one shoe or your toe; relax your head on your arm and relax the foot you are holding.

Neuromotor balance training: Perform the stretch while standing without holding on to a wall or other stabilizing object.

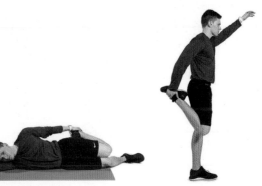

133

Back of Upper Leg and Rear Hip

Hamstrings and Gluteus Maximus

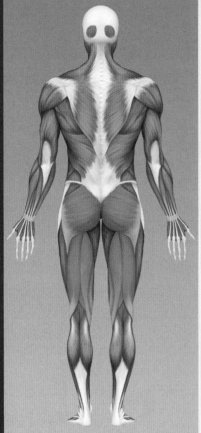

Daily activity use includes walking or running backward up a hill, stepping backward, and lowering items from a shelf.

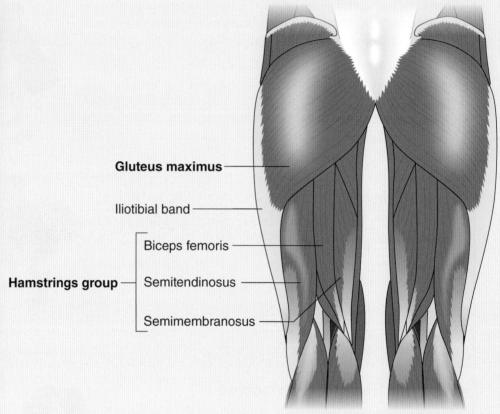

Gluteus maximus

Iliotibial band

Biceps femoris

Hamstrings group — Semitendinosus

Semimembranosus

Muscle Group:
Hamstrings (biceps femoris, semitendinosus, semimembranosus) and gluteus maximus

Muscle Action:
Hip extension 10 to 30 degrees and knee flexion 130 to 140 degrees

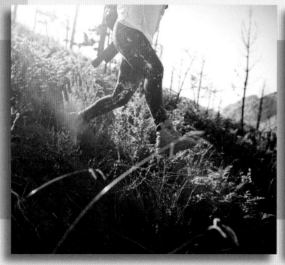

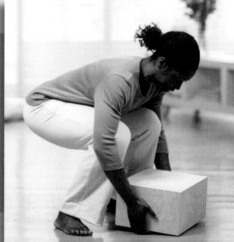

▶ Body Weight

Lie on your front side and extend the hip 10 to 30 degrees, keeping the hip bone on the ground, and then flex the knee 90 degrees to maximize strengthening.

Neuromotor balance training: Position yourself on your hands and knees and complete the same exercise but extend one arm forward.

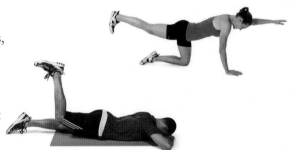

▶ Free Weights

Perform a squat, lifting a weight bar while simultaneously extending at the hips and knees. Maintain a neutral spine throughout the entire movement and lift the bar by contracting the hamstrings and glutes.

Neuromotor balance training: Hold a weight in one hand and extend the opposite leg behind you; slightly bend the standing knee and raise the weight straight forward. Progress to using the arm on the same side as the extending leg (e.g., left leg and arm).

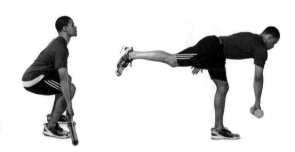

▶ Variable Resistance Machine

Options are standing hamstring curl and prone hamstring curl machines. Read placards carefully since there are many adjustments to make on both of these machines.

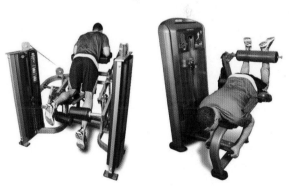

▶ Flexibility: Static Stretch

For the standing hamstring stretch, bend one knee and extend the other leg in front of you. Put all your weight on the bent knee, relaxing the straight leg. Tilt your hips backward to lengthen the hamstring muscle and keep the spine in alignment.

For the hamstring and gluteus maximus stretch, lie on your back and grasp the thigh of the raised leg with both hands. Keeping the knee of the opposite leg flexed, relax both the leg in your hands and your neck muscles to keep your head on the ground.

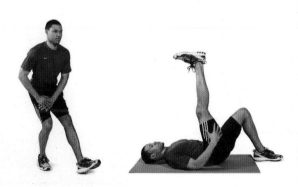

Trunk and Abdomen (Abs)

Rectus and Transversus Abdominis and Obliques

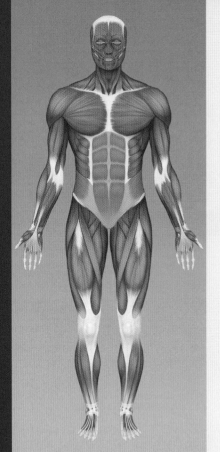

Daily activity use includes maintaining posture, getting up out of bed, carrying items, and rotating the torso with weight in your hands (e.g., golfing).

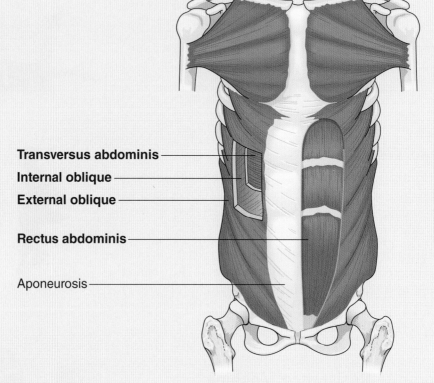

Transversus abdominis

Internal oblique

External oblique

Rectus abdominis

Aponeurosis

Muscle Group:
Rectus abdominis, transversus abdominis, internal oblique, and external oblique

Muscle Action:
Spine flexion 30 to 45 degrees, torso rotation 20 to 45 degrees, and abdominal compression

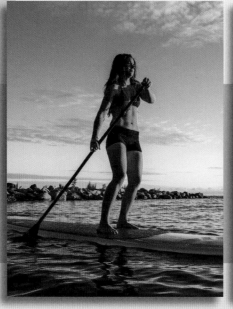

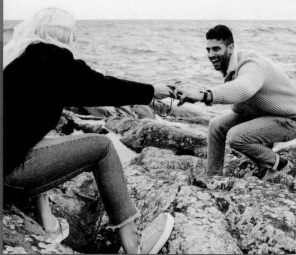

▶ Body Weight

Lie on your back with both hands behind the head and elbows out to the side (you should not be able to see your elbows), relax your head in your hands, and flex your spine 30 to 45 degrees.

Lie on your back; rotate your shoulder and point it toward the opposite knee, keeping the other shoulder on the floor. Continue by alternating the rotation to every other knee.

▶ Free Weights

Lie on your back on a stability ball with feet flat on the ground and knees bent at 90 degrees. Holding a weight (preferably a ball) on your chest or over your head, flex the spine 30 to 45 degrees. Holding the ball overhead is more difficult because it creates a longer lever.

Neuromotor balance training: Sit on the ground and recline 35 to 45 degrees (flexing the spine). Balancing with the heels on the ground, take a weight and rotate side to side 20 to 45 degrees. Keep the abdominals contracted as you rotate.

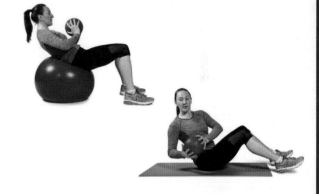

▶ Variable Resistance Machine

Use the abdominal flexion machine. Keep in mind that spine flexion is 30 to 45 degrees forward. Stay within appropriate range of motion.

Neuromotor balance training: Set the functional training machine for standing spinal rotation by placing elbows at your sides and biceps flexed; with knees slightly bent, rotate the spine side to side 20 to 45 degrees. Keep the abdominals contracted and knees slightly bent as you rotate.

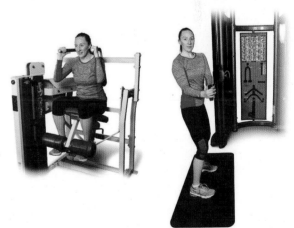

▶ Flexibility: Static Stretch

Lie on your back, point your toes, and slightly arch your back while extending your arms overhead to stretch your abdominals.

Lie on your front and prop yourself up on your elbows; hold this position, keeping the spine aligned and the hips on the ground if possible.

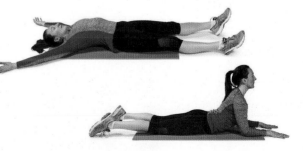

Lower Back

Erector Spinae

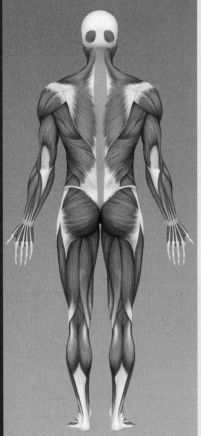

Muscle Group:
Erector spinae (iliocostalis lumborum, longissimus dorsi, and spinalis dorsi)

Muscle Action:
Spine extension 20 to 45 degrees

Daily activity use includes picking up a box from the floor and carrying a backpack over both shoulders.

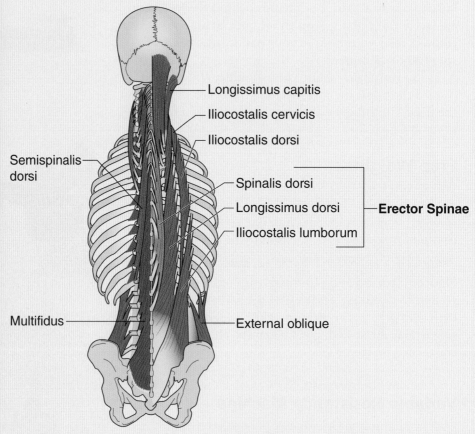

Longissimus capitis

Iliocostalis cervicis

Iliocostalis dorsi

Semispinalis dorsi

Spinalis dorsi

Longissimus dorsi — **Erector Spinae**

Iliocostalis lumborum

Multifidus

External oblique

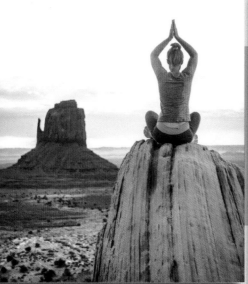

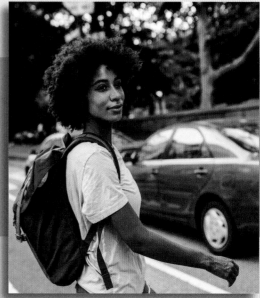

▶ Body Weight

Lie on your front on the floor. With your arm fully extended (like Superman), simultaneously lift the right arm and the left leg and keep the hip bone on the floor. Repeat with the left arm and the right leg.

Neuromotor balance training: Lie on your front on a stability ball with toes on the ground and extend the spine 20 to 45 degrees. For additional difficulty, raise the opposite hand and foot.

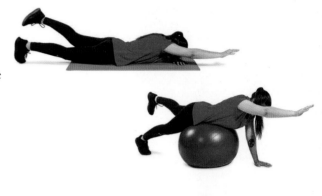

▶ Free Weights

Using a back-extension bench, flex the spine 20 to 45 degrees and then extend the lower back into an upright posture. Hold a weight to increase the challenge.

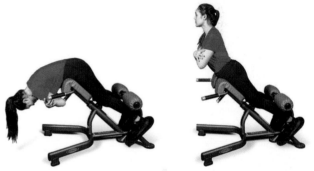

▶ Variable Resistance Machine

Use the lower back extension machine. Sit back into the seat before starting. Be careful to stay within the recommended range of motion for a back extension movement (20 to 45 degrees).

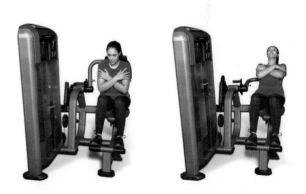

▶ Flexibility: Static Stretch

Lie on your back with knees bent and feet flat on the floor. Gently pull one knee toward your chest until you feel a stretch in your lower back. If you are comfortable, you can put your hands behind both knees, pull them to your chest, and hold.

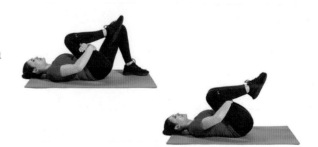

Outer Thigh and Upper Hip

Gluteus Medius and Gluteus Minimus

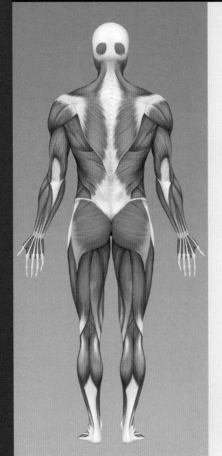

Daily activity use includes getting out of a car, keeping the hips in line when brisk walking, and stepping sideways.

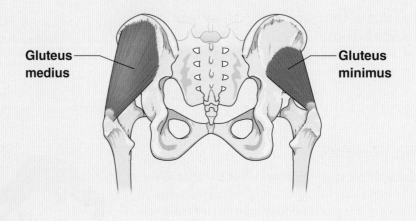

Gluteus medius

Gluteus minimus

Muscle Group:
 Gluteus medius and gluteus minimus

Muscle Action:
 Hip abduction 30 to 50 degrees (main action)

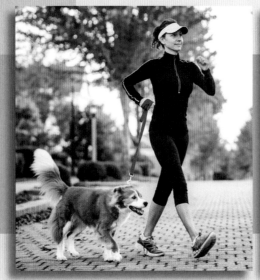

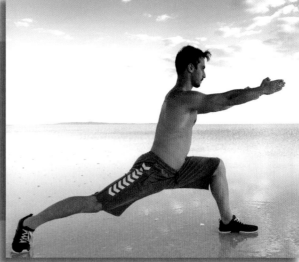

▶ Body Weight

Lie on your side with your head relaxed on your arm and your bottom leg bent, stacking the hips on top of each other to improve your base of support. Raise your leg 30 to 50 degrees and then lower it, leading with the heel.

Neuromotor balance training: Perform the same 30- to 50-degree hip abduction movement in a standing position.

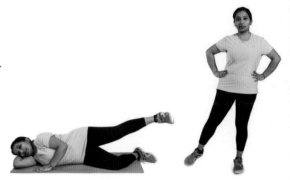

▶ Free Weights and Resistance Band

Lie on your side in the same position as for the body weight exercise and place a weight on your ankle or rest it on the outside or your thigh. Raise your leg 30 to 50 degrees and then lower it, leading with the heel. Another choice is to place a resistance band around both legs above the knee and sidestep in each direction 30 to 50 degrees.

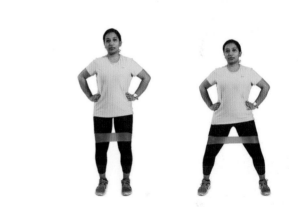

▶ Variable Resistance Machine

Sit in a variable resistance hip abduction machine. Perform a bilateral hip abduction movement to 30 to 50 degrees.

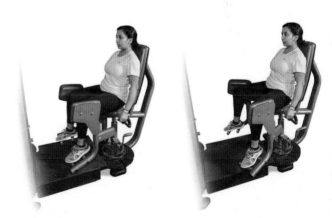

▶ Flexibility: Static Stretch

For this stretch, sit on a mat, and place your right foot to the outside of your left knee. Place your left hand outside of your right knee and turn your head to look back. At the same time, rotate your right thigh inward. To modify this exercise if you have less flexibility, hold your leg with your hand rather than placing your arm on the opposite side of your leg. Repeat on the other side.

For a variation, stand up tall and place one foot behind the front leg. Lean the outside hip slightly outward to feel a stretch in the hip abductor. Repeat the movement on the other side.

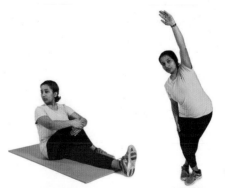

141

Inner Thigh (Hip Adductors)

Adductor Longus, Adductor Brevis, Adductor Magnus, and Gracilis

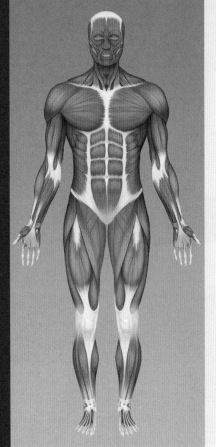

Daily activity use includes stabilizing the body laterally on a bike and picking up heavy objects from the ground.

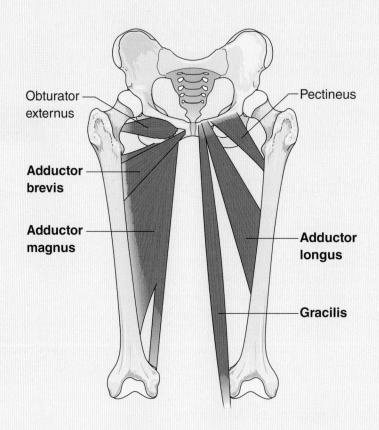

Obturator externus

Pectineus

Adductor brevis

Adductor magnus

Adductor longus

Gracilis

Muscle Group:
Adductor longus, adductor brevis, adductor magnus, and gracilis

Muscle Action:
Hip adduction 10 to 30 degrees

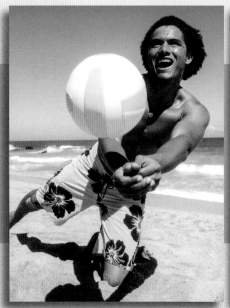

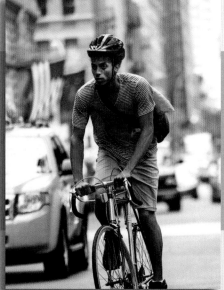

Inner Thigh (Hip Adductors)

▶ Body Weight

Lie on your side with your head relaxed on your arm. Line the hips up, bend the knee of the top leg, and place the foot on the ground to create a good base of support. Next, lift the bottom leg, adducting it 10 to 30 degrees.

Neuromotor balance training: Place a resistance band around one ankle and anchor the band to a heavy object. Stand with your shoulders over your hips and cross one leg in front of your body, adducting the hip 10 to 30 degrees. Alternate sides. Keep your spine in alignment and the range of motion to 30 degrees maximum. Lead with the heel and keep the toe forward.

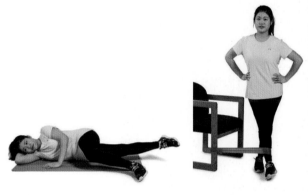

▶ Free Weights

Hold a weight (e.g., use a dumbbell and hold it like a goblet) and perform a squat with the toes turned out slightly to engage the adductors. Stabilize the weight in the center of the body.

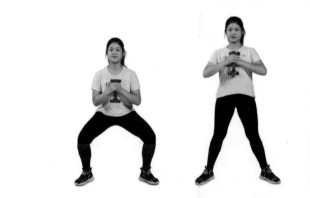

▶ Variable Resistance Machine

Use the hip adductor machine to perform hip adduction in a seated position.

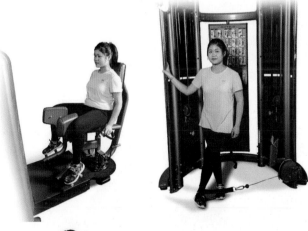

▶ Flexibility: Static Stretch

Put the soles of your feet together and let your knees relax to the sides, relax your elbows on your thighs, and keep your head up for proper posture. If your knees pop up, press them down slightly with your elbows.

For another option, move your legs to the straddle position and put your hands behind the buttocks; keep your head up. Lean your torso slightly forward and hold the position.

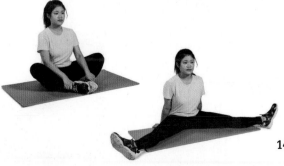

143

Chest and Front of Shoulder

Pectorals and Anterior Deltoids

Daily activity use includes putting something heavy on a high shelf, carrying and lifting items in front of you, and lifting yourself up off the floor.

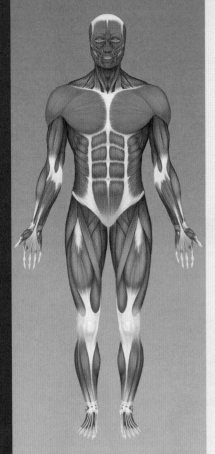

Muscle Group:
Pectoralis major and anterior deltoids

Muscle Action:
Anterior deltoid flexion and horizontal shoulder adduction 90 to 135 degrees

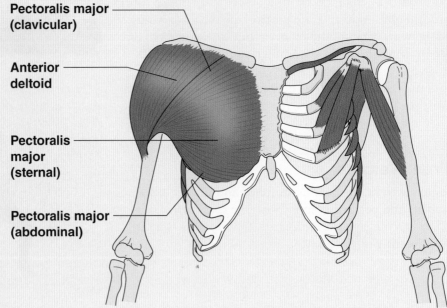

Pectoralis major (clavicular)

Anterior deltoid

Pectoralis major (sternal)

Pectoralis major (abdominal)

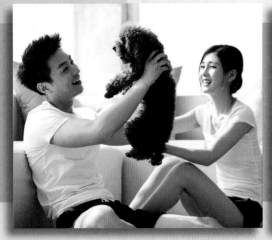

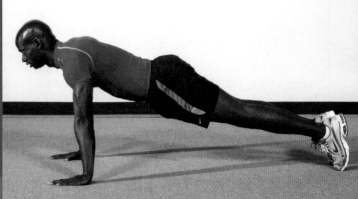

Chest and Front of Shoulder

▶ Body Weight

Stand in front of a wall and step back a few feet. Lift your elbows so they are level with your shoulders. Maintain that distance between the hands as you position them on the wall in front of you. Slowly bend your elbows and perform a push-up. Overload can be increased by doing the push-up from the knees or feet position.

Neuromotor balance training: Extend one leg behind you and balance while performing the same movement. Lifting one leg off the floor when performing a traditional push-up will increase the challenge further.

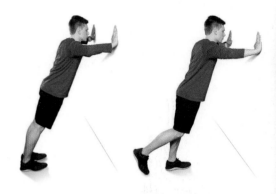

▶ Free Weights

Holding a weight in each hand, sit on a weight bench and keep the weights close to your body as you lie back on your lower back. Simultaneously press the weights straight up and return slowly. Make sure you do not let your elbows drop more than 10 to 15 degrees past a basic push-up position.

Neuromotor balance training: Hold a weight in each hand and lift both arms in front of you at the same time to 90 degrees, and then lower the weights. To increase the challenge to your balance, stand on one leg while you lift both arms. Progress in difficulty by performing the exercise one arm at a time and extend the opposite hip 10 to 30 degrees.

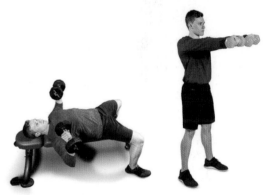

▶ Variable Resistance Machine

To perform a chest fly movement, adduct both arms simultaneously, keeping both feet on the ground, the chin and chest up, and the spine in alignment.

For the seated bench press machine, simultaneously press both arms forward, keeping the feet on the floor.

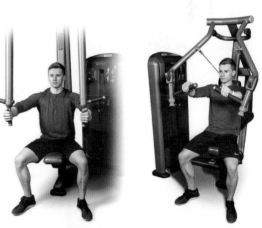

▶ Flexibility: Static Stretch

Stand and stretch both arms behind you. Clasp your fingers to stretch the pectoral and anterior deltoid muscles.

Standing in front of a doorway with knees relaxed, put one arm out to the side to hold onto the doorframe and lean slightly forward.

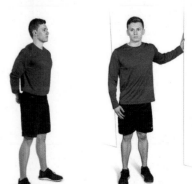

Upper Back and Shoulders

Rhomboids and Posterior Deltoids

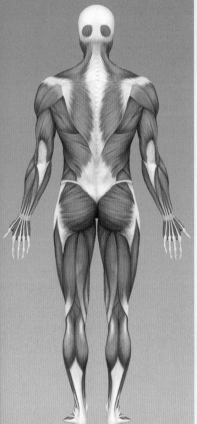

Daily activity use includes rowing activities such as sweeping or vacuuming the floor, sitting up tall at a desk, or tucking your shirt in your pants.

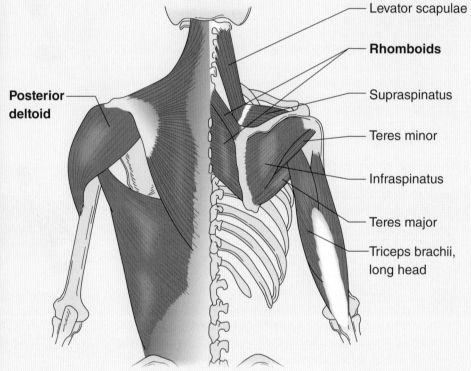

Levator scapulae

Rhomboids

Supraspinatus

Teres minor

Infraspinatus

Teres major

Triceps brachii, long head

Posterior deltoid

Muscle Group:
Rhomboids (rhomboid major, rhomboid minor) and posterior deltoids

Muscle Action:
Scapular retraction 15 to 20 degrees

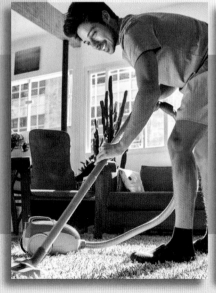

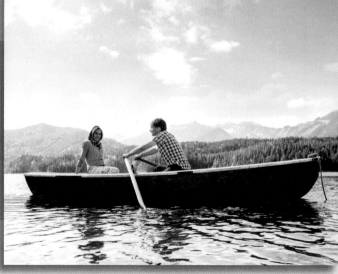

▶ Body Weight

Lie on your front on a mat or a pillow, relax your feet, and stretch both arms in a T position. Relax your lower body and lift your arms and torso off the ground, keeping your head facing down, hips on the ground, and feet relaxed.

Neuromotor balance training: Perform this same movement on a stability ball.

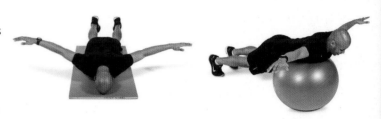

▶ Free Weights

Perform this exercise holding weights in each hand. Keeping the spine neutral, hinge at the hips to bend forward 45 degrees, bring arms out into a T position, and squeeze the shoulder blades together.

Neuromotor balance training: Perform the same movement, but slightly lift one leg off the floor and advance to extending one leg behind you.

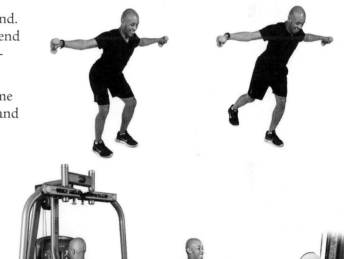

▶ Variable Resistance Machine

For the reverse fly variable resistance machine, adjust your trunk so you connect with the support pad and put your feet flat on the floor. Reach up and grab the handles, then retract your scapulae at the same time, squeezing the shoulder blades together.

For the seated cable high row, be sure not to lean back on the second part of the movement but rather start and end with good posture, letting the bar touch your chest as you squeeze the shoulder blades together.

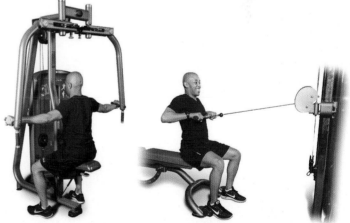

▶ Flexibility: Static Stretch

Stand and clasp both hands straight out in front of you. Round your middle back while slightly dropping your chin.

For the cat stretch on the floor, round your middle back. Inhale on the effort and exhale on the relaxation portion.

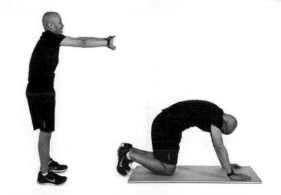

147

Middle Back (Lats)

Latissimus Dorsi

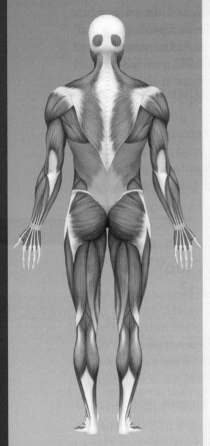

Daily activity use includes lifting up an object from the ground with one hand, performing a pull-up, and swimming.

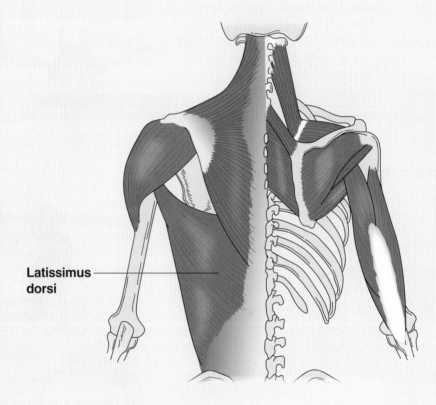

Latissimus dorsi

Muscle Group:
Latissimus dorsi

Muscle Action:
Shoulder adduction 80 to 100 degrees and shoulder extension 20 to 60 degrees

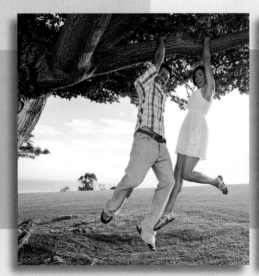

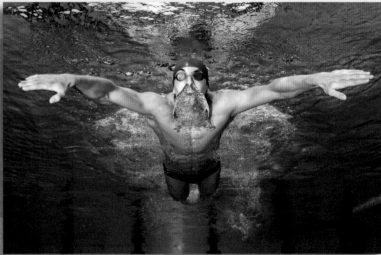

Middle Back (Lats)

▶ **VIDEO AVAILABLE**   **Latissimus Dorsi**

▶ Body Weight and Resistance Bands

Due to gravity, it can be challenging to overload the lats using body weight. If the equipment is available and you have the conditioning base, a chin-up is effective. For most people, bands can be used to provide an overload. Stand, holding a band overhead with approximately 6 to 8 inches of band between your hands. Anchor one arm overhead and adduct the other arm, bringing the elbow down to your side. Then alternate, bending one arm and then the other, bringing your elbow down to your side each time.

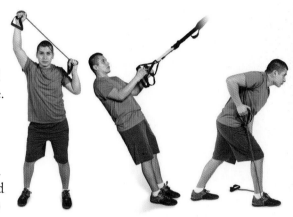

Neuromotor balance training: Perform this upper back exercise using TRX straps anchored to a rack or pull-up bar. Begin leaning back with your arms extended. Pull up toward the anchor using your upper back muscles. Slowly return to the starting position, keeping the back muscles activated. Another choice is to put a resistance band under one foot and hold the band with one arm. Pull the band up as if you are starting a lawnmower.

▶ Free Weights

Holding a weight in each hand, lie on your back on a stability ball. Extend arms overhead to 180 degrees (arms by ears), then bilaterally flex arms with weights as if you are closing a hatchback on a car; stop the movement when the weights are at eye level. The use of the stability ball also provides neuromotor balance training.

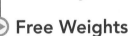

▶ Variable Resistance Machine

You can use a seated row machine or a lat pull-down machine. Using a seated row machine, perform a seated low row movement using a V-bar. Bend the knees slightly and row the arms, squeezing the middle back and lats while sitting upright. Using a lat pull-down variable resistance machine with either a bar or handles, stabilize the spine on the support pad and simultaneously adduct the arms to the sides.

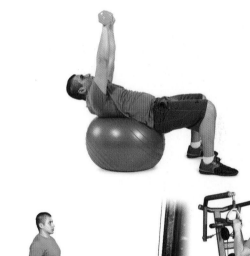

▶ Flexibility: Static Stretch

Kneel on the floor and extend both arms out in front of you, relaxing your hands on the floor. Look down and relax.

In a standing position, reach one arm over to the side and let one hip turn slightly inward.

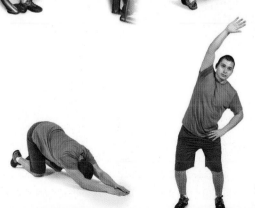

149

Front of Upper Arm

Biceps

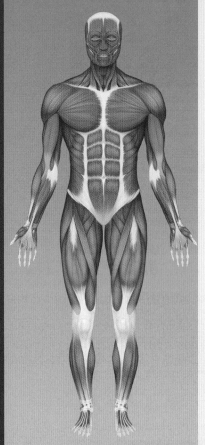

Daily activity use includes carrying groceries, picking up objects in front of you, and picking up objects from the floor and placing them on a table.

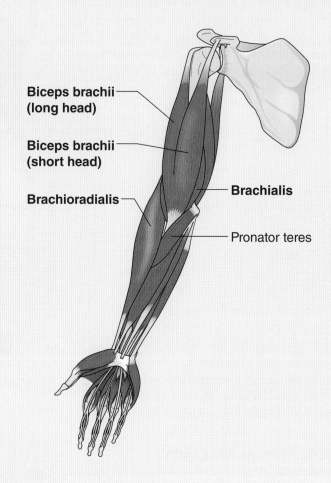

Biceps brachii (long head)

Biceps brachii (short head)

Brachialis

Brachioradialis

Pronator teres

Muscle Group:
Biceps (biceps brachii, brachialis, brachioradialis)

Muscle Action:
Elbow flexion, range of motion is 135 to 160 degrees

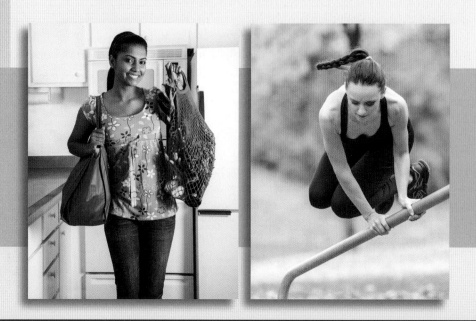

▶ Body Weight

Pull-ups and flexed-arm hangs from a bar are effective body weight exercises for the biceps. Because that equipment is not often readily available, we show biceps curls here, which you can do with weights or other heavy objects such as a backpack. Perform a bilateral biceps curl standing with feet shoulder-width apart and hold weights in the hands or put a band under one foot.

Neuromotor balance training: Sit on a stability ball with your feet placed together and perform a bilateral biceps curl, using the 135- to 160-degree range of motion of elbow flexion.

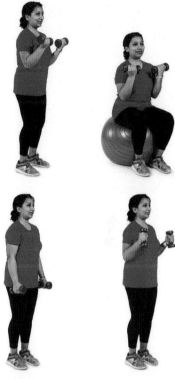

▶ Free Weights

Stand, holding weights in each hand. With your palms facing up, flex the elbow, using a 135- to 160-degree range of motion. You can also perform this with the palms facing the sides of your body to work your brachioradialis.

▶ Variable Resistance Machine

Using a straight bar and cable machine, or a biceps variable resistance machine, stabilize your shoulder joint on the pad and hold the handles to isolate the biceps. Curl your elbow 135 to 160 degrees and let the weight down slowly. Keep your abdominals contracted and your knees slightly bent.

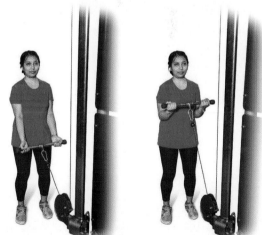

▶ Flexibility: Static Stretch

Extend arms straight out in front of you. Using one hand at a time, gently pull back the fingers of the other hand until a stretch is felt in the biceps.

Alternatively, clasp both hands behind your back to stretch both biceps at the same time. You can also stretch your biceps by reaching your arms behind the back without clasping your hands.

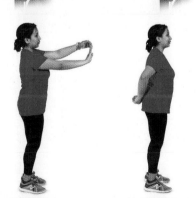

151

Back of Upper Arm

Triceps

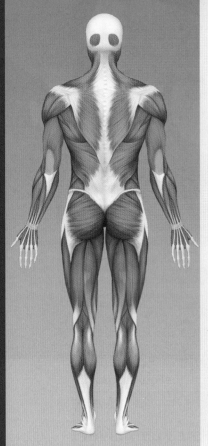

Daily activity use includes getting out of a chair, putting a box on a high shelf, and lowering a box from an overhead position.

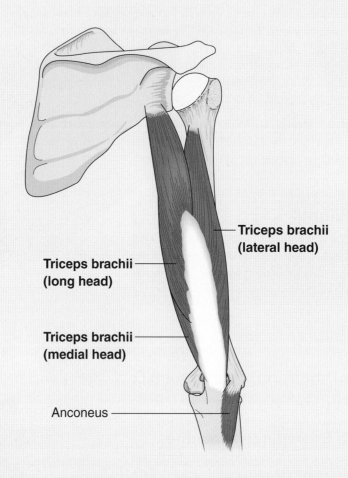

Triceps brachii (lateral head)

Triceps brachii (long head)

Triceps brachii (medial head)

Anconeus

Muscle group:
  Triceps (triceps brachii)

Muscle action:
  Elbow extension, range of motion is 135 to 160 degrees

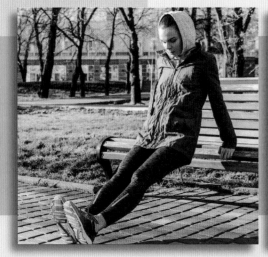

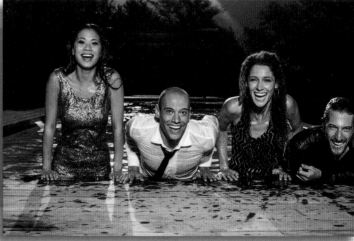

▶ Body Weight

Using a flat, stable bench, perform triceps dips. Flex and extend your elbows, keeping your knees bent and head up.

Neuromotor balance training: Lift one leg as you perform the triceps dips on a bench.

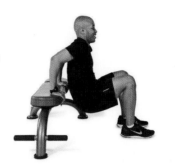
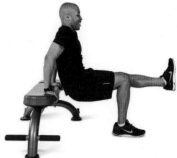

▶ Free Weights

Stand up tall with your knees slightly bent. Hold a weight overhead in both hands. Keeping your upper arms by your ears (perpendicular to the ground), bend your elbows, lowering the weight toward your neck until your elbows point straight up.

Neuromotor balance training: Perform the same movement while sitting on a stability ball.

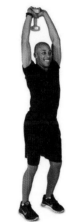
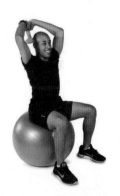

▶ Variable Resistance Machine

Adjust the handles on the triceps dip machine so you get the shoulders as close to the body as possible. Push down and straighten the arms.

Neuromotor balance training: Stand close to a cable machine and extend both elbows 135 to 160 degrees, then let the bar up slowly. Increase the balance challenge by standing on one leg or extending a leg backward.

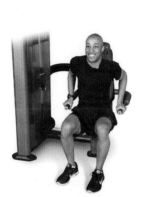
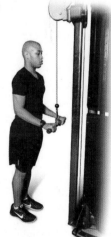

▶ Flexibility: Static Stretch

Point one elbow overhead, toward the ceiling. If the shoulder joint is not flexible, use a stretch band or a towel and slowly move your elbow upward. If you are more flexible, place the hand of that arm on your back after pointing your elbow up. Using the other hand, slightly press the elbow down and point your fingers down your back.

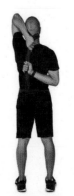
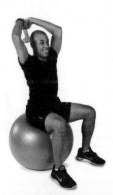

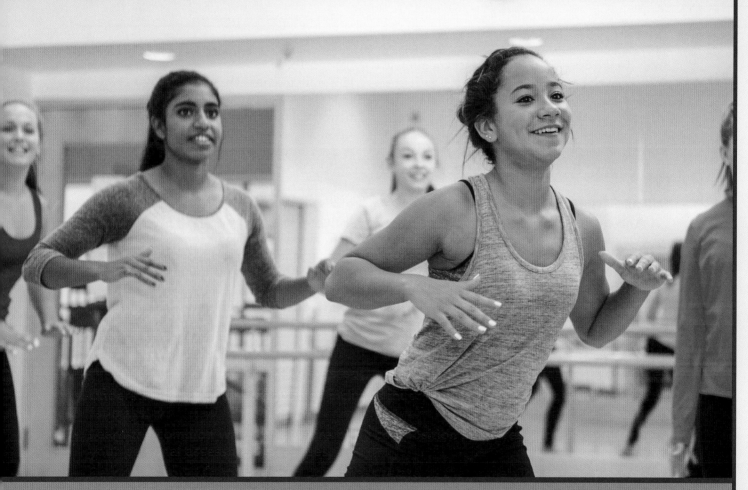

Body Composition

OBJECTIVES

- Understand that body composition includes muscle mass and bone mass in addition to fat mass.
- Learn the common ways to measure body composition in the research lab and for your personal assessment purposes.
- Recognize how fat, muscle, and bone mass relate to the primary diseases of obesity, sarcopenia, and osteoporosis.
- Understand how the "three-legged stool" of physical activity, nutrition, and hormones work together to influence your body composition.

155

KEY TERMS

adiposity	hydrodensitometry
air displacement plethysmography	intermuscular adipose tissue
bioelectrical impedance analysis (BIA)	magnetic resonance imaging (MRI)
body composition	osteoporosis
body mass index (BMI)	percent body fat
bone density T-score	sarcopenia
dual-energy X-ray absorptiometry (DEXA)	skinfold thickness
ectopic fat	subcutaneous fat
essential fat	visceral fat
female athlete triad	

Body composition is an important component of health-related physical fitness. As with the health-related physical fitness components discussed in previous chapters—cardiorespiratory fitness, muscular fitness, flexibility, and neuromuscular fitness—body composition is important for functional fitness and sport performance. If you successfully manage your body composition, you will enhance how you look, feel, and move.

In this chapter, we will discuss the three main components of body composition, how to measure your body composition, and the benefits of a healthy body composition, as well as the primary strategies for body composition management. The most important point to take away is that a healthy body composition is much more than body weight or body fatness. Please note that the concept of biological sex discussed in this chapter differs from the concept of gender. Your gender identity may differ from your biological sex, or you may identify as agender. In such a case, biological sex will provide the most accuracy for comparison with normative data, but you can make a selection according to what makes you most comfortable.

Body Composition Basics

Many people mistakenly think of **body composition** simply as body fat, but it is much more complex. Body weight can be divided into three major components: fat mass, lean (or muscle) mass, and bone mass. In earlier evolutionary times, fat was an efficient vehicle for energy storage, and life spans were so short that people did not contemplate chronic diseases and conditions of old age. Today, however, it is well accepted that the three major components of body composition are all important factors in your overall health. Most of us can also appreciate that in our modern times, a desirable body composition is often considered a social status symbol.

> Body composition is much more than body fat. Your weight can be divided into three major components: fat mass, lean or muscle mass, and bone mass.

A perspective of body composition that moves beyond body fat and aesthetics will help you design your personal program and successfully manage your body composition for a long, healthy life!

A Conceptual Model of Body Composition

The measurement of body composition has greatly evolved over the past several decades. Methods vary in complexity. All methods are highly accurate, but many also require specialized equipment and trained personnel and thus are conducted in specialized research laboratories. This chapter will therefore use the three-component model of body composition, which divides the body into fat mass, lean mass (includes muscle and water), and bone mass. This provides a useful conceptual model for body composition as it relates to health, especially for young adults.

Fat Facts

Although body fat is often thought of negatively in our society, it serves several important functions.

In addition to storing energy, fat cushions organs and helps regulate the body's temperature. Fat, or lipid, is also contained in all cell membranes. You may remember the lipid bilayer that surrounds all cells from biology class. Thus, we all need a certain amount of fat for healthy body function. This is called **essential fat**. The percentage of essential fat needed for health is approximately 3 to 5 percent for biological males and 8 to 12 percent for biological females. Growing children and older adults also need different levels of essential fat to remain healthy (Heymsfield et al. 2005).

Most of the fat available for stored energy purposes is in adipocytes (i.e., fat cells). When combined, these cells form adipose tissue. Hence, a common term to describe body fat is **adiposity**. The great majority of fat storage in the body is located either right beneath the skin (**subcutaneous fat**) or deep within the abdomen surrounding the organs (**visceral fat**). Visceral fat is often called *intra-abdominal fat* because it is located underneath the abdominal muscles. Fat storage can also occur in less typical locations, such as within the liver, around the heart, or near bundles of muscle fibers; this is termed **ectopic fat**. Minimal fat is stored in these locations in physically active healthy-weight adults.

Figure 7.1 illustrates the fat mass, lean mass (mainly muscle that contains protein and water), and bone mass components of the body composition of average healthy-weight biological male and female college-aged students. In the figure, the percentage of fat mass, or **percent body fat**, for the average young adult means the percentage of the total body mass (or weight) that is fat mass.

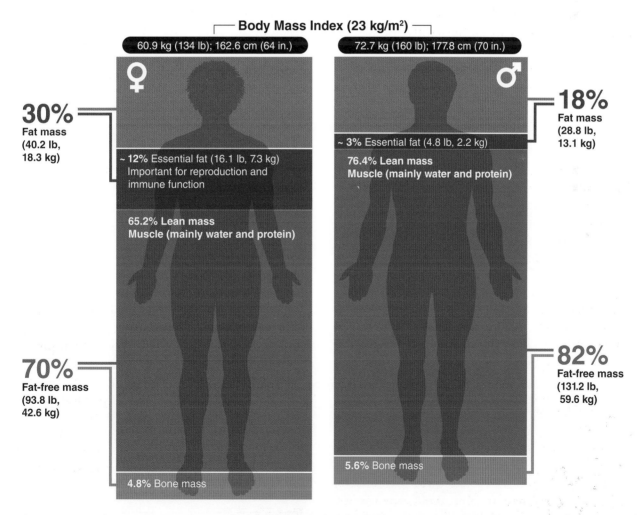

Body Mass Index (23 kg/m²)

60.9 kg (134 lb); 162.6 cm (64 in.)   72.7 kg (160 lb); 177.8 cm (70 in.)

30%
Fat mass
(40.2 lb,
18.3 kg)

~ **12%** Essential fat (16.1 lb, 7.3 kg)
Important for reproduction and
immune function

65.2% Lean mass
Muscle (mainly water and protein)

70%
Fat-free mass
(93.8 lb,
42.6 kg)

4.8% Bone mass

18%
Fat mass
(28.8 lb,
13.1 kg)

~ **3%** Essential fat (4.8 lb, 2.2 kg)

76.4% Lean mass
Muscle (mainly water and protein)

82%
Fat-free mass
(131.2 lb,
59.6 kg)

5.6% Bone mass

Figure 7.1   Body composition of a typical young biological male and female with a similar body mass index.

Interactions Between Fat, Muscle, and Bone

Because bones adapt in response to repeated muscle contraction, lean mass has a strong relationship to bone mass and density in adolescents and young adults (Weaver et al. 2016). Also, as you gain or lose weight, not all the weight change is due to increases or decreases in fat mass—you will also experience changes in lean mass and bone mass. The exact composition of weight change is influenced by many factors, including your age and overall health, how much you exercise and what type (e.g., cardiorespiratory or resistance training), and the quality of your diet, especially protein and bone nutrients like calcium and vitamin D (Shapses and Sukumar 2012).

Effects of Sex and Age on Body Composition

Both sex and the aging process influence body composition (Xiao et al. 2017). As depicted in figure 7.1, after puberty, the average biological male has greater lean mass (muscle and water) and bone mass and less fat mass than the average biological female. These differences do not exist in prepubertal children and are primarily due to sex-specific differences in testosterone and estrogen.

Distinct changes also occur in fat, muscle, and bone mass with aging. Essentially, as a person moves beyond middle age, fat mass increases and muscle mass and bone mass decrease (Kohrt 2010; Looker et al. 2009). These body composition changes are a natural part of the aging process that are mostly caused by changes in hormones. However, the degree to which body composition changes with age is highly influenced by lifestyle choices, including physical activity and intentional exercise, especially strength training, and dietary habits. Moving and eating well during your younger years helps you establish healthy habits that you will maintain throughout your life.

> Body composition is much more than body fat. Your weight can be divided into three major components: fat mass, lean or muscle mass, and bone mass.

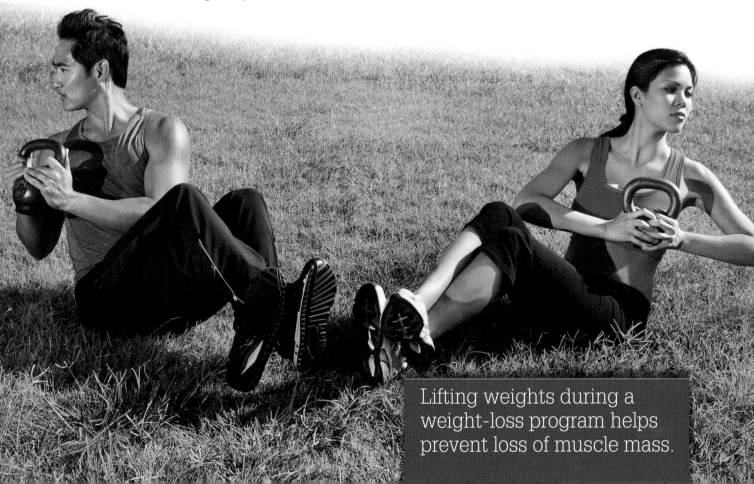

Lifting weights during a weight-loss program helps prevent loss of muscle mass.

Genetics Influence Your Body Type

Have you considered your family members' sizes and shapes? The question of nature versus nurture has been used to describe personalities, patterns of behavior, and body characteristics. Certainly, both factors play a role. One factor influenced by genetics is fat distribution (Bouchard and Perusse 1988). This is especially true for biological females, who vary in their fat patterning more than males do. For example, if you are biologically female and most females in your family store extra weight in their midsection, you are likely genetically inclined to have this android fat pattern, often called an "apple" shape. However, if these family members tend to store extra weight in the hips and thighs, they have a gynoid fat pattern, or a "pear" shape (figure 7.2). Some people are not an apple or a pear; their fat storage is more evenly distributed throughout their body regions. As will be discussed later, not all fat depots are created equal regarding their risk to your health.

As with fat distribution, genetics often play a role in determining your body type. Nearly 50 years ago researchers noted links between body composition or body type, called a *somatotype* (Slaughter and Lohman 1976). This term is still used today to describe the three fundamental elements of body type:

- *Endomorph.* This is the roundest body type, with wider shoulders and hips. This type tends to be pear shaped, easily regains weight after weight loss, excels at strength activities such as resistance training, and finds weight-bearing aerobic exercise (i.e., activities that require one to carry their own weight such as running as compared to cycling) more challenging.

- *Mesomorph.* The *m* in mesomorph is for muscle! This type is typically lean and muscular with broad shoulders and responds to exercise training with quick and very evident results. With their athletic build, they tend to excel at exercise and sport activities and manage their body composition very easily.

- *Ectomorph.* The ectomorph is thin and generally very linear, with narrow shoulders and hips. Regardless of their height, they

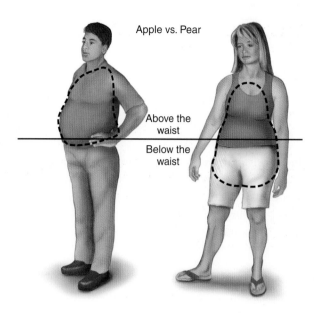

Figure 7.2   Do you have an apple or a pear body shape?
Reprinted by permission from K.E. McConnell, C.B. Corbin, D.E. Corbin, and T.D. Farrar, *Health for Life* (Champaign, IL: Human Kinetics, 2014), 70.

have little fat or muscle, relatively speaking. These light-framed individuals excel at sports or fitness activities that are aerobic and require them to carry their weight, such as distance running.

Most people have a blend of two different body types. All individuals can align with any of the three body types, regardless of their biological sex or sex hormone status. Some bodies do not match any particular type. Regardless of body type, everybody can benefit from meeting the guidelines described in previous chapters. However, if you are strongly aligned with one type, training adaptations might be more challenging. For example, a true ectomorph will struggle to gain a lot of muscle mass with resistance training compared to a true mesomorph.

Assessing Body Composition

Body composition can be measured in several ways. In general, the greater the resources available, the more accurate the results. Methods commonly used in clinics and fitness facilities measure the whole body or regional parts of the body and are based on two-component and three-component models.

Laboratory Methods

The following sections provide an overview of some common laboratory methods for assessing body composition. This methodology and expertise might be used in research labs or in a hospital setting.

Hydrodensitometry

Hydrodensitometry, commonly called *underwater weighing*, uses the density of the body to determine body fatness. Body density ranges from a theoretical 0.9 g/dL for a purely fat body to 1.1 g/dL for a purely fat-free body (i.e., lean) body (Heymsfield et al. 2005).

For example, if you were to put a pan that is greasy from frying hamburger into a sink full of water, the fat droplets from the meat would rise to the top and any lean meat that had been left in the pan would go to the bottom. Fat floats because it is less dense than water and meat sinks because is it denser than water. The same principle applies for hydrodensitometry. In the swimming pool, people with higher levels of body fat float easily, whereas very lean people must work harder to stay afloat.

Recall that density equals mass divided by volume. The difference between weight on land and weight underwater provides a calculation of body density. Underwater weighing requires a person to be completely submerged in a tank of water while their weight is obtained on a scale. Once body density is determined, a prediction equation is used to estimate relative adiposity, or percent body fat.

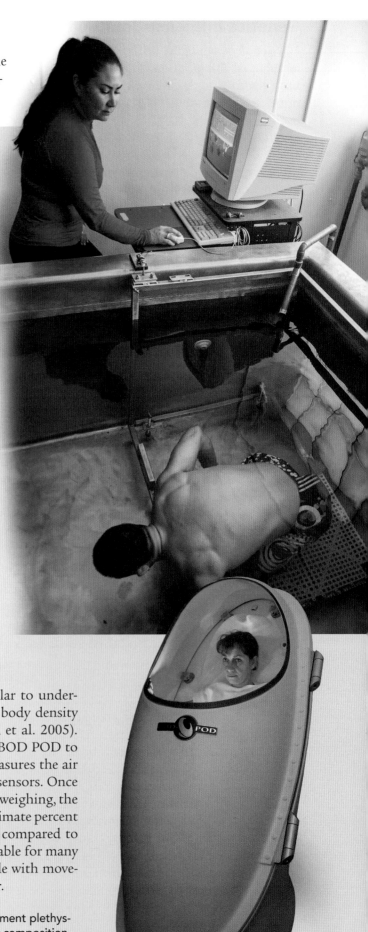

Underwater weighing, or the hydrodensitometry method, is used to measure body composition.

Air Displacement Plethysmography

Air displacement plethysmography is very similar to underwater weighing. However, instead of using water, body density is determined from air displacement (Heymsfield et al. 2005). This methodology uses a closed chamber called a BOD POD to acquire body density. The BOD POD chamber measures the air volume changes with sophisticated computerized sensors. Once body density has been determined, like underwater weighing, the body density value is entered into an equation to estimate percent body fat. The BOD POD offers many advantages compared to underwater weighing. It is safer and more comfortable for many individuals, especially children, older adults, people with movement disabilities, and those who are afraid of water.

The BOD POD uses air displacement plethysmography to measure body composition.

Dual-Energy X-Ray Absorptiometry (DEXA)

One of the best technological advances for body composition to date has been **dual-energy X-ray absorptiometry (DEXA)**. This equipment, available in many exercise science, kinesiology, and nutrition departments at universities and in nearly all hospitals, works by exposing the body to low- and high-energy X-rays. The computer software then maps the body's composition of fat, lean tissue, and bone mass (Heymsfield et al. 2005). DEXA provides both whole-body and regional (arms and legs) estimates of body composition as well as bone density. DEXA is a valid and reliable method for estimating body composition and only requires lying still on a scanning table for a few minutes. However, in addition to the high cost and expertise required, a small amount of radiation exposure is associated with DEXA scanning, though the actual amount of radiation depends on the type and number of scans a person undergoes.

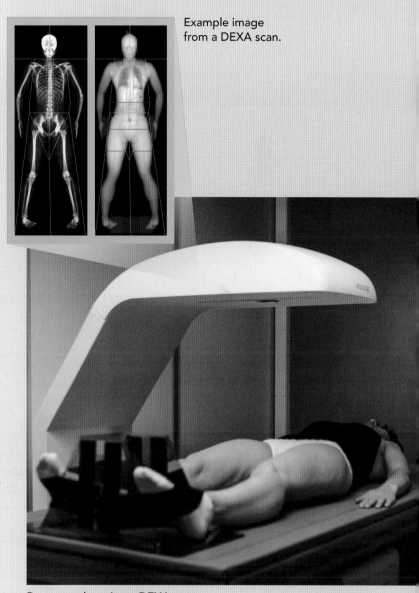

Example image from a DEXA scan.

Person undergoing a DEXA scan.

Magnetic Resonance Imaging (MRI)

Although it is not readily available, **magnetic resonance imaging (MRI)** is an important method for body composition assessment because it shows ectopic fat depots (the presence of fat in places where only very small amounts of fat should be stored) and visceral fat (fat stored deep in the abdomen), and both are associated with health risks. MRI is readily available in most hospitals and in many research centers. This technology can visually map the body by slices, or cross-sections. MRI is also used to assess fat infiltration into muscles, a specific type of ectopic fat of special importance in the leg muscles called **intermuscular adipose tissue**, which has been linked with a higher risk for metabolic diseases, physical functional limitations, and disability, especially in older individuals (Addison et al. 2014).

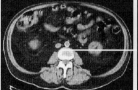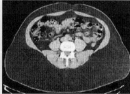

MRI images of visceral adipose tissue from a person with a large waist due to visceral fat and a person with a large waist due to subcutaneous abdominal fat.

Field Methods

For assessing body composition on the sports field, at a health fair, or anywhere else outside of the laboratory, the two most common field methods used are bioelectrical impedance analysis and skinfold measurements. Both methods require some level of expertise to acquire quality estimates of body composition.

You may also want to monitor your own body composition at home. At a minimum, you should monitor your weight and waistline if you do not have access to some of the more complex measurement methods and devices discussed in this chapter.

Bioelectrical Impedance Analysis (BIA)

Bioelectrical impedance analysis (BIA) is considered suitable for laboratory, field, and personal use. Because nearly all body water is contained within the lean (muscle) mass of the body, lean mass can be estimated from a measurement of body water. The difference in weight can be used to estimate fat mass and percent body fat (Heymsfield et al. 2005). A bioelectrical instrument sends a small electrical current through the body and measures the resistance to the current. Because water is a great conductor and fat is a good insulator, the balance between the two tissues determines the resistance to the current.

Based on previous research, the resistance to the current, and other factors such as height are used to estimate body water, which then can be used to estimate body composition based on research-established equations. Because this methodology measures water, the person being tested must be properly hydrated. Testing when you are dehydrated or, less commonly, overhydrated can greatly affect the accuracy of this testing method. The quality of BIA instruments ranges greatly. Research-grade multifrequency BIA instruments are more accurate and include measures of where the body water is located (i.e., inside or outside the cell). Lower-cost BIA instruments offer a less accurate measure of total body water and percent body fat.

Personal BIA instruments can also be purchased that range in price from $50 to several hundred dollars, including handheld devices and stand-on scales. The latter are higher quality, and many can also measure weight. Remember to standardize your measurement protocol using the four S's mentioned in the next section, especially for factors that influence hydration. If you are using a scale at home, be sure to place it on a flat surface to avoid an inaccurate reading. Finally, read the specific instructions for use, especially regarding equation selection. Like skinfold methodology, described next, the selection of prediction equations can affect quality.

Although many companies produce personal BIA instruments, two manufacturers that have been in the BIA instrumentation business for many decades are RJL Systems for research-grade instruments and Tanita for personal instruments. You are encouraged to visit their websites for more information.

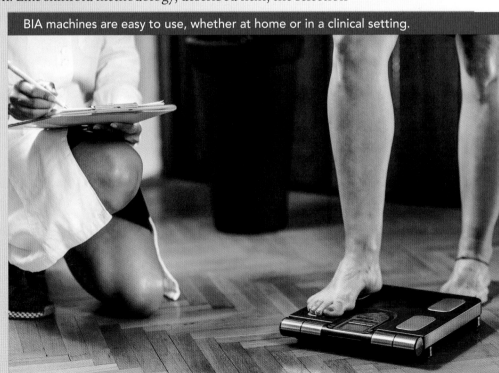

BIA machines are easy to use, whether at home or in a clinical setting.

Skinfolds

Skinfold thickness tests are sometimes used in the field to assess body composition (Heymsfield et al. 2005). Most stored fat is located just beneath the skin. Thus, once skinfold thicknesses have been obtained from several sites and summed, the total number reflects overall skinfold thickness, which represents percent body fat. Because standardized measures can be taken on the legs, arms, back, and abdomen, this method can also give a quantitative measure of where you store your fat and the degree of change in various fat depots.

Acceptable measurements of skinfold thickness are a bit more challenging to obtain than BIA measures. First, the instrument needed to measure the skinfold, called *calipers*, should be high quality. Research-grade calipers can cost several hundred dollars, and acceptable spring-loaded ones that are well calibrated are also expensive. Second, being able to obtain valid and reliable measurements requires extensive practice on many different body types. Finding a well-trained and experienced tester can be problematic. Third, having your skinfolds assessed requires a person to touch you on multiple parts of your body, which you may find uncomfortable. Finally, when converting the sum of skinfolds into a percent body fat estimate, the tester will need to choose from numerous prediction equations, which can influence the accuracy of the estimate. In summary, obtaining relatively accurate estimates from this method can be challenging, particularly when using the method to assess change in percent body fat.

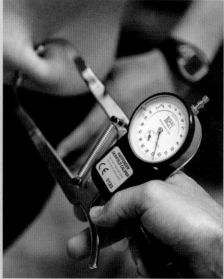

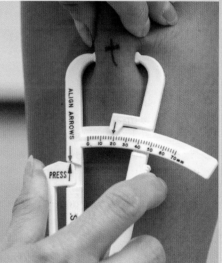

Research-quality calipers compared to low-quality calipers.

Personal Measurement of Weight Status and Body Composition

Whether you assess your body composition because you want to learn about your health risk or establish a baseline to help you track your progress, your choice of method will depend on your purpose, the availability of equipment, testing expertise, and your budget.

Weight status is evaluated primarily using **body mass index (BMI)**, which is a ratio of weight to height. Although limitations exist for the personal assessment of body composition from BMI, the measure does provide a well-established index for health risk. Waist circumference is highly related to visceral fat. As the chapter 7 labs on HK*Propel* describe in more detail, proper measurement of

your height, weight, and waistline is key to getting good baseline data and tracking changes over time. Therefore, investing in a good tape measure or consistently noticing your belt notch can help you understand your health status and keep your weight management on track. Be mindful of the four S's of monitoring your weight status:

- Same time of day
- Same day each week
- Same clothing (or none at all!)
- Same scale

Also, recognize that normal fluctuations in weight occur over the day and week as a result of changes in body water, especially after eating salty and starchy foods. Other factors can also affect your weight, such as the weather, stress, and hormonal changes, including those caused by the menstrual cycle.

Beyond regularly monitoring your weight and waistline and perhaps considering the purchase of your own BIA device for home use, another great option is to pay for quality assessment services that use one of the techniques described previously. Many colleges and universities provide body composition assessments through the campus health or recreation center. In addition, many departments and medical centers have DEXA capabilities and offer testing services for a fee. Finally, higher-quality fitness facilities often have respectable BIA instruments and trained staff. It is highly recommended that you select conventional established methods for body composition testing as described in this chapter.

> Measuring your waist is as important as tracking your weight. Your best tool for assessing your weight status is likely a simple tape measure!

Now and Later

Find Your Assessment Sweet Spot for Life

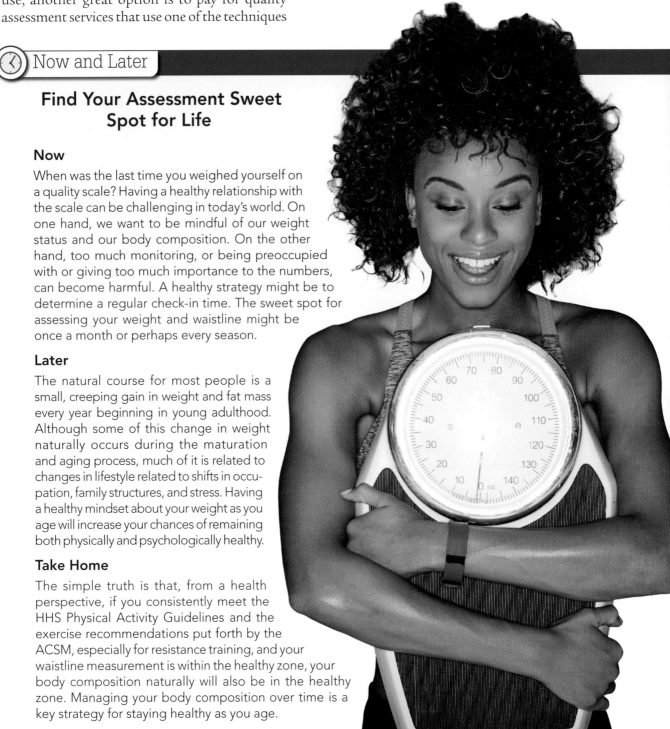

Now

When was the last time you weighed yourself on a quality scale? Having a healthy relationship with the scale can be challenging in today's world. On one hand, we want to be mindful of our weight status and our body composition. On the other hand, too much monitoring, or being preoccupied with or giving too much importance to the numbers, can become harmful. A healthy strategy might be to determine a regular check-in time. The sweet spot for assessing your weight and waistline might be once a month or perhaps every season.

Later

The natural course for most people is a small, creeping gain in weight and fat mass every year beginning in young adulthood. Although some of this change in weight naturally occurs during the maturation and aging process, much of it is related to changes in lifestyle related to shifts in occupation, family structures, and stress. Having a healthy mindset about your weight as you age will increase your chances of remaining both physically and psychologically healthy.

Take Home

The simple truth is that, from a health perspective, if you consistently meet the HHS Physical Activity Guidelines and the exercise recommendations put forth by the ACSM, especially for resistance training, and your waistline measurement is within the healthy zone, your body composition naturally will also be in the healthy zone. Managing your body composition over time is a key strategy for staying healthy as you age.

Using Body Composition Assessment Mindfully

As a starting point, work on having a healthy perspective toward getting your body composition assessed. Make sure to have a positive mindset whereby the process and results won't be counterproductive to your physical and mental health.

Purpose of Assessment

Before getting your body composition assessed, you should reflect on why you want to know the numbers. Do you want to know if you are in the healthy range? Are you trying to get a baseline so that you can track your response to a new exercise or dietary program? Or are you comparing yourself to a friend or celebrity? These groups are not appropriate for comparison. If the results will not help your physical or psychological health, you don't need to get your body composition assessed.

Body Composition Assessments Are Estimates!

You may have noticed when reading the preceding descriptions of body composition methods that they all provide *estimates* of percent body fat. Another way to think of this is that the values they provide all have a degree of error. The only way to truly know what your body composition is would require you to be assessed as a cadaver—and we all agree that this would not be a good idea! With methods for body composition assessment, you get what you pay for. This means that the more expensive equipment and sophisticated expertise will provide estimates that have lower levels of error. For example, DEXA can provide an estimate that has an error of only 1 to 2 percent. Alternatively, many BIA instruments on the market have an error rate of 4 to 5 percent (Heymsfield et al. 2005). Therefore, depending on your purpose for assessment, the availability of methods and expert testers, and your resources, the wiser choice might be to not get your body composition assessed, because the level of error may be too great to inform your program plans.

Weight Status, Body Composition, and Your Risk of Chronic Disease

The three body composition components—fat mass, lean (muscle) mass, and bone mass—are directly linked to primary diseases. Having too much fat mass (a high percent body fat), especially stored in certain places in the body, is defined as *overweight* or *obesity*. Overweight is linked to many chronic diseases and conditions that increasingly occur as a person enters middle age and beyond. However, having too little muscle mass and a low bone mass can also cause serious conditions and diseases that often arrive later in life.

Weight Status Classified

Table 7.1 lists the BMI classifications of underweight, healthy weight, overweight, and obese, along with the recommendations for a healthy waist circumference (Centers for Disease Control and Prevention 2022a). Recall that BMI is a ratio of weight to height: It is calculated by dividing your weight in kilograms by height in meters squared. The calculation is more complicated if you would like to use the units of pounds and inches, so we recommend you use an online BMI calculator to determine your BMI. Many people struggle with excessive weight. However, it should be recognized that a lower BMI is not always better: Being underweight can also compromise health, typically increasing risk for frailty and compromising bone health and immune function, especially with increasing age. Toward the other direction, because of the key link between waist size and visceral fat and the related risk for metabolic and cardiovascular diseases, it is also important to take note of your waist size. A person can have a healthy BMI but be at higher risk for disease due to an increased waist size, especially in middle-age and beyond. You might hear the slang expressions of a "beer belly" or a "muffin top" and chuckle. But seriously, an increased waist size is no laughing matter when it comes to your metabolic and cardiovascular health risk.

Table 7.1   Classification of Weight Status and Disease Risk by BMI and Waist Circumference for Biological Males and Females

| Weight status | BMI | DISEASE RISK[1] | |
		Waist circumference Male: ≤40 in. (102 cm) Female: ≤35 in. (88 cm)	Waist circumference Male: >40 in. (102 cm) Female: >35 in. (88 cm)
Underweight	≤18.5	Not Applicable	Not Typical
Healthy weight[2]	18.5-24.9	**None**	Increased ↑
Overweight	25.0-29.9	Increased ↑	Further Increased ↑↑
Obese[3]	≥30	Further Increased ↑↑↑	Greatly Increased ↑↑↑↑

Data from Centers for Disease Control and Prevention (2022a, 2022b, 2022c).
[1]Disease risk for metabolic and cardiovascular diseases relative to healthy weight and waist circumference.
[2]Increased waist circumference can increase risk of disease even in persons of healthy weight.
[3]BMI values above 35.0 and 40.0 are classified as Obesity Class 2 and 3, respectively (Centers for Disease Control 2022c), and increase disease risk further.
Data from Centers for Disease Control and Prevention (2022a, 2022b, 2022c).

BMI and Adiposity Relationships

A relatively strong relationship exists between BMI and percent body fat across all age groups, which is why it is used to assess health status at the medical clinic. Additionally, much research supports the fact that for a typical adult, BMI levels in the overweight and obese categories are linked to increased risk of chronic disease and death. However, these predictions are not perfect. Many other factors influence one's risk, such as physical activity, diet quality, smoking, alcohol and drug habits, and stress. In addition, BMI can misrepresent an individual's body composition. In the special cases that follow, interpret the BMI value with caution.

- *Heavily muscled athletes.* People who undergo a high intensity and volume of resistance training, typically males, often have a high BMI that is not attributable to increased fat mass. Their increased muscle mass increases their weight, thereby increasing their BMI as well.
- *Altered height.* Because height is included in BMI calculations, any situation where height is altered will introduce error into the relationship between BMI and percent body fat. For example, older adults lose several inches later in life. If their weight remains stable, it will appear that BMI has increased.

- *Reduced physical activity.* In individuals with reduced mobility due to illness, a spinal cord injury, or other health-related challenges, the relation between BMI and percent body fat can also be greatly altered as a result of reduced muscle mass. Even in people who can walk but choose to be very sedentary, reductions in muscle mass can cause the BMI to misrepresent percent body fat (i.e., as the person might not be as healthy as the BMI number suggests).

Percent Body Fat Health and Fitness Categories

Unlike those established for BMI, no universally accepted norms for percent body fat exist. Age, sex, and race may affect the level of percent body fat that is in the healthy range (Gallagher et al. 2000). Note that biological females have greater body percent fat compared to biological males. A slight increase in body percent fat (3 to 5 percent) is also a normal part of the aging process Table 7.2 highlights the percent body fat ranges corresponding to the healthy weight, overweight, and obese categories of BMI.

The ACSM also supports using percent body fat ranges to categorize body composition fitness for biological males and females into rankings of very lean, excellent, good, fair, poor, and very poor, with percentiles from 1 to 95 percent in 5 percent increments (American College of Sports Medicine 2022). Table 7.3 summarizes the main

Chapter 7   Body Composition   **167**

cut points within the categories for young males and females. Being excessively lean, which corresponds to a percent body fat below 3 to 5 percent for young males and 10 to 13 percent for young females, can be harmful to health.

Not All Fat Depots Are Equal

Where people store their fat influences their risk for many chronic conditions and diseases. Keep in mind that not all fat depots are created equal. Where you store fat as a healthy young adult depends on your genetics, sex hormones, and, to a lesser extent, your level of physical activity, diet quality, and your stress hormones.

As mentioned previously, changes in body composition occur with the aging process. The preferred storage depot shifts, particularly in biological females, to store more fat centrally and less in the lower body. In addition, with higher levels of adiposity and a very sedentary lifestyle, you increase intermuscular adipose tissue. In simple terms, muscles get "mushier"—that is, lower quality—with age.

Another important site of ectopic fat storage is the liver. A small amount of fat in your liver is normal, but once it gets beyond 10 percent of the organ weight, you may be at high risk for fatty liver disease. There are two main types of fatty liver disease: alcoholic fatty liver disease and nonalcoholic fatty liver disease. The latter occurs mainly in middle-aged obese individuals. As expected, if this person also heavily drinks alcohol, the risk of fatty liver disease greatly increases. Remember to treat your liver right!

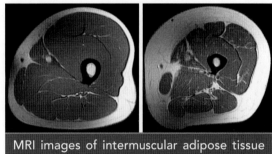

MRI images of intermuscular adipose tissue from a healthy, active young woman compared to a sedentary, obese older woman.

Table 7.2   Percent Fat Classifications Based on BMI

	AGE 20 TO 39		AGE 40 TO 59		AGE 60 TO 79	
BMI	Female	Male	Female	Male	Female	Male
18.5 (healthy weight)	20%-25%	8%-13%	21%-25%	9%-13%	23%-26%	11%-14%
25 (overweight)	32%-35%	20%-23%	34%-36%	22%-24%	35%-38%	23%-25%
30 (obese)	38%-40%	26%-28%	39%-41%	27%-29%	41%-43%	29%-31%

Data from Gallagher et al. (2000).

Table 7.3   Fitness Categories for Body Composition Levels for Young Adults (Ages 20 to 29)

		PERCENT FAT	
Percentile (%)	Category	Male	Female
95	Very lean	6.4	14.1
85	Excellent	10.5	16.1
60	Good	14.8	20.0
40	Fair	18.6	23.5
20	Poor	23.3	28.6
1	Very poor	33.7	38.4

Data from ACSM (2018).

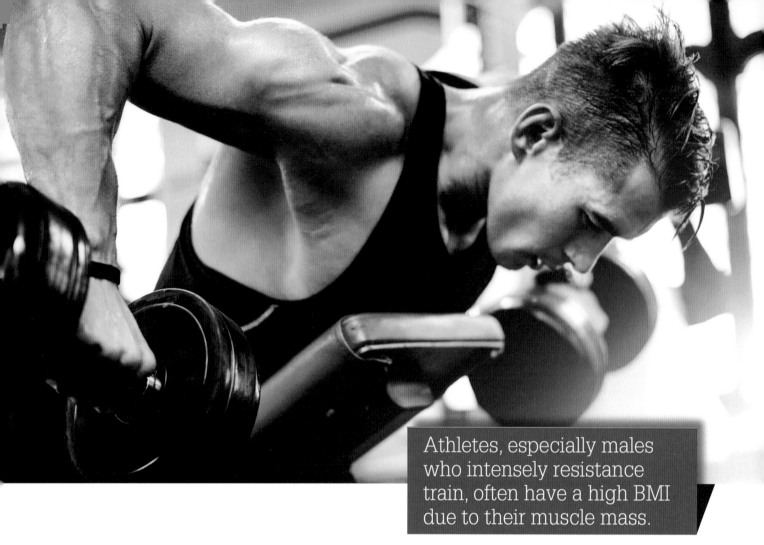

Athletes, especially males who intensely resistance train, often have a high BMI due to their muscle mass.

Preventing Sarcopenia: Keep Your Muscle Mass!

Relative healthy young adults have an adequate amount of muscle mass to meet the needs of their daily lives. However, during middle age (45 to 65 years old), muscle mass is lost at a greater rate. With advanced age, many older adults are at risk for **sarcopenia**, or age-related loss of muscle mass and strength. Sarcopenia is usually diagnosed using a DEXA scan to measure muscle mass of the arms and legs. Sarcopenia is one of the main causes of physical functional decline and loss of independence in older adults.

Although this sounds like bad news, the good news is that our muscles retain the ability to get stronger in response to resistance training well into our 90s. Much research documents that older adults of all ages and conditions can still safely strength train, which leads to physical functional benefits and affords them the ability to live independently. For an awesome life as an older adult, build the habit of incorporating resistance training into your weekly movement routine.

This single health behavior can pay great health dividends late in life!

Osteoporosis: Building the Bone Bank Early in Life Is Important

Osteoporosis (meaning "porous bone") is a bone disease where decreased bone strength and mass significantly increase the risk of fractures, especially from a nontraumatic injury such as a fall in the bathroom or on an icy sidewalk. Most people think of osteoporosis as a disease that affects older females. In fact, osteoporosis affects all types of people. It is very serious and costly to our health care system. Osteoporosis is also silent, which means you can be completely unaware of having it until you suffer a fracture. More important to you as a young adult, the risk for osteoporosis starts early in life! The good news is that it is largely preventable with good health behaviors.

How Is Osteoporosis Diagnosed and Who Gets It?

Typically, screening for osteoporosis occurs based on a person's age and health history. A medical evaluation to diagnose osteoporosis and estimate your risk of breaking a bone often involves a combination of clinical exams (medical history, physical examination, and laboratory tests), a bone density test, and a FRAX score evaluation, which estimates your 10-year risk of major osteoporosis fracture.

A DEXA scan, introduced earlier for measuring body composition, also measures bone mass and bone density. The **bone density T-score** value is the tool primarily used to diagnose osteoporosis. A T-score is simply the standard deviation below peak bone density of a young healthy person, typically of the same biological sex and race or ethnic group as the person tested. Figure 7.3 summarizes the Bone Health and Osteoporosis Foundation's (2022) definition of osteoporosis: a T-score below or equal to –2.5 (i.e., 2.5 standard deviations below the peak bone density of a young healthy person).

There are several primary uncontrollable risk factors for osteoporosis and several factors related to health behaviors that can be modified. Compare these factors to your personal demographics, health history, and behaviors. For more information, visit the Bone Health and National Osteoporosis Foundation at www.bonehealthandosteoporosis.org.

- *Age.* Being over the age of 50 increases the risk.
- *Biological sex.* Biological females have a greater risk of osteoporosis than biological males due to bone size and differing sex hormone profiles. Menopause and the loss of estrogen is an important factor for females.
- *Family history.* As with most diseases and conditions, genetics play an important role.

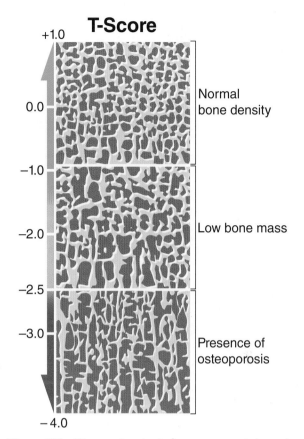

Figure 7.3 Diagnostic criteria for osteoporosis based on a DEXA T-score.

- *Race or ethnic group.* White and Asian people have greater risk of osteoporosis than African American people, likely due to both genetics and cultural behaviors.
- *Diseases or conditions.* Cancer, endocrine or hormonal disorders, autoimmune disorders such as lupus, and digestive disorders such as celiac disease are just a few health challenges that can increase the risk for osteoporosis.

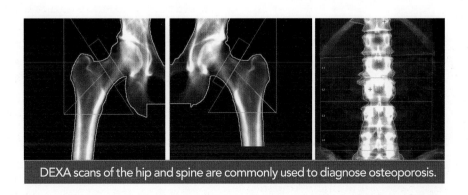
DEXA scans of the hip and spine are commonly used to diagnose osteoporosis.

- **Medications.** Many medications (e.g., steroids) can compromise bones.
- **Weight status.** Having a low body weight or small and thin frame increases risk for osteoporosis. Losing weight increases bone loss.
- **Nutrition.** Poor intake of calcium and vitamin D has a direct effect on bone health. High amounts of protein, sodium, and caffeine and low fruit and vegetable intake have also been linked to poor bone health.
- **Smoking and alcohol.** Smoking is a known risk factor for poor bone health. Drinking too much alcohol also increases the risk for osteoporosis.
- **Physical activity and exercise.** Being sedentary, especially bedridden, greatly affects bone health.

The Bone Bank: Deposits and Withdrawals

With the aging process, all people lose bone mass and density. If you stay alive long enough, it is very likely that you will develop osteoporosis.

When planning for retirement, the goal is to put money in the bank during your greatest earning years for the day when you retire and need to withdraw funds to support your life. If you planned correctly, you won't outlive your money to finance your lifestyle. In this same way, the goal with bone health is to maximize your deposits, because sometime around middle age—especially for people who undergo menopause—you will begin to withdraw bone mass and lose bone density. Therefore, the goal is to deposit as much as possible in your bone bank to maximize your peak bone mass and flatten the withdrawal curve as you age (figure 7.4). This two-part strategy will help ensure that your bone density stays out of the danger zone and that you do not suffer an osteoporotic bone fracture later in life, even if you live to be 90 or older!

> Maximizing your peak bone mass while you're young can reduce your fracture risk as an older adult. It pays to deposit in your bone bank early in life!

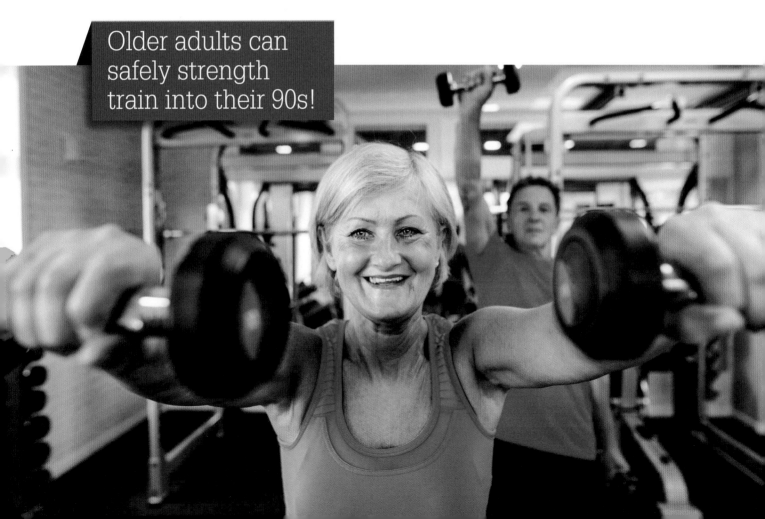

Older adults can safely strength train into their 90s!

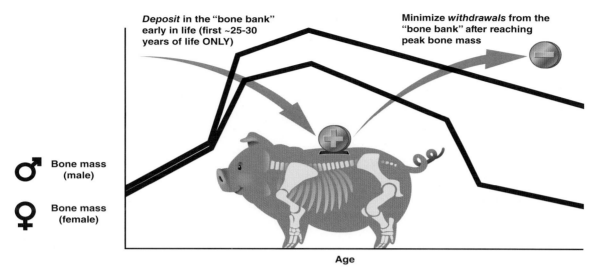

Figure 7.4 To keep your bones healthy for life, deposit more bone mass early in life and minimize withdrawals later in life.

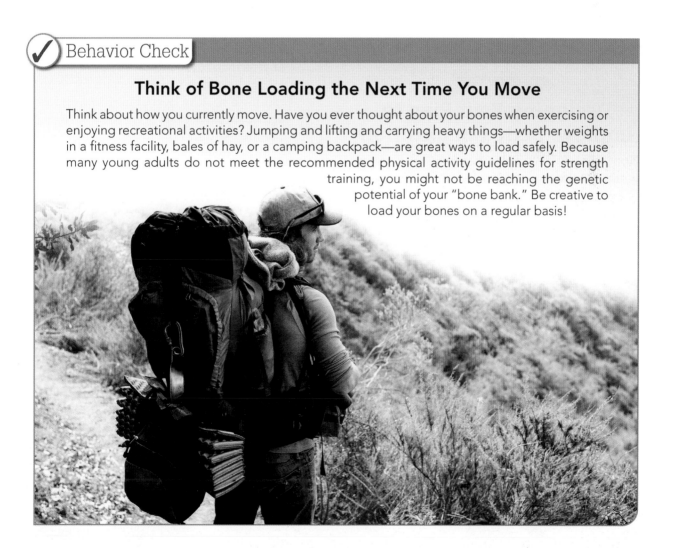

✓ Behavior Check

Think of Bone Loading the Next Time You Move

Think about how you currently move. Have you ever thought about your bones when exercising or enjoying recreational activities? Jumping and lifting and carrying heavy things—whether weights in a fitness facility, bales of hay, or a camping backpack—are great ways to load safely. Because many young adults do not meet the recommended physical activity guidelines for strength training, you might not be reaching the genetic potential of your "bone bank." Be creative to load your bones on a regular basis!

A Healthy Body Composition Benefits You— Today and in the Future!

If you meet physical activity guidelines and have good dietary habits, there is a high likelihood that you will adequately manage your body composition. A healthy body composition means maintaining a healthy level of fat mass, adequate muscle mass, and optimal bone mass and density for your stage of life. Although you won't be able to notice or feel your bone health status, having a good ratio of muscle to fat mass will give you many benefits. In addition to having enhanced physical function for work, recreation, or sport performance, you will also feel better in general. Importantly, you will help prevent conditions such as cardiovascular disease, diabetes, cancer, sarcopenia, and osteoporosis. Although these typically occur later in life, it bears repeating that the foundation of these health challenges begins in early adulthood, often silently. Invest in your future self by successfully managing your body composition.

Designing Your Plan to Improve Body Composition

Hopefully you now realize that body composition is much more than body fat and will consider how to manage all three components: fat mass, lean (muscle) mass, and bone mass. Although weight management is discussed in chapter 9, the following information can remind you of key program components to successfully manage your body composition.

The Plan Depends on the Goal

Your plan to have a healthy body composition is highly dependent on your goal. Your personal goals may be functional in that when you work or play, you want to perform well. Or you may be more concerned with looking good and feeling good about the way you look. We hope your goals will be about both your current and future self. Committing to a weekly routine of cardiorespiratory and muscle-strengthening exercises and physical activities, as well as managing your bone health, can reduce your risk for many diseases and conditions over your life span.

The Three-Legged Stool of Healthy Body Composition

An excellent conceptual model for a healthy body composition is the three-legged stool (figure 7.5). If any one of the legs is compromised, the stool will not function well. Regardless of the component—fat, lean, or bone—optimal health depends on the three primary factors of physical activity (and exercise), adequate nutrition, and appropriate hormones.

Physical Activity: Movement Mode Matters

Hopefully, the previous chapters have convinced you of the importance of regular physical activity and intentional exercise and provided information to guide you in developing a personalized program that keeps you safely moving on a regular basis. Regarding body composition, mode really does matter! Consider these aspects of body composition management.

- *Fat mass.* Because cardiorespiratory endurance activities expend lots of calories and energy balance is very important for maintaining a healthy level of fat mass, choose activities that use lots of energy. The higher the intensity and the longer the duration of the activity, the greater the amount of energy expenditure, relatively speaking.

- *Lean mass (mainly muscle).* Any movement is better than none when working the muscles, but relatively high-intensity strength training is the most effective mode for

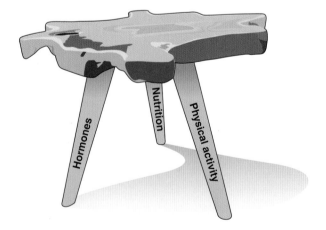

Figure 7.5   The three-legged stool for a healthy body composition: physical activity, nutrition, and hormones.

gaining and keeping muscle mass. Resistance training is also linked to reductions in fat mass.

- **Bone mass and density.** Bones must be loaded to adapt. The best loading for bone health comes from ground reaction forces (e.g., jumping, running), joint reaction forces (e.g., resistance training), and novel forces. Many sport activities offer a combination of loading forces. Your young adult years are a prime time for building bone!

Nutrition

Optimal nutrition is essential for a healthy body composition—and, of course, calories do count for weight management. However, other nutrients are also important for body composition. For example, adequate protein intake is important for muscle maintenance and bone health, especially later in life. Micronutrients that are critical for bone health include calcium and vitamin D. Unfortunately, poor dietary habits and physical inactivity are major reasons for the rising rates of obesity, sarcopenia, and osteoporosis in our contemporary society.

Hormones

Hormones also play a primary role in a healthy body composition. Sex hormones (testosterone and estrogen) and other growth hormones and factors play major roles in the differences in fat, muscle, and bone mass seen in biological males and females during and after puberty. Natural declines in these hormones that occur with aging are a key reason for changes in body composition, which include increases in fat mass and decreases in muscle and bone mass.

However, abnormal levels of hormones for a given life stage are also problematic for a healthy body composition. For example, many biological females, especially younger individuals, for a variety of medical reasons, do not have a regular monthly menstrual cycle. If a biological female does not start to menstruate by age 16, misses three consecutive periods, or has a cycle longer than 35 days, bone loss could be occurring. This reduced estrogen state can lead to bone loss like that seen in menopausal females.

Highly active females should be aware of the **female athlete triad**, which involves three dis-

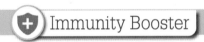

Resistance Training and Immune Function

Recall from chapter 4 that improved cardiorespiratory fitness has positive effects on the immune system. Most of the initial research conducted in this area evaluated cardiorespiratory modes of exercise. However, a recent review indicates that regular resistance training also decreases susceptibility to infections and improves the effectiveness of vaccines (Salimans et al. 2022). Importantly, resistance exercise benefited several aspects of immune cell function in both young and older individuals. Although some benefits were noted after a single exercise session, it appears that several weeks of resistance training are needed to obtain beneficial adaptations in immunity and reduced inflammation. In summary, resistance training is good for your functional fitness and posture, your body composition (especially your muscle and bone mass) and also your immunity. Just lift and carry something now and through your ages and stages to keep you functioning well!

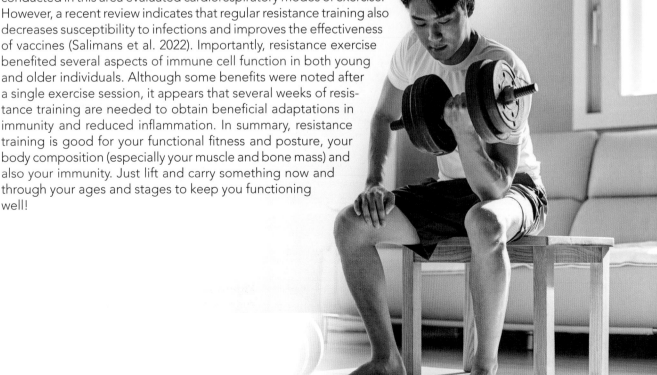

tinct and interrelated conditions: disordered eating (with a range of poor nutritional behaviors), amenorrhea (irregular or absent menstrual cycles), and osteoporosis (low bone mass and poor bone quality) (Joy et al. 2014). The triad occurs most often in

> If you are a female whose cycle is unexplainably irregular or absent, see your physician. You might be compromising your bone health.

highly trained athletes who excel in their sport by being very thin or lean (e.g., dancer, gymnast, distance runner). This provides a great example of the three-legged stool. The athlete greatly overloads the skeleton, but poor or inadequate nutritional intake disrupts the menstrual cycle and causes the estrogen levels to be much lower than what is normal. The stool now has only one optimal leg: physical activity. The triad, or any other reason for menstrual cycle disturbances, reduce the chance of reaching peak bone mass in young biological females.

Summary

Body composition is the final component of health-related physical fitness, joining cardiorespiratory and muscular fitness, flexibility, and neuromuscular fitness. Although body composition is generally thought of as fat mass, lean (muscle) mass and bone mass are also primary components. Accurate and adequate measurement of body composition can occur in both the research laboratory and the privacy of your home. Having optimal nutrition and participating in regular physical activity and intentional exercise can go a long way toward successfully managing your body composition. The benefits of your efforts will pay off today with better physical function in your daily life, including in your sports and active leisure activities. You will also look and feel great. However, the bigger payoff will occur in your future, with a decreased risk of chronic disease and a greater chance of feeling and functioning better as you age. Make the commitment to manage your body composition today!

(www) ONLINE LEARNING ACTIVITIES

Go to HK*Propel* and complete all of the online activities to further facilitate your learning:

Study Activities: Review the main concepts of the chapter.

Labs: Complete the labs your instructor assigns.

Videos: Look through the videos and choose which ones you want to try this week.

REVIEW QUESTIONS

1. Using a three-component model, list and describe the primary body composition components that can affect your health.

2. Describe the primary ways that body composition can be measured in the laboratory, in the field, and in the privacy of your home. Which method is the most accurate?

3. Body mass index (BMI) is a useful health index, but it does have limitations. When does caution need to be used when interpreting BMI to classify weight status?

4. Although chronic diseases often don't present until middle age, they often begin in young adulthood. Describe how the three body composition components relate to primary diseases that occur later in life.

5. List and describe the primary ways that a healthy body composition will make you both function better and feel better during your college years.

6. What are the three legs of the healthy body composition stool? What specific behaviors or factors do you need to address to apply these to your life as a young adult?

Dietary Guidelines for Healthy Fueling

OBJECTIVES

- Understand the primary dietary components of macronutrients, micronutrients, and fiber, and identify sources of each one.
- Understand why each dietary component is important for health.
- Realize that diet is much more than energy intake and that diet quality is important for health.
- Find high-quality resources, including endorsed government and agency guidelines, to assist you in designing a healthy eating plan that fits your lifestyle, budget, and tastes.
- Appreciate the key role that hydration plays in managing environmental stress and daily function.
- Gain strategies to be a smart consumer.

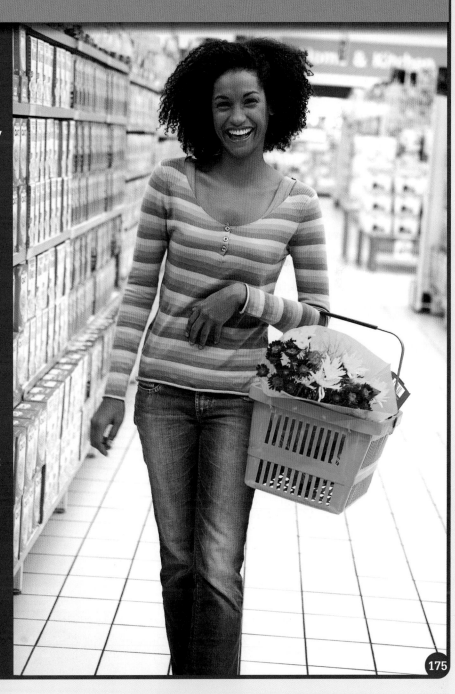

KEY TERMS

Unlike engaging in physical activity, which is almost optional in our contemporary society, you must eat and drink to survive. Therefore, you'll need different skills for managing your eating and drinking behaviors than for your movement behaviors. When it comes to a healthy diet, it may seem as though the advice is ever changing. To some extent, as more research emerges, this may be true, but the fundamentals of nutrition are not as confusing as you might think. A primary strategy for making consistent healthy choices is to find the time to plan so you have healthy foods that you enjoy readily available to you, helping you to stave off unhealthy temptations. This chapter will help you explore how to consistently consume a balanced and varied diet in a society that often promotes unhealthy choices.

Eating Well: Balanced and Clean

Although the expression *eating clean* doesn't have an official definition, this is a common term used to describe eating foods that are as close to their natural state as possible. The term *processed* has taken on a negative connotation. Many people associate processed foods with those that are high in added sugar, salt, fat, and preservatives, but this is not always the case. Processing is simply altering a food product before consumption. Methods include freezing, pasteurizing, cooking, canning, preserving, baking, and fortifying with vitamins and minerals. Thanks to processing, we can enjoy a safer and more varied diet. Although the idea to "eat clean" is theoretically good, being too rigid in this practice is often impractical and sometimes unsafe.

Beyond Calories to Fuel Quality

Many people reduce nutrition down to a food's energy content, or calories. However, the quality of your food also matters. If you put low-quality fuel into your car, it won't run very well. The same is true for your body—if you don't consistently provide it with high-quality fuel, you won't run very well either. Running in this case goes beyond exercise to include productive mental concentration, motivational energy, and mood management. Running well in the long term also includes reducing the risk for the metabolic big three (cardiovascular disease, type 2 diabetes, and cancer), introduced in chapter 4, osteoporosis and sarcopenia, introduced in chapter 7, and other chronic health conditions.

Essential Nutrients

A useful way to consider your healthy diet is to start thinking beyond the good taste and pleasure of food and drink to the nutrients they can provide. Your diet should provide about 45 essential nutrients. These are deemed essential because your body cannot provide them, at least not without causing other conditions or diseases. The six main classes of essential nutrients include carbohydrates, fats, and proteins (or **macronutrients**); vitamins and minerals (**micronutrients**); and water. Figure 8.1 lists the three primary macronutrients in order of energy density. Note that although alcohol is neither a macronutrient nor considered essential, it does contribute calories to daily energy intake.

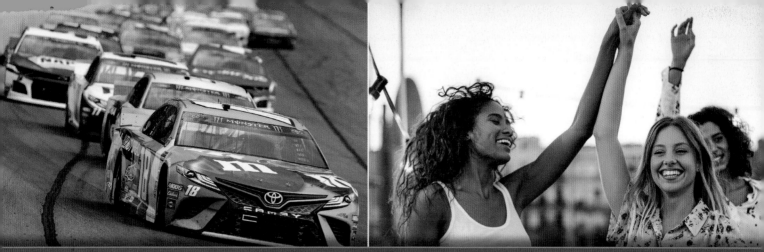

Just as race cars require high-quality fuel to run properly, your body needs high-quality food and drink to give you optimal energy.

Calories

A calorie is a unit of energy used to describe many scientific processes. When the word *calorie* is mentioned, what comes to mind? Something that can lead to unwanted weight gain? Something you require for energy to make it through the day? Do you think of this term when reading nutrition labels? A **calorie** (or, more correctly, a **kilocalorie**) is the way that energy from foods and drinks is expressed. Because most people are familiar with the term *calorie*, which is also used on food labeling, we will use it in this book rather than *kilocalorie*.

Energy Needs

An individual's energy needs are influenced by age, biological sex, height, weight, exercise or physical activity, and health conditions. In addition, a need or desire to lose, gain, or maintain weight can affect how many calories you need. The dietary guidelines in this chapter provide an estimate of energy needs based on age and biological sex, as well as physical activity levels. Chapter 9 explores energy needs more fully in the context of weight management.

Carbohydrates: Great Energy Sources

Carbohydrates are the body's main source of energy. During digestive processes, carbohydrates are broken down into glucose for immediate use as fuel or stored for later use in the liver and muscles in the form of glycogen. To say that carbohydrates are essential for healthy living is an understatement: Glucose is the sole energy source for the brain. Carbohydrates provide working muscles

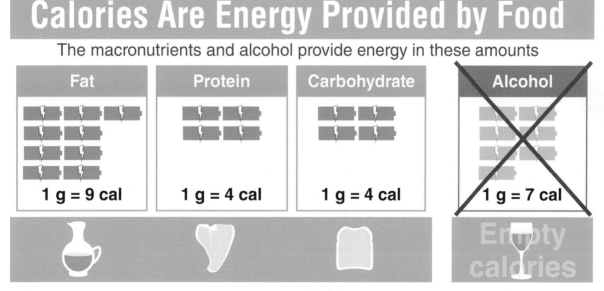

Figure 8.1 Macronutrients and alcohol vary in the number of calories they provide per gram.

with a readily available energy source, especially during high-intensity exercise. Compared to fat and protein, only a small amount of carbohydrate is stored in the body.

What foods can you think of that contain carbohydrates? If you think of bread, potatoes, pasta, and cookies, you are certainly correct, but other main sources are fruits and vegetables. Compared with the other macronutrients, carbohydrates typically contribute the most energy in terms of daily caloric intake. In fact, the current recommendation is that 45 to 65 percent of your total daily caloric intake should be from carbohydrates (see figure 8.3 later in the chapter; U.S. Department of Agriculture and U.S. Department of Health and Human Services 2020). Table 8.1 summarizes the types of carbohydrates that are classified as **simple carbohydrates** or **complex carbohydrates**, the latter of which is further divided into **refined carbohydrates** and **whole grains** (Institute of Medicine 2005a).

Simple Carbohydrates

Your taste buds identify simple carbohydrates because they add sweetness to our foods. Although they are found naturally in fruits and milk, simple carbohydrates are also added to soft drinks, fruit drinks, candy, desserts, yogurt, condiments, and plant-based milks such as soy milk, as some examples.

Beware of Added Sugars

Added sugars are those that do not occur organically in foods but are added by the food manufacturer or the consumer. Sugars that naturally occur in fruits or milk are not considered added. If, on the other hand, you put brown sugar in your oatmeal, honey in your tea, or sugar in your morning coffee, you have added sugars to your diet. Although most people generally recognize these intentional additions of sugar and other obvious sources like soda and cookies, hidden sources in packaged foods are more challenging to identify. These may include yogurt and peanut butter, processed fruit blends or punches, energy drinks, salad dressings and spaghetti sauces, and most processed snack goods. Many foods that are high in added sugars are low-quality fuel, providing unneeded calories and minimal nutrients. In addition to increasing your risk for obesity and other metabolic diseases, added dietary sugars are also linked with tooth decay. Because added sugars in the diet are a major public health concern, there are specific guidelines to limit the amount of added sugar in the diet; these will be outlined later in this chapter. In addition, the U.S. Food and Drug Administration (FDA) recently updated its Nutrition Facts label requirements to clearly identify the amount of added sugar to help the consumer make healthy decisions. You will learn about food labeling later in this chapter.

> With the recently revised Nutrition Facts label, it is easier than ever to detect added sugars in food.

Complex Carbohydrates: Refined Carbohydrates and Whole Grains

Whole grains are complex carbohydrate sources that include the germ, endosperm, and bran of

Table 8.1 Types of Carbohydrates

Simple carbohydrates (sugars): Lack vitamins, minerals, and fiber	Complex carbohydrates: Provide vitamins, minerals, and fiber
Monosaccharides: Single-sugar molecules • Glucose • Fructose • Galactose	Starches: Long, complex chains of sugar molecules • Grains (wheat, rice, oats) • Legumes (beans, peas, lentils) • Tubers and vegetables (potatoes, yams, corn)
Disaccharides: Double-sugar molecules • Sucrose or table sugar (fructose + glucose) • Maltose or malt sugar (glucose + glucose) • Lactose or milk sugar (galactose + glucose)	Fiber: Nondigestible carbohydrates • Soluble (oats and barley, beans, peas, and lentils; some fruits and vegetables) • Insoluble (wheat bran, vegetables, whole grains)

Data from Institute of Medicine (2005a).

the grain (figure 8.2). Compared to processed carbohydrates, whole grains are often more energy dense and contain more nutrients, including fiber, B vitamins, and minerals (Whole Grains Council n.d.). When whole grains are refined, the germ and bran are often removed, mainly leaving behind the starchy endosperm. This processing is how brown rice becomes white rice and whole-wheat flour becomes white flour. Foods made from refined grains are often enriched and fortified with vitamins and minerals, but not all nutrients lost during the refinement process are replaced. For this reason, the Dietary Guidelines for Americans recommends that consumers choose half of their grain sources from whole grains. Some examples include brown rice, whole-wheat or whole-grain bread, whole-wheat pasta, quinoa, and popcorn. Whole grains play an important role in weight management and gastrointestinal health due to their fiber content (U.S. Department of Agriculture and U.S. Department of Health and Human Services 2020).

Fiber: Beyond Bathroom Business

If the discussion of fiber makes you snicker because of its well-known link to essential bathroom business, you are not alone—but the benefits of fiber are no laughing matter. Unlike the starchy, digestible component, fiber is the nondigestible carbohydrate in plants. As fiber moves through the intestinal tract, it provides bulk for fecal matter in the large intestine, which ultimately assists in elimination—a technical way to describe that essential bathroom business. Depending on the type of fiber you consume, the bacteria processing in the large intestine results in gas. Bothersome and sometimes painful gas can result from consuming too much fiber, especially when it is not consumed regularly (Institute of Medicine 2005a).

Two types of dietary fiber exist, both of which are important for health. The first, soluble fiber, delays stomach emptying, slows glucose uptake into the blood after eating, and reduces absorption of cholesterol. Good sources of this type of fiber are oat bran and some fruits and beans, peas, and lentils. The second, insoluble fiber, increases fecal matter bulk and prevents constipation, hemorrhoids, and other digestive disorders. This type of fiber is found in wheat bran or psyllium seed, the latter being found in some cereals and fiber supplements and laxatives. Even though humans cannot digest

> Keep your bathroom business in order by meeting the recommendation for fiber intake for young adults: 28 grams per day for females and 34 grams per day for males (U.S. Department of Agriculture and U.S. Department of Health and Human Services 2020).

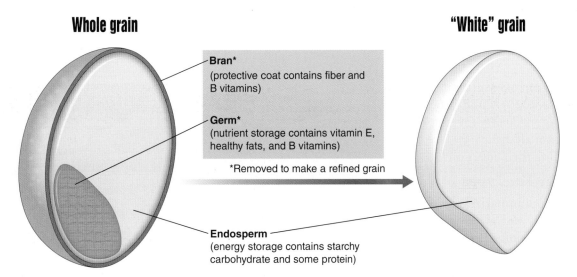

Whole grain   **"White" grain**

Bran*
(protective coat contains fiber and B vitamins)

Germ*
(nutrient storage contains vitamin E, healthy fats, and B vitamins)

*Removed to make a refined grain

Endosperm
(energy storage contains starchy carbohydrate and some protein)

Figure 8.2 Whole grains include the germ, endosperm, and bran of the grain, whereas refined grains have only the endosperm.

fiber, it is critical to aid digestion of other foods. See table 8.1 for food choices that provide good sources of both soluble and insoluble fiber (Institute of Medicine 2005a; U.S. Department of Agriculture and U.S. Department of Health and Human Services 2020).

Fats: Unsaturated, Saturated, and Trans Fats

Dietary fats have a complicated reputation. In fact, you might think of them as the good (unsaturated), the bad (saturated), and the ugly (trans fats). High levels of certain fats in the diet can increase risk for cardiovascular disease. Fats also pack the most calories per gram, so intake is usually limited by those attempting to lose weight. However, as explained in chapter 4, dietary fats can also help with energy balance, especially under conditions of intense physical exertion or labor. Dietary fats assist your body in absorbing fat-soluble vitamins and add flavor and texture to foods. If you have ever eaten a low-fat cookie, you probably have noticed how dry it is compared to a conventional higher-fat option.

Dietary Fat Recommendations

As illustrated in figure 8.3, the current recommendation for dietary fat is 20 to 35 percent of your total daily caloric intake (U.S. Department of Agriculture and U.S. Department of Health and Human Services 2020). Like carbohydrates, there are several different types of dietary fats (e.g., animal based versus plant based). A few fats—linoleic acid and alpha linoleic acid, for example—are essential fatty acids, so they must be consumed in the diet (Institute of Medicine 2005a; U.S. Department of Agriculture and U.S. Department of Health and Human Services 2020). Food processing often alters dietary fat properties. Thus, not all dietary fats are equal regarding their effect on health.

Dietary Fat Types

Table 8.2 summarizes the types of fatty acids and gives examples of foods that contain them. Although many foods contain a combination of **saturated fatty acids** and **unsaturated fatty acids**, you can typically tell the main source by the characteristics of the food. Saturated fats are primarily contained in animal products, such as fatty meats and butter; however, they are also contained in oils from tropical plants, including coconut and palm oils. They are easy to identify because they are solid at room temperature. Alternatively, unsaturated fats most often come from plant sources and are typically liquid at room temperature. Fatty fish, such as salmon, are also a source of unsaturated fats. Unsaturated fats are often further described by their chemical structure as monounsaturated fats (MUFAs) and polyunsaturated fats (PUFAs). PUFAs are further classified by their chemical structure into omega-3 and omega-6 sources (Institute of Medicine 2005a; U.S. Department of Agriculture and U.S. Department of Health and Human Services 2020).

Because the food industry is on a quest to bring products to the marketplace that offer taste at a lower price with a longer shelf life, food scientists have discovered processes to change naturally occurring fats. One common process is hydrogenation, which takes an unsaturated vegetable oil and converts it to a mixture of saturated fatty acids that creates a more solid fat from a liquid fat. What is the benefit of **hydrogenated oils**? Hydrogenation increases stability of oils so that they can be reused for deep frying, a practice common in restaurant businesses. Hydrogenation also improves the texture of many foods—for example, making pie crusts flakier. Finally, hydrogenation is the critical process that makes a margarine or vegetable shortening from a liquid oil.

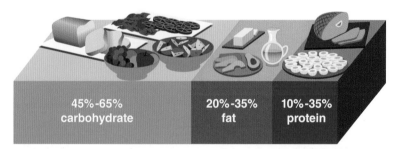

Recommended Intake of Calories for Healthy Adults

Figure 8.3   Recommended macronutrient distribution for young adults (U.S. Department of Agriculture and U.S. Department of Health and Human Services 2020).

Table 8.2 Types of Fatty Acids

Type of fatty acids	Common sources
Saturated	Animal fats, especially fatty meats (e.g., beef steaks) and poultry fat and skin Butter, cheese, and other high-fat dairy products Palm and coconut oils
Trans (avoid, if at all possible)	Partially hydrogenated oils (banned from the food supply in 2018) Small amount occurs naturally in animal fats such as beef and dairy
Monounsaturated	Olive, canola, and safflower oils Avocados and olives Peanut butter (without added fats) Many nuts such as almonds, cashews, and pecans
Polyunsaturated: Omega-3	Fatty fish such as salmon, white albacore tuna, anchovies, and sardines Walnuts, flaxseed, soybean oils, dark green leafy vegetables
Polyunsaturated: Omega-6	Corn, soybean, cottonseed oils (used in margarines and salad dressings)

Data from Institute of Medicine (2005a); U.S. Department of Agriculture and U.S. Department of Health and Human Services (2020).

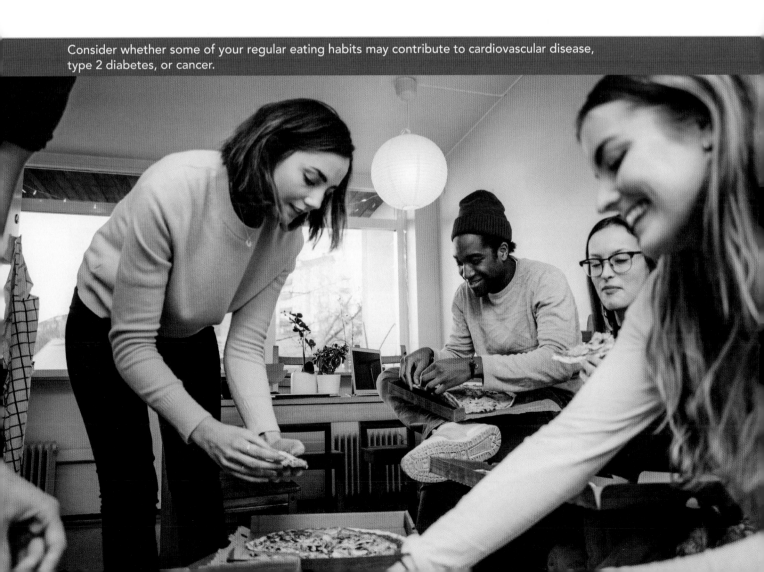

Consider whether some of your regular eating habits may contribute to cardiovascular disease, type 2 diabetes, or cancer.

The hydrogenation process also changes some unsaturated fatty acids into **trans fatty acids** (trans fats). Although very small amounts of trans fats occur naturally in animal fats, including beef and dairy products, the great majority of trans fat consumed in the American diet in recent years came from artificial trans fats in packaged and commercially available foods (e.g., fast food) that contain partially hydrogenated oils. In response to the discovery that the consumption of trans fats is linked to a significant increase in coronary heart disease, the U.S. Food and Drug Administration (FDA) banned the use of partially hydrogenated oils in the food supply in 2018 (U.S. Food and Drug Administration 2018).

Protein: Building Blocks of Muscle and Tissue

Of the macronutrients, protein is a popular dietary topic. However, for most Americans, protein contributes the least amount to their daily calories. Most people think about muscles when they think about protein. However, protein is also important for bones, blood, enzymes, cell membranes, some hormones, and optimal immune function. The building blocks of proteins are amino acids, 20 of which exist in food. Nine of these are essential, which means they cannot be synthesized by the human body and must be consumed. The remaining 11 amino acids can be created through various metabolic processes (Institute of Medicine 2005a). Being protein deficient can be harmful to many systems within the body; thus, having adequate protein intake in your diet is clearly important for health.

Protein Foods

Like carbohydrates and fats, protein can originate from both animal and plant sources, including meat, poultry, eggs, seafood, nuts, seeds, and soy products. Dairy can also be an important source of protein, as can beans, peas, and lentils. However, some sources of protein are considered less healthy than others because they are also high in saturated fat and negatively influence heart health. Table 8.3 highlights common protein sources. As discussed in chapter 13, the healthier choices may improve blood pressure and blood cholesterol levels, whereas the less healthy choices can be harmful to your heart and, as a general daily rule, should be limited (Academy of Nutrition and Dietetics 2022).

Get the Right Amount of Protein

Because protein is good for muscles, we often think that eating more is better. As depicted earlier in figure 8.3, the recommended range for protein is 10 to 35 percent of total daily calories (U.S. Department of Agriculture and U.S. Department of Health and Human Services 2020). Most healthy adults should aim for the recommended dietary allowance of protein for their age and sex. For females aged 19 to 30, 5.5 ounce-equivalents are recommended. For males aged 19 to 30, 6.5 ounce-equivalents are recommended. However, if

Table 8.3 Protein Sources in Daily Dietary Intakes

👍 Healthy protein sources	👎 Less healthy protein sources
Meat: Lean cuts of beef, lamb, goat, pork loin	Meat: Bacon, chorizo, hot dogs, lunch meats, organ meats, processed meats
Poultry: Skinless chicken and turkey	Poultry: Chicken fried steak, fried chicken
Fish and seafood: Salmon, tuna, cod, shrimp, mackerel, lobster, catfish, crab	Fish and shellfish: Breaded and fried options
Low-fat or fat-free dairy: Yogurt, milk, cheese, cottage cheese	Whole-fat dairy: Whole milk or other whole-fat dairy products (e.g., cottage cheese)
Legumes: Beans, peas, and lentils	
Nuts and seeds: Walnuts, almonds, chia seeds, pumpkin seeds, pistachios, cashews, peanuts	

Adapted from Academy of Nutrition and Dietetics (2022).

a person is very physically active or has certain medical conditions, they may need more protein. People who are pregnant or breastfeeding also may need additional protein. Varying protein sources from those among the healthier choices listed in tables 8.3 and 8.4 is also recommended. In general, most Americans would benefit from shifting their protein intake to include seafood twice a week and legumes (beans, peas, lentils) more often in place of other meat or poultry (Academy of Nutrition and Dietetics 2022).

Note that the recommendations for protein foods are expressed in ounce-equivalents. One ounce-equivalent is equal to 1 ounce of cooked meat, poultry, or fish; 1/4 cup of cooked beans; 1 egg; 1 tablespoon of peanut butter; or 1/2 ounce of nuts or seeds. Many common servings provide more than 1 ounce of protein. For example, both a small chicken breast and a can of tuna provide 3 ounce-equivalents of protein.

Nearly all Americans consume adequate levels of protein in their diets. Consuming more than the recommended amount of protein is typically not harmful, except potentially in the following situations:

- *Kidneys and dehydration.* The metabolic processing of dietary protein challenges kidney function and increases urine excretion, which is not a problem if your kidney function and protein intake are in normal ranges. However, if your kidneys are compromised, which often happens with age or with unique medical conditions, or if your protein intake is excessive, you could be damaging your kidneys and causing dehydration.

- *Calories.* Excessive protein, if not incorporated into muscle or tissue growth or repair, will be stored as excess energy in the form of adipose (fat) tissue. Many dietary protein sources are high in fat.

- *Disordered eating.* Being very rigid with eating routines, including with protein foods and supplements, can be a sign of disordered eating. Having quality protein in your diet is important, but if this aspect of your diet is starting to compromise your social relationships and ability to enjoy a variety of foods in a variety of settings, take care to explore your relationship with dietary protein.

- *Financial considerations.* High-quality protein sources can also tax your budget. Protein powders and bars and other packaged foods can be expensive.

Dietary protein is provided by both animal and plant sources, including meats, dairy, beans, peas, and lentils.

Table 8.4   Foods Commonly Selected for Protein Content

Food	Serving size	Energy (calories)	Grams of protein
Meat, poultry, and seafood			
Ground beef (cooked; 90% lean)	3 oz (85 g)	184	22
Pork chop (boneless, broiled)	3 oz	144	22
Chicken breast (grilled)	3 oz	128	26
Salmon	3 oz	156	23
Egg (cooked, poached)	1	72	6
Dairy			
Milk (nonfat or skim)	1 cup	83	8
Yogurt (plain skim milk)	6 oz (170 g)	95	9.8
Yogurt (Greek, plain nonfat)	6 oz	100	17
Cheese (cheddar)	2/3 oz (20 g); 1 slice	78	4.6
Cottage cheese (1% milk fat)	4 oz (110 g)	81	14
Beans, peas, and lentils			
Lentils	1 cup	230	18
Black beans (boiled)	1 cup	227	15
Chickpeas (boiled)	1 cup	269	14.5
Peas (boiled)	1 cup	230	16.4
Soy foods			
Tofu*	1/2 cup	190	20
Soy milk* (light, plain)	1 cup	70	6
Seeds and nuts			
Pumpkin seeds (dried)	1/4 cup	180	9.75
Peanut butter* (smooth)	2 tbsp	191	7
Almonds (dried)	1/4 cup	206	7.25
Walnuts (black, dried)	1/4 cup	194	7.5

*Varies by manufacturer.

Micronutrients: Vitamins and Minerals

Although they provide no calories, **vitamins** and **minerals**, which are obtained through foods or supplements, are key to health. Most notably, fruits, vegetables, and grains are rich in vitamins and some key minerals. Many processed foods such as flour and breakfast cereals contain added vitamins and minerals. Because of the availability of these foods, vitamin or mineral deficiencies that are advanced enough to present noticeable signs and symptoms are rare. However, many Americans consume fewer vitamins and minerals than are recommended, which can predispose them to chronic conditions later in life. You can determine specific recommended intakes of vitamins and minerals based on your age, biological sex, body size, and physical activity from sources such as WebMD (www.webmd.com), the Academy of Nutrition and Dietetics (www.eatright.org), and the USDA's interactive website (www.nal.usda.gov/legacy/fnic/dri-calculator/index.php).

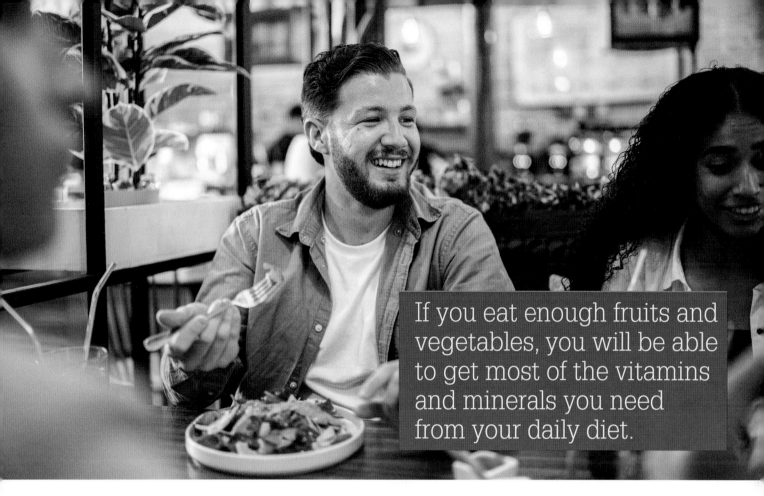

If you eat enough fruits and vegetables, you will be able to get most of the vitamins and minerals you need from your daily diet.

Vitamins

Vitamins are organic substances required in small amounts to assist with chemical reactions within the body. They are essential to produce red blood cells and for maintenance of key systems, including the nervous, skeletal, and immune systems. Vitamins E and C and the precursor to vitamin A (beta-carotene) are also considered **antioxidants**, which block the formation and action of **free radicals**, substances produced during regular metabolic processes that are known to promote aging and cancer. Antioxidants are part of a broader class called **phytochemicals**, located in plant foods, that prevent chronic diseases. In addition to the vitamins that are contained in food and supplements, a few vitamins are made in the body, including vitamins D and K, although consumption of these vitamins is still needed for optimal health (U.S. Department of Agriculture and U.S. Department of Health and Human Services 2020; Institute of Medicine 2005b).

The 13 vitamins required for human health are divided into fat- or water-soluble categories based on how they are absorbed, transported, and stored in the body. The four fat-soluble vitamins (A, D, E, and K) are carried by special protein carriers in the blood and stored in the liver and adipose tissues (hence the name *fat-soluble*). The nine water-soluble vitamins (B_6, B_{12}, biotin, C, folate, niacin, riboflavin, thiamin, and pantothenic acid) are absorbed directly into the bloodstream, where they travel freely. Water-soluble vitamins are removed by the kidneys and excreted in urine. Because of these differences, you are less likely to retain excessive water-soluble vitamins in your system than fat-soluble vitamins (U.S. Department of Agriculture and U.S. Department of Health and Human Services 2020; Institute of Medicine 2005b).

Minerals

Minerals are nonorganic elements that are required for human health, primarily to regulate body processes, grow and maintain bodily tissues, and produce energy. Of the 17 essential minerals, the key minerals that are needed in amounts greater than 100 milligrams per day are calcium, chloride, phosphorous, magnesium, potassium, and sodium. The essential trace minerals needed in very small amounts are copper, fluoride, iodine, iron, selenium, and zinc (U.S. Department of Agriculture and U.S. Department of Health and Human Services 2020; Institute of Medicine 2005b).

Too Much and Too Little

Unless an individual has abnormal or disordered eating patterns or inappropriately supplements vitamins and minerals in pill or powder form, excessive intake of vitamins and minerals is rare. Fat-soluble vitamins are of greatest concern because they are stored in the body, which can increase the risk of toxicity. On the other hand, inadequate intake of vitamins and minerals is very common.

> Colorful fruits and vegetables provide many key vitamins and minerals as well as fiber and energy!

Chronically poor nutritional habits are more common than nutritional deficiencies. Poor habits can result in an increased risk for chronic diseases later in life, including heart disease and osteoporosis. A varied and nutritionally balanced diet is usually sufficient to obtain adequate amounts of vitamins and minerals without supplementation (see table 8.5). Relying on supplements to gain most of your vitamins or minerals also makes you miss other important substances contained in food, such as fiber.

The Importance of Hydration

Hydration is an underappreciated health behavior. Compared to other nutrients, water is by far the most important. Water makes up 50 to 60 percent of our body weight. It is essential because it is the medium for chemical reactions and temperature regulation and is the main component of blood. Generally speaking, the human body can live several weeks to months (depending on body size and reserves) without food but only a few days without water. We lose water on a continual basis through urine and feces, evaporation from breathing processes, and, of course, from sweat.

Fluid recommendations for a young adult female is approximately 2.7 liters per day, with 2.2 liters (9 cups or 72 ounces) coming from beverages and a small amount being contained in foods. For an adult male, the recommended intake is around 3.7 liters per day, with 3.0 liters (13 cups or 104 ounces) coming from beverages (Institute of Medicine 2005b). All fluids, including coffee and tea, count toward total daily amounts. Your need for fluids is highly dependent on exertion and sweat rate, which are greatly affected by

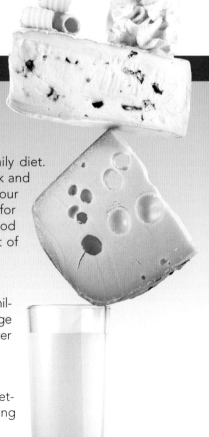

 Now and Later

Calcium Intake

Now

Few people meet their recommended calcium intake through their daily diet. Some of the best calcium sources are low-fat dairy products such as milk and yogurt. If dairy is not an option, try to get calcium from other sources in your diet, such as broccoli or fortified orange juice. The intake recommended for young adults (ages 19 to 30) is 1,000 milligrams per day; this includes food and supplements (U.S. Department of Agriculture and U.S. Department of Health and Human Services 2020).

Later

After the age of 51, the calcium recommendation increases to 1,200 and 1,000 milligrams per day for older females and males, respectively. Because of the change in hormones that occurs with the aging process, bone loss rapidly increases after middle age. People with low calcium intake have accelerated bone loss.

Take Home

To reduce your risk of bone fracture later in life, build your bone bank by getting an adequate amount of calcium in your diet. If you have trouble getting enough calcium from food, consider a supplement.

Table 8.5   Key Vitamins and Minerals

Vitamin or mineral	Common dietary source	Major function
Vitamin A	• Milk and cheese • Carrots, spinach, and other dark green and orange vegetables	• Maintenance of vision • Skin health • Health of linings of mouth, nose, and digestive tract • Function of immune system
Vitamin C	• Citrus fruits • Peppers, broccoli, brussels sprouts, tomatoes, and strawberries	• Maintenance and repair of connective tissue, bones, teeth, and cartilage • Promotion of healing • Assistance of iron absorption
Vitamin D[1]	• Fortified milk and butter • Fish oils • Egg yolks	• Development and maintenance of bones and teeth • Promotion of calcium absorption
Folate	• Green leafy vegetables and oranges • Whole grains and legumes	• Metabolism of amino acids • Synthesis of RNA and DNA • Synthesis of new cells
Calcium[1]	• Milk and milk products • Tofu • Fortified products (orange juice, bread) • Green leafy vegetables	• Formation of bones and teeth • Control of nerve impulses • Muscle contraction • Blood clotting
Iron[1]	• Meat and poultry • Fortified grain products • Dark green vegetables • Dried fruit (raisins)	• Formation of hemoglobin and myoglobin • Supports enzyme activity • Immune function
Magnesium[1]	• Grains and legumes • Nuts and seeds • Green vegetables • Milk • Water supply (except soft water)	• Nerve function • Energy production • Enzyme activation
Sodium[2]	• Table salt • Soy sauce • Fast and processed foods, especially lunch meats, canned soups, and vegetables	• Body water balance • Acid–base balance • Nerve function
Potassium[1]	• Meats and milk • Fruits and vegetables • Grains and legumes	• Body water balance • Nerve function

[1]Many young adults do not obtain enough vitamin D, calcium, iron, magnesium, or potassium in their diets. [2]Many young adults have too much sodium in their diets.

Data from U.S. Department of Agriculture and U.S. Department of Health and Human Services (2020); Institute of Medicine (2005b)

temperature, humidity, and exercise intensity. For example, a marathoner who runs for several hours in the heat and humidity in direct sunlight will lose much more water from sweat than someone exercising in an air-conditioned facility.

Hydration guidelines include prehydrating, hydration during the exercise session, and postexercise hydration. Monitoring body weight is a valid method to gauge hydration. It is important to avoid severe dehydration (a loss of 2 percent or more body weight), which causes weakness and can lead to death—fortunately, this is rare except in emergency situations or in response to a major illness such as the flu. However, many people suffer from chronic minor dehydration, which often does not lead to thirst. In addition to the color of your urine (see figure 8.4), other signs of mild dehydration are headaches, tiredness, lack of mental focus, and dizziness when standing up rapidly. Get in the habit of drinking a large glass of water when you get up in the morning, with each of your meals, and right before you go to bed.

Simple water is usually best for fluid replacement. However, in some situations, replacement with beverages that contain electrolytes and carbohydrates is warranted. Because hydration needs can be very individualized, consultation with a sports nutritionist or an athletic trainer may be necessary (American College of Sports Medicine 2007).

Nonessential Components: Alcohol and Caffeine

Alcohol and caffeine are not nutrients; however, both are common dietary components (U.S. Department of Agriculture and U.S. Department of Health and Human Services 2020). If you choose to consume alcohol and caffeine, like other aspects of your diet, you should strive to make wise choices.

Alcohol

Alcohol is a drug and must be respected for its many body-altering effects and its risk of addiction. However, the role that it plays in terms for energy balance and chronic disease is also important. Although it contains 7 calories per gram, alcohol is not considered a nutrient because it is not needed by the body. If alcohol is mixed with fruit or a sugar-sweetened beverage, the caloric content is increased. Chronic overconsumption of alcohol is a risk factor for many chronic diseases,

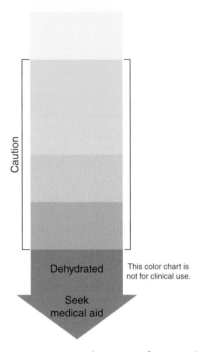

Figure 8.4   An easy way to determine if you are hydrated is to check the color of your urine.

including breast and stomach cancers, cardiovascular diseases, obesity, and fatty liver disease.

If you choose to consume alcohol, think about your alcohol consumption as a potential risk to your metabolic health and consider the recommendation of one drink or less per day for females and two drinks or less per day for males. (See figure 11.10 for what qualifies as one drink.) Remember that alcohol is a diuretic, which means it will dehydrate you. Finally, alcohol use and physical activity are not a good combination. Although many entertainment activities are centered around the interaction between alcohol and sports, slowed reaction times and impaired judgment increase the risk of injury. If these events take place out in the hot sun, the dehydration effects of the alcohol and the environment can result in heat illness. Just don't do it.

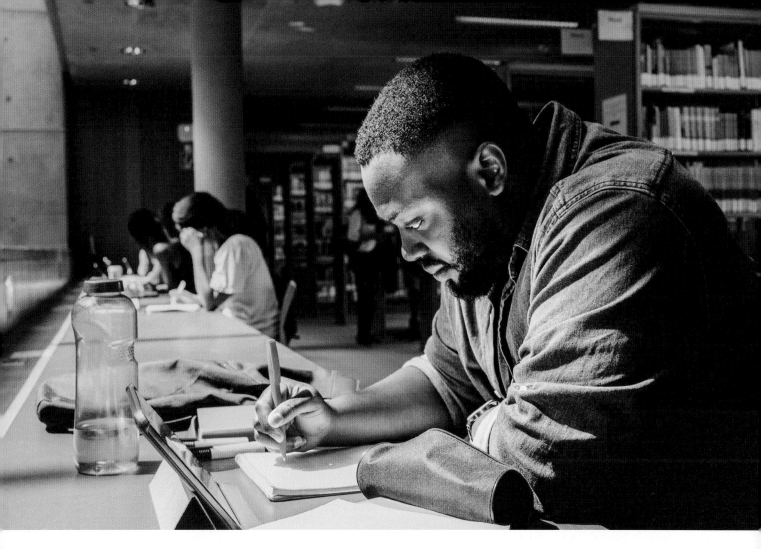

Caffeine

Like alcohol, caffeine is also a part of our social and cultural lives. As a stimulant, many individuals choose caffeine to start the day and aid in performance, both mentally and physically. Caffeine is not a nutrient and does not contribute to your caloric intake; however, it is the most widely used drug worldwide. Caffeine is typically consumed in coffee, tea, and soda. Do you consume your caffeine in sugary energy drinks, heavily sweetened coffee, or black tea? Be aware of the calorie content and added sugar in many tea and coffee drinks, not to mention caffeinated sodas. More caffeine is not necessarily better for energy or mental focus; depending on your tolerance, excessive caffeine intake can reduce your ability to focus. Caffeine abuse is also related to anxiety. In moderation, which can be defined as three to five cups of coffee per day (up to 400 milligrams), caffeine can be safe and part of a healthy diet (Academy of Nutrition and Dietetics 2020a).

Common caffeinated beverages include drip or brewed coffee, which contains 12 milligrams of caffeine per fluid ounce (mg/fl oz), instant coffee (8 mg/fl oz), espresso (64 mg/fl oz), brewed black tea (6 mg/fl oz), brewed green tea (2 to 5 mg/fl oz), and caffeinated soda (1 to 4 mg/fl oz). Energy drinks have the greatest variability of caffeine content (3 to 35 mg/fl oz). If caffeine is added to a food, it must be included in the listed ingredients on the Nutrition Facts label. Online sources, such as the Center for Science in the Public Interest (2021), have provided comprehensive resources for caffeine in common foods and beverages. Beverages can vary widely in their caffeine content, so read labels carefully.

The Many Benefits of a Healthy Diet

Now that you have been introduced to the primary considerations on your quest to have a balanced and high-quality diet, let's discuss motivational reasons for managing your eating and drinking behaviors. Why is eating healthy important to you? Contemplate what factors (e.g., family traditions, college friends, mood, stress, budget) influence your daily food and drink choices. Whatever your reasons, there are many benefits to consuming a healthy diet that can benefit you now so you can be a healthier version of yourself in the future.

Weight Management

Energy balance can be a challenge. Without understanding calorie counting and recognizing where calories are hidden in your diet, you may struggle to manage your weight. For example, many people do not recognize how many calories in their daily diet come from their drinks in the form of sweetened sodas, sport beverages, coffees, and teas. Learning about macronutrients and their associated calorie counts will help you understand the energy-in side of the energy balance equation, as explored in chapter 9.

Feeling and Performing Better

Fuel quality and hydration matter when it comes to performance, whether physical, mental, or social. Feeling sluggish because you are dehydrated can reduce the quality of your day. Skipping breakfast can give you low blood sugar and a headache by your midmorning classes—recall that your nervous system, especially your brain, uses glucose as its primary fuel source. Too much caffeine can also increase your anxiety. How you eat and drink can directly influence how you feel and how you perform academically.

Investment in a Healthier Future Version of Yourself

Over and above the link between dietary intake and weight management, diet has major implications for your risk of many chronic diseases, including the metabolic big three and other diseases related to body composition explained in chapter 7. Although these diseases and conditions do not typically develop until later, your choices today have direct implications for the risk factors.

Dietary Guidelines for Americans

The many food options available today can make it challenging to consistently make healthy choices. How do we know what and how to eat and drink to be healthy? Fortunately, scientists and governmental agencies have collaborated to provide recommendations and resources to aid the design of your personal nutrition program, helping you build a healthy and balanced diet to accommodate your food preferences and budget. A very accessible summary of these recommendations is provided within the Dietary Guidelines for Americans (DGA), as described next. Importantly, the DGA provides quantitative dietary guidance to prevent chronic disease and promote health for the average person; it does not provide dietary guidelines for disease treatments. Finally, in addition to using the DGA, you are encouraged to consult a **registered dietitian nutritionist** or **licensed dietitian (LD)** if you have unique dietary challenges such as food allergies or a chronic health condition such as an inflammatory bowel disease.

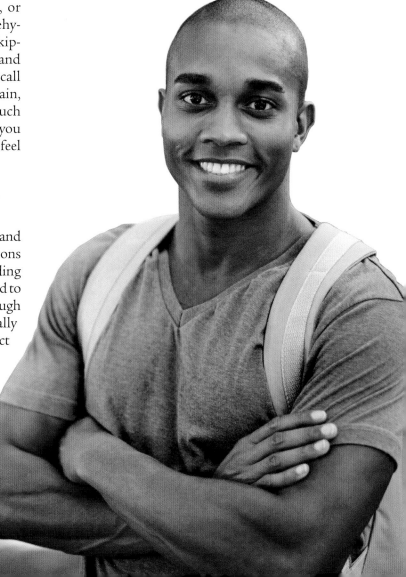

Goal Sources

The DGA provides goals for all macronutrients, minerals, and vitamins based on age, biological sex, and life stage. Key recommended intakes and optimal safety guidelines include the following:

- The recommended dietary allowance (RDA)
- The acceptable macronutrient distribution range (AMDR; see figure 8.3)
- Adequate intake (AI)
- Chronic disease risk reduction level (CDRR)
- The dietary guideline itself

The DGA document provides a wealth of information from many government and expert sources in one freely accessible document (www.dietaryguidelines.gov).

Framing Guidelines

Although you are highly encouraged to review the complete DGA, we will summarize four guidelines from the latest version to get you thinking about healthy eating and drinking, especially from a pattern perspective. Recall that your physical activity and sitting behaviors are best managed if they are thought of in terms of daily and weekly patterns (e.g., FITT). Similarly, the following four guidelines can help you manage your eating occasions (i.e., meals and snacks) across your busy days and weeks to improve the chances that you will make healthy choices that add up to a healthy dietary pattern.

Guideline 1: A Healthy Dietary Pattern Is Important for All Life Stages

The DGA defines *dietary pattern* as the combination of foods and beverages that make up a person's dietary intake over time (days, weeks, years, etc.). In other words, a dietary pattern is the totality of what a person typically eats or drinks, not individual foods or nutrients. It is important to recognize that it is never too late to change your eating patterns. However, every life stage—infancy, toddlerhood, childhood, adolescence, young adulthood, and older adulthood—brings different nutritional concerns and recommendations. In the emerging adult stage, meeting nutrition needs can help achieve a healthy body weight and reduce the risk of future chronic diseases.

The DGA provides several detailed examples of different dietary patterns that contain nutrient-dense options and appropriate portions. For example, the healthy U.S.-style pattern is based on the types and proportions of foods typically consumed by Americans, such as meat and dairy. It also provides a healthy Mediterranean-style dietary pattern that includes frequent consumption of unsaturated fats, such as seafood, olive oil, and plenty of fruits and vegetables. The Mediterranean diet has been associated with many positive health outcomes.

A healthy vegetarian dietary pattern is also detailed in the DGA and includes recommendations to provide all protein from plant sources. These diets tend to be lower in calories, saturated fats, and cholesterol and higher in whole grains and fiber. In practice, various vegetarian diets exist. Adherents may eat only plants (vegan); plants and dairy products (lacto-vegetarian); plants, dairy products, and eggs (lacto-ovo vegetarian); or plants, dairy products, eggs, and fish or seafood (pescatarian). People may select vegetarian diets for health reasons, religious preferences, ethical reasons, or environmental concerns, among others.

Guideline 2: Food Is Personal and Pleasurable

A healthy dietary pattern can benefit every person regardless of their age, race, ethnicity, or current health status. The DGA provides a framework for healthy eating with the flexibility to easily allow customizations based on personal preferences, cultural traditions, and budgetary constraints. It is recognized that meals are often social events grounded in family and cultural traditions. There are many options to have a healthy dietary intake! The DGA are intentionally not prescriptive and encourage people to "make it their own."

Guideline 3: Nutrient Density Is Critical for All Food Groups and Energy Balance

A cornerstone concept in the DGA is that nutritional needs should be met primarily by nutrient-dense foods and beverages across all food groups in the recommended amounts and within calorie limits. Nutrient-dense foods provide macronutrients, vitamins and minerals, and other health-promoting components (e.g., fiber) yet have little or no added sugars, saturated fat, and sodium. The core elements of a healthy dietary pattern include the following:

- Vegetables of all types, including dark green leafy vegetables and broccoli; red and orange vegetables; beans, peas, and lentils; and starchy vegetables
- Fruits, especially whole fruit
- Grains (recommended ≥50 percent whole grains)
- Dairy and fortified soy alternatives (fat-free or low-fat options recommended)
- Protein foods, including lean meat, poultry, and eggs; seafood; and nuts, seeds, and soy products (e.g., tofu and soy flour products)
- Oils, including vegetable oils and oils in food (e.g., seafood and nuts)

Guideline 4: Limit Added Sugars, Saturated Fat, Sodium, and Alcohol

A healthy dietary pattern meets nutrient recommendations and calorie needs to keep you in energy balance (assuming weight maintenance is the goal; see chapter 9). To meet these goals, follow the 85-15 guide: Consume 85 percent of your daily calories from nutrient-dense foods—that is, in forms that have the least amounts of added sugars, saturated fat, sodium, and alcohol—and the remaining 15 percent of daily calories can be "spent" on other food or drink. This equates to about 250 to 350 daily calories for most Americans. Specific recommendations for these dietary components of concern for adults includes the following:

- *Added sugars.* Added sugars should comprise less than 10 percent of daily calories, or about four and six tablespoons of sugar for females and males, respectively.

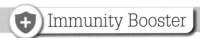 Immunity Booster

The Impact of Diet Quality on Immune Function

Like the effects of regular exercise, your diet quality also influences your immune function. For example, adherence to the Mediterranean diet is known to be protective against chronic low-grade inflammatory diseases, including cardiovascular disease, type 2 diabetes, and cancer, and is also associated with reduced cognitive decline and depression symptoms (Casas, Sacanella, and Estruch 2014). Relatedly, with respect to the recent pandemic, recent research suggests that a dietary pattern that includes more healthy plant-based foods is also linked to lower risk and severity of COVID-19 (Merino et al. 2021).

The take-home message is that healthy fueling habits have benefits beyond helping you feel energetic and managing your weight in your college years. This important health behavior also helps prevent chronic disease, improves brain health, and directly impacts your ability to fight off viruses, including COVID-19. Just another motivational reason to eat your veggies!

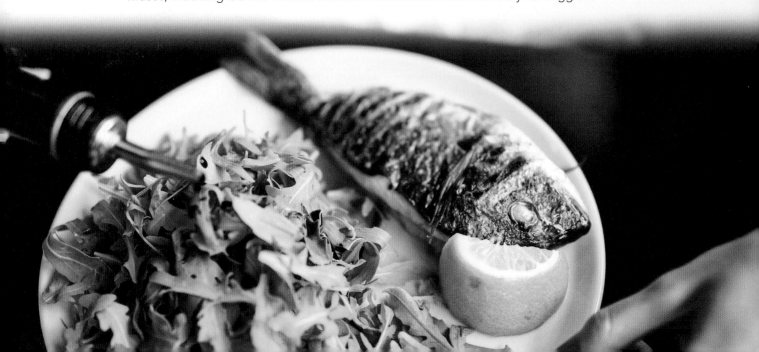

- *Fats.* Saturated fats should be limited to less than 10 percent of daily calories.
- *Sodium.* Less than 2,300 milligrams of sodium per day should be consumed.
- *Alcoholic beverages.* As discussed previously, adults of legal drinking age can choose not to drink or to do so in moderation. Males should limit drinks to two or fewer per day and females should limit drinks to one or fewer per day. Drinking less is always healthier than drinking more. Individuals with certain health conditions should not drink alcohol, including those who are pregnant.

Replacing foods that are high in added sugars, fats, and sodium with more fruits, vegetables, whole grains, and low-fat dairy foods will go a long way toward improving your diet quality. Try to find opportunities to practice subbing in healthy foods.

Can MyPlate Be Your Plate?

Even though you may completely understand the recommendations for healthy eating, it still can feel overwhelming to put your knowledge into practice. A picture is worth a thousand words. MyPlate is the USDA's visual teaching tool for helping Americans meet their recommended nutrient intake (figure 8.5). This online source provides a wealth of information on how to make the healthy choice the easy choice. A major theme of this tool is personalization—you can customize the recommendations to fit your goals, health needs, tastes, and other factors. The key message of MyPlate is that selecting moderate portions of a variety of nutrient-dense foods will provide a strong framework for your balanced dietary plan. The chapter 8 labs in HK*Propel* will provide an opportunity to determine your basic knowledge of nutritional practices using the interactive ChooseMyPlate website.

Reading Nutrition Facts Labels

One way to meet the recommendations highlighted in MyPlate is to select unprocessed foods. Dried beans and nuts, fresh or frozen fruits and vegetables, low-fat dairy, whole grains such as brown rice and oatmeal, and lean, fresh meats are all examples of nutrient-dense foods that likely do not have an extensive Nutrition Facts label, although you can find nutrient information for

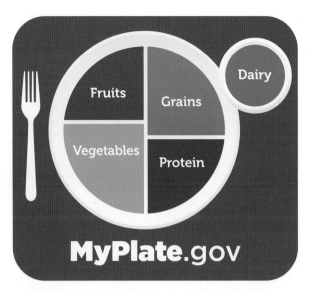

Figure 8.5   Search MyPlate.gov for information to calculate a personalized food plan.

Reprinted from U.S. Department of Agriculture (2020).

these foods on the USDA website. However, the FDA does require labeling for all packaged foods for the consumer to make informed food choices (U.S. Food and Drug Administration 2014).

Nutrition Facts Label

The five mandatory requirements for all food labels are statement of identity (what is the product), net contents of package, nutrition information, list of ingredients (in order of percentage from largest to smallest), and manufacturer information. The FDA recently updated the Nutrition Facts label on packaged foods and beverages, the first major update to the label in over 20 years. The updated Nutrition Facts label includes several important values, as shown in figure 8.6:

1. The serving size and servings per container
2. The amount of calories per serving
3. The macronutrients (total fat, total carbohydrate, and protein), nutrients and components of concern (added sugars, saturated fat, sodium, and fiber), and vitamins and minerals of concern (vitamin D, calcium, iron, and potassium)
4. Percent of daily value (%DV) of each component
5. An explanation of %DV based on a 2,000 calorie diet

The FDA provides an excellent resource about how to understand and use the Nutrition Facts label (U.S. Food and Drug Administration 2020). The chapter 8 labs on HK*Propel* will give you an opportunity to practice your Nutrition Facts label reading skills.

Food Package Nutrient and Health Claims

Understanding food labels can also greatly assist you on your grocery shopping trips. Food-labeling regulations by the FDA require that products meet very distinct definitions before they can make the following types of food-packaging claims.

✓ Behavior Check

Do You Make the Grade?

The Healthy Eating Index (HEI) is a measure of diet quality that has been used to assess compliance with the DGA based on U.S. population data (U.S. Department of Agriculture and U.S. Department of Health and Human Services 2020). A perfect HEI score of 100 indicates that the recommendations, on average, were met or exceeded. Although all age groups scored poorly, the groups that were the unhealthiest were adolescents aged 9 to 13 and 14 to 18, with HEI scores of 51 and 52, respectively. The group with the best score was older adults: Those aged 60 years or older scored a 63. For adults aged 19 to 30, years that typically span college and early adulthood, the HEI score was 56. This failing score is alarming. Within food groups, this cohort did not meet recommendations for vegetables, fruits, or dairy intake. Although recommendations were met for total grains, intakes for whole grains were low and refined grains were high. Females met and males exceeded total protein intake recommendations; however, both sexes could benefit from increased seafood intake.

Table 8.6 illustrates that the great majority of young adults exceed recommended limits for added sugars, saturated fats, and sodium described in guideline 4. By increasing fruit and vegetable intakes and reducing added sugars, saturated fats, and sodium to be within the recommended limits, you can greatly improve your healthy fueling grade. The chapter 8 labs will help you determine if you are getting a passing HEI grade for your diet quality.

Table 8.6 Healthy Fueling Report Card

Dietary component	Limit recommendation	Males	Females	Top three sources
Added sugars	10% of total daily energy	62% exceed	66% exceed	1. Sugar-sweetened beverages 2. Desserts and sweet snacks 3. Coffee and tea
Saturated fats	10% of total energy	76% exceed	71% exceed	1. Sandwiches 2. Desserts and sweet snacks 3. Rice, pasta, and grain-based mixed dishes
Sodium	2,300 mg	97% exceed	84% exceed	1. Sandwiches 2. Rice, pasta, and grain-based mixed dishes 3. Meat, poultry, and seafood mixed dishes

Note: Current HEI score for Americans ages 19 to 30 (on a scale of 0-100): 56 = F.

Adapted from U.S. Department of Agriculture and U.S. Department of Health and Human Services (2020).

1. Serving Size

This section is the basis for determining the number of calories, amount of each nutrient, and percent Daily Value (%DV) of a food. Use it to compare a serving size to how much you actually eat. Serving sizes are given in familiar units, such as cups or pieces, followed by the metric amount, e.g., number of grams. The serving size reflects the amount people typically eat and drink today. It is not a recommendation of how much to eat.

2. Amount of Calories

If you want to manage your weight (lose, gain, or maintain), this section is especially helpful. The key is to balance how many calories you eat with how many calories your body uses.

3. Nutrients

You can use the label to support your personal dietary needs—look for foods that contain more of the nutrients you want to get more of and less of the nutrients you may want to limit.

- Nutrients to get more of: Dietary Fiber, Vitamin D, Calcium, Iron and Potassium. The recommended goal is to consume at least 100% Daily Value for each of these nutrients each day.
- Nutrients to get less of: Saturated fat, Sodium, and Added Sugars. The recommended goal is to stay below 100% Daily Value for each of these nutrients each day.

4. Percent Daily Value

This section tells you whether the nutrients (for example, saturated fat, sodium, dietary fiber, etc.) in one serving of food contribute a little or a lot to your total daily diet: 5%DV or less is low and 20%DV or more is high.

5. Footnote

The footnote explains that the %Daily Value (DV) tells you how much a nutrient in a serving of food contributes to a daily diet. 2,000 calories a day is used for general nutrition advice.

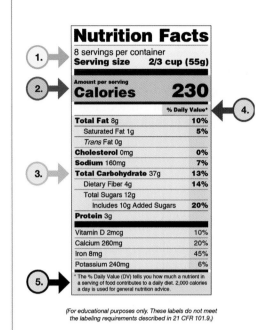

Figure 8.6   Everything you need to know about the FDA Nutrition Facts Label.
Reprinted from U.S. Food and Drug Administration (2019).

- ***Authorized health claims and qualified health claims.*** Authorized health claims indicate that significant scientific evidence has been shown to link the food or ingredient in question to a decreased risk of a disease or health-related condition (e.g., "Adequate calcium throughout life may reduce the risk of osteoporosis"). A qualified health claim is supported by some scientific evidence but does not meet the standards required by the FDA for an authorized health claim and must include a disclaimer or other qualifying language.

- ***Structure or function claims.*** These indicate how a nutrient or ingredient influences the normal structure or function of the body (e.g., "Calcium builds strong bones").

- ***Nutrient content claims.*** Most claims on food packages are nutrient content claims, which make a statement about the level of a nutrient in a product (e.g., "Excellent source of calcium"). These claims can be very confusing. Commonly used terms include *free, low, reduced* or *less, healthy, light, high, good source, more, lean* or *extra lean, high potency, modified, fiber source,* and *antioxidants.* Many of these terms can be applied to different products or foods targeting calories, fat, cholesterol, or sodium.

For current information about labeling requirements, go to the FDA website and review the Nutrition Labeling and Education Act (U.S. Food and Drug Administration 2014).

Common Dietary Limitations: Allergies and Intolerances

Having allergies or intolerances to various food sources is common. Food allergies often start early in life and may be outgrown, whereas about 15 percent develop in adulthood. They occur when your body's immune system reacts to a substance, most often a protein within a food. Signs of a food allergy are similar to other allergies, ranging from a runny nose or itchy eyes to a major life-threatening anaphylactic event. A food intolerance is not the same as a food allergy. The symptoms of food intolerance generally include abdominal cramping and diarrhea, which are not life threatening, although this could lead to dietary deficiencies if left untreated. Although many types of food allergies are known, nearly 90 percent are related to what are commonly thought of as the *big eight* (Academy of Nutrition and Dietetics 2020b):

1. Milk
2. Eggs
3. Shellfish (shrimp, lobster, crab)
4. Fish (pollock, salmon, cod, tuna, snapper, eel, tilapia)
5. Peanuts
6. Tree nuts (walnuts, cashews)
7. Wheat
8. Soy

Gluten, a protein found in common cereal grains (mainly wheat, barley, rye, and spelt), also deserves a special mention given its recent public attention. The gluten-sensitivity spectrum ranges from a mild allergy to severe celiac disease. Symptoms depend on the degree of sensitivity, ranging from mild allergy symptoms and diarrhea to more intensive digestive distress to a cluster of more subjective symptoms such as headaches, muscle and joint pain, and fatigue. Increased research and public attention to gluten sensitivity has created greater awareness, and

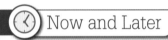
Now and Later

Sustaining You and the Earth

Now

Choosing a dietary pattern like a vegetarian or Mediterranean diet can save you saturated fat calories and money, especially if you prepare your food at home. For example, a large pot of bean soup can be relatively inexpensive to make in your slow cooker compared to a similar amount of a beef stew.

Later

Small choices add up over time for your waistline, your arteries, and your pocketbook. These small choices also add up for our environment. For example, beef and dairy cattle are very environmentally expensive in terms of land use, water use, greenhouse gas emissions, and ultimately ecosystem disruption. You could easily reduce your environmental footprint by eating less meat and dairy.

Take Home

On your way to being a healthier you, remember to think socially when acting personally. Food choices affect your health, but they also have major long-term effects on our planet. This does not mean that everyone should be a vegetarian; however, by making small changes, you can be healthier and help our planet, too. For example, try meatless Mondays or eat only plant-based foods for one day per week. This could not only increase your fruit and vegetable intake but help you discover some new favorite dishes as well.

gluten-free products are now more widely available. However, the research regarding the benefits and potential adverse effects of avoiding gluten remains inconclusive. Although a gluten-free diet is currently very popular, it is neither intended for weight loss nor is it nutritionally superior to one containing gluten. Moreover, following a gluten-free diet can often be more expensive and can cause social and psychological barriers (Aljada, Zohni, and El-Matary 2021). If you suspect you have a gluten intolerance, consult your personal physician.

If you suspect or know you have a food allergy or intolerance, several steps can improve your quality of life:

- *Meet with a registered dietitian nutritionist.* An RDN can assist you with designing an eating plan that is nutritionally adequate and meets your lifestyle.

- *Learn about ingredients in your food.* Navigating menu items and dishes, especially when foods include a combination of ingredients, can be challenging. Ask questions and do your research.

- *Read labels carefully.* The FDA has mandated that food companies specify on product labels if foods contain any of the big eight allergens.

- *Inform friends and family.* Explain your food allergy so that your friends and family can accommodate your food requirements during social gatherings. This is especially critical if your allergy causes a life-threatening reaction.

Dietary Supplements

Supplement sales are a big business. Dietary supplements include vitamins, minerals, herbals and botanicals, amino acids, enzymes, and many other products. They can also come in a variety of forms: traditional tablets, capsules, and powders, as well as drinks and energy bars. Before supplementing, think carefully about your needs and check with your physician or an RDN. Remember that some supplements can cause damage to your health.

When Is a Supplement Needed?

Although a balanced dietary plan is the best way to meet your optimal vitamin and mineral needs, a supplement is needed in certain situations:

- Individuals of childbearing age who are pregnant or planning to become pregnant should consume adequate amounts of folate or folic acid (synthetic form) to prevent neural tube defects. This may require a supplement, often termed a *prenatal vitamin.*

- People who are older than 50 often have a reduced ability to absorb B_{12}. In addition to eating foods that supply this important vitamin, they may need supplements.

Although you may choose a gluten-free diet for a variety of reasons, it is not necessarily nutritionally superior.

- Individuals with heavy menstrual cycles may need additional iron to prevent anemia.
- Older people, those with dark skin, or people who do not receive enough natural sunlight may need vitamin D supplementation.
- Vegans may need B_{12}, calcium, and iron supplementation.

Supplement Quality

The FDA does not regulate dietary supplements (U.S. Food and Drug Administration 2019). In fact, manufacturers do not have to prove a supplement is safe or effective before selling it. The FDA can take action to remove or restrict the sale of a supplement from the market only if it has been proven unsafe. For this reason, consumers should exercise caution when choosing to use any supplements.

Manufacturers of supplements can voluntarily test their products for quality control. Those that meet the USP Dietary Supplement Verification Services are awarded the USP verified mark, which assists suppliers and consumers in determining quality. For more information, see www.usp.org/about.

Protein Supplements

Many people, typically biological males, on the quest for bigger muscles resort to protein supplements in the form of protein powders, bars, or drinks. Adequate protein can be obtained in the diet through whole foods for most healthy, recreationally active adults with good dietary habits. However, there might be exceptions to the protein recommendations. For example, research suggests that older adults do not metabolize protein the same way that younger individuals do and may need additional protein to get the same muscle-enhancing effects. Some highly trained strength-based athletes may also require higher levels of protein for peak performance (Phillips, Chevalier, and Leidy 2016). Remember that too much protein can be hazardous to your health.

Protein supplements are typically delivered in bars or powders and come from either soy or whey protein. Soy protein powder contains protein isolated from the soybean and made from the soybean meal. Whey is obtained from dairy milk processing. For people who are lactose intolerant or struggle to digest dairy products, whey isolate

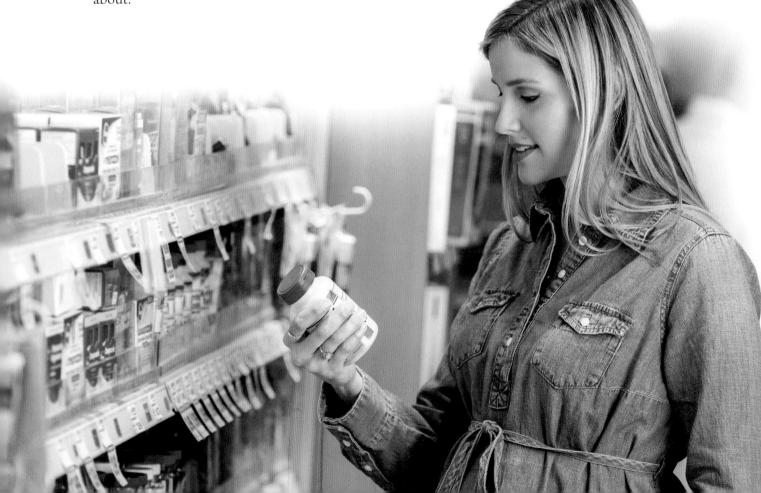

may provide benefits because it is low in lactose. Protein isolates and concentrates differ in terms of protein content as well as carbohydrate and fat.

In addition, many food protein sources are not very portable and require refrigeration. Protein powders, bars, and drinks can be a great option for a busy athlete or nonathlete alike; thus, some protein supplements and products may have a place in your dietary plan. Notably, dietary supplements are not regulated like food products in the market and can lead to excessive protein intake that can be dangerous to your health. If you decide to use protein supplements, do your research and read labels carefully; many protein bars on the market have a lot of added sugar. Also, it might be a good idea to consult a registered dietitian nutritionist (RDN) or licensed dietitian (LD) with expertise in sports performance or medical nutrition for your individual needs.

Food Safety Basics

Food allergies and intolerances are a concern for some people, but food safety is everyone's concern. If you have ever suffered from food poisoning, you understand how sick you can get from contaminated food. The federal government provides excellent resources to help keep you safe using good food practices. They advocate these four simple steps for food safety (see www.foodsafety.gov for more information):

1. *Clean.* Wash your hands and surfaces often! Illness-causing bacteria can survive in many places around the kitchen. Unless you wash your hands, utensils, and surfaces the correct way, you could spread these bacteria.

2. *Separate.* Don't cross-contaminate! Raw meat, poultry, seafood, and eggs can still spread illness-causing bacteria to ready-to-eat foods unless you keep them separate, which includes in your grocery cart and your refrigerator.

3. *Cook.* Cook to the right temperature! The danger zone for bacteria that cause food poisoning is between 40 and 140 degrees Fahrenheit (4 to 60 degrees Celsius). Bacteria multiply quickly, so knowing the right temperatures for various foods and cooking methods is essential.

4. *Chill.* Refrigerate promptly! Illness-causing bacteria can grow in foods within two hours, especially in a warm environment. Therefore, cooling foods promptly is critical. Keep meat and dairy consistently cool by placing them near the back of fridge.

See figure 8.7 for tips on planning wisely and choosing carefully to keep you on the right path as you design your personal nutritional plan.

Healthy Choices Require Planning

The more you plan ahead in terms of willpower, food purchasing, and preparation, the more you will be able to stick to a healthy diet. Making the healthy choice on a routine basis while managing a complicated daily schedule will require you to invest some thought and action into your nutritional plan.

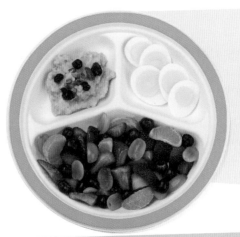

Start With Breakfast

Healthy fueling should be part of your planning. An important fuel of the day is typically breakfast. Know yourself. If you need a good breakfast to feel and perform well, plan the time to invest in this behavior.

Plan Your Fuel To-Do List

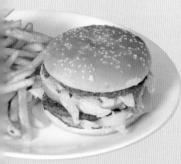

Stressful week of exams coming up! My main goals:

- Eat out only once this week. Eat homemade meals or at the dining hall the rest of the time.
- Plan all my meals so I don't overeat or overspend.
- Stay in budget at the grocery store.
- Pack healthy snacks and water in my backpack.

Plan for Healthy Eating at the Dining Hall

- Plan ahead of time what you will eat and make up your mind to stick with that plan.
- If you know you will be spending a long time at the dining hall, make a plan for how much you will eat and at what times. This will help you avoid mindless eating.
- Apply the knowledge you have gained from this chapter to your choices of food in the dining hall.

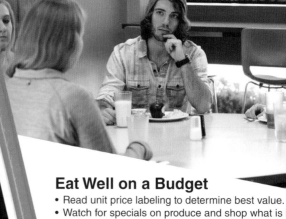

Eat Well on a Budget

- Read unit price labeling to determine best value.
- Watch for specials on produce and shop what is in season.
- Try frozen vegetables: They are just as nutritious as fresh and decrease likelihood of spoiling if they are not consumed right away.
- If storage is available, purchase frequently consumed foods in bulk.
- Make a grocery list and avoid shopping when you are hungry.
- Share spices, condiments, and other pantry staples with roommates and alternate preparing meals.
- Invest in a slow cooker so you can make large batches of food to refrigerate or freeze for later meals.
- If you notice that some fruits are not getting used, wash and dry them thoroughly, and freeze for later use in smoothies, pancakes, breads, or oatmeal.
- Buy meat in bulk and freeze what you won't be able to use right away.
- Choose water instead of soda, sweet tea, or fruit-flavored beverages.

Avoid Fast-Food Foibles

Fast food is generally not a healthy choice, but we turn to that option when we haven't planned ahead. In addition, fast food can cost two or three times more than eating at home. Plan ahead by buying ingredients to make quick and easy food. For example:

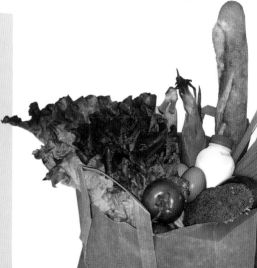

- Tortillas, shredded cheese, and sausage to make breakfast burritos
- Fresh vegetables put into containers for grab and go with hummus or cottage cheese dip
- Baked potatoes stuffed with salsa, broccoli, and low-fat cheese or cottage cheese
- Canned black or red beans heated and eaten over rice with low-fat cheese sprinkled on top

Eating out has a place in your life, but it should be the treat for the week, not a daily occurrence.

Figure 8.7 Plan wisely and choose foods carefully to create the best healthy dietary pattern for you.

Be Informed to Make the Best Food Decisions

No one diet is best. Most of the time, eating well really means making high-quality fuel choices. This starts with accessing quality information. The food marketplace can be overwhelming with the choices and marketing strategies. Be a smart consumer by consulting trusted and reliable sources and knowing the difference between trends and facts.

Consult sources endorsed by scientific and government agencies for the highest quality information.

- United States Department of Agriculture (USDA)
- Food and Drug Administration (FDA)
- The Food and Nutrition Board
- The Academy of Nutrition and Dietetics

Are Whole Foods Better?

It depends. Some food processing is healthy because it increases shelf life. However, packaged or processed foods often give you more of the bad stuff and less of the good stuff.

Read food labels. Compared to a processed food, eating the whole food version typically provides more vitamins and minerals, fiber, and healthy fats and less sodium, added sugars, and preservatives. If the ingredient list is long, chances are there are healthier alternatives.

Who Should I Trust to Advise Me?

It is important to know the difference between a "nutritionist" and a registered dietitian (RD) or licensed dietitian (LD), which are sometimes abbreviated as a registered dietitian nutritionist (RDN).

Registered Dietitian	Nutritionist
Education and training established by the Accreditation Council for Education in Nutrition and Dietetics	
Bachelor's degree with a specifically designed curriculum	Anyone can call themselves a nutritionist
Must complete an extensive internship	
Must pass a rigorous registration examination	

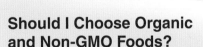

Should I Choose Organic and Non-GMO Foods?

Before you spend the extra money on an organic and non-GMO product, are these foods healthier than conventional foods?

Organics
Although it is intuitive that organic foods might be healthier and prevent chronic diseases, at this time research does not support organic foods as being more nutritionally healthful than conventional foods. However, a consumer may choose to purchase organic foods due to other perceived benefits such as supporting small farms and decreasing overall pesticide use in the environment.

GMOs
Non-GMO foods have recently become a major consumer demand. Genetic modification techniques allow for introduction of new traits or greater control of other traits to increase the efficient use of natural resources, resistance to diseases, or nutrient profiles. There is no scientific consensus that currently available GMO crops pose any health risk compared to conventional food. However, public concerns are ongoing. The longer term effects have not been studied as GMO foods have only been on the market for a few decades.

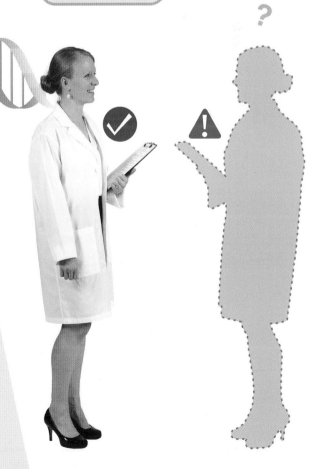

Summary

Having a healthy dietary pattern will require you to have a fundamental understanding of your personal macronutrient (protein, carbohydrate, and fat), micronutrient (vitamins and minerals), fiber, and hydration needs. Eating a high-quality diet can greatly influence how you feel and perform academically and socially, as well as prevent many chronic diseases and conditions later in life. The government and other organizations provide many guidelines and quality resources to assist you in planning and adhering to a healthy dietary pattern. Being able to identify quality foods, supplements, and resources as a smart and informed consumer will be essential to maintaining your health. Finally, beyond physiological needs, food is meant to be enjoyed as a source of pleasure and is an important part of our social lives. Practice the primary principles of moderation, variety, and balance to ensure a healthy diet.

www ONLINE LEARNING ACTIVITIES

Go to HK*Propel* and complete all of the online activities to further facilitate your learning:

Study Activities: Review the main concepts of the chapter.

Labs: Complete the labs your instructor assigns.

Videos: Look through the videos and choose which ones you want to try this week.

REVIEW QUESTIONS

1. List the three macronutrients along with the recommended daily intake of each (as a percent of caloric intake). List three food sources that best represent each macronutrient group.

2. List the two primary types of fiber and two food sources of each type, then explain why fiber is so important for health.

3. List several factors that influence daily water intake needs. Describe three strategies that can enhance your daily hydration levels. What is an easy test to determine if you are adequately hydrated?

4. Do you need a vitamin or mineral supplement to be healthy? Describe a few situations where a supplement might be needed to enhance health.

5. List and describe key resources that you might access to obtain quality information based on scientific evidence to inform your dietary selections.

6. Being a smart consumer spans health and budget concerns. Describe several strategies for designing a healthy dietary pattern that will also allow you to stay on budget.

Weight Management

OBJECTIVES

- Recognize that obesity is the greatest health challenge of our modern times and understand how it affects health.
- Know the primary factors that contribute to weight status.
- Learn energy balance principles that influence weight status.
- Become familiar with weight-management strategies that are useful for all weight statuses and life stages.
- Respect that regular exercise and physical activity are critical for weight management for most people.
- Understand that weight status and management can cause psychological distress and that a healthy body image is important for long-term physical and mental health.
- Recognize when professional help may be needed for weight-management issues and learn the resources that are available.

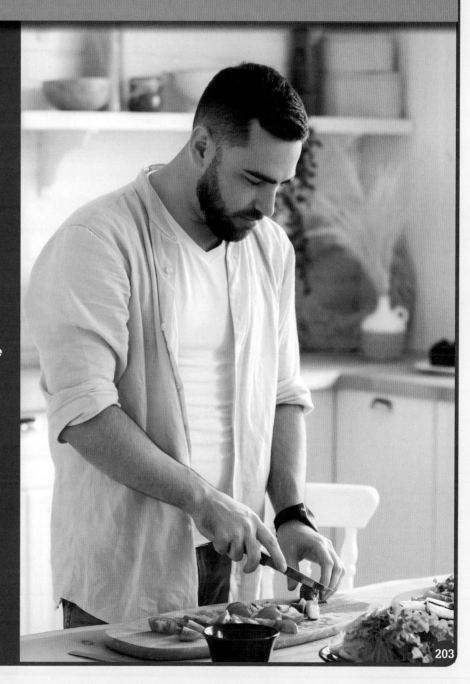

anorexia nervosa

binge-eating disorder

body dysmorphic disorder

body image

bulimia nervosa

energy balance

energy density

exercise addiction

glycemic index

muscle dysmorphia disorder

obesity

obesogenic environment

overweight

resting metabolic rate (RMR)

satiety

thermic effect of activity (TEA)

thermic effect of meals (TEM)

Most people think about weight management a lot. Weight management is not only a critical public health issue, but it can also cause a significant amount of psychological distress. Whether you are trying to prevent weight gain, lose weight, or maintain weight loss, managing both sides of the energy balance equation can be a struggle. Weight management means far more than looking good or feeling good about the way you look. Being overweight or obese is linked to a long list of physical and mental conditions and diseases. This chapter provides a sociocultural perspective of weight management that can be applied to your life. It also discusses weight-management strategies to help you balance your personal energy balance equation, with a special highlight on the importance of energy expenditure. Our final focus is on psychological concerns regarding weight management, including specific information about how to get help for yourself or a friend if needed.

Weight Management: Our Greatest Modern Health Challenge

Current data reports indicate that the prevalence of **obesity** has increased significantly among adults in the United States in the past decades, with data now indicating that greater than 40 percent of all adults are obese. As displayed in figure 9.1, obesity rates are alarmingly high for all adult age cohorts and both biological sexes. Figure 9.1 shows the prevalence of obesity in adults in the United States by sex and age. On average, obesity prevalence rates increase from young adulthood (40.0 percent) through middle age (44.8 percent), then decline among adults aged 60 and over (42.8 percent). Of interest is the fact that across the life span, females have greater obesity rates than males. Finally, there are known racial and ethnic differences in obesity prevalence rates, with non-Hispanic Black (49.6 percent) and Hispanic (44.8 percent) origin groups having greater risk for obesity compared to non-Hispanic white (42.2 percent) and non-Hispanic Asian (17.4 percent) origin groups (Hales et al. 2020).

Importantly, on a personal level, when people become overweight or struggle with obesity early in life, they will likely continue to be challenged with weight management, although a sustained change in lifestyle can alter this course. The **energy balance** equation, discussed in depth later in this chapter, is very simple in concept: Energy in – energy out = weight status. However, the causes of obesity are multifactorial. The factors that influence our eating and movement habits and metabolic rates are very complicated, and what causes one person to be overweight compared to another is unique and personal. This chapter reviews some of these factors to help you make healthy decisions about weight management.

If about 70 percent of the population is overweight or obese, why is 30 percent able to maintain a normal weight? Beyond inheriting good genes, most people who are successful in managing their weight eat a balanced diet and regularly expend energy by being physically active (Hill and Wyatt 2013).

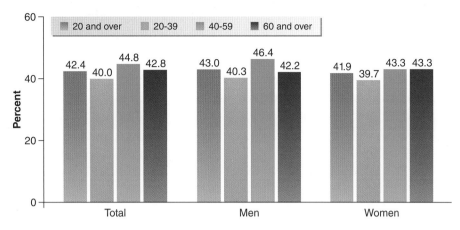

Figure 9.1 Prevalence of obesity among U.S. adults, 2017-2018.

Notes: Estimates for adults aged 20 and over were age adjusted by the direct method to the 2000 U.S. Census population using the age groups 20 to 39, 40 to 59, and 60 and over. Crude estimates are 42.5 percent for total, 43.0 percent for men, and 42.1 percent for women.

Access data table for this figure at https://www.cdc.gov/nchs/data/databriefs/db360_tables-508.pdf#1.

Source: NCHS, National Health and Nutrition Examination Survey, 2017-2018.

Reprinted from NCHS Data Brief, no 360 (2020).

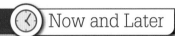 Now and Later

Obesity, Functional Fitness, and Quality of Life

Now

Hopefully, you continue to ponder what it means to have optimal daily function. As introduced in earlier chapters, although the concept of functional fitness can apply to various aspects of life (e.g., cognitive, psychosocial), it very clearly links to physical aspects of functional fitness for your daily activities. Just as physical activity and exercise play key roles in functional fitness, obesity affects your ability to function daily with zest and joy.

Later

Obesity at any age is problematic for health. However, for older adults, obesity has major implications for physical function, especially of the lower body, which leads to reductions in walking function and increases risk for physical disability. Obesity in older adults is a major risk factor for admission to an assisted care facility because they lose the ability to care for themselves. Do you have a grandparent or other relative who is in an assisted care facility? Why did they end up there? Do they have heart disease, arthritis, or uncontrolled diabetes? Are they unable to live independently because they cannot get out of a chair and walk easily?

Take Home

Although it can be challenging to think about and manage your weight, doing so now will go a long way toward preventing physical disability and perhaps even retaining your independence later in life.

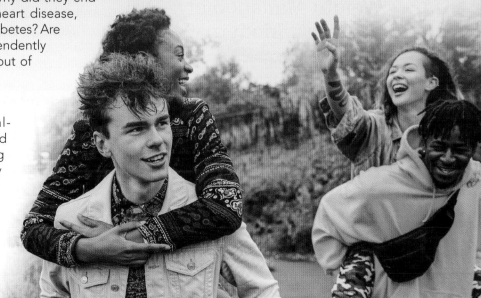

Obesity: A Disease Linked to Many Other Diseases and Conditions

Obesity has been defined as a disease by the American Medical Association. **Overweight** and obesity are typically diagnosed using body mass index (BMI) (see table 7.1), and the state of being obese, as assessed with height and weight (i.e., BMI), is strongly associated with being overfat or having an unhealthy level of fat mass. In addition, as chapter 7 explains, the storage of too much fat, especially in the abdominal region, is strongly linked to many other chronic health conditions. Therefore, the behaviors that lead to the state of being overweight or obese—typically poor nutrition and a sedentary lifestyle, in addition to the excess fat storage in the body—are linked to many diseases and conditions spanning both physical and psychosocial domains (Centers for Disease Control and Prevention 2021), as shown in figure 9.2.

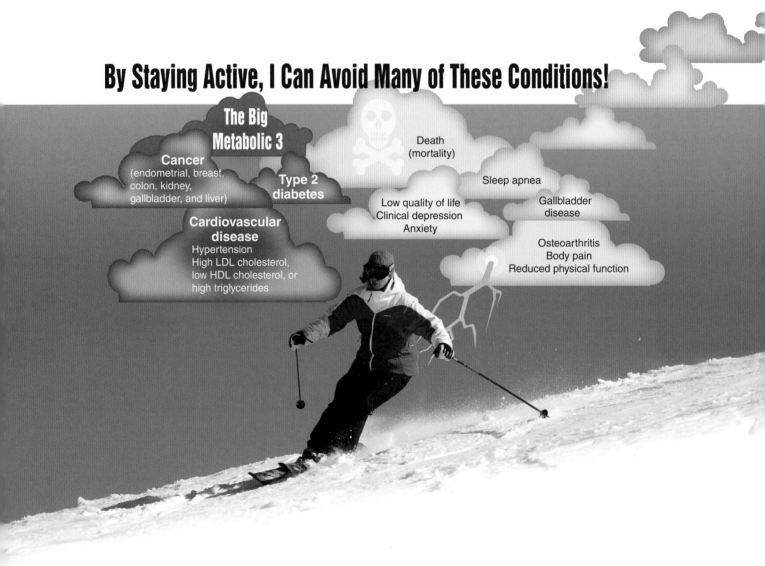

Figure 9.2   Invest in your health and manage your weight to prevent obesity and these related consequences.

Think Socially, Act Personally

The struggle to manage weight causes a great deal of emotional distress and human suffering. Inadequate weight management is often caused by a mismatch between our genetics and our ability to adapt to societal changes. With all its comorbidities, obesity has major direct and indirect negative impacts on our health care costs. From a social perspective, two major demographic shifts in our modern society over the past 50 years have influenced our health care system.

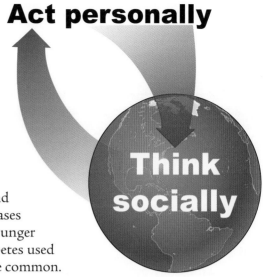

1. Because more people have unhealthy behaviors and are becoming obese at a young age, chronic diseases and conditions are also becoming prevalent at younger ages. For example, hypertension and type 2 diabetes used to be very rare in young adults but now are more common.

2. Older adults are predicted to outnumber young adults in the decades to come. This demographic shift, coupled with an increase in early-onset obesity, will lead to a significant percentage of the population living with an unhealthy weight status and related chronic conditions.

Figure 9.3   As you work to manage your weight, consider how your personal actions affect those around you.

Poor lifestyle choices that result in obesity, when coupled with an aging society, will greatly strain our health care resources. How do we not only act personally but also think socially? As you work to manage your weight, consider the benefits to yourself, as well as your country and the world (figure 9.3). We are all in this weight-management struggle together.

Genetics + Modern Society = Energy Imbalance

Long ago, our food supply was unpredictable and sometimes scarce, requiring us to be physically active to seek food and shelter and avoid being someone else's lunch. However, our environment has undergone enormous changes since those hunter–gatherer days, and now we have complicated social structures and a built environment. Obesity scholars believe we are challenged to manage our weight because this mismatch between our genetics and our technologically advanced society creates a so-called **obesogenic environment** (Bouchard and Katzmarzyk 2010). This environment makes it very easy (behaviorally speaking) to overeat high-calorie food, perform minimal physical activity, and sit too much. Our biological predisposition to engage in these behaviors creates a positive energy balance, so keeping our weight in a healthy range can be a constant challenge.

If you struggle with weight management, think of your challenge as a global problem as well as a personal challenge. This does not mean you should not take personal responsibility for your weight-management behaviors but recognize that you are not alone in your struggles. There are very valid evolutionary reasons for your current situation.

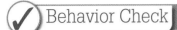

Help End the Stigma of Obesity

People with obesity are commonly subject to social stigma and often face discrimination in the workplace, schools, health care settings, and even their own homes. This discrimination not only causes serious psychological harm to the individual but also impacts the level of care sought and received. Thus, weight stigma damages personal health, undermines health and social rights, and simply is not acceptable in our modern society.

Weight stigma is often reinforced by misconceived ideas that have been debunked by modern science. Most people think that obesity is a choice and that it can be entirely reversed by voluntary decisions (i.e., eat less and move more), thereby implying that a person who is obese has a character flaw (e.g., "low willpower," "laziness," or "gluttony"). The biological and clinical evidence accumulated in the past few decades clearly supports that there are many other factors completely out of a person's control that contribute to overweight or obesity, including genetics, epigenetics, sleep deprivation, psychological stress, medications, and intrauterine and intergenerational effects. It should also be appreciated that obesity was quite rare just 100 years ago. The social, technological, and environmental changes of the last century, though wonderful in many ways for our daily lives, have essentially altered our energy balance abilities.

If you are a person who rarely struggles to manage your weight, resist the urge to be smug. Although you live in the same social and built environment as your overweight and obese friends, chances are that you do not have the biological predisposition to overeat or remain inactive. Perhaps you have a relatively high metabolic rate, or you learned behavior-management techniques at an earlier age. Although highly valued in our society, managing one's weight does not make one morally superior. Indeed, try to maintain compassion for others who may be struggling to keep their weight within a healthy zone. To reduce obesity stigma, we need to work together to change the narrative. Do your part. Check your weight biases, both explicit and implicit. Challenge your beliefs and those of others, when given the opportunity to do so. You are encouraged to review the Joint International Consensus Statement for Ending Stigma of Obesity, written by a 36-member expert panel (Rubino et al. 2020).

Your Family Tree: Nature and Nurture

The heritability of BMI is estimated to be 40 to 70 percent, which means that about half of your weight status and body composition can be attributed to your genes and the other half to environmental influences (Bray et al. 2016). Genetic links have been discovered for body size, body fat distribution (e.g., are you an apple or a pear?), resting metabolic rate, and how challenging it is to gain or lose weight, among many other factors. However, you probably know families in which the parents are obese, and the children are not, or vice versa, which suggests that although some of the risk of obesity is inherited, it can be altered through lifestyle behaviors and choices.

> We have engineered physical movement out of our daily lives by creating a built environment that includes more buildings, less green space, and a heavy reliance on automobile transportation.

Prevention of Obesity Is Critical

Much research and public health efforts have targeted obesity prevention in younger people. This helps to reduce the risk of associated comorbidities occurring at an earlier age and prevent various social issues such as low self-esteem. However, another important reason to prevent obesity in adolescents is because once a person is obese, it becomes challenging to regain a healthy weight status. This challenge only increases the longer a person is obese, so that a person who has been obese since childhood will likely still be challenged by weight management as a middle-aged or older adult (Reinehr 2018).

The normal trajectory for weight change is to gain a small amount of weight each year after young adulthood (see figure 9.4). Most adults gain a small amount of weight every year, ultimately moving into a higher BMI category (e.g., normal weight to overweight or overweight to obese) by middle age. Thus, many normal weight young adults are overweight by the time they reach middle age (Malhotra et al. 2013). These weight changes can fluctuate because of many life events that affect hormones (e.g., pregnancy, menopause), health status (e.g., cancer), or psychosocial well-being (e.g.,

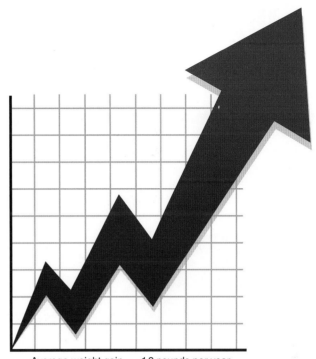

Average weight gain = ~1.2 pounds per year

Figure 9.4 Weight-gain trajectory.

grief, stress). Any major weight change (gain or loss) that cannot be explained by intentional behavior changes such as a new exercise program or dietary program should be checked by a physician to rule out other diseases or conditions.

A sweet spot exists in weight and weight behavior monitoring that needs to be acknowledged. Because weight gain is the normal pattern in our obesogenic society, it is important to intentionally monitor your weight status, as described in chapter 7. However, being hypervigilant about your weight and related behaviors suggests an eating disorder or exercise addiction, which can compromise your physical and mental health. Try to stay in the sweet spot of weight monitoring where you are aware of your weight-management behaviors but are not obsessive about them. That way, when you get off track, you can notice it in a relatively short period of time and make corrections to get back in energy balance.

Energy Balance Math

Trying to remain in energy balance is challenging without a firm understanding of the fundamentals that influence the equation (see figure 9.5).

Boost Your Immunity by Managing Your Weight and Waist

Energy Balance Is the Key to Weight Management

FUEL QUALITY MATTERS

Eating "clean" on most days—whole foods with little added sugar and fats—is important for weight management.

Remember the 85/15 rule: 15% energy intake is discretionary for most adults.

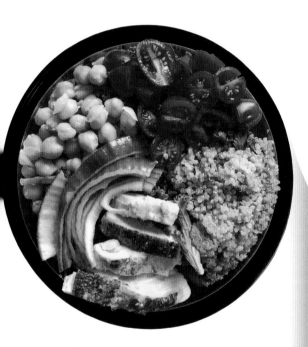

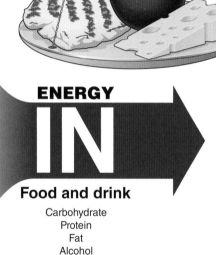

ENERGY
IN
Food and drink

Carbohydrate
Protein
Fat
Alcohol

More energy OUT gives you more discretionary energy bucks!

Obesity and COVID-19

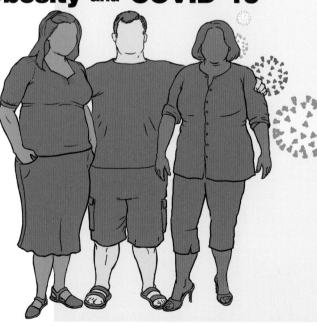

Figure 9.5 Weight management, which requires balancing energy in and energy out, is important to prevent metabolic syndrome and type 2 diabetes, cardiovascular diseases, and cancer. Weight management is also critical to enhance immune function, including the ability to prevent and recover from COVID-19.

"Adverse Effects of Obesity" adapted by permission from B.M. Popkin, S. Du, W.D. Green, M.A. Beck, T. Algaith, et al., "Individuals with Obesity and COVID-19: A Global Perspective on the Epidemiology and Biological Relationships," *Obesity Reviews* 21, no.11 (2020): e13128. https://doi.org/10.1111/obr.13128. Distributed under the terms of the Creative Commons Attribution 4.0 International License (http://creativecommons.org/licenses/by/4.0/).

Energy expenditure has three components

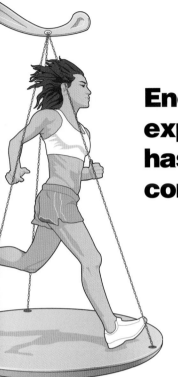

TEA (thermic effect of activity)

TEA is generally accepted as energy expended for voluntarily muscle contraction and is the easiest factor to adjust on the energy expenditure side of the equation. The components of FITT (Frequency, Intensity, Time, Type) greatly influence the energy expenditure of movement.

Age
Hormones
Environment
Exercise/physical activity
Weight change

FITT:
Frequency
Intensity
Time
Type

RMR (resting metabolic rate)

RMR is the energy expended to maintain all vital functions in the body at rest. It is the largest contributor to daily energy expenditure, using ~60%-75% of daily calories. Many factors influence RMR...

TEM (thermic effect of meals)

The energy cost to process and digest food can be altered by food choices but is so small in its contribution to energy OUT that it is not typically considered an important player in energy balance.

ENERGY OUT

RMR
TEA (Move!)
TEM

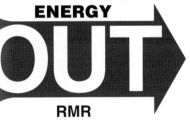

Weight management prevents the metabolic big three in the long term and provides immune function in the short term!

Overweight and obesity and physical inactivity negatively affect COVID-19 outcomes!

True for adults <65 years old too! (CDC 2023)

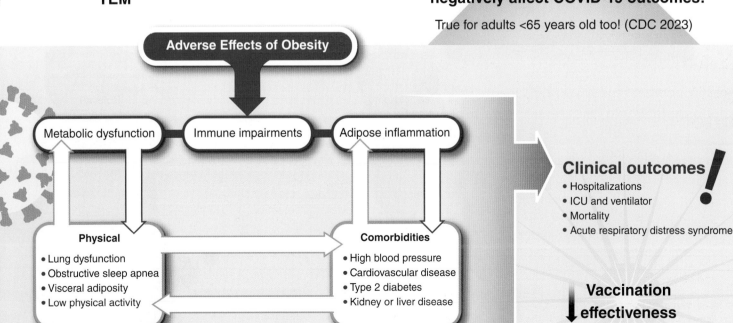

Adverse Effects of Obesity

Metabolic dysfunction — Immune impairments — Adipose inflammation

Physical
- Lung dysfunction
- Obstructive sleep apnea
- Visceral adiposity
- Low physical activity

Comorbidities
- High blood pressure
- Cardiovascular disease
- Type 2 diabetes
- Kidney or liver disease

Clinical outcomes !
- Hospitalizations
- ICU and ventilator
- Mortality
- Acute respiratory distress syndrome

Vaccination ↓ effectiveness

Most people understand the energy-in side of the equation, at least conceptually. The energy-out part is a bit more complicated. Losing weight requires a disruption of the energy balance equation; more energy needs to be going out than coming in. Alternatively, gaining weight requires a greater amount of energy coming in than going out. Keep in mind that how you unbalance the energy balance equation can have a major effect on your body composition, including your muscles and bones. As you start to assess the math of your personal energy balance equation, it is important to recognize that it is highly variable among individuals.

Energy In

As discussed in chapter 8, the energy content of macronutrients—carbohydrate, protein, and fat—varies from 4 to 9 calories per gram. And alcohol also provides 7 calories per gram. On your quest to balance calories in with calories out, don't forget about diet quality, especially macronutrient balance. For example, diets that are higher in fiber, higher in protein, or have a lower **glycemic**

index are linked to **satiety**, which theoretically should help align your energy intake with your energy expenditure (Tremblay and Bellisle 2015). Certain carbohydrates are higher on the glycemic index, which means they raise your blood sugar more quickly than other carbohydrate foods. In general, refined sugars and breads have a higher glycemic index than vegetables and whole grains. Relatedly, carbohydrate foods that are found in nature have a much lower glycemic index than those within processed and packaged foods (see figure 9.6).

Energy density, the number of calories per gram of food, is also a major factor to consider (figure 9.7). Regularly consuming foods with a greater energy density makes weight management more challenging. Foods with a low energy density have a higher water content, such as soups or foods that absorb water during cooking like rice. Foods with a high energy density are typically high in fat and sugar and have a low water content, such as cheese, peanuts, and sweets. If you choose foods relatively low in calories, you can have larger portions and more of them.

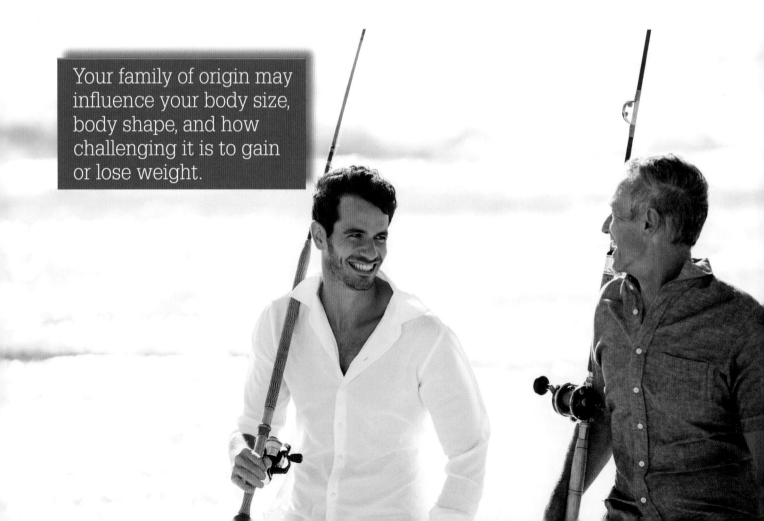

Your family of origin may influence your body size, body shape, and how challenging it is to gain or lose weight.

Obesity and Physical Inactivity Negatively Impact COVID-19 Outcomes

The past few years have brought many new breakthroughs in health research as a result of the COVID-19 pandemic. Although the research continues to inform what we know about risk factors for and complications of the COVID-19 disease, several important factors influence your risk as a college-aged young adult. First, although older adults are more impacted by COVID-19 than younger individuals, being overweight or obese increases the risk of contracting, suffering long-term complications, and dying from COVID-19. The mechanisms for these adverse outcomes are complicated (see figure 9.5) but involve dysfunction in metabolic and immune systems influenced by inflammation (to be explained in chapter 13). Importantly, emerging evidence suggests that being obese also compromises the effectiveness of the COVID-19 vaccine (Popkin et al. 2020). Second, the CDC added those who are physically inactive to the list of individuals who require extra precautions against COVID-19. Simply, those who are not physically active have a greater chance of getting very sick from COVID-19 (Centers for Disease Control and Prevention 2022).

Weight management requires balancing energy in and energy out on a relatively routine basis. As discussed in chapter 4, regular exercise and physical activity have positive effects on the immune system, even if you are overweight investing in your weight-management program will enhance your immune function and help protect you from illness—whether the common cold or COVID-19.

GLYCEMIC INDEX

High glycemic index foods are those that raise blood sugar more quickly, like refined sugars and breads. It's better to choose foods with a lower glycemic index, like vegetables and whole grains. Foods with a lower glycemic index help you balance your blood sugar better and avoid low blood sugar, which typically triggers eating.

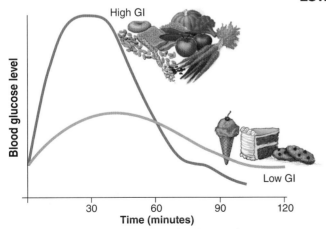

Figure 9.6   Choosing foods with a lower glycemic index can help you manage blood sugar and feelings of hunger.

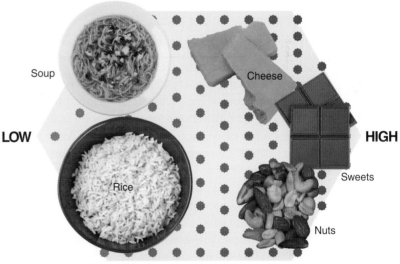

ENERGY DENSITY

Energy density refers to the number of calories per gram of food. Consuming lower energy density foods means you can have higher portions with a relatively low calorie content.

Figure 9.7   Eating lower energy density foods and beverages can help you feel full but consume fewer calories.

As chapter 8 describes, fuel quality matters. Eating healthy (on most days) is very important for long-term weight management. Compared to energy expenditure, most people find it easier to reduce their dietary intake than to expend the same amount of energy engaging in exercise or physical activity. This is a key strategy for weight loss, but because most foods and beverages are mixed in their macronutrient content, counting calories can be challenging. It requires education, attention, discipline, and maybe even a great app!

Energy Out

Energy expenditure can be categorized into the three components of resting metabolic rate; thermic effect of activity (TEA), which requires skeletal muscle contraction and movement; and food processing costs. Excluding highly trained endurance athletes, most people spend most of their daily energy through resting metabolic rate. However, we have the most control over muscle contraction and movement, so this area is a key target for energy balance on the energy-out side. The energy cost of processing and digesting food can be altered by food choices, but this component contributes so little to energy out that it is not typically considered an important player in energy balance.

Resting Metabolic Rate

Resting metabolic rate (RMR) is the largest contributor to daily energy expenditure, using 60 to 75 percent of daily calories. Simply put, maintaining vital functions when the body is at rest takes a lot of energy—your body must keep the heart beating and the lungs inflating, maintain body temperature and blood pressure, and so on. The higher your RMR, the more energy your body is using while at rest. Many factors influence individual RMR, including genetics and daily fluctuations. The main factor consistently influencing RMR is muscle mass, which is highly metabolically active compared to fat or bone mass. This is one reason that the average biological male can eat more calories than the average biological female without gaining weight. Other factors that influence RMR include the following:

- **Hormones.** Several hormones influence RMR, primarily those connected with the thyroid. Sex hormones also influence RMR (e.g., RMR changes throughout the menstrual cycle).
- **Age.** As a result of many factors, RMR decreases with age.
- **Environment.** Very cold or very hot environments can influence RMR.
- **Exercise and physical activity.** Exercise can influence RMR. Intense sessions elevate RMR for many hours. RMR is also consistently elevated in highly active people, primarily as a result of their increased lean body mass.
- **Weight change.** RMR decreases with weight loss. This is one reason it is more challenging to keep losing weight without continuing to adjust energy balance by reducing energy intake or expending more energy.

Thermic Effect of Activity (Muscle Movement)

The **thermic effect of activity (TEA)** refers to all muscle contractions that use energy over and above RMR, including walking for active transportation and intentionally exercising. TEA is the most easily adjustable factor on the energy expenditure side of the equation. Body size, especially lean mass, also affects the amount of energy used during a given session. For example, a large person with a great deal of lean mass will spend more energy than a smaller person running the same distance at a given intensity. The components of FITT, introduced in earlier chapters, also greatly influence the energy expenditure of movement.

- **Frequency.** The more you move, the more energy you use.
- **Intensity.** The higher the intensity, the greater the caloric expenditure during and after the session due to elevations in RMR.
- **Time.** The longer the activity is performed, the more energy is used. Energy expenditure charts typically express energy as calories used per minute for this reason.
- **Type.** This factor is critical because aerobic endurance activities use more energy than strength, flexibility, and neuromotor types of movement.

Table 9.1 provides examples of average energy expenditure for common activities, illustrating how different expenditure can be depending on mode, intensity, body size, and biological sex. Remember that some activities are not performed at a constant rate. For example, weightlifting uses a similar rate of kilocalories per minute compared to cycling at 10 miles per hour (16 km/h); however, the exertion portion of the weightlifting session is not constant, nor does it last very long on a percentage of time basis.

Thermic Effect of Feeding

The **thermic effect of feeding (TEF)**, sometimes referred to as the thermic effect of meals or food, represents the small energy cost of food processing—that is, chewing, digesting, transporting, metabolizing, and storing ingested calories. The exact cost depends on the amount of food or drink and its caloric and macronutrient content. Protein is the most expensive to digest and process, meaning it requires more energy than other foods. Many factors influence thermic effect of

feeding energy costs; however, the total amount of energy used is minimal. Hence, for a person in energy balance, TEF only contributes about 10 percent to their energy expenditure.

Weight-Management Strategies

Although most people think of weight management as reducing weight, energy balance principles also apply to gain weight. However, because people are more commonly trying to lose or maintain weight than to gain weight, the focus in this section is on applying the energy balance equation to weight loss. It is useful to think of weight management in phases: weight-gain prevention, weight loss, and weight-loss maintenance. For most people, it is easier to prevent weight gain than to lose weight. Relatedly, maintaining weight loss is often the most challenging phase of all

Table 9.1   Average Values for Energy Expenditure During Various Physical Activities

Activity	Males (kcal/min)	Females (kcal/min)	Relative to body mass (kcal/kg/min)
Basketball	8.6	6.8	0.123
Cycling			
11.3 km/h (7.0 mph)	5.0	3.9	0.071
16.1 km/h (10.0 mph)	7.5	5.9	0.107
Handball	11.0	8.6	0.157
Running			
12.1 km/h (7.5 mph)	14.0	11.0	0.200
16.1 km/h (10.0 mph)	18.2	14.3	0.260
Sitting	1.7	1.3	0.024
Sleeping	1.2	0.9	0.017
Standing	1.8	1.4	0.026
Swimming (crawl), 4.8 km/h (3.0 mph)	20.0	15.7	0.285
Tennis	7.1	5.5	0.101
Walking, 5.6 km/h (3.5 mph)	5.0	3.9	0.071
Weightlifting	8.2	6.4	0.117
Wrestling	13.1	10.3	0.187

Note: The values presented are averages for a 70-kilogram (154 lb) male and a 55-kilogram (121 lb) female. These values will vary depending on individual differences.

Reprinted by permission from W.L. Kenney, J.H. Wilmore, and D.L. Costill, *Physiology of Sport and Exercise*, 8th ed. (Champaign, IL: Human Kinetics, 2022), 142.

because of alterations to RMR and the permanent changes in lifestyle that must occur.

If you are currently at a healthy weight, it is in your best interest to try to remain this way (using healthy practices!), especially as you age. If you are interested in losing weight and motivated to do it, don't think that it is impossible to lose weight and keep it off, but know that it might prove to be more challenging than preventing weight gain. Small choices over many days, months, and years really do add up. Most people have a slow, steady weight gain throughout their adult life. To successfully manage your weight in our obesogenic environment, you will need to create a lifestyle that respects energy balance principles on most days.

Healthy Strategies for Tipping the Energy Balance Scale

To change your weight status, you need to unbalance your energy balance equation over a given period. Three general principles should always be respected for healthy weight management:

1. Try not to lose more than about 2 pounds (1 kg) per week. Rapid weight loss is harder to maintain long term because it can potentially disrupt your RMR and often causes greater muscle and bone mass loss.

2. Include both sides of the energy balance equation. By reducing both your energy intake and increasing your energy expenditure, the total energy deficit is usually more behaviorally manageable in both the short and longer term, at least for many people. For example, if your goal is to cause a daily deficit of 500 calories, you could reduce energy intake by 300 calories and increase energy expenditure by an additional 200 calories in physical activity.

3. Remember that small changes in weight pay big health benefits. Although the path to weight loss can be long, challenging, and frustrating, small reductions in weight (around 3 to 5 percent of body weight) can reduce your risk for several chronic diseases if accomplished by improving your diet quality and engaging in physical activity on a regular basis (Jensen et al. 2014).

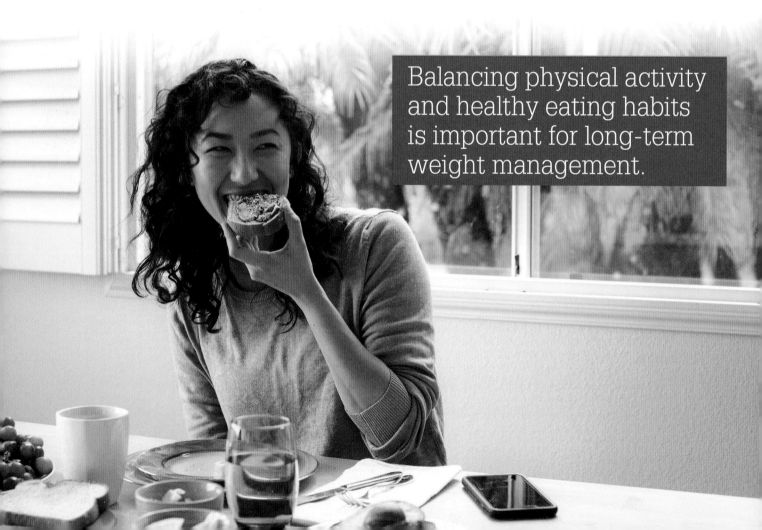

Balancing physical activity and healthy eating habits is important for long-term weight management.

Reducing Energy Intake

In our society, *diet* is both a noun and a verb. Everyone has a diet, but not everyone is dieting. Managing caloric intake can be challenging because we live in a world of plenty. Several key strategies exist for reducing calories in without making you feel deprived; however, to make it work well, you will probably need to mix and match these strategies depending on your social situation. A word of caution is in order. Your precise caloric needs depend on your body size, activity level, age, and other factors. On your quest to unbalance your energy balance equation, be careful not to take in fewer than about 800 calories per day unless you are under medical supervision. Your body requires a certain amount of high-quality fuel to perform well. Without it, you will have low energy and difficulty concentrating, and you may suffer from lack of required nutrients (as described in chapter 8). Very-low-calorie diets are unsustainable; you are setting yourself up for failure. Table 9.2 highlights a few key strategies for reducing energy intake and how you might apply them to daily living.

Move More: Expend More Energy

Previous chapters provide details about how to move more and sit less. All modes of exercise and types of physical activity play a role in health; however, two modes are key to managing the energy balance equation. First, as indicated previously, aerobic endurance activities not only improve the health of your cardiorespiratory systems but also use up a lot of energy. The higher the intensity and the longer the duration of the activity, the more energy that is spent and the greater the influence on RMR. Remember that cardiorespiratory activities can be very intentional (e.g., going out for a run) or they can be woven into your daily life in the form of active transportation.

Second, resistance training is critical for keeping your muscle mass as metabolically active as possible. This is important during all phases of

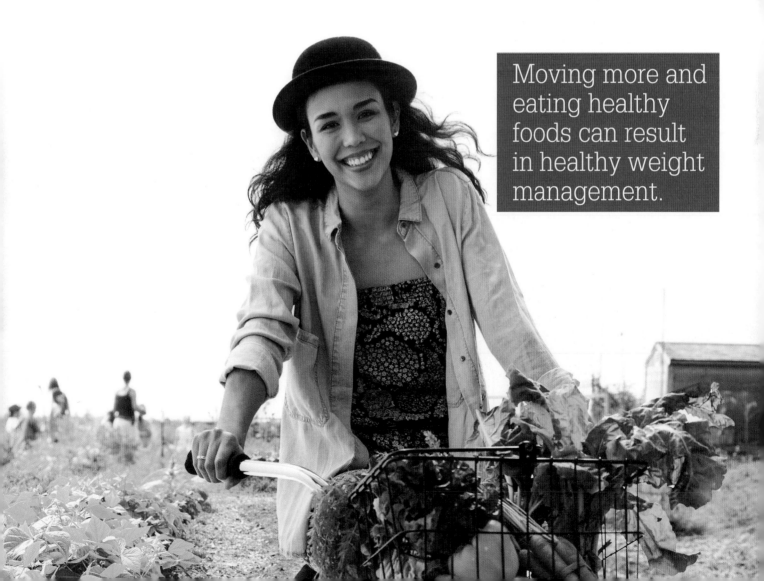

Moving more and eating healthy foods can result in healthy weight management.

weight management (preventing weight gain, weight loss, and maintenance), but it may be especially critical during the active weight loss phase to prevent a decline in RMR. From the perspective of your future healthiest self, regular strength training is the key to preserving your muscle mass and RMR as you age, especially through middle age and beyond.

Think about incorporating these daily strategies into your life:

> One primary key to sustained weight loss is to crank up your fat-burning metabolic machinery. This is best accomplished through a high level of physical activity and exercise and good dietary choices.

Table 9.2   Strategies for Reducing Energy Intake by Altering Dietary Intake

Energy intake reduction strategy	Implementation of strategy
Portion sizes	Overconsumption of total calories is linked to portion sizes. • Order the smaller meal, split a meal, or use smaller plates and bowls.
Energy density	Weight or bulk of food helps with feeling of fullness. • Substitute fruits and vegetables for chips and crackers because they have a lower energy density (i.e., fewer calories per gram).
Fiber	High-fiber foods make you feel fuller. • Add or substitute fruits and vegetables for many options at meals, including your dessert or appetizers.
Macronutrient balance	Having a protein and healthy fat source at each meal or snack might assist with satiety. • Add nuts or Greek yogurt to your cereal; avoid pure carbohydrate meals such as orange juice and a banana for breakfast.
Meal timing	Skipping meals can make it hard to manage your blood sugar and sabotage your efforts to make good choices and manage your portion sizes. • Try to eat smaller meals or snacks throughout the day.
Dietary fat	At 9 kcal/g, fat provides many calories, often hidden in foods such as salad dressings. • Select low-fat options when available; avoid fried foods as much as possible.
Added sugars and sweets	Added sugars over the day can really add up. • Reduce intentionally added sugars (e.g., sugar in coffee) and minimize sweets, saving them for a special treat after a long week or for an event such as a celebration.
Processed foods	Processed foods have many hidden calories in terms of added fat and sugar. • Eat processed foods sparingly and select those that have minimal processing and additives; know how to accurately read Nutrition Facts labels.
Physical activity	If you regularly expend extra energy on physical activity, you can afford a few "indulgence" calories. • Try to move at least 30 minutes per day at a moderate intensity to keep your metabolism healthy (Hill and Wyatt 2013).

- Ban the bus and any other step-saving device, such as elevators, escalators, and moving sidewalks. Don't let anyone steal your steps. Start to think of them as ways to spend your energy bucks.

- Load your backpack as much as possible. This will increase the intensity of your transportation walk. Be sure to use good posture to avoid back or shoulder pain or injuries.

- When planning your cardiorespiratory exercise, try to work hard for longer periods of time to really stimulate your metabolism.

- Stand when possible and take planned breaks for movement. For example, if one of your buildings has stairs, try to get up and walk the stairs for a few minutes every hour. Think of these breaks as energy-buck spenders even if they spend just a few cents per break.

- Consistently do resistance training with loads beyond your body weight. This is especially important for females, who often focus exclusively on cardiorespiratory activities for weight management. Don't underestimate the key role that muscle mass can play in energy balance.

Buyer Beware: Be a Smart Consumer

The weight-management business is a booming industry. Because so many people struggle to manage their weight, the marketplace has responded with countless plans, programs, pills, supplements, and aids. Most products on the market claim to either curb the appetite or increase RMR. However, most of these products are ineffective and many can actually be dangerous. Remember that the FDA does not regulate dietary supplements. A good source of information is the FDA website, which informs the public of products with hidden active ingredients that are potentially harmful (go to www.fda.gov and click on Food and then Dietary Supple-

> Weight management is a lifestyle choice. A product that is advertised as a quick fix is likely too good to be true.

ments, where there is a wealth of general educational information). If a product sounds too good to be true, it likely is. To safely manage your weight, you need to keep your energy balance equation in check by following the principles described in this chapter, which can be implemented over a lifetime. Unfortunately, when the struggle for weight management gets frustrating—and subsequently emotional—many people get desperate, which may lead them to make bad decisions.

Prescription Drugs and Surgery

Certain medical options are available for weight management. Prescription drugs have been developed over the years that influence energy consumption and energy expenditure or interfere with energy absorption. A complete review is beyond the scope of this book; however, recognize that all prescription drugs on the market have a limited effect on weight status in the long term, and many have numerous side effects. Also, many people regain any weight lost when stopping the medication. All medications work best in conjunction with a behavioral modification program reinforcing the importance of managing lifestyle habits for long-term weight management success.

Surgical treatment of obesity, known as *bariatric surgery*, is often considered a last resort, although it is growing in prevalence worldwide. It is typically recommended only for people who have morbid obesity (BMI > 40, or 35 with other major obesity-related health risks). Essentially, bariatric surgery involves reducing the size of the stomach to reduce the amount of food a person can eat. Although it is very effective, there are major risks associated with this procedure, including nutritional deficiencies, chronic nausea and vomiting, and serious postoperative complications that can result in death. For long-term success, behavioral modification strategies are essential. For more information, see www.webmd.com (search "gastric bypass surgery") or https://asmbs.org/patients.

Potential Interactive Implications of Stress, Sleep, and Alcohol

Alcohol, stress, and sleep have important implications for weight management. Many people have good intentions to adhere to healthy weight-management behaviors but fail to do so for a variety of reasons, especially those related to stressful lifestyle issues. The chapter 9 labs on HK*Propel* will help you utilize SMART goal planning to set effective long- and short-term goals for healthy eating practices.

1. **Stress.** Emotional and psychosocial stressors play major roles in the health of our society. Our 24/7 go-go-go world alters our cardiovascular and neuroendocrine systems and often challenges our psychosocial well-being.

   - Energy in: Stress has been shown to increase the selection of starchy, sweet foods (junk food). Feeling pressed for time can lead you to select more fast food and processed foods.

   - Energy out: High levels of stress can cause fatigue, which then can reduce your motivation to move, resulting in more sitting and less activity.

2. **Sleep.** Many people are chronically sleep deprived, which not only disrupts the neuroendocrine system but can also lead to many behavioral changes.

   - Energy in: Fatigue may reduce your motivation to stick with healthy food choices. It might also increase your intake of caffeine, which can increase your energy intake in the form of soda or sweetened coffees.

   - Energy out: As with stress, fatigue reduces your interest in moving.

3. **Alcohol.** In addition to the substance abuse concerns discussed in chapter 11, alcohol can have negative effects on your weight management.

   - Energy in: At 7 calories per gram, alcohol can affect your weight-management plan. Depending on how much and often you indulge, especially if you drink heavy beer or sweet mixed drinks, the calorie intake can be substantial.

   - Energy out: Consuming too much alcohol can cause fatigue and reduce your interest in adhering to your exercise plan or engaging in active transportation or recreation. Recall that alcohol is a diuretic, so it can also dehydrate you, which influences your movement performance. Finally, the metabolism of alcohol, if consumed excessively, will reduce the use of fat as a fuel source.

Daily Movement Is Essential for Weight Management

Regular exercise and physical activity are essential for all three phases of weight management. How-

---

✓ Behavior Check

Do You Spiral Up or Down?

Your behavior choices can help you spiral either up or down in terms of your overall health. Have an honest conversation with yourself about how you manage pressure and stress. For example, when you are tired from your hectic schedule and stressed about a major exam, do you eat lower-quality foods such as fast foods, processed snacks, or candy? Do you reach for sugary sodas or sweet coffees to give you energy to power through? Alcohol may also play a role in your stress management. Alternatively, do you make sure to adhere to your exercise routine because you know it will help you manage your stress? Try to recognize and manage your triggers.

Make a plan to replace behaviors that will have a negative effect on your health with positive behaviors. For example, if you binge on chocolate when you are stressed, plan for a healthier replacement: You might plan to go for a walk, take a hot bath or shower, or listen to relaxing music. Find a plan that will work for you so that when life issues arise, you are prepared to deal with them.

ever, how much exercise you will need to perform and why you need to do it might change.

Prevention of Weight Gain

The role of energy expenditure in preventing weight gain is not well established because of challenges with research study designs. However, we can assume that the role that energy expenditure plays is important, especially when RMR begins to decline with age. High levels of activity, especially resistance training, lessen this RMR decline by maintaining muscle mass and keeping existing muscle mass metabolically active.

Weight Loss and Healthy Body Composition Change

Incorporating both cardiorespiratory and resistance training into your weight-loss program is essential. First, it will allow you to eat more (i.e., restrict energy less) while meeting the same energy deficit goals, which will help you stick with your program. Second, it will promote the healthiest body composition change. When we try to lose weight by restricting calories alone, more of the weight loss comes from lean (muscle) mass than when exercise and physical activity are included in the program. Loading your bones when undergoing weight loss will also help reduce bone loss, which typically occurs with caloric restriction and weight loss. Finally, physical activity, especially higher-intensity cardiorespiratory and strength training, will help protect against reductions in RMR that occur with weight loss.

With specific attention to FITT guidelines for weight loss, the ACSM suggests performing moderate- to vigorous-intensity (as tolerated) aerobic activities that use large muscle groups for a minimum of 30 minutes per day, progressing to 60 minutes per day, on at least five days per week. Resistance exercises are also recommended two or three days per week with two to four sets of 8 to 12 repetitions for each major muscle group being performed. Finally, a flexibility program (as described in chapter 6) is also recommended (American College of Sports Medicine 2022).

Weight-Loss Maintenance

If exercise and physical activity are important during weight loss, they are even more important for weight-loss maintenance. However, unlike weight loss, specific recommendations for physical activity to maintain weight loss are not well defined. The ACSM endorses research suggesting that an increased amount of cardiorespiratory activity is needed for weight-loss maintenance, with weight loss generally not maintained by following the regular FITT guidelines (American College of Sports Medicine 2022). Some studies support 200 to 300 minutes per week, with more activity being better to improve the chances of weight-loss maintenance; this could be obtained with intentional exercise or physical activity related to lifestyle choices (e.g., active transportation) if they are of a moderate intensity.

Some of the best evidence for the importance of energy expenditure for weight-loss maintenance comes from the National Weight Control Registry, a longitudinal study of individuals who have successfully lost weight and maintained weight loss. The primary successful strategies include using a macronutrient balance approach to eating (see table 9.2) and a high level of physical activity (Hill and Wyatt 2013).

Psychological Concerns Regarding Weight Management

We live in an environment that makes it challenging to manage weight using healthy behaviors. On top of that, our society values being thin and fit. As a result, many people live in a constant state of psychological distress related to body image issues. Nearly all body image issues stem from a lack of congruence between what people look like (or think they look like) and what they feel they should look like based on cultural messages, family pressures, and individual belief systems. Unfortunately, it is becoming increasingly rare to find any person who is content with their body image.

Although an in-depth review of these issues is beyond the scope of this textbook, you are encouraged to seek professional resources if you or someone you care about struggles with these issues. Weight management should take place in a positive and supportive atmosphere, including from within. With few exceptions, most people can be relatively healthy at any weight. Moreover, being content in one's own skin—regardless of appearance—and being self-confident is an attractive feature in our culture.

Developing and Maintaining a Healthy Body Image

Body image is the perceptions, images, evaluations, and emotions regarding one's appearance that may span the entire body or target a certain body part. Developing a positive body image is essential to psychosocial well-being and successful weight management. A negative body image can cause great mental anguish, damage self-esteem, interfere with healthy relationships and social activities, and lead to depression. When extreme, it is often termed **body dysmorphic disorder**. The chapter 9 labs in HK*Propel* will help you explore your personal body image.

Eating Disorders and Exercise Addiction

Negative body image and unhappiness with weight status can lead to more serious issues such as eating disorders and other unhealthy weight-management behaviors. Unfortunately, eating disorders are becoming increasingly common among all ages and sexual and gender identities. The most common disorders related to a negative body image are **anorexia nervosa**, **bulimia nervosa**, **binge-eating disorder**, and **exercise addiction**:

- *Anorexia nervosa.* Although often expressing interest in food, people who suffer from anorexia nervosa do not eat enough to maintain a normal weight and often have a very low BMI. Historically, this condition has mainly afflicted young females, but it is getting more common among other groups. Sadly, this starvation condition can result in death.

- *Bulimia nervosa.* A person with bulimia nervosa engages in recurrent episodes of binge eating followed by purging, typically through vomiting or using laxatives and diuretics. Bulimia is more challenging to identify because these behaviors are performed in private, and those with the disorder often have a normal weight. However, fluctuations in weight can be a sign. The binge–purge cycle greatly stresses many systems of the body, including the teeth, esophagus, liver, kidneys, and heart.

- *Binge-eating disorder.* People who binge eat often do so in response to stress, strong emotions, or conflict. The uncontrolled eating episode is followed by shame, depression, and ramped-up efforts in weight management. People with this disorder are almost always obese, and this behavior compromises their health. In

Seeing yourself differently in a mirror than how others see you is called body dysmorphic disorder.

addition, they also live with higher rates of anxiety and depression.

- *Exercise addiction.* Note that although the previous behaviors center on energy intake, obsessive or excessive exercise may also be used to achieve weight control.

Muscle Dysmorphia

Although eating disorders often bring to mind a stereotype of young females on a quest to be very thin, another type of struggle with eating and exercise behaviors can take the form of **muscle dysmorphia disorder**. In this situation (sometimes called *bigorexia*), individuals strive to be ever-larger and more muscular. Even though the goal of people who struggle with this condition is the opposite of that of people with conventional eating disorders (i.e., trying to become bigger as opposed to smaller), the root cause is often the same—a poor body image that results in unhealthy eating and exercise behaviors. The mental anguish can be just as serious and lead to life-endangering behaviors, including steroid use.

When Professional Help Is Needed

Sometimes the best course of action in life is to recognize you need help and wisely secure quality resources for yourself. Weight management is no exception to this rule.

Psychologist or Therapist

Although you or someone you know may not suffer from a diagnosed eating disorder, many people have symptoms of an eating disorder or a body image disturbance severe enough to compromise their quality of life. Having an honest conversation is the first step to improving your well-being. Most college campuses have counselors who can provide quality assistance with these issues or a referral to a professional in the community. Working with a professional counselor can help address both problematic eating disorders and the misuse of food and activity to manage stress and emotions. Anxiety or depression are often key underlying issues that cause further problems with weight-management behaviors.

> If you are worried about yourself or a friend, a great resource for eating disorders is the National Eating Disorders Association (www.nationaleating-disorders.org).

Registered Dietitian Nutritionist (RDN)

As mentioned in chapter 8, an RDN can help with personal dietary plans. This is especially important if you have special dietary needs caused by a chronic illness or a food allergy. A few sessions may be all you need to understand some key principles and get on your way to healthier fueling.

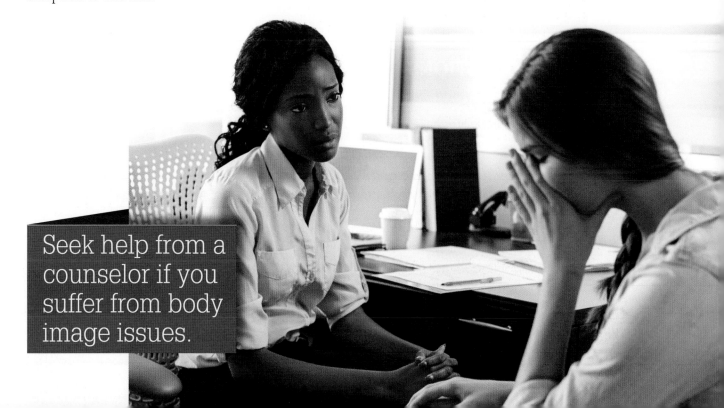

Seek help from a counselor if you suffer from body image issues.

Certified Fitness Trainer

Although the fundamentals of the established physical activity guidelines have been discussed extensively, sometimes you need additional assistance to set up a program or improve your adherence as you get started. When selecting a professional fitness trainer, look for someone who is certified by the National Commission for Certifying Agencies (NCCA) and who aligns with your goals and personality. Just as you would not go to a doctor who has not passed a medical board examination, you would be wise to select a fitness trainer who has been nationally certified by an organization that has gone through the NCCA accreditation process.

Medical Evaluation

Finally, if your weight changes for no apparent reason or does not change in response to your intentional manipulation of energy intake or expenditure, you are encouraged to see a physician. Unexplained weight change is always cause for concern. Although you are young and the risk is minimal, conditions such as hyper- or hypothyroidism or cancer can alter your weight.

Summary

Weight management is a challenge in our obesogenic society, where we have so much easily accessible, highly palatable food and minimal need to use energy to survive. To manage weight, we need to constantly balance our energy intake with our energy expenditure. Movement, especially cardiorespiratory and resistance training, can enhance your weight-management success by expending energy and maintaining or enhance your resting metabolic to keep you closer to energy balance. You can gain many strategies for remaining in energy balance by educating yourself and paying attention to your daily behaviors. Managing weight can be very emotionally challenging, and disordered eating and exercise behaviors can greatly damage mental and physical health. Knowing when to seek professional assistance may be a key part of your weight-management program.

ONLINE LEARNING ACTIVITIES

Go to HK*Propel* and complete all of the online activities to further facilitate your learning:

Study Activities: Review the main concepts of the chapter.

Labs: Complete the labs your instructor assigns.

Videos: Look through the videos and choose which ones you want to try this week.

REVIEW QUESTIONS

1. How do relatively recent changes in our social and built environments contribute to our ongoing public health challenge with weight management?

2. List the three primary components of energy expenditure. Which factor explains the greatest amount of daily energy expenditure for most people? Which factors can be manipulated in the short term to cause an energy deficit to lose weight?

3. Describe three strategies you could use to manage energy intake without feeling greatly deprived.

4. Which primary modes of exercise should be incorporated into your weight-loss program? Justify their use from a mechanistic perspective.

5. Briefly explain the signs and symptoms of an eating or exercise disorder.

6. List and explain how various professionals might be able to help you with your goals related to a healthy and sustainable weight-management program.

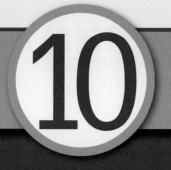

Stress Management

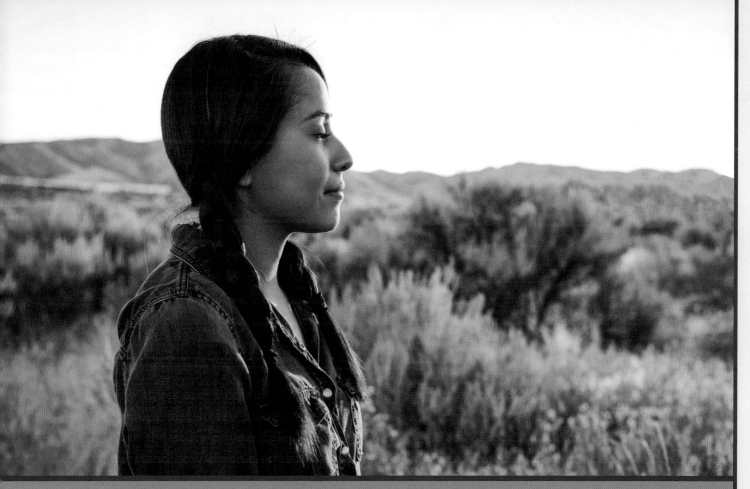

OBJECTIVES

- **Define** *stress* **and** *stressor* **and recognize that perception of both is personal.**
- **Recognize that stress is not always bad and spans from eustress to distress.**
- **Explain the acute physiological and psychological stress response.**
- **Understand how chronic stress, if unmanaged, can cause physical and emotional health problems.**
- **Recognize the primary stressors for college students.**
- **Describe key strategies, especially sleep and physical activity, that can help manage stress.**

KEY TERMS

adrenal glands

allostasis

allostatic load

autonomic nervous system (ANS)

cortisol

depression

distress

endocrine system

epinephrine

eustress

fight-or-flight response

generalized anxiety disorder

hypothalamus-pituitary-adrenal axis (HPA axis)

mantra

mindfulness meditation

norepinephrine

panic disorder

parasympathetic nervous system

personality

pituitary gland

social anxiety disorder

stress

stressor

sympathetic nervous system

time management

Transcendental Meditation

Do you ever feel overwhelmed by your to-do list? Are your days full of constant hassles? Stress is a natural part of our lives, but how you react to it can have major implications for your health and well-being. This chapter targets stress management, beginning with an overview of the stress response. Importantly, it emphasizes the implications of mismanagement of stress for your health, now and in your future. Common sources of stress for the college student are highlighted, including work habits and academic performance. Finally, this chapter explores key strategies for managing stress, especially physical activity, and quality sleep.

The Contemporary Stress Experience

The primary sources of stress for most people are related to social and psychological challenges, including our relationships and job performance. For college students, performing well academically is equivalent to full-time employment and has many of the same stressors. Regardless of the source of stress, it is important to recognize when you are stressed, the sources of the stress, and how to manage these stressors so that they do not negatively affect your health and life. As with most health habits, this will take intentional strategies and effort.

Stress Defined

Most people view **stress** as some unpleasant threat defined along the lines of a "physical, mental, or emotional strain" or "feelings that occur when a person perceives that a demand exceeds their personal or social resources." Thus, stress is generally considered a negative experience and something to be avoided. A few major myths are that stress is the same for everyone and that it is always bad for you. However, if there is no healthy tension, most people become bored and lose motivation to engage in life. Therefore, stress can be helpful because it motivates us to be productive, try new things, and engage in our social world.

This brings us to another important stress concept: It is very useful to differentiate the stimulus from the response. The stress stimulus is considered the **stressor**. You probably know that not all stressors produce the same response for everyone (see figure 10.1). A given stressor may be very distressing only if it occurs under specific conditions—for example, when you are short on sleep, hungry, or very pressed for time. An important concept discussed in this chapter is that you cannot always control the stressors in

> How an event or situation is viewed is highly individual; one person's awful stressor is another person's adventure.

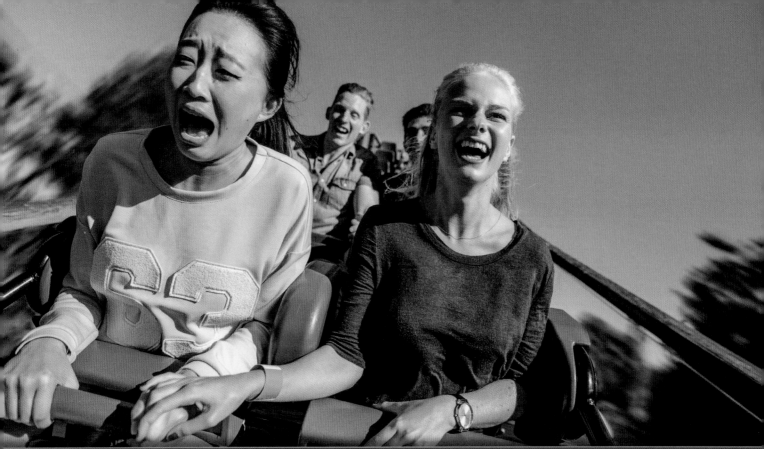

Being stressed and not having coping techniques can be like running a marathon and never crossing the finish line.

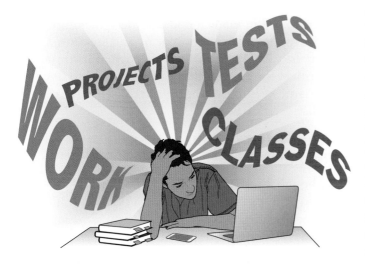

Figure 10.1 College students have many stressors related to their academic courses and employment obligations. Develop a personal stress-management plan to prevent adverse health outcomes.

your life (e.g., your midterm exams all landing on the same day), but you can alter the way you *perceive* and *react to* the stressors, which will greatly alter your physiological and emotional experiences of stress.

Eustress Versus Distress

Stress can be thought of as existing on a continuum. The good stress, **eustress**, occurs when you experience something new or different or you are anticipating a positive experience. Examples of eustress might include going on a long-awaited vacation, learning how to drive, or going to college. **Distress** occurs when you are exposed to negative circumstances that are often out of your control. Examples of distress include failing a major exam, enduring a physical injury, or breaking off your relationship with your romantic partner. Distress, especially if it is ongoing, is the type of stress that negatively affects your health and well-being. Figure 10.2 depicts a conceptual model of how eustress and distress interact on a continuum.

The Stress Response

How do you feel when you are stressed? How does your body know how to react when faced with a stressor? Understanding how the body responds to stressors, both physiologically and psychologically, will help you develop stress-management skills.

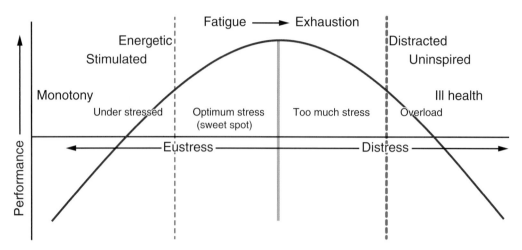

Figure 10.2 The stress curve: Eustress versus distress.

Physiological Response

When the body is exposed to a stressor, the nervous and the endocrine systems work together to initiate the **fight-or-flight response**. Earlier in our evolution, this response was necessary because without it, many humans would have been killed by predators. Nowadays we rarely need to run away or physically fight a predator, but this same response system is set in motion when we are confronted with stress or danger (or even by the anticipation of stress or danger).

The **parasympathetic nervous system**, a primary arm of the **autonomic nervous system (ANS)**, is in control during relaxed states. The **sympathetic nervous system**, the other primary arm of the autonomic nervous system, is a key player in the stress response. Its nerves release **norepinephrine** (also called *noradrenaline*) to signal nearly every organ, sweat gland, blood vessel, and muscle to prepare your body to move in the fastest, most efficient manner possible (to run or prepare to fight!). The coordinated stress response occurs because your **endocrine system** works with your nervous system to release a hormonal cascade often summarized as the **hypothalamus-pituitary-adrenal axis (HPA axis)**. This cascade results in the release of key hormones **epinephrine** (also called *adrenaline*) and **cortisol** (the primary hormone).

Activation of the HPA axis is like a short-term crisis in the body, shifting resources from any longer-term bodily functions, such as digestion, immune function, or reproduction (see figure 10.3). When the stressful situation is over, the parasympathetic nervous system returns the body to its resting prestress state (e.g., the heart rate returns to resting levels). Longer-term projects now begin to take priority again, including digestion and energy storage. The immune system can now repair any injuries to prepare for the next threat. Changes in the function of the HPA axis are involved in many mood disorders, including anxiety disorders, depression, and insomnia (Sapolsky 2004). Learning to manage your stress is critical for protecting the health of your HPA axis and keeping it appropriately sensitive to realistic stressors.

What Affects Your Stress Response?

Although we all experience physiological and psychological stressors and exhibit the same cascade of bodily changes in response to them, the magnitude of the stress response varies greatly from person to person and for an individual in different situations. A few of the primary factors that influence the stress response are your cognitive evaluation of the situation and your emotional reaction to it. Your personality might also influence your specific reactions to a given stressor and your stress response in general.

Cognitive Evaluation: Can I Cope?

When presented with a stressor, most people immediately assess the situation—that is, you think it through. Although several well-established psychological theories exist, most align with the idea that the level of stress experienced is highly dependent on a few key questions you ask yourself (Lazarus and Folkman 1984):

1. Is there potential for harm or threat?
2. If so, will my resources to protect myself be enough?
3. If my resources are not enough, can I cope with the resulting situation?

The cognitive evaluation of the threat and your ability to cope will be greatly influenced by your perception of control. For example, knowing the date of a course's final exam, the structure of the exam, and the material to be covered will make the exam less stressful than one for which you have been given no guidance on how to prepare. Also, having a bad experience will nearly always result

in more stress in similar situations in the future (Sapolsky 2004). If you have been successful with comprehensive exams in the past, the next round of exams will be less stressful.

Emotional Responses: Does It Matter to Me?

Psychological stress is often thought of as our emotional response to an event or situation that we perceive as a threat to our well-being. If you don't care much about the outcome, you won't perceive the event as a threat and therefore will have a minimal stress response. However, if the stakes are high, the situation will pose a significant threat or challenge, triggering a larger stress response (Sapolsky 2004). Therefore, you would probably perceive a minor quiz in an elective class as less stressful than a comprehensive final exam

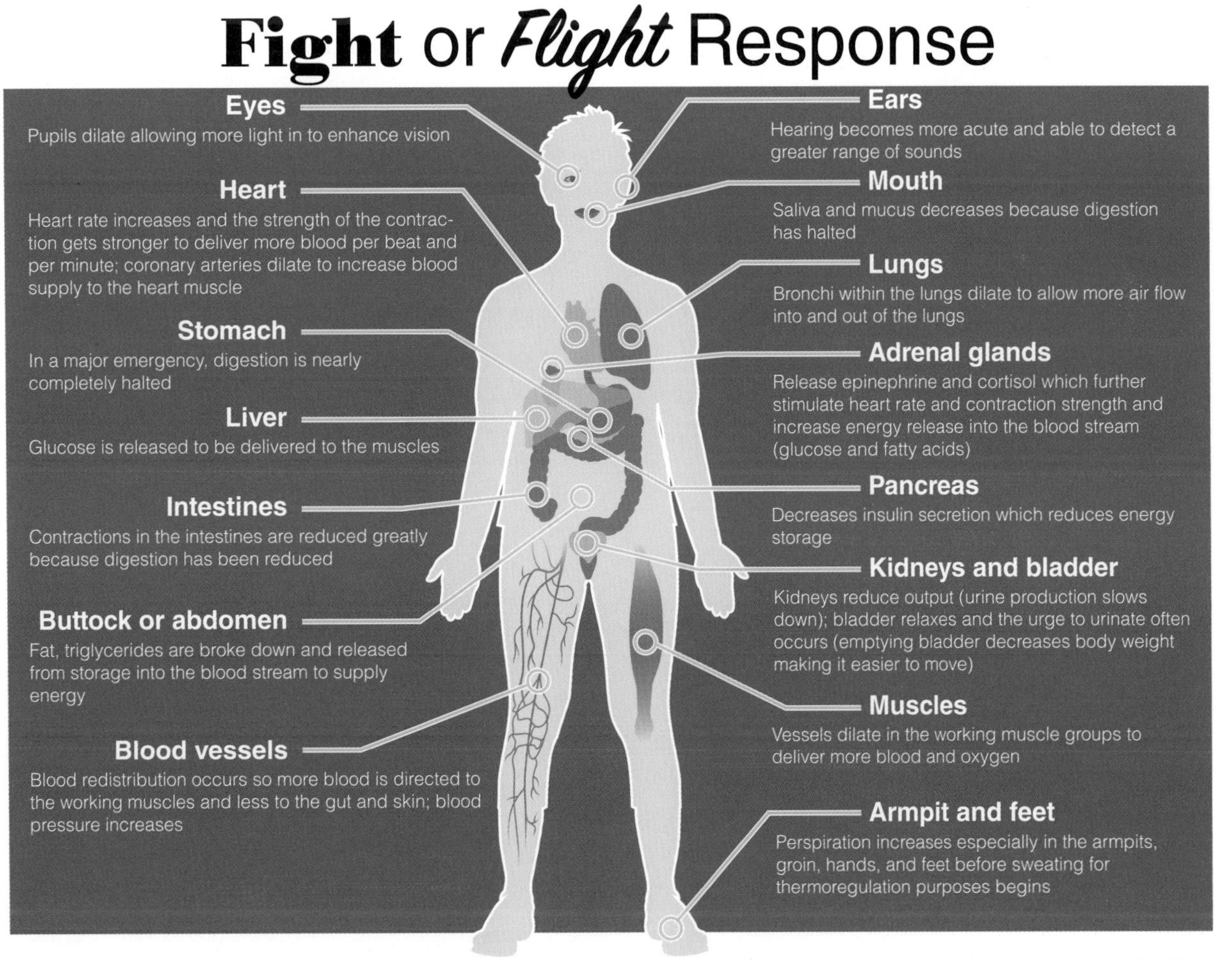

Fight or *Flight* Response

Figure 10.3 The physiological responses of your body to stress.

in a core class in your major, especially if the latter could affect your chance of getting into a competitive graduate program. This is also why hearing the news of a stranger passing will likely not cause a stress response, whereas losing a loved one can be a significant stressor.

Personality Type

Think about the personalities of your family members and close friends. Some people seem very calm and able to handle anything that comes their way, whereas others are anxious about anything that disrupts their daily routine. These traits are aspects of **personality**. Personality can influence how you perceive and respond to stressors. There are many ways to characterize personality, and many researchers have attempted to classify personality into types (search for "personality types" in your favorite browser and you are sure to find many results). The important thing is not to determine the most accurate personality theory that applies to you, but rather appreciate that your personality influences your behaviors and reactions to certain situations.

The most well-known type is a Type A personality. In general, people with Type A personalities are competitive and impatient. They are hardworking overachievers who are highly concerned with time management. In contrast, Type B personalities are more relaxed and less competitive. Research has shown that being Type A can increase the risk for coronary artery disease, especially if it is linked to being hostile, time pressured, and socially insecure. Other personality types, such as the chronic worrier who sees danger everywhere, also tend to have a chronically activated stress response and a higher risk for anxiety and depression.

> Learning to manage your stress is critical for protecting your health.

Although most people do not fit neatly into one personality type, the important point is that your personality can influence your perception of stressors as well as your physiological and psychological responses to them. Some personalities chronically activate a stress response that is much higher than it should be for a given stressor (Sapolsky 2004).

Modern Life and the Stress Response Mismatch

Allostasis is an organism's process of achieving internal stability, or homeostasis, through physical or behavioral changes. Therefore, a stressor is anything that throws your body out of allostatic balance, and the stress response is your body's attempt to return to homeostasis. Whether the stressor is physical, psychological, or social, or even an anticipation of a challenge, the body responds with the same physiological cascade. Thus, being too hot or too cold, hungry, or worried about an important exam can all activate the stress response.

For the great majority of nonhuman animals on the planet, the physiological stress response is about managing a short-term crisis. If you are a lion chasing your lunch—or a zebra trying not to become a lion's lunch—this response is wonderfully adapted and appropriate for these situations. Unlike species that are less cognitively advanced, however, humans can turn on the stress response just by thinking about potential stressors. Because of our advanced thinking capabilities, complicated social environment, and technological advances, humans get very stressed about many things that have no relevance to other mammals, such as a failing course grade, a text that ends a relationship with a romantic partner, or a low bank balance. This worry can throw our systems out of homeostatic balance even if the event will occur far in the future, or maybe not even occur at all (Sapolsky 2004).

The physiological stress-response system evolved to assist us in short-term physical emergencies, but for many people, the stress response is being set off multiple times per day or nearly all day long as we worry about issues such as our relationships, finances, employment, and social status. This is the conceptual basis of stress-related disease.

Allostatic Load

A contemporary theory of how chronic stress causes disease is the concept of **allostatic load**, which is defined as wear and tear on the body caused by the neuroendocrine response to chronic stress. Another way to understand this concept is that repeated stress can be managed; however, getting back into allostatic balance after each stress response takes a great deal of effort and having to constantly rebalance eventually wears a person down.

In his book *Why Zebras Don't Get Ulcers*, Robert Sapolsky (2004) explains this concept well. He calls it the "two elephants on a seesaw" model of stress-related disease. Figure 10.4a shows two small children balancing on a seesaw, representing the low levels of stress hormones in your system easily achieving allostatic balance when nothing stressful is occurring in your life. In contrast, Figure 10.4b shows two elephants trying to

balance on the seesaw. The size of the elephants represents the huge amount of stress hormones in your system in response to some stressor (whether real, anticipated, or even theoretical). As you can see, the elephants can balance, but costs and consequences are involved in achieving this, including the following effects:

- ***Allocation of effort.*** It takes an enormous amount of energy to balance two elephants on a seesaw. This means that energy must be diverted from longer-term investments like reproduction and immune functions to handle the chronic short-term emergencies.

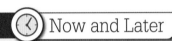

Now and Later

Personality and Stress

Now

By this stage of life, you are likely aware of your main personality traits. Without getting too caught up in the alphabet of personality typing, you might be able to align yourself with one of the types described in this chapter. When you understand factors you cannot change—such as genetic contributions to your personality or aspects of your temperament formed in your childhood—you can better choose the strategies that might help you manage your stress.

Later

Many students assume that their stress level will go down after they graduate. This is not typically the case—life gets even more complicated, with multiple social roles and professional and family demands. Continual unmanaged stress has been linked to chronic conditions such as cardiovascular disease, anxiety disorders, and depression (Sapolsky 2004). Many of these stress-related diseases and conditions begin to show up during midlife.

Take Home

You may not be able to change your basic personality, but you can learn how to manage your stress response by practicing stress-management techniques, including positive thinking. Stress management is a key health behavior that will help you feel better now and have a long, happy, and healthy life.

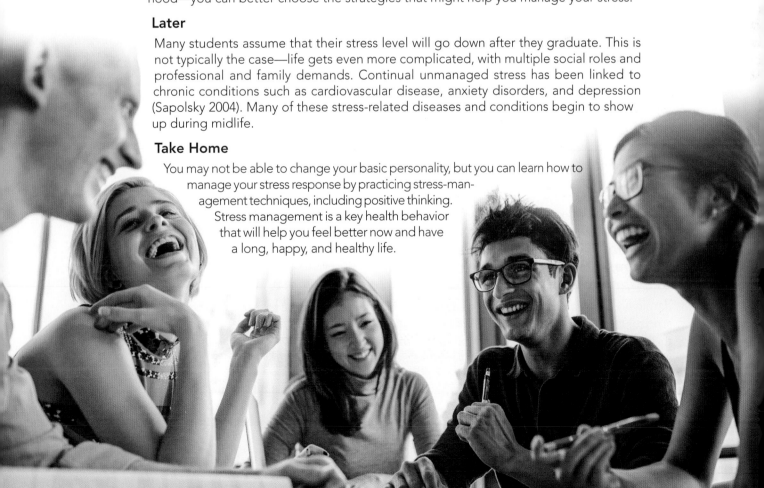

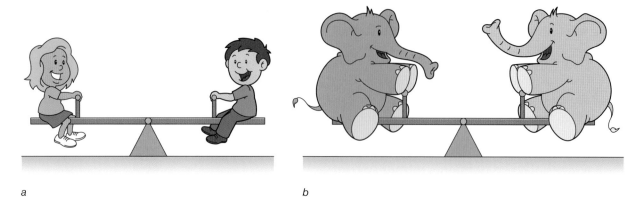

Figure 10.4   The "two elephants on a seesaw" model of stress-related disease (Sapolsky 2004). *(a)* Allostatic balance, with the children representing low levels of stress hormones. *(b)* Allostatic load, with the elephants representing the abundance of stress hormones responding to chronic stress. The elephants can balance but not without creating conditions for chronic diseases.

- *Collateral damage.* Although the seesaw might be able to balance, other damage will occur because the elephants cause a lot of wear and tear. Balancing your elephants (huge levels of stress hormones) for extended periods of time can be done, but it will negatively influence other systems in the body. This, essentially, is allostatic load.
- *Complicated dismount.* When these elephants are no longer needed because the stress has decreased, they will have a hard time getting off the seesaw gracefully. For example, if only one jumps off, the other will crash to the ground—in other words, some hormones will be high while others are low, even though they should generally run parallel. This illustrates how stress-related disease can be caused by the stress response turning off too slowly or by different components responding at different speeds. This effect also has negative health implications.

Conditions and Diseases Affected by the Stress Response

Repeatedly turning on the stress response can damage your health. In other words, it is not the stressor that makes us sick, it is the stress response itself—especially if it is purely psychological—that predisposes us to certain conditions and diseases. Table 10.1 summarizes the main systems that are adversely affected by chronic activation of the stress response, along with a brief description of their mechanisms (Sapolsky 2004).

Common Stressors and Hassles of College Life

Activation of the stress response typically occurs in three situations. First, an acute physical crisis can occur (e.g., accidentally stepping off a curb in front of a speeding car). Second, a chronic physical challenge can occur, which might include a major injury, chronic condition, or extended illness. Third, we encounter psychological and social disruptions, the primary causes of modern stress described earlier in the chapter. Essentially, the basic needs of humans are usually covered, but we create lots of stressful challenges in our own minds! Some of these concerns are legitimate (e.g., deadlines or being worried about a loved one's health); however, our stressful challenges are often not realistic or within our control, suggesting that we should not be activating our stress response to fight or flee from them.

Big Stressors and Little Stressors

Stress-response activators can be broken down into major life events and daily hassles. Major life events can be further divided into unforeseen environmental or societal events, such as living through a hurricane, witnessing a terrorist attack like the events at the World Trade Center in 2001, or living through the COVID-19 pandemic; and personal events, such as death of a loved one, divorce, disability, or a life-threatening illness (Lazarus and Folkman 1984).

Although we usually don't consider them as important as major life events, daily hassles—like

Table 10.1 Primary Systems Affected by Chronic Activation of the Stress Response

System	Primary mechanism	Symptoms or related diseases
Cardiovascular	Increases in resting heart rate and blood pressure Chronic systemic inflammation	Hypertension Coronary artery disease
Metabolic	Elevated levels of glucose and fat in the bloodstream	Atherosclerosis Type 2 diabetes
Digestion	Change in appetite (majority of people eat more, but some eat less) Changes in acid levels and blood flow in stomach	Weight loss or obesity Irritable bowel syndrome Ulcers (stress makes some types worse)
Immune	Mechanisms not well established	Colds and flu Cancer (potentially)
Sex and reproductive	Menstrual cycle irregularity Erection difficulties Loss of interest	Infertility Impotence
Brain	Neuron networks altered Less neurogenesis (fewer new neurons produced)	Reduced concentration and memory performance Dementia (potentially)

being stuck in traffic, having an argument with someone, and worries about money and relationships—are a significant contributor to our stress response. These minor but common events lead to frustration, annoyance, anger, and distress and are highly linked to other psychological and physical symptoms of stress (Lazarus and Folkman 1984).

Signs and Symptoms of Excessive Stress

The numerous signs of excessive stress span physical, emotional, and behavioral categories (table 10.2). Not all people experience all symptoms all the time, and a given symptom may show up in response to different stressors. Being able to recognize your personal stress symptoms will help you act quickly to make behavioral changes before your stress becomes an anxiety disorder or depression. Think of your personal stress signs as a glowing orange "check engine" light on your dashboard. In the chapter 10 labs on HK*Propel*, you will identify your main life stressors and develop a plan to cope with the effects of these stressors in your life.

Specific Stressors of College Life

Over and above the general stressors of life, college can involve specific stressors, especially during your first year. As you review the following categories, recall that one person's stress is another person's thrill. Although you might dread the first day of class because you don't know anyone, your more extroverted roommate might bounce out the door looking forward to meeting new people.

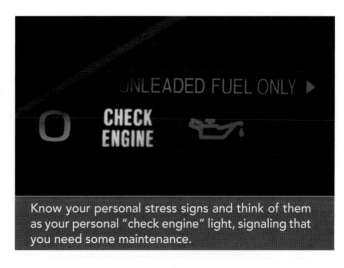

Know your personal stress signs and think of them as your personal "check engine" light, signaling that you need some maintenance.

Stress and the Aging Process: Before and After Serving in Office

Look at some photos of U.S. presidents taken when they were sworn into office and compare them to photos taken near the end of their terms. What do you notice? Chronic activation of the stress response is implicated in the aging process. The pictures of presidents when they took office compared to when they departed office suggest that highly stressful careers accelerate aging.

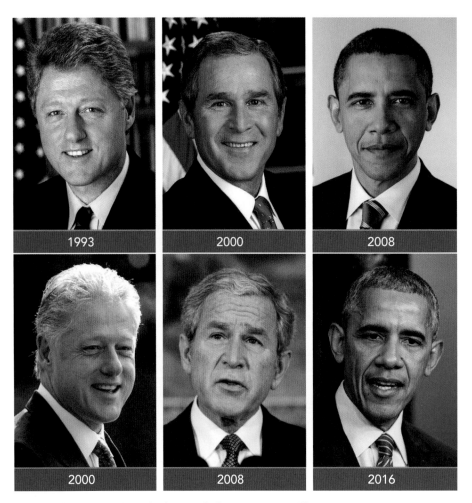

Photos of U.S. presidents before and after serving in office.

Academic Challenges

The heavy workload in college can be a challenge. Many students who attend college were very good students in high school; however, they may find college more challenging with its increased academic rigor and expectations. There is also much less structure in college than in high school, with fewer homework assignments, more comprehensive final exams, and classes and exams that are scheduled independently of one another.

Changing Social Roles, Relationships, and Identity

The transition to independence can be stressful even if it is welcome. Many challenges are interrelated, including the following examples:

- *Family.* Moving away from home can cause relationships with your family to change. Moving away can be welcome or cause great homesickness if your family is one of your primary social supports.

Table 10.2 Potential Signs of Excessive Stress

Physical	Emotional	Behavioral
Headaches	Easily angered, short tempered	Difficulty falling or staying asleep
Muscle tension; neck or back pain	Feeling depressed or down	Increased alcohol and substance abuse
Upset stomach, including nausea, constipation, and diarrhea	Feeling jittery	Loss of appetite or overeating comfort foods
Dry mouth and difficulty swallowing	Crying	Changes in connections with friends and family
Chest pains and rapid resting heartbeat	Becoming easily frustrated	Avoidance techniques with devices
Fatigue, low energy	Feeling overwhelmed	Reduced performance in job or school
Frequent colds and infections	Feeling bad about yourself (low self-esteem)	
Excessive sweating		
Clenched jaw and grinding teeth		

From Center for Diseases Control (2017a); American Psychological Association (n.d.); Sapolsky (2004).

- *New friends and relationships.* Meeting different people can be exciting but also a source of strain or even overwhelming, depending on your personality. Navigating your new social dynamics can be stressful.
- *Roommates.* Sharing space with new living partners can be challenging, especially if you had your own room and bathroom at home.
- *Self-image.* As you leave high school, you may need to adjust your self-image. Maybe you were thought of as the smart one, the talented athlete, or captain of the cheerleading team. Transitioning to college life can be a struggle as you get to know many different new people.
- *Larger social issues and choices.* College can also be a time when you are exposed to many different lifestyle choices, including sexual activity, alcohol use, and other issues such as sexual or gender orientation, religious beliefs, and political affiliations. You may experience stress as you begin to question or explore your own beliefs and choices.

Environment Changes

The transition to college will come with many changes in your physical environment, especially if you are living in the residence halls. You will sleep in a new bed in a new room with a new bathroom arrangement. You will eat in the dining halls rather than your own kitchen. The amount of noise may be different compared to your home, which may disrupt your sleep. Transportation on campus and around town will be different. Finding out where to go for classes and other requirements can be a source of stress.

Financial Pressures and Future Worries

College costs continue to rise, which stresses both students and their families. There are also many hidden and unplanned costs in college, including course fees, textbooks, and fees to join organizations. Many students now work part time to offset these rising costs, which can be stressful due to the added fatigue and time constraints. Accumulating student loan debt can also be a source of chronic stress and worry.

Many students who struggle to find a major and settle into a career path are stressed because

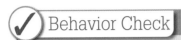

Behavior Check

What Are Your Top Stressors?

Recent representative data from college students indicated that only 27 percent reported no or low psychological distress. The balance reported moderate (50 percent) and serious (22 percent) psychological distress. Of a long and varied list of reported stressors, the top two challenges were procrastination (73 percent) and academics (52 percent) (American College Health Association 2021). Clearly, well-being is being compromised by mental health struggles, perhaps caused in part to the COVID-19 pandemic and the unique challenges it has brought to college campuses.

Take a few minutes to do a stressor inventory and determine your top two stressors. If you have minimal stressors, your life may be lacking challenge. If you have lots of stressors, you might be on overload. Remember that what constitutes a stressor is very personal. Try to determine if these top stressors are temporary or chronic. A temporary stressor might be a challenging course that will be finished at the end of the term. A chronic stressor might be having to balance a full academic load and a part-time job to pay for college for the next few years. At the end of the chapter, you will revisit these stressors and develop a stress-management plan to help you cope with and reduce the negative effects of stress in your life.

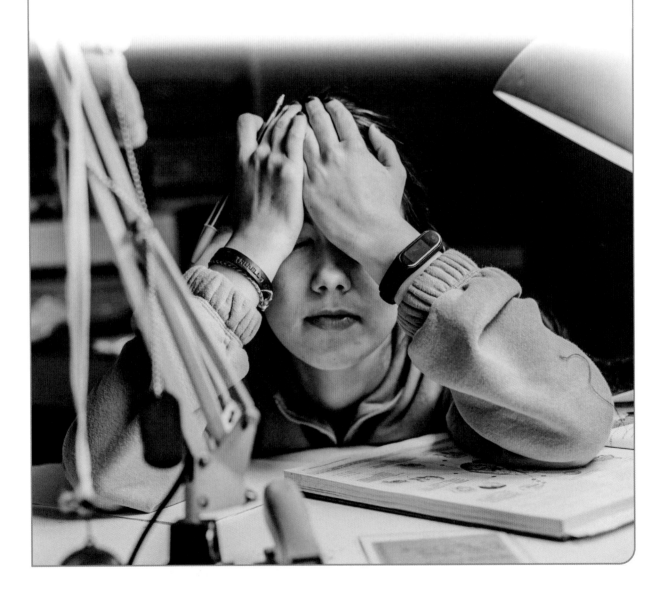

they know a good education is also supposed to prepare them for the workplace and put them on the path to financial independence. Although managing your life, including managing your money, is an essential component of becoming an independent person, the pressures of this process can be overwhelming.

Time Management

Many students struggle to manage their time and often complain that there is not enough time in the day. College adds tremendous freedom to your daily schedule. However, this lack of structure can also be a source of stress because you will need to learn how to simultaneously manage your academic, social, and (potentially) work lives. Figure 10.5 shows how college students use their time on an average weekday. However, note that this data has likely shifted in recent years as more people moved to remote working and online activities because of the COVID-19 pandemic. How our use of time has been permanently altered postpandemic will require more research in the next few years.

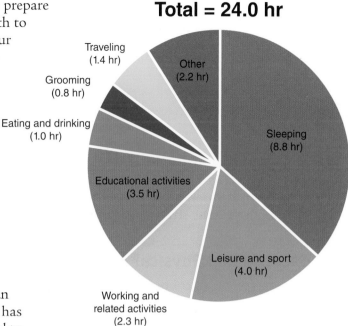

Total = 24.0 hr

- Traveling (1.4 hr)
- Other (2.2 hr)
- Grooming (0.8 hr)
- Eating and drinking (1.0 hr)
- Sleeping (8.8 hr)
- Educational activities (3.5 hr)
- Leisure and sport (4.0 hr)
- Working and related activities (2.3 hr)

Figure 10.5   Time use on an average weekday for full-time university and college students.

Note: Data include individuals aged 15 to 49 who were enrolled full time at a university or college. Data include nonholiday weekdays and are averages for 2011 to 2015.

From Bureau of Labor Statistics (2016).

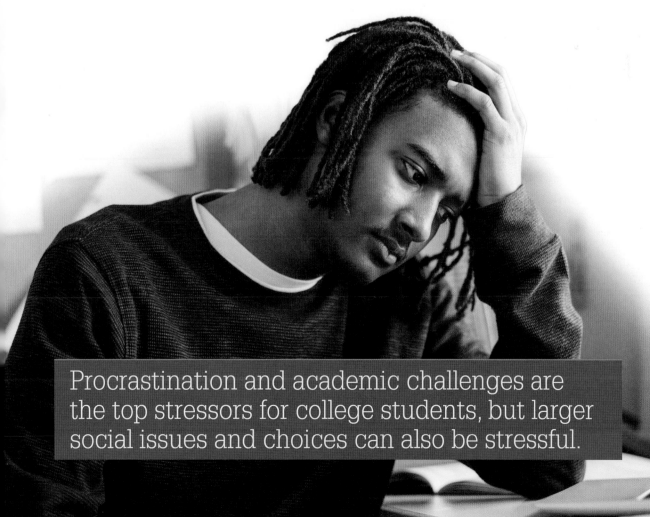

Procrastination and academic challenges are the top stressors for college students, but larger social issues and choices can also be stressful.

Key Stress-Management Strategies

Because we all have stressors in our lives, and there are times when these stressors are more significant and debilitating than others, it's important to learn how to put these life events into perspective and to have a coping plan in place. Like stressors, strategies for managing stress are personal. One tactic may help you more than your roommate, and some strategies will work better for combatting certain stressors than others. The primary stress-management strategies are summarized next.

Exercise and Physical Activity

As this textbook describes in detail, exercise and physical activity have many benefits for your health, including your mental health. Exercise can help you manage stress and anxiety and is used to help prevent or treat mild depression (U.S. Department of Health and Human Services 2018). Many modes of exercise are important, but most of the research on stress management is focused on cardiorespiratory activity. Regular daily movement of at least a moderate intensity can prevent the "check engine" light from going on (i.e., prevent stress from getting out of control).

You can also temporarily increase the amount of exercise you do when you are facing a short-term stressor, such as during finals week.

Fuel Your Body

Stress can have effects on dietary intake (Sapolsky 2004). Coping by eating for comfort—typically by overconsuming calories or increasing your intake of foods with more added sugars, saturated fats, and sodium—is often termed *stress eating*. When pressured for time, you may take in excessive caffeine, which can increase stress and anxiety in both the short and long term. Conversely, many people have a reduced appetite in response to stress, which can lead to low blood sugar. People also commonly skip breakfast due to stress, which can then cause low blood sugar during prime productive hours in the morning. Stress hormones can also cause your blood sugar to be less balanced, which can further contribute to stress levels. Making healthy fuel choices throughout the day is therefore important to help you manage stress (see chapter 8 for more information on nutrition).

Social Support

Social support is also a primary strategy for reducing your response to life's stressors. Being supported as well as being a support to others in

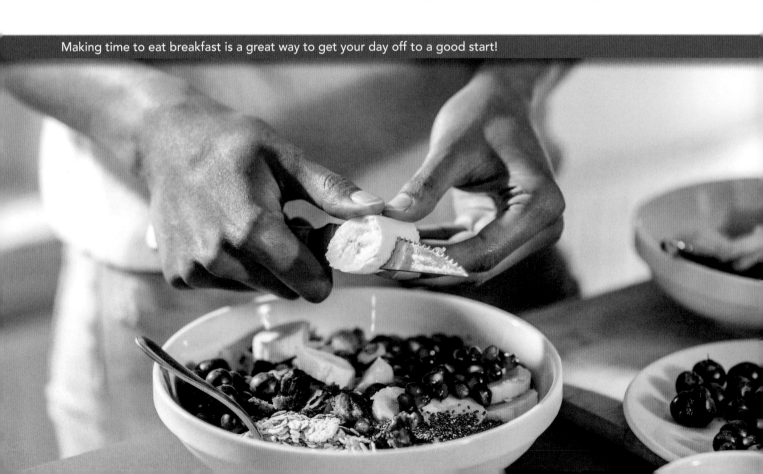
Making time to eat breakfast is a great way to get your day off to a good start!

times of need reduces the stress response, especially to psychological stressors (Sapolsky 2004). It is important to get social support from the right person, the right network of friends, and the right community. (We all know people who would increase our stress response if we asked them for help!)

Instead of placing the management of friendships, which take time and energy, into the "fun" category, start thinking of these activities as a health behavior. Fostering new friendships, maintaining established relationships, and investing effort to keep family connections healthy are all critical to your health. College presents opportunities to join many different clubs and organizations, ranging from church, sports, political, and volunteer experiences. Many of these are offered as registered student organizations at your institution. Finally, if you are struggling with relationship issues or are suffering from loneliness, most campuses offer counseling services for free or at a reduced cost. Good relationship skills are an important investment in your health. Invest in yourself.

Relaxation Techniques and Meditation: Quieting the Mind

Relaxation techniques often combine breathing and focused thoughts and images to calm the mind and the body. Common examples of relaxation response techniques are biofeedback, deep breathing, guided imagery, progressive relaxation, and self-hypnosis. Mind and body practices, such as meditation and yoga, are also sometimes considered useful for relaxation (National Institutes of Health 2022). When performed on a regular basis, meditation has been shown to reduce the negative effects of psychological stress (Goyal et al. 2014) and to reduce stress hormones (Sapolsky 2004).

Many different types of meditation exist, but most are focused on adopting positive and affirming thoughts. Two common methods are mindfulness meditation and Transcendental Meditation. **Mindfulness meditation** reduces psychological stress and the stress response by learning how to be mindful of the present moment, as opposed to thinking about the past or future. **Transcendental Meditation** emphasizes using a **mantra**, which is a word or phrase that is repeated to reach a point where your attention is no longer focused on the distressing thoughts.

Managing Your Life and To-Do List

Setting goals and priorities to keep you organized and prepared can help you manage your stress level. Oversleeping, running late for class, and rushing through your morning will almost cer-

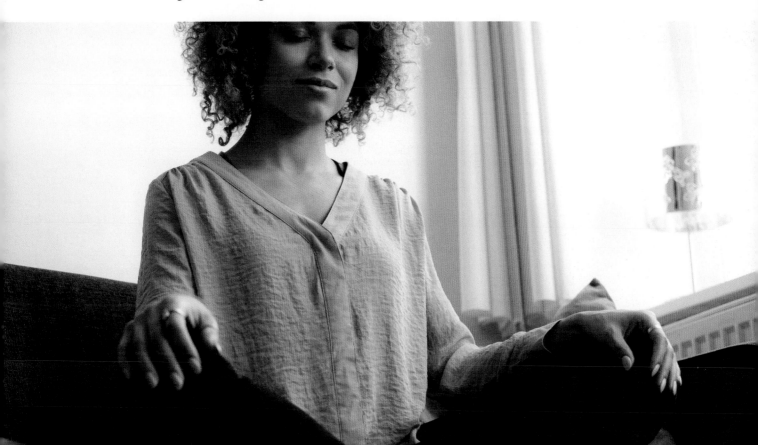

tainly cause a stress response. Arriving to class and realizing that you forgot about the exam scheduled for that day will cause your cortisol levels to increase. Consciously thinking through what must get done and what can wait for another day so you can prioritize your work *and* your rest is critical. **Time management** means successfully and efficiently prioritizing and scheduling one's time. Figure 10.6 illustrates steps that might offer some insights to increase your skills in managing your time and your life. Recall that the top challenge reported by college students is procrastina-

tion. How can you avoid procrastination? If you are struggling to find solutions, campus resources include trained professionals who can help you identify causes and workable solutions to reduce procrastination habits.

Managing Stress Through Sleep

Not only can the stress response can cause sleep disturbances, but lack of quality sleep greatly increases the stress response to life's challenges. For optimal health, it is important to make sure you get the quantity and quality of sleep you

Learn to Manage Your Time

1 **Set goals and priorities:** Write a "To-Do List" to help you stay focused.

Make a plan: Determine the milestones you want to accomplish and by when. **2**

3 **Divide big tasks into smaller tasks:** Chip away at the bigger task by breaking it up into smaller, more manageable pieces.

Set a deadline: Determine realistic deadlines so you can see your accomplishments. **4**

5 **Take breaks:** Determine a set time you will work on a project without any distractions (including your phone). Set a timer and work until the alarm goes off, and then reward yourself by taking a break.

Be organized: Have a place for all of your belongings so you don't have to take extra time in your day to search for them. **6**

7 **It's OK to say no!:** Recognize your limitations and realize it is okay to say no and focus on your priorities.

Enlist the help of friends and colleagues: Ask others to help you. **8**

9 **Anticipate the unexpected:** Allow extra time to complete your projects as problems may arise that are not under your control.

Record everything in a journal or calendar: Record all appointments, project due dates, and events in your calendar, and keep it updated. **10**

11 **Prioritize:** Focus on what is most critical and needs your attention.

Determine when you are the most productive: Are you a morning person, night person, or middle-of-the-day person? Notice when you have the most energy and complete your most demanding projects at this time of the day. **12**

Figure 10.6 Use these tips to successfully manage your time and lower your stress.

require to function properly. In today's society, regular, good-quality sleep is often thought of as a luxury reserved for days off. Your sleep behaviors are just as important for your health and academic performance as your diet and physical activity behaviors.

Sleep Quantity and Quality

As figure 10.7 depicts, sleep is an important health behavior, and many people struggle to get enough quality sleep (Watson et al. 2015). College students need 7 hours or more of sleep per night; however, the amount of sleep a person needs varies, especially with age. Infants, children, and adolescents need the most sleep. Most adults require 7 to 8 hours per night. However, some people function well on 5 hours, whereas others need 10 hours of sleep to feel their best (American Sleep Association n.d.).

Beyond quantity, uninterrupted (i.e., not fragmented) sleep is also very important for sleep quality so that each of the five stages of sleep can be experienced, especially stages 3 and 4 and REM (rapid eye movement) sleep. Typically, if uninterrupted, a healthy sleeper will pass through all five stages of sleep in a cycle of 90 to 110 minutes, with the length spent in the stages changing through the night (American Sleep Association n.d.).

- Stage 1 sleep:
  - Light sleep occurs.
  - You drift in and out of sleep but can be awakened easily.
  - Your eyes move slowly, and muscle activity slows.
  - You often experience a sense of falling or muscle spasms or jerks.
- Stage 2 sleep:
  - Your eye movements stop.
  - Your brain waves become slower.
  - Rapid brain waves occur occasionally.
- Stages 3 and 4 sleep:
  - In stage 3, slow brain waves appear called delta waves.
  - By stage 4, delta waves are the only brain waves.
  - Stages 3 and 4 are deep sleep with no eye or muscle activity.
  - If awakened, you are groggy and may be disoriented.

- REM sleep:
  - Your breathing becomes rapid, irregular, and shallow.
  - Your eyes jerk rapidly in random directions.
  - The muscles in your arms and legs become temporarily paralyzed.
  - Your heart rate increases, and blood pressure rises.
  - If awakened in this stage, you may recall bizarre or illogical dreams or thoughts.

If you feel drowsy during the day, you likely are not getting enough sleep. If you routinely fall asleep within five minutes of lying down, you likely have major sleep deprivation (American Sleep Association n.d.). Inability to fall asleep or stay asleep and sleep disorders such as sleep apnea are also a concern.

Therefore, it's important to get regular sleep instead of skipping sleep for many days and then planning to catch up on weekends or holiday breaks (figure 10.7). An excellent sleep resource is the American Sleep Association (www.sleepassociation.org). Speak with your personal physician if you are concerned about your sleep patterns.

> Thirty-three percent of the U.S. population reports being chronically sleep deprived, which is regularly sleeping for less than 7 hours in a 24-hour period (Centers for Disease Control and Prevention 2020).

Health Risks Associated With Poor Sleep

Regular, good sleep is essential for optimal health and a high quality of life. Without it, we experience adverse physical and mental consequences. These include an increased risk of accidents, injuries, cardiovascular and metabolic diseases, and mental health afflictions such as anxiety and depression. Lack of sleep also negatively affects mental alertness and focus and contributes to poor behavioral choices in general. Chronic sleep deprivation stimulates the stress systems, contributing to allostatic load. If you have poor sleep habits, you are at risk of developing numerous chronic health conditions that will negatively affect your life, now

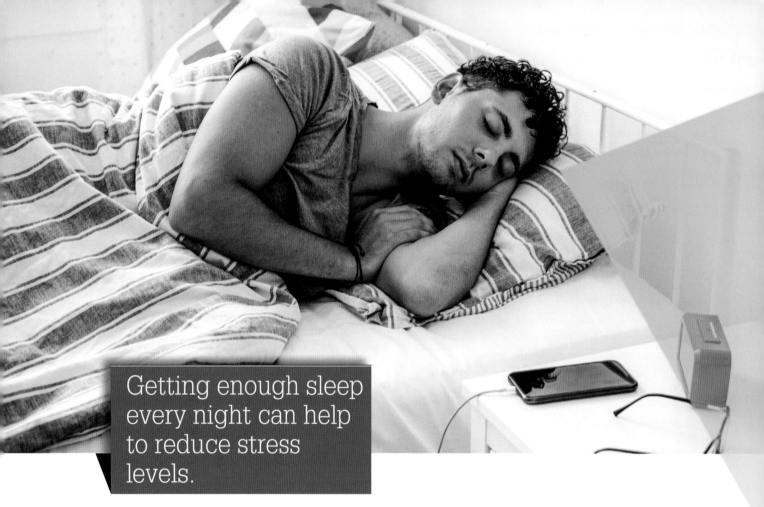

Getting enough sleep every night can help to reduce stress levels.

and in the future (American Sleep Association n.d.; Watson et al. 2015).

Strategies for Enhancing Sleep and Energy Levels

Like most health behaviors, sleep is a habit. Therefore, having good sleep habits can help you get a good night's sleep on a regular basis. The chapter 10 labs on HK*Propel* will help you assess your sleep quantity and quality and craft a personal plan for getting the sleep you need. The following main considerations will help you explore your sleep habits. For more detailed information, visit the sleep education site of the American Academy of Sleep Medicine (2020).

- Be consistent: Get up and go to bed at about the same time every day. This includes weekends, holidays, and breaks from school.

- Make sure your bedroom is cool (not too hot), peaceful, and quiet. Your mattress and pillows should be comfortable.

- Install dark curtains or blinds over your bedroom windows or wear an eye mask.

- Make your bedroom a screen-free zone. Do not share your bed with your computer and cell phone.

- Eat small meals before bedtime and resist the temptation to have pizza, tacos, and other spicy foods a few hours before bed. Some foods can cause indigestion, or acid reflux, which worsens when lying down.

- Limit your caffeine in the late afternoon or early evening (this includes chocolate and energy drinks) and limit alcohol and other fluids before bed to reduce the chances of having to use the bathroom during your sleep cycle.

- Get more physical activity during the day to help you fall asleep more easily at night.

- Talk to your health care provider about any medications you are taking and their effect on your sleep. You may be able to take medications that cause drowsiness before bed so you can stay awake for class and sleep at night.

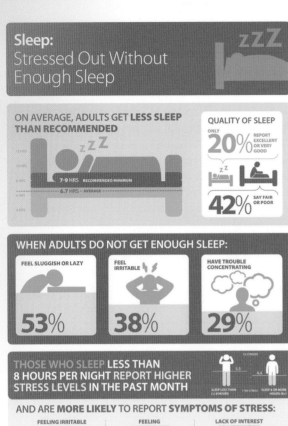

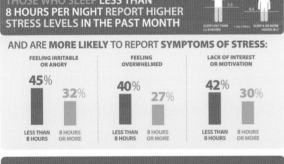

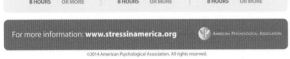

Figure 10.7 Where do you fall in this illustration? If you're not getting enough sleep, can you identify with some of the consequences?

Reprinted from American Psychological Association. www.apa.org/Images/2013-sia-Sleep-Infographic-1024_tcm7-166594.jpg

Social, Stressed, and Sleepless

The college years, especially the early ones, can be stressful, which affects sleep quality. The new relationships and environment of campus can also cause your social life to gear up significantly. You may find that the three factors of social life, stress, and sleep are intertwined. Social lives can cause stress, but social support is also very important for stress management. If you give more hours to your social life, you will have less time for academic work and sleep. Being pressed for time and sleep-deprived can also cause stress. Learning to balance the competing demands of all that you have to do and all that you want to do is a challenge that you will likely have for all of your working years. Learning this balance will serve you well, both now and in the future. Two important keys are keeping the positive energy and getting professional help if needed.

Keeping the Positive Energy: Habitual Movement Is Key

Of all of the stress-management strategies outlined in this chapter, a relatively high level of exercise and physical activity is one of the most important. Being regularly physically active at a moderate to high intensity, especially through cardiorespiratory and resistance training, can help manage stress and reduce the risks for anxiety disorders and mild depression. This level of activity is also linked with improved sleep quality (U.S. Department of Health and Human Services 2018). Finally, regular activity can also help you maintain mental and physical energy (Puetz, O'Connor, and Dishman 2006), which can help you accomplish the *have to do* and the *want to do* tasks on your list. In this way, your daily movement is the cornerstone of your plan to keep your stress responses in check.

Know When to Get Help

Although triggering your stress response can be unpleasant, experiencing stress now and again is not a problem for most of us. But for some people, repeated or sustained stress-response activation can lead to more serious mental health challenges, including anxiety disorders and depression.

Anxiety Disorders

Chronic stress can progress to an anxiety disorder (National Institutes of Mental Health 2023a). For example, **generalized anxiety disorder** is a condition where a person displays excessive anxiety and worry for months, with several relatively intense symptoms that do not go away and can get worse with time. **Panic disorder** presents with recurrent panic attacks, which are sudden periods of intense fear that might include heart pounding (palpitations), sweating, trembling, sensations of choking, shortness of breath, and sometimes a feeling of impending doom. People

Immunity Booster

Mind Your Exposome for Immune Health

The COVID-19 pandemic has altered our lives in countless ways, including the way we think about our health. The importance of our immune health has come to the forefront, and a growing literature is supporting the importance of lifestyle and environmental factors—the so-called *exposome*—for immune health (Morales et al. 2021). The main exposomes are lifestyle choices that have already been introduced in this textbook: physical activity; weight management; a high-quality diet rich in fruits, vegetables, and omega-3 fatty acids; adequate vitamin D; managed psychosocial stress; and adequate restorative sleep. Collectively, these behaviors greatly reduce systemic inflammation, which is a key factor in the metabolic big three and compromised immune function. Finally, minimizing exposure to environmental pollutants (e.g., air and water quality) are also important.

Studies with twins suggest that nonheritable factors (i.e., exposomes) play a greater role in immune responses than genetics do. Importantly, these factors not only impact the immune response, but they also influence individual response to vaccination. An important takeaway is that factors within the exposome interact over time to influence your defense against viruses. Although the COVID-19 pandemic is slowing as of this writing, most experts predict there will be similar viral pandemics in our future.

Behavior Check

Are Your Devices Hurting Your Sleep and Relationships?

We live in a world where we have access to news, weather, celebrity trends, and what our friends are doing 24 hours a day. Social media and technology have opened the world to us, allowing us to stay connected and work anywhere. Although these technological advances have improved our lives in many ways, they also have the potential to hurt our health. First, using devices too close to bedtime disrupts the sleep cycle because the blue light can potentially invoke the stress response, which keeps the brain engaged. Second, relying on technology for entertainment and social reactions may reduce the quality of your in-person relationships.

For your health, make a conscious effort to disconnect from email, the Internet, and social media and post an "out of office" reply every now and then. Plan screen-free days once a week or during a holiday or vacation. If you are uncomfortable with tuning out completely, consider how you can limit your screen time. Evaluate your notifications: Which ones can you do without? Try to check your phone for messages just once an hour while studying.

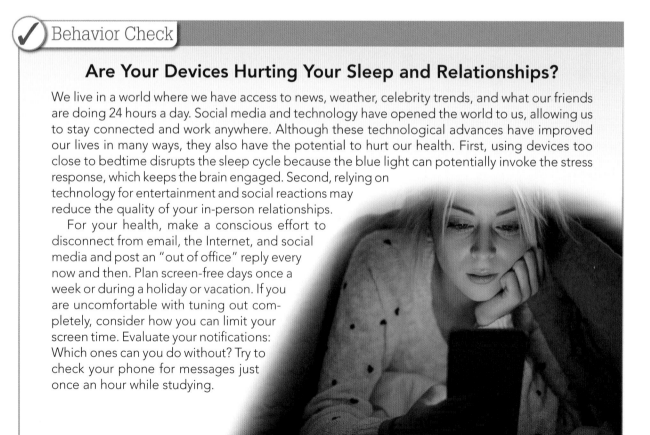

with **social anxiety disorder** have a marked fear of social or performance situations, with worries of embarrassment, judgment, or rejection triggering a stress response. Anxiety disorders can greatly reduce your quality of life, causing great distress, straining class or work performance, and hindering relationships.

Depression

Also related to stress and a close cousin to anxiety disorders is **depression**. Many different types of depression exist, and the most concerning type is major depressive disorder or clinical depression. Symptoms include persistent sadness, feelings of hopelessness, changes in sleep patterns (difficulty sleeping, early morning awakening, or oversleeping), changes in appetite or weight, decreased energy, and aches and pains that occur for at least two weeks (National Institutes of Mental Health 2023b). This is not a mild case of the blues in response to a temporary event; a defining feature of depression is loss of pleasure. Unfortunately, depression is highly linked to suicide.

Professional Help

If you are experiencing sustained symptoms of stress that you are unable to manage through the strategies described in this chapter, you may need to get some help to prevent longer-term health issues. Sometimes there are medical reasons for anxiety or depression. For example, some medications have side effects that can mimic anxiety disorders or depressive symptoms. Low blood sugar can also cause feelings of anxiety. Seeing a health care professional can help you sort through the various physiological, situational, or emotional reasons for your struggle. Nearly all colleges and universities have a student health center that offers services for both medical and psychological challenges that students routinely face. Know your resources and get help sooner rather than later.

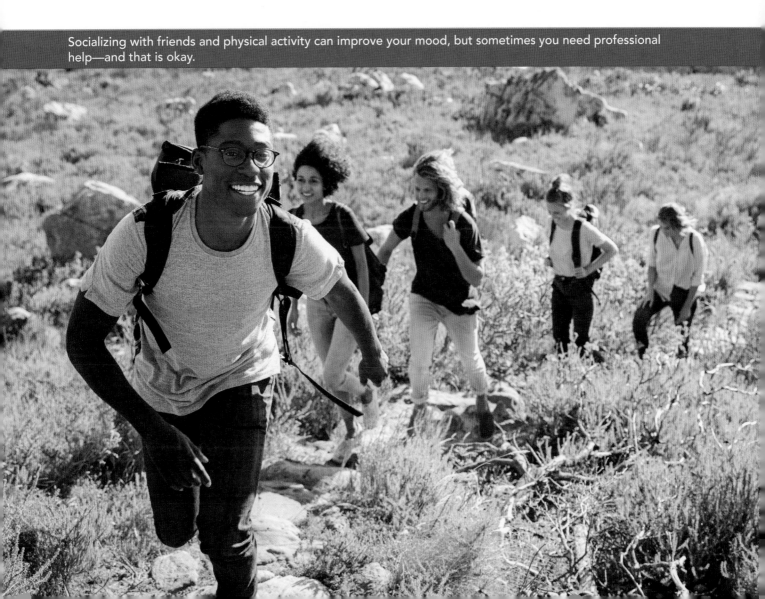

Socializing with friends and physical activity can improve your mood, but sometimes you need professional help—and that is okay.

Summary

We all experience stressors, especially psychological and social challenges. Although many stressors are good because they keep you engaged and challenged, too much challenge, especially for extended periods of time, can be overwhelming. Managing your stress response is important to prevent long-term negative health effects. Understanding your personal stressors, learning to read your "warning light," and practicing good stress-management strategies can help you cope. A regular moderate- to high-intensity physical activity program and healthy sleep practices are both foundational to managing your stress response and maintaining a high energy level to meet the demands of your busy schedule.

(www) ONLINE LEARNING ACTIVITIES

Go to HKPropel and complete all of the online activities to further facilitate your learning:

Study Activities: Review the main concepts of the chapter.

Labs: Complete the labs your instructor assigns.

Videos: Look through the videos and choose which ones you want to try this week.

REVIEW QUESTIONS

1. Define eustress and distress and provide typical examples of each for a college student.
2. What is the stress response and how do the neural and endocrine systems work together to cause it?
3. Define allostatic load and describe its link between chronic stress and health.
4. Describe three systems that are negatively influenced by chronic stress. By what mechanisms does stress affect the system, and what are the resulting conditions or diseases?
5. Describe common stressors for college students.
6. Stress symptoms are a "check engine" light for your health. Describe five common symptoms of chronic stress.
7. List the six key stress-management strategies described in this chapter and provide an example of each that might be used by a college student.

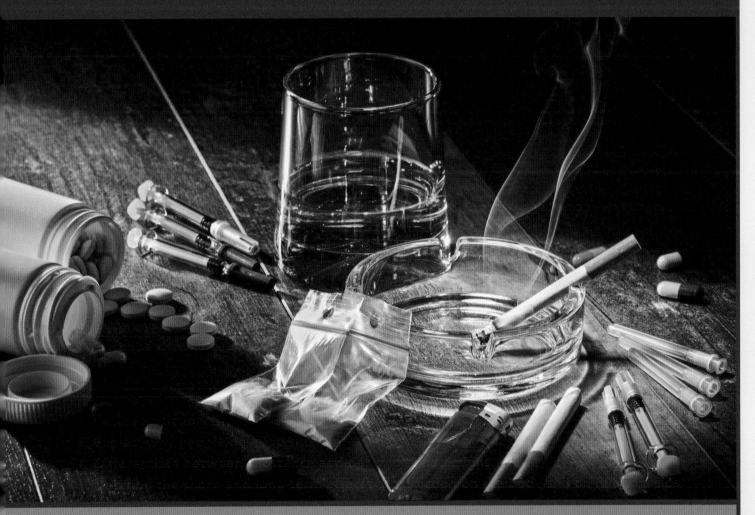

Remaining Free From Addiction

OBJECTIVES

- Define addiction.
- Explain why people develop substance and behavioral addictions.
- Differentiate between substance and behavioral addictions.
- Describe the short- and long-term effects of addiction on the body and on relationships with others.
- Identify treatment options for addiction.

KEY TERMS

addiction	illegal drugs
behavioral addiction	illicit drugs
binge drinking	marijuana
blood alcohol concentration (BAC)	methamphetamine
club drugs	neonatal abstinence syndrome (NAS)
cocaine	nicotine
dependence	opioids
depressants	psychoactive drugs
drug abuse	stimulants
drug misuse	substance addiction
heroin	vaping

Substance and behavioral addictions can take over a person's life, leading to an inability to care for themselves, debilitating disability, and even death. You may know someone who is struggling with an addiction: In 2018, 20.4 million Americans were diagnosed with a substance abuse disorder (Substance Abuse and Mental Health Services Administration 2019). Addictions are most likely to begin during adolescence and young adulthood (Grant et al. 2010). Addiction is a complex issue that is neither caused by a lack of willpower nor a sign of weakness. Research has shown that addiction influences the brain in ways that make quitting difficult, even for those who have a great desire to do so. This chapter focuses on how and why people become addicted to drugs and other harmful behaviors. It also provides information about resources for treatment and prevention of the most abused substances.

Types of Addictions

Two primary types of addictions exist: substance addiction and behavioral addiction. Both types can lead to serious health and social outcomes, such as poor decision making, loss of relationships, being arrested, increased risk of sexual assault (as the victim or the perpetrator), memory loss, and unemployment. Addiction can have fatal consequences if treatment is not sought or is not successful.

Substance Addictions

Substance addiction can be considered a dependence on a substance that, when stopped or reduced, leads to psychological and physiological tolerance and withdrawal symptoms. Figure 11.1

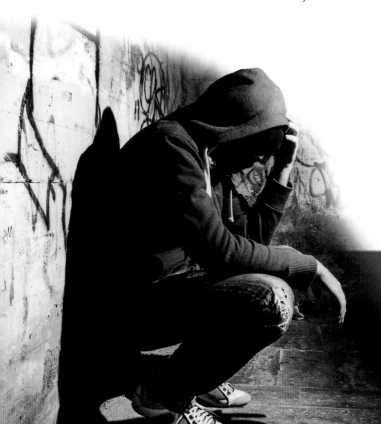

Addictions are complex and are not the result of a lack of willpower.

shows that in 2019, an estimated 60.1 percent of Americans aged 12 and older surveyed had used a substance within the past month. The most used substance was alcohol, followed by tobacco. It is important to keep in mind that not all people represented in figure 11.1 are considered to be addicted to substances; this represents how often per month people use these substances.

Alcohol and tobacco were included in the data regarding substances used within the last month by those ages 12 and older but will be discussed in further detail later in this chapter. For now, we will turn our focus to other substances. Drugs may be either used as intended or prescribed, or they may be misused or abused. **Drug misuse** occurs when a drug is taken for reasons other than intended by the manufacturer—for example, taking an antihistamine to feel high rather than to relieve allergy symptoms. **Drug abuse**, or taking a drug not as prescribed or intended consistently and over a long period of time, causes chemical changes to the brain that lead the individual to seek more drugs because of the euphoric and pleasurable effects. The primary chemical that causes these feelings is dopamine, the release of which motivates an addicted person to continue taking these drugs over and over. After a long period of taking drugs, the brain produces less dopamine, and the addicted person develops a tolerance that diminishes the euphoric feelings. This results in the need to take the drug in higher doses to achieve the same effects. Long-term use of drugs affects the brain's ability to process simple functions such as learning, judgment, decision making, adapting to and dealing with stressful situations, and memory (National Institute on Drug Abuse 2020a). Although many addicts are aware of the negative effects of abusing drugs, this knowledge alone is not enough to help them stop—this is the reality of addiction.

Figure 11.2 shows the total number of drug overdose deaths in the United States from 1999 to 2021 (National Institute on Drug

Abuse 2021h). In 2021 alone, more than 100,000 Americans died from overdose; this includes deaths from both illicit drugs and prescription opioids (National Institute on Drug Abuse 2021h).

Treatment of Substance Addictions

The good news is that, like many diseases and illnesses, addictions can be treated. Although there is always the possibility of relapse, many people in recovery succeed at managing their addiction for the rest of their lives. In 2017, 10.4 percent of people with substance abuse disorder received treatment (McCance-Katz 2019). The majority of those sought help for alcohol abuse, followed by marijuana abuse (Substance Abuse and Mental Health Services Administration 2014). The most common type of treatments used by those seeking help were self-help groups (e.g., Alcoholics Anonymous, Narcotics Anonymous) and outpatient rehabilitation facilities (McCance-Katz 2019). The best chance of success is a combination of

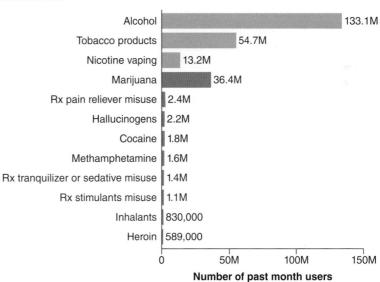

Figure 11.1 Number of past-month substance use among people aged 12 or older, 2019.

Note: Substance use includes any illicit drug, kratom, alcohol, and tobacco use. The estimated numbers of current users of different substances are not mutually exclusive; people may have used more than one type of substance in the past month.

From Substance Abuse and Mental Health Services Administration, *Key Substance Use and Mental Health Indicators in the United States: Results from the 2021 National Survey on Drug Use and Health,* (HHS Publication No. PEP22-07-01-005, NSDUH Series H-57), Center for Behavioral Health Statistics and Quality, Substance Abuse and Mental Health Services Administration (2022), https://www.samhsa.gov/data/sites/default/files/reports/rpt29394/NSDUHDetailedTabs2019/NSDUHDetTabsSect1pe2019.htm.

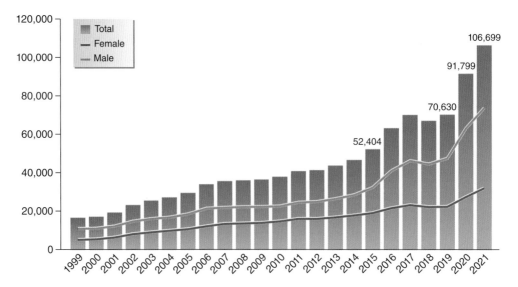

Figure 11.2   U.S. overdose deaths involving any illicit or prescription opioid drug, 1999-2021. The lines over the bar graphs depict the number of deaths by gender.

Reprinted from Centers for Disease Control and Prevention, National Center for Health Statistics, *Multiple Cause of Death 1999-2021* on CDC WONDER Online Database (2023).

https://www.drugabuse.gov/drug-topics/trends-statistics/overdose-death-rates.

addiction treatment medication with behavioral therapy that is specific to the needs of the patient.

Treating drug abuse and addictions may require the use of medications; however, all treatment options must include behavior therapies specific to the patient's needs to have the best chance at success. FDA-approved medications exist to treat addictions to cocaine, heroin, and methamphetamines. Examples of behavioral treatment options include cognitive behavior and skills therapy, couples and family therapy, community-based therapies, contingency management, rational emotive behavioral therapy, motivational interviewing, and 12-step therapy (Fifield 2021). Unfortunately, in 2019, the reasons people with substance use disorder reported for not receiving treatment at a specialty facility—despite believing they needed help—were that they were not ready to stop using the substance (39.9 percent), they did not know where to go for help (23.8 percent), or they did not have health care coverage and were not able to pay for the costs (20.9 percent) (Substance Abuse and Mental Health Services Administration, 2020).

Behavioral Addictions

Although not often a topic of discussion compared to substance addiction, the desire to get a high from certain behaviors is very common

and can lead to **behavioral addiction** (see figure 11.3). People with behavioral addictions experience similar highs to people with substance abuse problems because the brain releases dopamine during the addictive behavior (as it does when taking drugs), and the results can have equally negative consequences.

Examples of behavioral addictions include compulsive shopping, gambling, Internet addiction, video or computer game addiction, sexual addiction, excessive tanning, plastic surgery addiction, binge eating disorder (food addiction), exercise addiction, and risky behavior addiction (e.g., skydiving, rock climbing). See chapter 9 for information on addictions related to exercise and food.

People with behavioral addictions spend excessive amounts of time engaged in that behavior and are unable to stop or reduce that time. Eventually the addictive behavior leads to the inability to carry out normal daily activities and maintain positive relationships with others. A common characteristic of behavioral addictions is the inability to resist the temptation to engage in the behavior despite causing harm to oneself or others, like the inability to resist the urge to drink or use drugs. Many people with behavioral addictions report experiencing intense cravings prior to

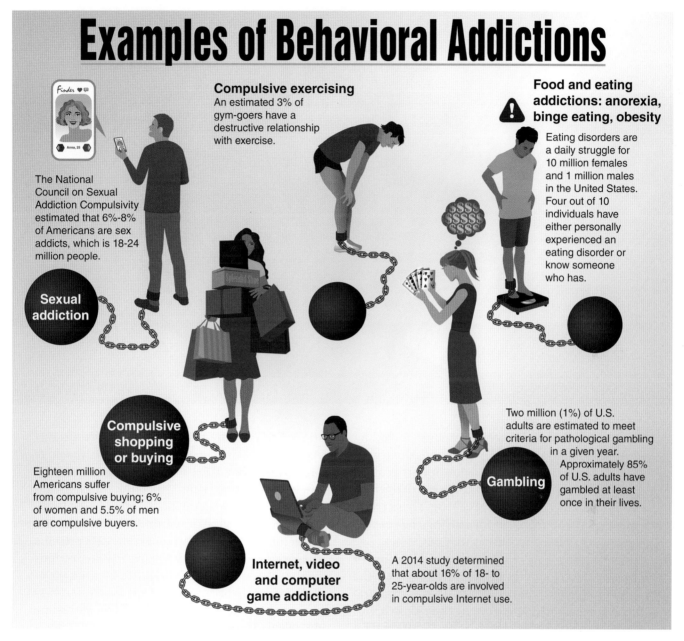

Examples of Behavioral Addictions

Compulsive exercising
An estimated 3% of gym-goers have a destructive relationship with exercise.

Food and eating addictions: anorexia, binge eating, obesity
Eating disorders are a daily struggle for 10 million females and 1 million males in the United States. Four out of 10 individuals have either personally experienced an eating disorder or know someone who has.

The National Council on Sexual Addiction Compulsivity estimated that 6%-8% of Americans are sex addicts, which is 18-24 million people.

Sexual addiction

Compulsive shopping or buying

Eighteen million Americans suffer from compulsive buying; 6% of women and 5.5% of men are compulsive buyers.

Gambling

Two million (1%) of U.S. adults are estimated to meet criteria for pathological gambling in a given year. Approximately 85% of U.S. adults have gambled at least once in their lives.

Internet, video and computer game addictions

A 2014 study determined that about 16% of 18- to 25-year-olds are involved in compulsive Internet use.

Figure 11.3 Behavioral addictions occur when the desire to get a high through certain behaviors becomes chronic and out of control.

Data from Bragg (2009); Koran et al. (2006); National Council on Problem Gambling (2014); Addiction Hope (2017); BBC News (2014); Eating Disorder Hope (2017); National Eating Disorders (2016).

the behavior. Once they engage in the behavior, they feel a sense of relief, somewhat like the high that is experienced with drug or alcohol abuse. The pleasure and gratification that accompanies the addictive behavior prevents the individual from recognizing its destructive effects (Grant et al. 2010).

Treatment of Behavioral Addictions

Many people with behavioral addictions experience numerous relapses and have a difficult time stopping these behaviors without professional help. Treatment options for behavioral addictions

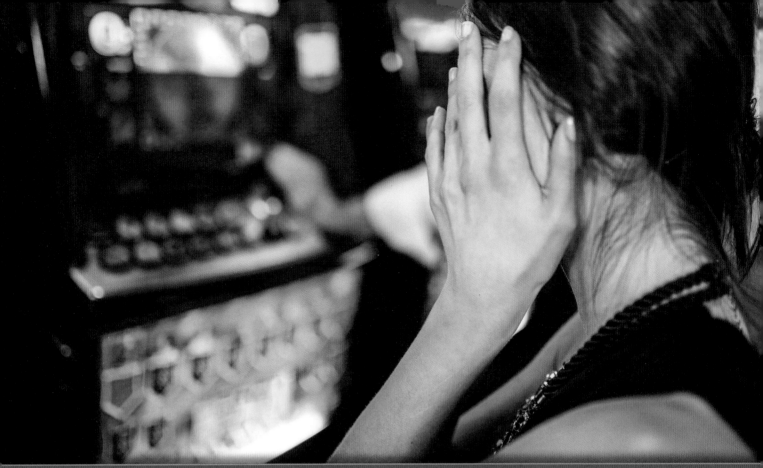

If a desire to get a high from any activity becomes chronic or out of control, it has become an addiction.

are much like those for substance abuse, including psychosocial support and medication, along with the traditional 12-step self-help support groups, motivational enhancement, and cognitive behavioral therapies (Grant et al. 2010). These treatment methods focus on identifying the specific behaviors that led to the negative outcomes (e.g., financial ruin, loss of close relationships, loss of employment) for the individual. They also help the person cope with the need for feelings of euphoria experienced when engaging in these destructive behaviors. These therapies provide alternative coping mechanisms for when addicted individuals are in high-risk situations and help them develop a plan that specifically identifies healthier behaviors they can implement for life.

What Is Addiction?

Consider for a moment how you would define drug addiction. Would your definition include how frequently a person uses a substance, how much is used, or a combination of those factors? Would it include other aspects, such as not being able to stop or always wanting more? In the chapter on Substance-Related and Addictive Disorders

in the 5th edition of the American Psychological Association's *Diagnostic and Statistical Manual of Mental Disorders* (2022) 10 separate classes of drugs are identified and include alcohol; caffeine; cannabis; hallucinogens; inhalants; opioids; sedatives, hypnotics, or anxiolytics; stimulants; tobacco; and other (or unknown) substances. The APA presents these classifications of drugs in separate sections of the DSM-5, but they are not to be thought of independently because all drugs taken in excess activate the brain's reward circuitry, and some people use more than one of these drugs concurrently (Grant and Chamberlain 2016). A common result of these substances when taken in excess is a disruption of the brain reward systems. Instead of reward system activation through adaptive behaviors, these substances produce such an intense activation of the reward system that normal activities may be neglected (Koob and Volkow 2016).

The DSM-5 provides criteria that indicate when someone has a substance abuse disorder based on the number of symptoms (Addiction Policy Forum 2022). Two or three symptoms indicate a mild substance use disorder; four or five symptoms indicate a moderate substance use disorder, and six or more symptoms indicate a severe substance use disorder (SUD). A severe SUD is classified as having an **addiction.**

The four categories are (1) impaired control, (2) social problems, (3) risky use, and (4) physical dependence. The symptoms per category include the following (Addiction Policy Forum 2022):

Impaired Control

- Using a substance for a longer time, or more often, or using more of the substance than intended
- Being unable to reduce the amount of substance use or stop using the substance, despite having the desire to do so

Social Problems

- Failing to give attention to work and other responsibilities like paying bills on time, scheduling medical appointments, etc.
- Stop engaging in activities that once were a priority, or not wanting to participate in social activities like sports, events with friends, volunteering, etc.
- Struggling to complete or follow through on responsibilities at work, home, or school

Risky Use

- Using the substance in unsafe situations and putting others in danger, like driving a car or using machinery after substance use
- Using the substance knowing it impairs cognitive and physical functioning and can cause long-term complications

Physical Dependence

- Adapting to the body's need for an increased use of the substance, and using more of it and more often to get the same effects because there is an increased tolerance effect
- Experiencing withdrawal symptoms when the substance is not in the body

Addiction becomes a concern when a person is not able to attend to daily responsibilities (e.g., not paying bills on time, neglecting relationships, arriving late to work, not attending school, or missing appointments). The addiction begins to consume the individual's life, which often leads to taking more of the drug and using it longer than intended.

Risk Factors: Why Do Some People Develop Addictions?

Many factors can lead to an addiction. It can be hard to predict whether someone has an addictive

---

 Behavior Check

Your Attitudes About Drug Use

Think about whether you agree or disagree with each of these statements (Centers for Disease Control and Prevention 1988):

1. Drug dependence happens when using drugs every day.
2. Most people who use drugs have financial problems.
3. Smoking cigarettes helps people control their emotions.
4. Using illegal drugs prevents people from being responsible.
5. Marijuana helps people cope with life stressors.
6. Smoking can cause people to age prematurely.
7. Cocaine can help reduce sleeping problems.
8. Drugs help people to be more creative.
9. Using drugs can lead to the loss of self-control.
10. Alcohol use can negatively affect relationships with family and friends.
11. People can remain relatively healthy even if they use illegal drugs.

personality and will develop dependence on drugs or behaviors that are harmful to themselves or others. Drugs influence the brain in a way that hinders the ability to stop taking them, causing many people to have a very difficult time quitting despite their desire to stop.

> Signs of addiction include the need to use more of a substance than before to get the desired effects and the inability to cut down or stop using it.

The more risk factors a person has, the more likely an addiction is to occur. The primary factors are as follows (National Institute on Drug Abuse 2020e):

- *Biology and genetics.* Genetics account for about half of a person's risk for developing an addiction; sex, ethnicity, and mental health also play a role. Males and individuals with mental disorders have a higher risk of drug use and addiction. People of color also experience an increased incidence of substance abuse because of barriers to appropriate treatment, stigma, bias, and socioeconomic status (PEW Trusts 2020).

- *Environment.* Family, friends, peers, socioeconomic status, and quality of life affect the likelihood of addiction. Lower socioeconomic status, pressure from peers to use drugs or participate in risky behaviors, significant stress, early exposure to drugs, physical and sexual abuse, and parental guidance all influence the risk.

- *Development.* The earlier drugs are introduced, or the risky behavior is initiated, the more likely an addiction is to develop. The teenage years are when most addicts experiment with drugs and risky behaviors. These years are critical for brain development, so teens are less likely to demonstrate good judgment and exhibit self-control.

College Students and Addictions

The use of **illicit drugs** among college students has increased in recent years. Unfortunately, a change in this trend does not appear to be on the horizon. In 2020, 43 percent of college students used illicit drugs (National Center for Drug Abuse Statistics 2021). Although there are many illicit drugs used by college students, alcohol remains the most commonly used substance (Schulenberg et al. 2020).

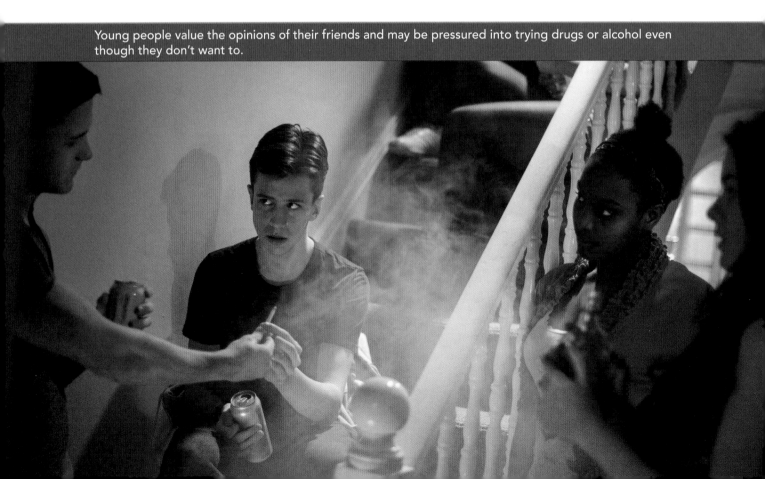

Young people value the opinions of their friends and may be pressured into trying drugs or alcohol even though they don't want to.

The types of drugs most used among college students include marijuana, amphetamines, heroin, inhalants, cocaine, and club drugs. Since 1980, researchers have been tracking substance abuse on an annual basis among college students and non-college students and reporting the results in the Monitoring the Future (MTF) National Survey Results on Drug Use. In 2019, the prevalence of use of any illicit drug was about the same for college students (47 percent) and for non-college students (46 percent) in 2019 (Schulenberg et al. 2020). Figure 11.4 shows the prevalence of various types of drug use by college students in 2019 (Schulenberg et al. 2020). Marijuana continues to have a high prevalence rate among college students; this percentage (43 percent) was unchanged between 2018 and 2019. Other noteworthy data include the increased rates of college students vaping marijuana and nicotine. The percentage of college students who vaped marijuana in the past 30 days increased from 5.2 percent in 2017 to 14 percent in 2019, whereas vaping nicotine for the same time period jumped from 6.1 percent in 2017 to 22 percent in 2019. According to Schulenberg et al. (2019), the increases in the use of vaping marijuana and nicotine are among the largest increases in use for any substance during the over 45-year history that the MTF study has been collecting data from college students.

> The use of marijuana, amphetamines, cocaine, hallucinogens, and MDMA are highest among people in their early to mid-20s, and rates among males are typically higher than females aged 19 to 30 (Schulenberg et al. 2020).

Psychoactive Drugs

Psychoactive drugs include both illegal and prescription **opioids**, **stimulants**, and **depressants**. Commonly abused illicit drugs include marijuana and other cannabinoids, heroin, cocaine, methamphetamine, anabolic steroids, inhalants, certain prescription and over-the-counter medications, and a variety of club drugs. This section presents facts about many of these drugs, including their alternate names, incidence of use, mechanism of action, and short- and long-term effects.

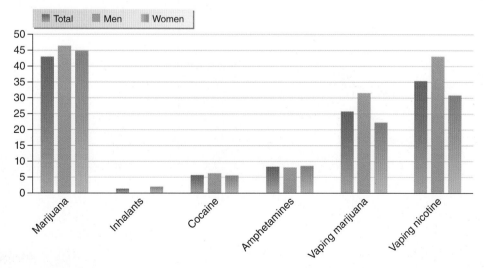

Figure 11.4 Annual prevalence of use of various types of drugs among full-time college students by sex, 2019.

Note: Entries are percentages.

Data from Schulenberg et al. (2020).

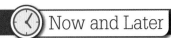 **Now and Later**

Substance Abuse and a Lifetime of Negative Consequences

Now

The best way to prevent substance abuse is to never try illicit drugs. There are many ways to avoid drugs in college (Kilpatrick 2016). Review the following information to stay drug free, now and for life:

- Become involved in extracurricular activities.
- Attend all classes and take advantage of assistance from professors to do well.
- Make a commitment to get at least eight hours of sleep a night, get some physical activity every day, and maintain a healthy weight.
- Hang around people who do not use illicit drugs or drink alcohol. Attend social events where these substances are not offered.
- Take courses or attend events to learn more about the dangers of drugs and alcohol, signs of addiction, and the connection between these substances and the prevention of sexual assault.
- Contribute to substance abuse prevention on your campus by volunteering to be part of alternative, responsible ways to have fun.

Later

Addictions to drugs and alcohol become chronic conditions that are very difficult to control despite the harmful and potentially fatal outcomes. Review the following facts about addiction to help you understand the negative consequences that may occur:

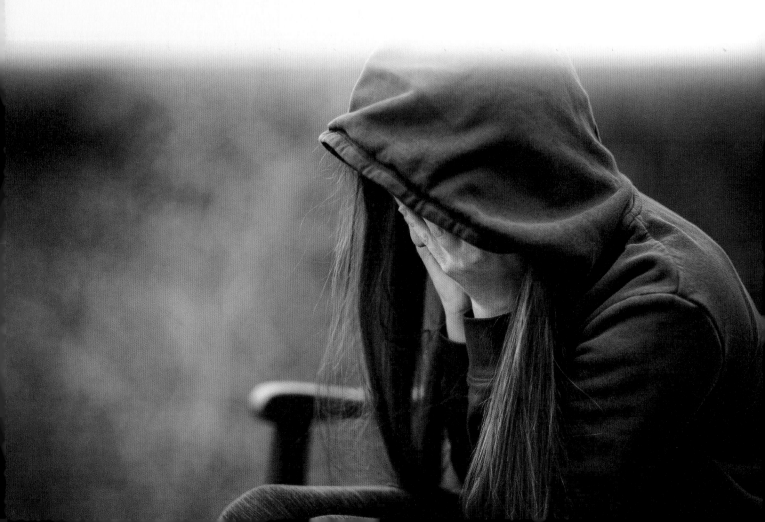

- Alcoholics are more likely to get divorced (Cranford 2014).

- In 2014, every 15 minutes, a baby was born with *neonatal abstinence syndrome (NAS)*, which is a group of conditions related to drug withdrawal experienced by an infant who was exposed to opioids or other addictive drugs during pregnancy (Jilani et al. 2019). The number of opioid-related diagnoses documented at the time of delivery increased by 131 percent between 2010 and 2017 (Hirai et al. 2021).

- Staying on the job is more difficult. Addicts are 2.7 times more likely to have injury-related absences (National Council on Alcoholism and Drug Dependence 2015).

- Accidents can occur at work. Among workplace-related deaths, 11 percent of the victims had been drinking alcohol (National Council on Alcoholism and Drug Dependence 2015).

- Addiction makes it difficult to keep a job. Workers who had three or more jobs in the previous five years are about twice as likely to be current or past-year users of illegal drugs as people who have held a single job (National Council on Alcoholism and Drug Dependence 2015).

Take Home

No single factor can predict whether a person will become addicted to drugs; many circumstances related to genetics, environment, and development can cause an addiction. The best way to prevent addiction is never to try illicit drugs. It's always good to have a plan in place to help you and your friends avoid using drugs and alcohol. Should you find yourself addicted to drugs or alcohol and want information to help you stop, contact your university's drug and alcohol center, or call the national hotline at 800-662-HELP (4357). The Substance Abuse and Mental Health Services Administration's national helpline is a free, confidential, 24/7, 365-day-a-year treatment referral and information service (in English and Spanish) for individuals and families facing mental health or substance use disorders. You can also call the Drug and Alcohol Abuse Hotline: 888-328-2518.

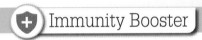 Immunity Booster

Pregnancy and Cannabis

Having a baby now may not be in your plans, but do you realize that preparing for a healthy pregnancy in the future starts now? Research shows that females who use cannabis could have a more difficult time conceiving a child than those who do not (Mumford et al. 2021). Research also shows that pregnant people who use illicit drugs are more likely to use cannabis than other drugs such as cocaine, heroin, or methamphetamine due to the belief that cannabis may be less harmful to the developing embryo and fetus compared to other drugs. However, this fetal exposure during pregnancy can lead to a weakened immune system and an increased risk of cancer later in life (Dong et al. 2019). Of current concern is the abuse of potent synthetic cannabinoids, which are more easily accessible and contain chemicals that can cross the placental barrier and affect the fetus.

Therefore, if you plan on having a child in the future, keep your immune system at peak performance to support conception, and continue to refrain from using during pregnancy so you can give your baby the best start to life. When it comes to pregnancies (either current or future), it is simple—do not use cannabinoids of any kind, and if you are currently using, stop. Finally, it is important to note that marijuana use among males and the subsequent impact on conception rates is an area of current research efforts.

ILLEGAL DRUGS

Illegal drugs are limited in their production and use by governments. In the United States, commonly used illegal drugs include marijuana, heroin, inhalants, cocaine, and methamphetamine. Inhalants can be purchased legally as household substances, but it is illegal to use these substances for getting high. Most states have penalties for selling or providing common inhalants to minors.

MARIJUANA

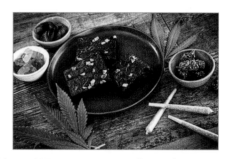

Marijuana is derived from the *Cannabis* plant. The active ingredient that causes changes in the brain is THC, or delta-9-tetrahydrocannabinol. Although research shows some benefits of their use for certain health conditions, cannabinoids are the most abused illicit drugs worldwide.

Alternate names. Blunt, dope, grass, herb, pot, skunk, weed.

Incidence of use. Marijuana is the most commonly used drug in the United States (National Institute on Drug Abuse 2020c). There is a four to seven times increased risk of developing marijuana use disorder among people who begin using marijuana before the age of 18 (National Institute on Drug Abuse 2021c). Figure 11.5 shows that marijuana use among college-aged adults is at about 43 percent, which is the highest in over three decades (Sherburne 2019).

Mechanism of action. Typically smoked in a rolled cigarette (joint) or with pipes or a bong (a device that uses water); can also be ingested in foods like brownies, cookies, or candy.

Short-term effects. Altered senses (for example, seeing brighter colors), a distorted sense of time, mood swings, inability to have normal body movements, difficulty with thinking and problem solving, and impaired memory (National Institute on Drug Abuse 2021e).

Long-term effects. Leads to impairments related to thinking, memory, learning, and how the brain makes connections between these cognitive functions. These impairments can be permanent (National Institute on Drug Abuse 2021e).

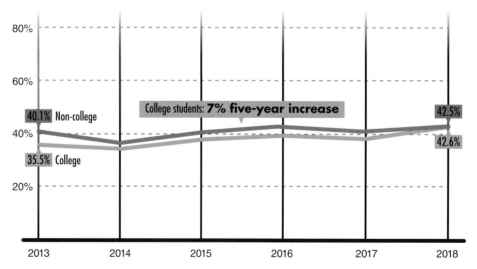

Figure 11.5   Marijuana use among full-time college students and non-college peers, 2018.
Reprinted from National Institute on Drug Abuse (2019b).

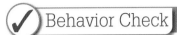

Behavior Check

Legalization of Marijuana

Marijuana is currently an illegal drug in the United States as a whole. However, cannabis products are legal for medical use in 37 states, including the District of Columbia, Guam, Puerto Rico, and the U.S. Virgin Islands (National Conference of State Legislators 2022).

One of the primary reasons given for why marijuana should be legalized is because of its medicinal uses in helping with pain and nausea; however, most physicians are not trained in the prescription of marijuana or the best methods of administration for their patients (e.g., smoking, ingesting, or vaping). Marijuana use during college can have an impact on educational achievement among college students. A study conducted by Arria et al. (2015) showed that students who used

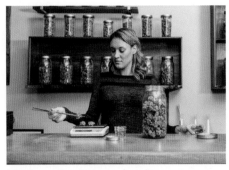

Marijuana has become legal in some states. These specialty stores are making marijuana more easily accessible.

marijuana more frequently during the first year of college were more likely to not attend classes leading to earning lower grades and delaying graduation for several years. Increases in marijuana use over time resulted in a lower GPA.

- What are your attitudes and values about the use of marijuana for recreational reasons?
- What are your attitudes and values about the use of marijuana for medical reasons?
- Does the legalization of marijuana lead to increased use?

HEROIN

Heroin is an opioid made from morphine, which is extracted from the seed pod of the Asian poppy plant. Heroin has no accepted medical use in the United States (Substance Abuse and Mental Health Services Administration 2015).

Alternate names. Smack, dope, mud, horse, junk, H, black tar, brown sugar.

Incidence of use. According to the Substance Abuse and Mental Health Services Administration (as cited in Strain, Saxon, and Friedman 2021), in 2019, it was estimated that 5.7 million Americans or about 2.1 percent of the population age 12 and older,

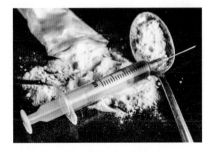

have used heroin at some time during their lives. An alarming statistic is that between 2002 and 2018, the rates of heroin use and heroin use disorder almost doubled (Substance Abuse and Mental Health Services Administration 2019 as cited in Han, Volkow, Compton, and McCance-Katz 2020). There has also been an increase among young adults aged 18 to 25 living in urban areas, an age group that is also seeking treatment at an increased rate (National Institute on Drug Abuse 2021k).

Mechanism of action. Injected, inhaled by snorting or sniffing, or smoked.

Short-term effects. Alters areas in the brain that affect pain, arousal, blood pressure, and breathing (National Institute on Drug Abuse 2021k).

Long-term effects. Deterioration of sections of the brain that affect decision making and responses to stressful situations, severe pulmonary complications like pneumonia, infections of the heart lining and valves, abscesses, constipation and gastrointestinal cramping, and liver and kidney disease. Chronic use of heroin leads to physical dependence so that a chronic user will experience severe symptoms of withdrawal within a few hours of stopping; these include restlessness, muscle and bone

> The risk is high: Almost one-fourth of people who use heroin become dependent on it.

pain, insomnia, diarrhea and vomiting, cold flashes with goosebumps, and kicking movements. During withdrawal, users also experience severe cravings for heroin that often lead to relapse (National Institute on Drug Abuse 2021l). Overdosing causes breathing complications that result in brain damage or coma.

✓ Behavior Check

Syringe Services Programs

People who inject drugs are at high risk of contracting life-threatening blood-borne infections, including HIV, hepatitis C (HCV), and hepatitis B (HBV) (National Institute on Drug Abuse 2021j). Many intravenous drug users share their syringes, thus increasing the risk of acquiring these fatal diseases through blood or other bodily fluids remaining in the needle or syringe. Engaging in unprotected sex with an intravenous drug user may increase the risks of acquiring these blood-borne infections.

Many communities have initiated needle exchange or syringe services programs to help reduce the chances of intravenous drug users spreading these diseases. These programs provide free access to sterile syringes and injection equipment, vaccinations, disease testing, safe disposal of used needles and syringes, counseling on risk reduction and safer sex practices, and substance abuse treatment (National Institute on Drug Abuse 2021j). These programs have been shown to be effective in preventing and tackling outbreaks of HIV and HCV in communities.

In 2015, there was an outbreak of HIV and HCV in a rural southern Indiana county that resulted in over 200 people infected. The state health department's syringe services program dramatically decreased the transmission rate and saved taxpayers $120 million in health care costs (Sightes et al. 2018).

- What do you think about syringe services programs? Are they effective? Why or why not?
- Does a syringe services program contribute to the problem of addiction?
- Does a syringe services program prevent the spread of fatal diseases like hepatitis B or HIV?
- Do you believe that syringe services programs give the message that it is okay to use intravenous drugs?
- What are other ways communities can prevent the use of illegal intravenous drugs besides implementing syringe services programs?

INHALANTS

Inhalants are chemical vapors that cause a mind-altering effect when breathed in. These include the following:

- **Volatile solvents.** Liquids from common household and industrial products that vaporize at room temperature.
- **Aerosols.** Sprays that contain propellants and solvents, such as those found in spray paints, deodorant, hair sprays, vegetable oil sprays, and fabric protector sprays.
- **Gases.** Vapors from medical anesthetic gases used in household or commercial products.
- **Nitrites.** Liquids from pain medications for heart conditions that are used primarily as sexual enhancers.

Alternate names. Laughing gas (nitrous oxide), snappers (amyl nitrite), poppers (amyl nitrite and butyl nitrite), whippets (fluorinated hydrocarbons), bold (nitrites), and rush (nitrites) (National Institute on Drug Abuse 2021b).

Incidence of use. In the United States, approximately 21.7 million

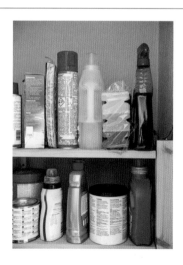

people aged 12 and older have used inhalants at least once during their lives, and 13.1 percent of eighth graders have tried inhalants (National Institute on Drug Abuse 2020b).

Mechanism of action. Users sniff or "snort" fumes from containers, spray aerosols directly into the nose or mouth, "bag" fumes by sniffing the inside of a plastic or paper bag where substances have been sprayed or deposited, "huff" from an inhalant-soaked rag stuffed in the mouth, or inhale from balloons filled with nitrous oxide (National Institute on Drug Abuse 2021b). After being inhaled through the nose or mouth, chemicals quickly pass into the bloodstream and then travel to the lungs, brain, and other body organs.

Short-term effects. Volatile solvents, aerosols, and gases affect the central nervous system (CNS). Nitrites dilate the blood vessels and relax the muscles. Inhalants alter one's mood by producing pleasurable effects; however, they can also result in dizziness, drowsiness, slurred speech, lethargy, depressed reflexes, general muscle weakness, and stupor (National Institute on Drug Abuse 2021b).

Long-term effects. Toxic chemicals can remain in the body for a long period of time. They are absorbed by the fatty tissues in the brain and central nervous system, causing muscle tremors and spasms that affect daily activities like walking, bending over, and talking. Users may experience difficulties having conversations with others and solving complex problems, as well as clumsiness (National Institute on Drug Abuse 2021b). Sporadic or single use of inhalants can cause death from cardiac arrest due to the sudden disruption of the heart rhythm or can reduce oxygen levels enough to lead to suffocation (National Institute on Drug Abuse 2020b).

COCAINE

Cocaine is a very powerful and addictive stimulant that is derived from coca leaves that grow in South America. Initially developed to treat illnesses and serve as a local anesthetic, it has detrimental effects on the brain when used repeatedly (National Institute on Drug Abuse 2021a).

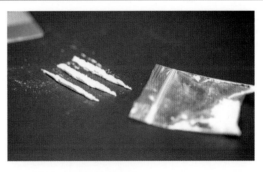

Alternate names. Blow, candy, coke, crack, rock, snow (National Institute on Drug Abuse 2021a).

Incidence of use. In 2021, people aged 12 or older, 1.7 percent (or 4.8 million people) used cocaine in the previous year. The percentage was highest, 3.5 percent, among young adults aged 18 to 25 (Substance Abuse and Mental Health Services Administration 2022).

Mechanism of action. Inhaled, smoked, or mixed with heroin (speedball) and injected into a vein.

Short-term effects. Enlarged pupils, increased energy and alertness, violent behavior, heart attacks, strokes and seizures, euphoria, anxiety, paranoia, psychosis, and an increase in body temperature, heart rate, and blood pressure (National Institute on Drug Abuse 2021a).

Long-term effects. Permanent loss of sense of smell, nosebleeds, damage to the nose, difficulty swallowing, and a decreased appetite that leads to poor nutrition and significant weight loss (National Institute on Drug Abuse 2021a).

METHAMPHETAMINE

Methamphetamine is an extremely addictive stimulant drug that is a white, odorless, bitter-tasting crystalline powder. The effects of the drug can last up to 24 hours, with an average duration of 6 to 8 hours (Foundation for a Drug-Free World n.d.). Meth produces an immediate, intense euphoria, but because of the short-acting power of the stimulant, users quickly adopt a binge-and-crash pattern in order to sustain the high.

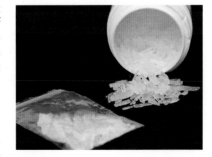

Methamphetamine has become a highly abused drug because it can be manufactured in concealed laboratories with ingredients such as pseudoephedrine, a common ingredient in cold medicines. For this reason, products containing pseudoephedrine are now kept behind the pharmacy counter, and stores limit the number of these products that individuals may purchase in a day (National Institute on Drug Abuse 2021f).

Alternate names. Meth, crystal, chalk, ice.

Incidence of use. Between 2015 and 2018, among Americans aged 18 years and older, an estimated 1.6 million had reported past-year methamphetamine use; 52.9 percent had a methamphetamine use disorder, and 22.3 percent reported injecting methamphetamine (Jones, Compton, and Mustaquim 2020).

Mechanism of action. Taken orally, smoked, snorted, or dissolved in water or alcohol and injected; the drug gets to the brain the fastest when it is smoked or injected.

Short-term effects. Anxiety, confusion, insomnia, mood disturbances, violent behaviors, psychosis (e.g., paranoia, hallucinations, and delusions), increased wakefulness, increased physical activity, decreased appetite, increased respiration, rapid heart rate, irregular heartbeat, increased blood pressure, and increased body temperature (National Institute on Drug Abuse 2021f).

Long-term effects. Reduced motor skills, impaired verbal learning, emotional and memory problems, extreme weight loss, severe dental problems ("meth mouth"), skin sores caused by scratching, increased risk of contracting infectious diseases like HIV and hepatitis B and C (National Institute on Drug Abuse 2021f).

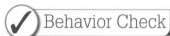 Behavior Check

Treatment for Drug Abuse and Addiction

Medications available to help addicts wean off opioids include buprenorphine, methadone, and naltrexone. Buprenorphine and methadone work by binding to the same cell receptors that heroin does with less of an effect, helping reduce cravings so the user can wean off the drug. Naltrexone blocks opioid receptors and prevents the drug from having an effect. Some patients have trouble complying with naltrexone treatment, but a new long-acting version given by injection in a doctor's office may increase this treatment's efficacy.

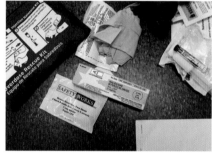

Emergency medication is also available for overdoses (National Institute on Drug Abuse 2017). Naloxone effectively reverses opioid and heroin overdoses. It is an inexpensive, quick-acting medication that restores breathing within minutes and only reverses overdose in individuals

This is an example of an overdose rescue kit that can be used to assist someone who is experiencing an opiate overdose.

who have opioids in their bodies (National Institute on Drug Abuse 2021g). Health care providers can administer naloxone and physicians can prescribe it to someone at risk of an overdose.

- What do you think about providing overdose rescue kits to addicted individuals or a family member or friend of the drug user?
- Would you want this kit if you had a friend or family member addicted to opioids or heroin? Why or why not?
- Do you think providing the kits to addicts keeps them from seeking treatment for their addiction because they know they have a safety net in case of an overdose?
- Does this medication save a life or enable an addiction?

Meth and Future Life Plans

Now

Methamphetamines are pervasive in our country, and much of it comes from other countries or is imported into the United States. Figure 11.6 shows the number of meth seizures in the United States between 2013 and 2019, and figure 11.7 shows methamphetamine lab sites, including dumpsites and seizures of chemicals and equipment.

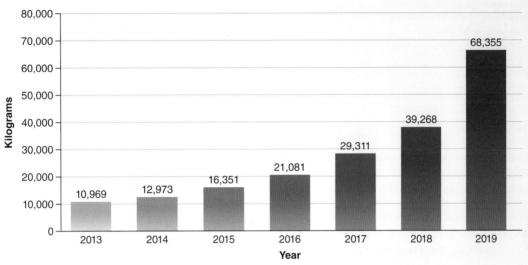

Figure 11.6 Methamphetamine seizures at the southwest U.S. border, 2013-2019.

Reprinted from Drug Enforcement Administration (2020).

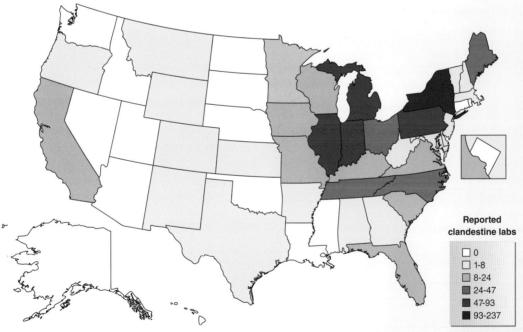

Figure 11.7 Methamphetamine lab sites (including dumpsites and chemical/equipment seizures), by state, 2019.

Reprinted from Drug Enforcement Administration (2020); Drug Threat Assessment (2021).

Later

How does the increased availability of meth coming into our country influence where you would want to go to graduate school, look for employment, engage in recreational activities, raise a family, and eventually retire?

Take Home

The choices we make, such as geographic location or the friends we spend time with, can influence our ability to remain free from addiction.

PRESCRIPTION DRUGS

Prescription drugs are prescribed to treat common disorders, but when they are obtained without a prescription and consumed in higher doses than prescribed, they can become addictive. Commonly abused prescription medications include opioids, depressants, and stimulants. The most common prescription drugs that are abused by teens and college-age students include Adderall, Ritalin, cold medicine with codeine and without codeine, and oxycodone.

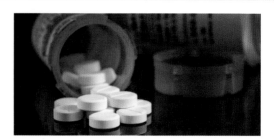

College students use prescription medications like Adderall illegally to help them focus on their academic responsibilities.

ADDERALL AND RITALIN (STIMULANTS)

Alternate names. Bennies, black beauties, crank, ice, speed, and uppers (Drug Enforcement Administration 2020).

Incidence of use. Approximately 20 percent of college students are abusing prescription stimulants, either recreationally or to help them study for longer periods of time (Kennedy 2018). Adderall seems to be more frequently misused by 19- to 30-year-olds than Ritalin (Schulenberg et al. 2019).

Mechanism of action. Swallowed, snorted, smoked, injected, or chewed.

Prescribed use. Prescribed to treat attention-deficit hyperactivity disorder (ADHD) or certain other conditions, such as narcolepsy.

Short-term effects. Increased alertness, attention, and energy; increased blood pressure and heart rate; narrowed blood vessels; increased blood sugar; opened-up breathing passages.

Long-term effects. Heart problems, psychosis, anger, paranoia (National Institute on Drug Abuse 2018).

High doses. Dangerously high body temperature and irregular heartbeat; heart failure; seizures.

COLD MEDICINES

Not all cold medicines that are abused contain a depressant called codeine, and cold medicines with codeine are not available over-the-counter (OTC) and require a prescription by a health care provider.

Alternate names. C-C-C, triple C, Orange Crush, Dex, Drex, DXM, robo, robo-dosing, robo-fizzing, velvet, vitamin D, syrup head (Stop Medicine Abuse 2021b).

Incidence of use. One in 31 teens reports using OTC cough medicine to get high (Stop Medicine Abuse 2021a).

Mechanism of action. Orally via tablet, capsule, or syrup; sometimes mixed with alcohol or soda.

Prescribed use. Used to treat lower and upper respiratory congestion and symptoms associated with colds and flu.

Short-term effects. Hallucinations, sedation, euphoria, impaired motor functions, increased heart rate and blood pressure, extreme agitation.

Long-term effects. Addiction, liver damage, central nervous system depression, respiratory depression, lack of oxygen to the brain (National Institute on Drug Abuse 2017).

OXYCODONE (OPIOIDS)

Alternate names. Hillbilly heroin, blues, kickers, OC, Oxy.

Incidence of use. Opioid-related overdose deaths more than doubled in the United States between 2010 and 2017 (see figure 11.8) and continued this trend through 2019. By the end of 2021, the number of deaths increased to over 80,000 annually (National Institute on Drug Abuse 2021h).

Mechanism of action. Swallowed, snorted, injected.

Prescribed use. Prescribed to treat moderate to severe pain.

Short-term effects. Pain relief, drowsiness, nausea, constipation, euphoria, confusion, slowed breathing, death.

Long-term effects. Unknown (National Institute on Drug Abuse 2021i).

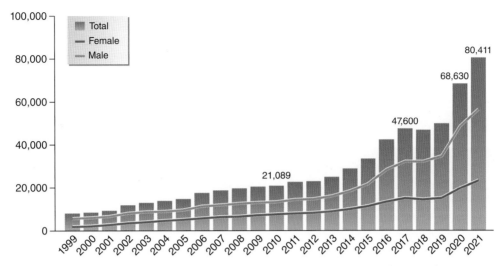

Figure 11.8   U.S. drug overdose deaths involving any opioid, 1999 to 2021. There was a significant increase in overdose deaths between 2010 and 2021. The lines over the graph bars show deaths by sex (National Institute on Drug Abuse 2023).

Reprinted from Centers for Disease Control and Prevention, National Center for Health Statistics, *Multiple Cause of Death 1999-2021* on CDC WONDER Online Database (2023), https://www.drugabuse.gov/drug-topics/trends-statistics/overdose-death-rates.

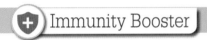 Immunity Booster

Opioids and COVID-19

As COVID-19 continues to spread around the world, we are still learning about how opioids may affect patients' prognosis for a full recovery. Chronic opioid use at high doses can suppress parts of the immune system, as well as decrease respiratory function and increase the risk of pneumonia, all of which can cause complications for a COVID-19 patient. Because COVID-19 impacts the respiratory system, the use of opioids through inhalation may significantly impact the lungs and cause organ damage. Epidemiologic studies show an increase in mortality rate in people with opioid use disorder with COVID-19. Overall, people who misuse opioids are likely to receive a poor prognosis if diagnosed with COVID-19.

To increase your odds of surviving COVID-19, avoid using opioids of any kind. If you are prescribed opioids by your health care provider, discuss your increased risk of compromised respiratory and immune function and these effects on COVID-19 so you can take the necessary steps for a full recovery (Ataei et al. 2020).

OTHER COMMONLY ABUSED DRUGS

Table 11.1 outlines the most abused club drugs. **Club drugs** tend to cause hallucinogenic or dissociative effects and lowered inhibitions. Use of these drugs cause altered states of perception and feeling, hallucinations, nausea, impaired body movements, long-term feelings of anxiety, tremors, numbness in hands or feet, and memory loss.

Table 11.1   Commonly Abused Club Drugs

Facts	MDMA (methylene-dioxymethamphetamine)	GHB (gamma-hydroxybutyrate)	Rohypnol (flunitrazepam)	Ketamine (ketalar SV)	LSD (lysergic acid diethylamide)	Mescaline
Street names	Ecstasy, Adam, Eve, lover's speed, uppers	Georgia home boy, liquid ecstasy	Forget-me pill, Mexican Valium, R2, roofies	Cat Valium, K, Special K, vitamin K	Acid, blotter, cubes, micro-dot	Buttons, cactus, mesc, peyote
Administration	Swallowed, injected, snorted	Swallowed	Swallowed, snorted	Injected, snorted, smoked	Swallowed, absorbed through mouth tissues	Swallowed, smoked
Short-term effects	Mild hallucinogenic effects, lowered inhibitions, anxiety, chills, muscle cramping	Drowsiness, nausea, headache, disorientation, loss of coordination, memory loss	Sedation, muscle relaxant, confusion, memory loss, dizziness, impaired coordination	Numbness, impaired memory, respiratory depression, cardiac arrest	Increased body temperature, heart rate, and blood pressure; loss of appetite; sweating; weakness; impulsive behavior	Increased body temperature, heart rate, and blood pressure; loss of appetite; sweating; weakness; impulsive behavior
Long-term effects	Sleep problems, depression, impaired memory, hyperthermia, addiction	Unconsciousness, seizures, coma	Addiction	Death	Flashbacks, hallucinogen persisting perception disorder	NA

Adapted from National Institute on Drug Abuse (2019a).

Alcohol

Alcohol is often used in social situations, to celebrate events and milestones, and to relax after a long day. It affects people differently depending on how much and how often alcohol is consumed, as well as age, health status, and family history (National Institute on Alcohol Abuse and Alcoholism 2020). Excessive drinking is a preventable leading cause of death in the United States and accounts for an average of 261 deaths per day (Esser et al. 2020). Research has shown that children of alcoholics are close to four times more likely to develop a drinking problem; this risk increases if the alcoholic parent is depressed, if the

In the United States, 95,000 people die every year due to excessive drinking—an average of 261 deaths per day (Centers for Disease Control and Prevention 2021a).

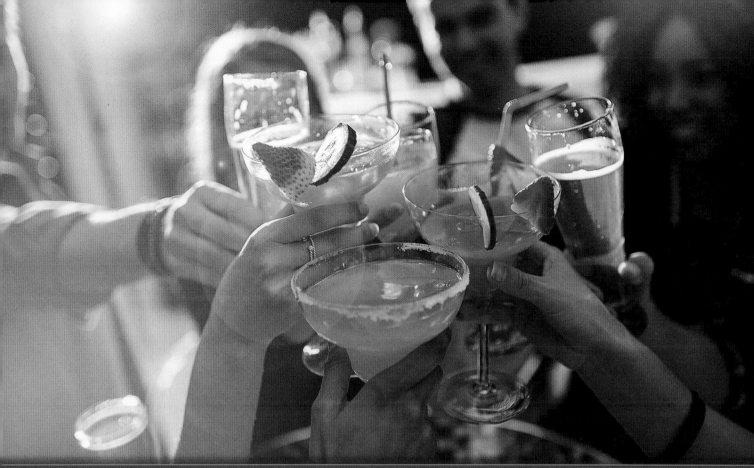

College students can drink responsibly by planning their activities with friends in advance, including knowing when to stop drinking to keep the blood alcohol levels within legal limits and developing a plan to keep each other safe (e.g., using designated drivers, getting a taxi, making sure no one in the group is left alone).

alcohol abuse is severe, if both parents abuse drugs and alcohol, or if there is aggression and violence in the home (National Institute on Alcohol Abuse and Alcoholism 2012).

In general, consuming limited amounts of alcohol and in moderation is not typically of great concern. However, it becomes a problem when one drinks too much, becomes dependent, and can no longer manage everyday activities such as attending classes, going to work, paying bills, and attending to family responsibilities. As a result, the alcohol abuser experiences lost productivity and wages, potential legal problems (e.g., driving while under the influence of alcohol), relationship and family problems, increased health care costs because of conditions or diseases caused by alcohol abuse, and early death.

Alcohol use and abuse on college campuses are common despite the number of alcohol-related illnesses, injuries, and deaths among college students. It is important to learn about the negative consequences of alcohol use as a moderate drinker, binge drinker, or heavy drinker. It is never

too late to quit using alcohol or to learn how to drink responsibly.

According to the 2019 Monitoring the Future study (Schulenberg et al. 2020), young adults reported increased alcohol use after high school through at least their mid-20s. This same study addressed **binge drinking**, which is defined as having five or more drinks in a row on at least one occasion. The results showed that rates of binge drinking increase as young adults age into their 20s—from 14 percent of 18-year-olds to 21 percent of those aged 19 to 20, to 32 percent of those aged 19 to 30. These data also indicate that binge drinking declines after age 30. Figure 11.9 shows the pattern of binge drinking among college students and their non-college peers in 2018.

Excessive drinking is associated with health and social issues that include liver disease, cancer, heart disease, impaired driving, violence, risky sexual activity, and unintended pregnancies (Centers for Disease Control and Prevention 2021b). For college students to reduce their risk of these outcomes, they should first avoid underage drinking—those

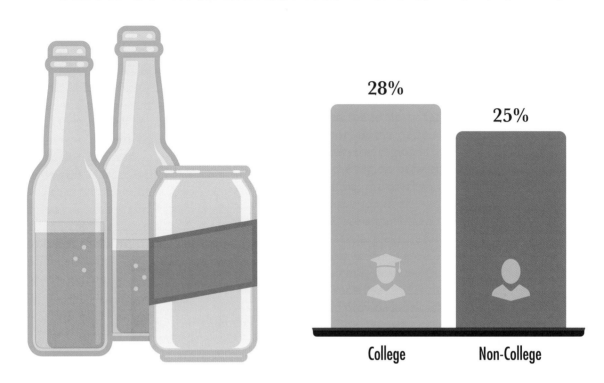

BELOW 30% FOR THE FIRST TIME AMONG COLLEGE STUDENTS

28%

25%

College   Non-College

5+ Drinks in a row in last 2 weeks

Figure 11.9   Monitoring the Future survey results, 2018. Binge drinking declined among college students (28 percent) and non-college adults (25 percent). This is the first time binge drinking fell below 30 percent among college students aged 19 to 22.

Reprinted from National Institute on Drug Abuse (2019).

who begin drinking at a younger age are more at risk for alcoholism. Second, college students who are of legal age should only drink in moderation and continue this behavior well into adulthood. Practicing drinking in moderation reduces the chances of becoming an alcoholic and reduces the risks of other social issues and diseases, such as drinking and driving, violence, personal trauma, liver disease, brain damage, and cancer (National Institute on Alcohol Abuse and Alcoholism 2021).

Effects on the Body

Alcohol can have detrimental effects on the body, and the intensities of these effects are dependent on the frequency, duration, and amount of consumption (figure 11.10). Drinking in moderation, and even binge drinking, has been associated with short-term effects on the body, meaning that alcohol can affect typical functioning and these results are not always the result of excessive use over years or decades: It does not take long for the adverse effects of alcohol to result in negative effects on the body. These include arrhythmia of the heart, hypertension, cardiomyopathy, damage to the lining of the stomach, gastritis, ulcers in the stomach, and dehydration. Some of the more serious diseases that result from heavy, long-term alcohol use include cirrhosis of the liver, alcoholic hepatitis, alcoholic cardiomyopathy, strokes, hypertension, severe dehydration, and pancreatitis (National Institute on Alcohol Abuse and Alcoholism n.d.b). Many of these diseases are irreversible but can be prevented by not drinking excessively.

> Alcohol can damage your liver, brain, stomach, and heart and lead to high blood pressure, stroke, and heart attack.

Blood Alcohol Concentration

The effects of alcohol on the body are directly related to the amount of alcohol in the blood, typically referred to as **blood alcohol concentration (BAC)**. It is measured from .01 to .40 (death). The higher the level of alcohol detected in the blood, the more significant and serious the impairment. Specific factors that affect BAC include the type and amount of alcohol consumed, the time over which the alcohol was consumed, the sex and

weight of the individual, and the amount of food in the stomach. An individual who weighs more and has eaten before consuming alcohol will have a lower blood alcohol level. Figure 11.11 illustrates the physical effects of blood alcohol concentration on driving.

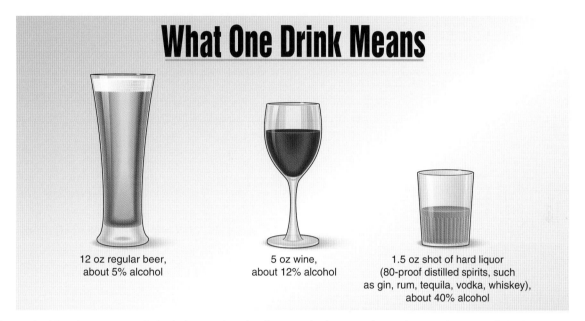

What One Drink Means

12 oz regular beer, about 5% alcohol

5 oz wine, about 12% alcohol

1.5 oz shot of hard liquor (80-proof distilled spirits, such as gin, rum, tequila, vodka, whiskey), about 40% alcohol

Figure 11.10   The amount of alcohol considered to be one drink varies depending on the type of alcohol.

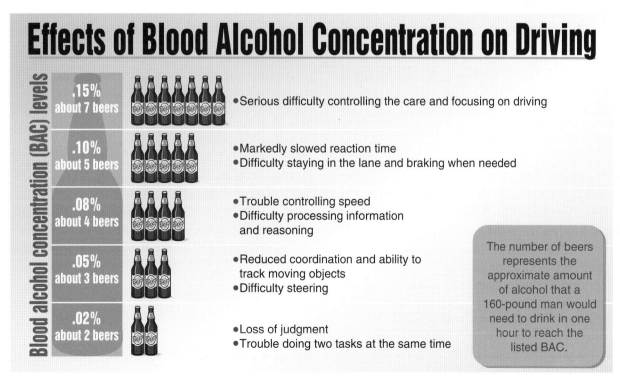

Effects of Blood Alcohol Concentration on Driving

Blood alcohol concentration (BAC) levels

.15% about 7 beers
• Serious difficulty controlling the care and focusing on driving

.10% about 5 beers
• Markedly slowed reaction time
• Difficulty staying in the lane and braking when needed

.08% about 4 beers
• Trouble controlling speed
• Difficulty processing information and reasoning

.05% about 3 beers
• Reduced coordination and ability to track moving objects
• Difficulty steering

.02% about 2 beers
• Loss of judgment
• Trouble doing two tasks at the same time

The number of beers represents the approximate amount of alcohol that a 160-pound man would need to drink in one hour to reach the listed BAC.

Figure 11.11   Physical effects of BAC levels on impaired driving.

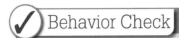

What's the Truth About Alcohol?

Which of the following statements about alcohol are myths (National Institute on Alcohol Abuse and Alcoholism n.d.a)?

1. People can drink alcohol and still be in control.
2. Drinking alcohol isn't dangerous.
3. People can sober up very quickly after drinking too much alcohol.
4. Beer has the least amount of alcohol per serving when compared to liquor or wine.
5. A few beers will not impair someone enough that he or she shouldn't drive.

The facts are as follows:

1. Alcohol impairs judgment and could lead to engaging in behaviors that could have serious consequences, like a car accident, risky sexual activities, or vandalism.
2. Alcohol use is dangerous. It can lead to injuries and deaths, sexual assault, or poor academic performance.
3. Sobering up takes about two hours. Nothing, not even coffee or a cold shower, can quickly eliminate alcohol from the body.
4. A 12-ounce (355 mL) glass of beer has the same amount of alcohol as a shot of 80-proof liquor or 5 ounces (148 mL) of wine (see figure 11.10).
5. Impaired driving can begin at .05 BAC, so you should not drive after drinking any amount of alcohol.

Mixing Energy Drinks and Alcohol

Although consumption of moderate amounts of caffeine is considered safe for adults, when highly caffeinated energy drinks are combined with alcohol, the effects could be fatal. According to the Institute for the Advancement of Food and Nutrition Science (2021), 85 percent of the U.S. population consumes at least one caffeine-containing beverage per day. Caffeine is not only found in energy drinks and coffee but is an added ingredient in many food products such as carbonated waters, maple syrup, energy bars, and chewing gum. A daily dose of up to 400 milligrams, which is about four cups of brewed coffee, seems to be safe for most healthy adults. However, keep in mind that the actual caffeine content in beverages and foods varies widely, especially in energy drinks (Mayo Clinic 2020), which contain significantly more caffeine than a regular soft drink.

Although experts advise against mixing energy drinks and alcohol (U.S. Department of Health and Human Services 2015), many college students continue to consume this mixture (Marczinksi and Fillmore 2014). When alcohol and energy drinks are combined, the caffeine can mask the depressant effects of the alcohol. Additionally, the caffeine does not affect the metabolism of alcohol by the liver, which increases blood alcohol concentration. Those who report mixing alcohol and energy drinks have a higher prevalence of binge drinking, sexually assaulting someone or being the victim of a sexual assault, and getting in a car as the passenger with someone who has been drinking.

✓ Behavior Check

What Is Alcoholism?

Alcoholism, or alcohol dependence, includes four symptoms. Do you have any of these? Think about each of these and your behaviors related to the use of alcohol. If you answered yes to more than one of these symptoms, seek the help of a counselor on your campus or in your community (National Institute on Alcohol Abuse and Alcoholism 2012):

- Craving—having a strong need, or urge, to drink.
- Loss of control—not being able to stop drinking once you've started to drink.
- Physical dependence—experiencing withdrawal symptoms such as an upset stomach, shakiness, and anxiety after drinking.
- Tolerance—experiencing the need to drink more alcohol to get that buzzed or drunk feeling.

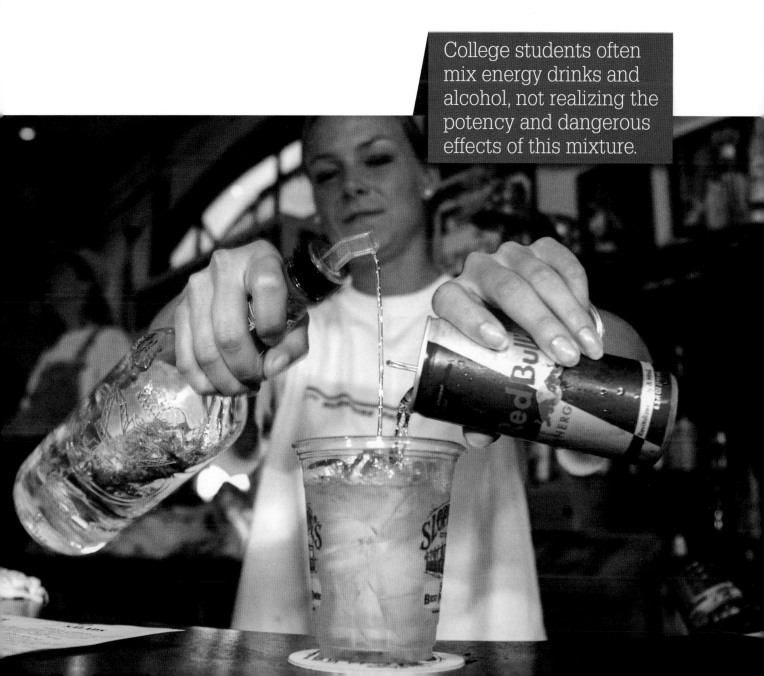

College students often mix energy drinks and alcohol, not realizing the potency and dangerous effects of this mixture.

Tobacco

Despite the efforts to reduce tobacco use in the United States, the use of these products continues to remain steady. Cigarette smoking continues to be a preventable cause of disease, disability, and death (see figure 11.12), although the good news is that the rates of smoking declined from 29.9 percent in 2005 (U.S. Department of Health and Human Services 2014) to 12.5 percent in 2020 (Cornelius et al. 2022). In 2020, nearly 13 of every 100 U.S. adults aged 18 years or older (12.5%) currently smoked cigarettes (Cornelius et al. 2022), meaning that approximately 30.8 million people in the United States smoke cigarettes and more than 16 million live with a smoking-related disease (U.S. Department of Health and Human Services 2014). Cornelius and colleagues (2022) reported that about 12.5 percent of adults aged 18 or older currently smoke cigarettes. Smoking trends are lower among college students and their non-college peers and continue to decline: In 2019, 7.9 percent of college students and 16 percent of their non-college peers reported having smoked in the past month (Substance Abuse and Mental Health Services Administration 2020).

Overall, cigarette smoking is down but remains high among certain groups. Many public health policies and strategies are aimed at helping people quit, reduce their use, or never start smoking (figure 11.13).

Chemicals in Cigarettes

Cigarettes contain over 7,000 harmful chemicals known to cause cancer (American Lung Association 2017b). **Nicotine**, originally intended for use as an insecticide (American Lung Association 2017b), is the chemical in tobacco products that causes addiction. It is found in cigars, smokeless tobacco, pipe tobacco,

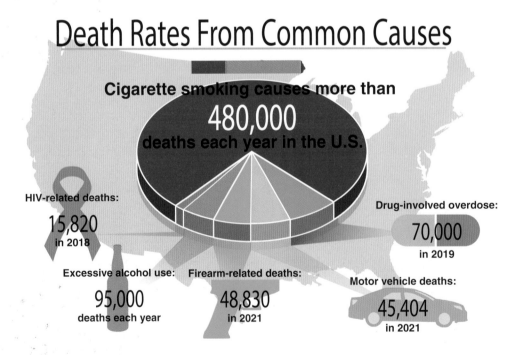

Figure 11.12   Death rate from smoking compared to other common death rates.

Data from United States Department of Health and Human Services (2014); Esser (2020); Centers for Disease Control and Prevention (2023); and Centers for Disease Control and Prevention (2019b).

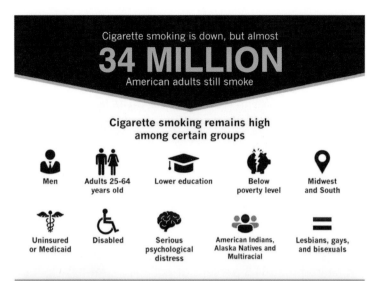

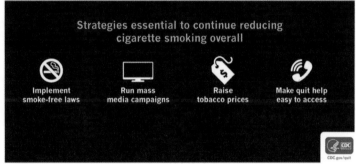

Figure 11.13   Cigarette smoking is down, but about 34 million American adults still smoke.

Reprinted from the Centers for Disease Control and Prevention (2021c).

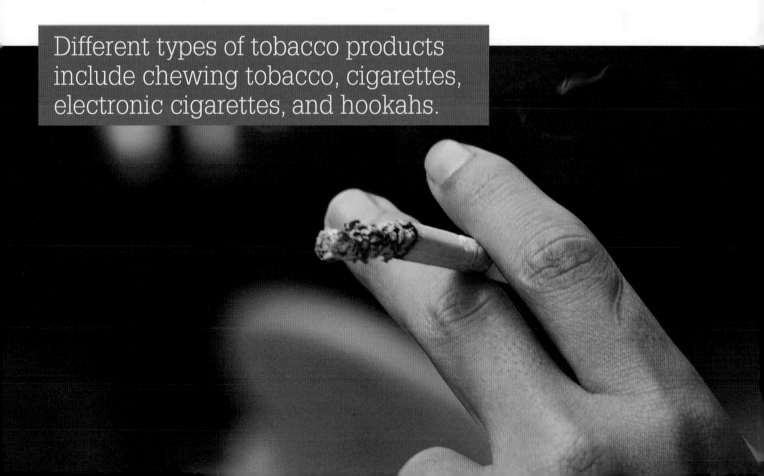

Different types of tobacco products include chewing tobacco, cigarettes, electronic cigarettes, and hookahs.

What Are Hookahs?

A hookah is a water pipe used to smoke flavored tobacco that is typically shared by passing the mouthpiece from person to person. Hookah smoking transmits many of the same harmful chemicals as cigarettes do, including nicotine and tar, and carries the same negative health risks as smoking a cigarette (Centers for Disease Control and Prevention 2021e). In fact, hookah users may absorb more toxic substances than cigarette smokers: In a one-hour hookah-smoking session, users may inhale 100 to 200 times the amount of smoke as from one cigarette (U.S. Department of Health and Human Services 2012).

- *Alternate names.* Narghile, argileh, shisha, hubble-bubble, and goza.
- *Incidence.* About 1 in every 8 young adults between the ages of 19 and 30 use a hookah as a method to smoke tobacco (Schulenberg et al. 2019). The National College Health Assessment, conducted by the American College Health Association (2019), stated that 84.8 percent of college students have never used hookah.
- *Health effects.* Lung, bladder, and oral cancers; clogged arteries and heart disease; infections caused by sharing the same mouthpiece; having babies with low birth weight; and decreased fertility.

and e-cigarettes. When smoked in a cigarette or absorbed through the mucous membranes, the effects of nicotine are experienced quickly, including increased heart rate and blood pressure and feelings of euphoria. These elevated feelings do not last long; therefore, the user seeks more nicotine to maintain this level of stimulation. In high doses, nicotine can be poisonous—children have died ingesting the nicotine-containing liquid in e-cigarettes. The risks of smoking negatively affect almost every part of the body, both physically and emotionally (figure 11.14).

Quitting smoking and tobacco use can be very difficult because the addiction to nicotine is significant. The withdrawal symptoms, even within 24 hours, include irritability, mood swings, aggression, and hostility. Despite the tremendous withdrawal symptoms, the body begins to heal itself within the first 24 hours after the last cigarette (see figure 11.15).

E-Cigarettes

E-cigarettes, or electronic cigarettes, are frequently used as an alternative to traditional smoking by allowing the user to inhale an aerosol that contains nicotine instead of smoking a cigarette.

Vaping is the term used to describe the act of inhaling and exhaling the water vapor produced by the electronic cigarette. E-cigarettes are battery operated and have a heating system that heats the e-liquid from a refillable cartridge and releases the nicotine-filled aerosol (American Lung Association 2016). Figure 11.16 shows the internal components of an e-cigarette.

Although the nicotine is not introduced into the body by a cigarette, e-cigarettes can still be harmful. The cartridges include ingredients used in antifreeze and formaldehyde, as well as additional chemicals such as carbonyl compounds and volatile organic compounds that can lead to negative health effects (American Lung Association 2016; U.S. Department of Health and Human Services 2016). Accidental poisoning, acute toxicity, and death can occur when the liquid is ingested; this is a particular danger to young children.

Quitting Tobacco Use

Quitting smoking can be very difficult: Nicotine can be as addictive as heroin, cocaine, and alcohol (American Lung Association 2017a). Various methods for quitting include gum, patches, inhalers, nasal spray, and tablets, which provide low

Risks from Smoking

Smoking can damage every part of your body

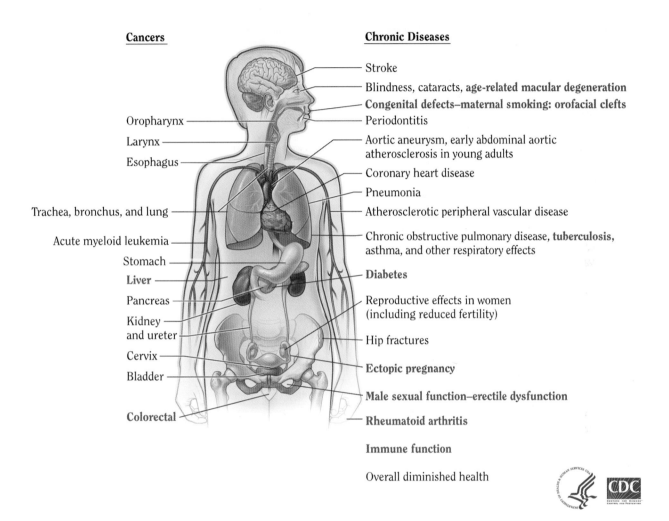

Cancers

- Oropharynx
- Larynx
- Esophagus
- Trachea, bronchus, and lung
- Acute myeloid leukemia
- Stomach
- **Liver**
- Pancreas
- Kidney and ureter
- Cervix
- Bladder
- **Colorectal**

Chronic Diseases

- Stroke
- Blindness, cataracts, **age-related macular degeneration**
- **Congenital defects–maternal smoking: orofacial clefts**
- Periodontitis
- Aortic aneurysm, early abdominal aortic atherosclerosis in young adults
- Coronary heart disease
- Pneumonia
- Atherosclerotic peripheral vascular disease
- Chronic obstructive pulmonary disease, **tuberculosis,** asthma, and other respiratory effects
- **Diabetes**
- Reproductive effects in women (including reduced fertility)
- Hip fractures
- **Ectopic pregnancy**
- **Male sexual function–erectile dysfunction**
- **Rheumatoid arthritis**
- **Immune function**
- Overall diminished health

Figure 11.14 Effects of smoking on the body.

Each condition presented in bold text is a new disease causally linked to smoking in the 2014 Surgeon General's Report, *The Health Consequences of Smoking—50 Years of Progress.*

Reprinted from Centers for Disease Control and Prevention (2021d).

levels of nicotine that help the smoker gradually reduce the level of nicotine in the system and reduce withdrawal symptoms. Behavior modification programs provide access to support groups, counseling, and follow-up support to help participants sustain a nonsmoking lifestyle. QuitLine is a toll-free call resource for tobacco users who want to quit smoking. This resource is staffed by trained health care professionals and tobacco counselors who respond to questions about staying smoke free. In addition, counselors assist smokers in developing a personalized plan. The National Cancer Institute (NCI) operates 800-QUIT-NOW, a toll-free number that will connect you directly to your state's tobacco quit line. Note that these are valuable resources for smokers trying to quit, but they do not replace the medical advice of a physician or health care provider.

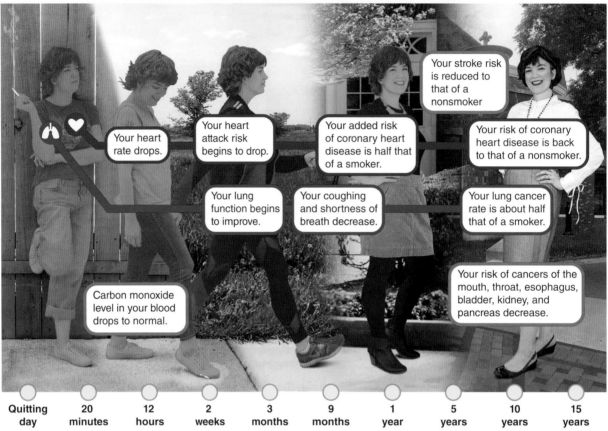

Figure 11.15   The benefits of quitting smoking are overwhelmingly positive and begin soon after quitting.
Data from Centers for Disease Control and Prevention.

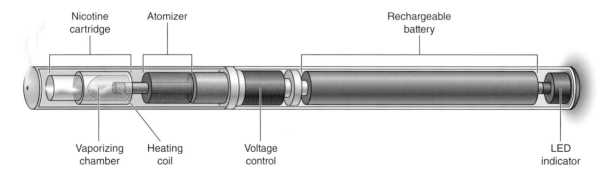

Figure 11.16   The internal parts of an e-cigarette.

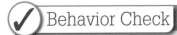 **Behavior Check**

The Path to Quitting Smoking

If you currently smoke, quitting is the best thing you can do for your overall health—your body will begin to heal immediately after that last cigarette. Quitting can be difficult and may take more than one attempt, so do not give up. Make sure you have a plan you can stick to (American Lung Association n.d.). Ask for support from former smokers or friends and family who will be able to help you quit.

1. List the reasons you want to quit (e.g., to avoid getting cancer, to save money, to stop smelling like cigarettes).
2. List the benefits of quitting smoking (e.g., breathe easier, improve blood pressure, reduce chance of getting cancer).
3. List campus and community resources that can help you quit smoking (e.g., American Cancer Society, American Lung Association—Freedom from Smoking, QuitLine, American Non-smokers' Rights Foundation list of smokefree and tobacco-free colleges and universities).
4. List specific support resources you can access (e.g., nicotine replacement therapy).
5. List the potential withdrawal symptoms and challenges and how you will handle them (e.g., choose healthy snacks to combat weight gain; go for a walk when feeling anxious).
6. List social media outlets for support (e.g., #quitbettertogether).

Summary

Alcohol, tobacco, and marijuana are the most abused substances among young adults. The more often people use these substances, the more likely they are to develop a tolerance for and dependency on these substances, leading to long-term use. This can lead to serious negative health effects on the body, which may include cancer, respiratory illnesses and diseases, mental health issues, violent behaviors, and poor judgment that leads to risky behaviors. Additionally, drug dependency can cause loss of jobs, failing in school, the inability to meet daily responsibilities like paying bills and keeping up with hygiene, and problems in personal relationships.

Individuals can reduce their chances of becoming dependent on drugs or alcohol by choosing not to spend time around people who use drugs or in places where drugs and alcohol are easily accessible. For you, develop a plan for how to handle peer pressure when these substances are available and to learn how to cope with stressful situations by choosing healthier alternatives. Many community and campus resources are available for assisting students with the decision to be substance free and helping students who are dependent on substances get the help they need for recovery. Staying away from drugs, tobacco, and alcohol is a key component of living a wellness lifestyle. It's important to be present in life—to not escape it, but rather face challenges head on. This is how you learn and grow as a college student.

www ONLINE LEARNING ACTIVITIES

Go to HK*Propel* and complete all of the online activities to further facilitate your learning:

Study Activities: Review the main concepts of the chapter.

Labs: Complete the labs your instructor assigns.

Videos: Look through the videos and choose which ones you want to try this week.

REVIEW QUESTIONS

1. What are ways to avoid developing a substance or behavioral addiction?
2. What are the criteria that are used to diagnose someone with a drug dependency?
3. What are some of the more common behavioral addictions among young adults?
4. What are the short- and long-term health effects of the following substances: marijuana, heroin, cocaine, club drugs, alcohol, and tobacco?
5. What are the physical effects of combining alcohol and energy drinks?
6. What are effective treatment options for individuals with a substance or behavioral addiction?
7. How does opioid use affect the prognosis of someone diagnosed with COVID-19?

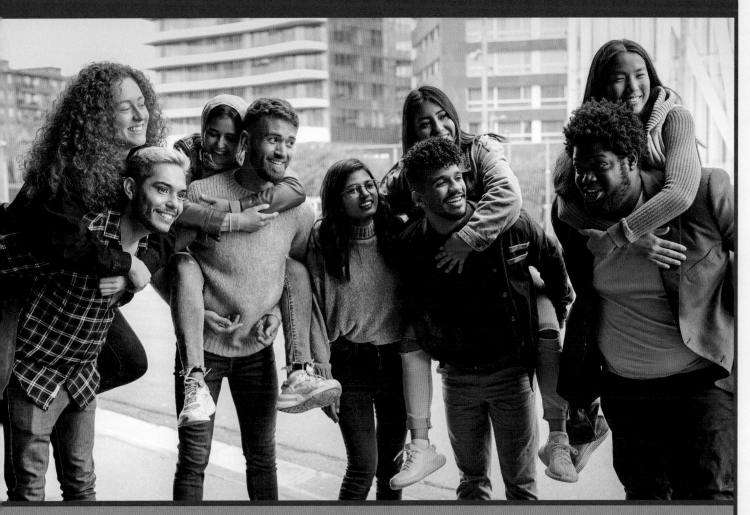

Sexuality and Health

12

OBJECTIVES

- List the internal and external parts of the female and male reproductive systems.
- Explain how the most commonly used birth control methods prevent pregnancy, and list their advantages and disadvantages.
- Explain the symptoms, diagnosis, treatment, prevention, and transmission of the most common bacterial and viral STIs.
- Define consent as it relates to sexual assault.
- Identify resources on college campuses that assist students in preventing and addressing sexual assault.

279

KEY TERMS

abstinence

areola

barrier birth control methods

birth control methods

bulbourethral glands

circumcision

clitoris

contraception

ectopic pregnancy

ejaculation

ejaculatory duct

embryo

endometrium

epididymis

erection

Fallopian tubes

fertility awareness–based contraception
  methods (natural family planning)

fertilization

fetus

gonads

hormonal birth control methods

hymen

labia majora

labia minora

mammary glands

mons pubis

ovaries

ovulation

ovum

pelvic inflammatory disease

penis

perfect use

prostate gland

scrotum

semen

seminal vesicles

seminiferous tubules

sperm

spermicide

sterilization

testes

typical use

urethra

uterus

vagina

vas deferens

withdrawal

zygote

This chapter includes an overview of the reproductive system, the variety of birth control and family planning options available to you, common sexually transmitted infections (STIs) and their prevention strategies and treatment options, and information about sexual assault and education and prevention initiatives. Throughout this chapter, you will notice that there has been a conscious effort to acknowledge that gender identities are diverse, and the words used are intended to be inclusive. However, the research and sources referenced in this chapter—particularly research conducted in previous decades—may not have used data collection methods that provided subjects a full range of gender options to select from; we encourage you to keep this in mind as you learn about sexual health despite the limitations of language to reflect the terminology used.

Sexuality as a Dimension of Health

Your sexual health is just as important as every other dimension of your health. Your sexuality is a critical and central component of who you are that emerges and evolves over your lifetime. Although your sexuality is evident throughout your life, there are pivotal sexual health milestones related to developmental, emotional, and physical changes. At times, these milestones require having uncomfortable conversations. Some of these milestones include puberty, first sexual experiences

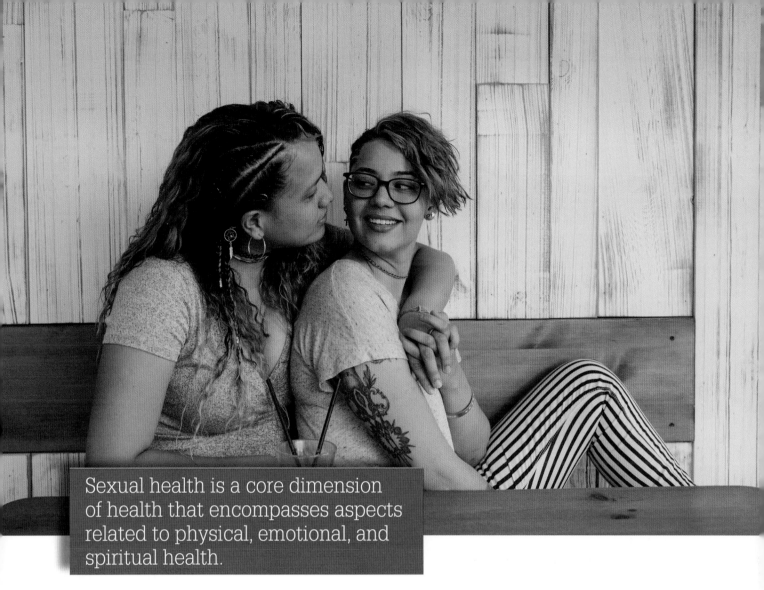

Sexual health is a core dimension of health that encompasses aspects related to physical, emotional, and spiritual health.

with self and others, having children, and changes during aging. A personal goal for young adults should be to seek out reliable and medically accurate sources for sexual health information and to become more comfortable and confident learning about and discussing these issues. This does not necessarily happen overnight; it may take time to learn about and understand the context of these issues and decide how to apply them to your life.

Over time, and with the addition of life experiences, you will develop specific beliefs, attitudes, feelings, morals, and behaviors that define your sexuality and how you want to express yourself. As you develop relationships with others, whether they are intimate or platonic, think about what you find physically and emotionally attractive in a partner, how to communicate effectively regarding your likes and dislikes, what it means to be sexually intimate, and how to develop empathy and understanding toward others who are not exactly like you.

This chapter focuses on the pressing and contemporary issues that are central in your life as a college student, how these issues affect you, and what you can do to become more confident and comfortable with expressing your own sexuality and understanding others' expression of their sexuality.

Reproductive System

The reproductive system comprises the mature sexual organs, cells, and hormones needed to contribute to the next generation. In utero, the reproductive organs of both female and male bodies develop from the same embryonic tissues; therefore, it is difficult to identify using ultrasound whether the fetus has female or male genitalia until approximately the 20th week of gestation. Genetic testing can be used to determine the sex of the baby sooner; however, ultrasound is

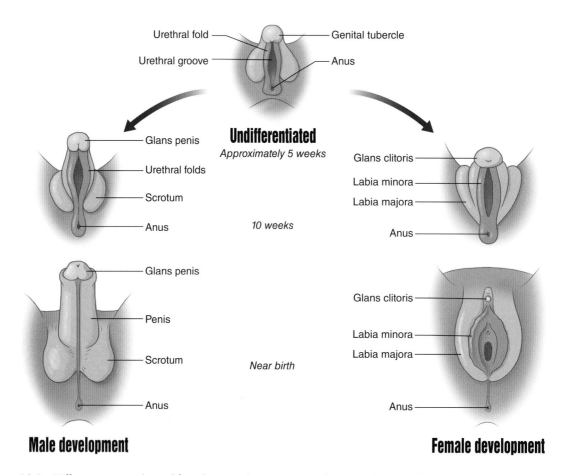

Figure 12.1   Differences in male and female reproductive organs during embryonic development.

the most common and inexpensive method. The homologous structures in male bodies and female bodies are the penis and clitoris and the scrotum and labia majora, respectively. Figure 12.1 shows the differences between male and female reproductive organs during embryonic development. Note the similar tissue development between the fetuses and how there are more similarities than differences in the early stages of development.

Additional similarities that both reproductive systems share are structures called **gonads**, which are the ovaries in female bodies and the testes in male bodies. These organs manufacture the sex hormones that produce the ova (sometimes referred to as the eggs) in the ovaries and **sperm** in the testes. Males can produce sperm beginning at puberty, whereas females are born with a defined number of ova that are released during the reproductive years. Ovulation ends when a female enters menopause. Puberty typically begins between ages 8 and 11 for females and 9 and 12 for males.

During penile-vaginal sexual intercourse, **fertilization** of the **ovum** by the sperm typically occurs in the Fallopian tubes. The Fallopian tube has millions of microscopic cilia that pull the ovum toward the uterus after it has been released from the ovary. The muscular wall of the Fallopian tube contracts to assist the ovum in moving expeditiously to meet the sperm. The uterus is the intended site for implantation and provides nourishment for the zygote as it develops into an **embryo** and then a **fetus**. If this sequence of events fails, implantation of the zygote may happen outside the uterus; this is called an **ectopic pregnancy**. A common site for an ectopic pregnancy is in the Fallopian tube; this is called a tubal pregnancy.

Female Reproductive System

The female reproductive system is composed of internal and external organs that work together to produce the necessary hormones for typical sexual development and reproduction. Figure 12.2 shows organs of the internal and external female reproductive system. Notice that the external organs are known as the vulva, not the vagina; the vagina is an internal structure.

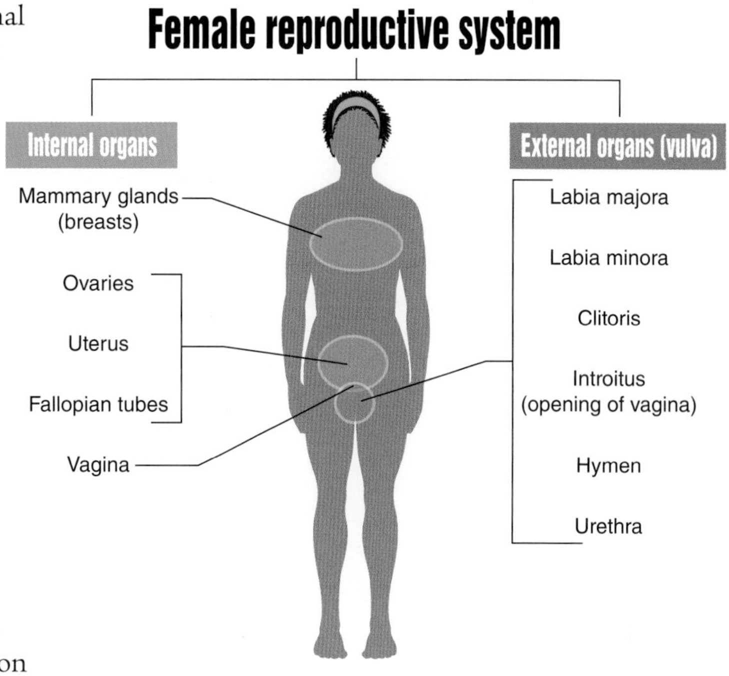

Female Internal Organs

The primary function of the female reproductive system is to produce the ova and hormones necessary to support a successful pregnancy The primary sex organs are the ovaries, in which the ova are produced and stored until **ovulation**, or the release of an ovum roughly once a month. The sex organs that support the transportation of the ovum out of the ovary to either unite with sperm (to create a zygote) or be expelled from the body during menstruation (if unfertilized) are the Fallopian tubes, uterus, and vagina. The **ovaries** are oval-shaped organs, each about the size of a walnut, that are positioned in the upper portion of the pelvic cavity on either side of the uterus. They are kept in place by strong, muscular ligaments. Each **Fallopian tube** is approximately 8 to 14 centimeters long. The end that hovers over the ovary has fingerlike projections called fimbriae, which aid the ovum by leading it into the Fallopian tube and down to the uterus (see figure 12.3).

The **uterus** is a thick-walled, pear-shaped muscular organ about the size of a fist. At the base of the uterus is the cervix. The functions of the uterus are menstruation, pregnancy, and labor. The uterus is where a fertilized egg, or **zygote**, typically implants.

Female reproductive system

Internal organs

- Mammary glands (breasts)
- Ovaries
- Uterus
- Fallopian tubes
- Vagina

External organs (vulva)

- Labia majora
- Labia minora
- Clitoris
- Introitus (opening of vagina)
- Hymen
- Urethra

Figure 12.2 The internal and external organs of the female reproductive system.

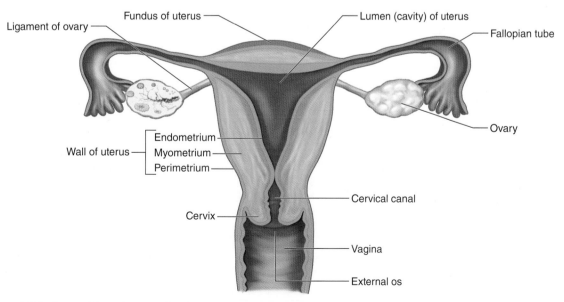

Figure 12.3 Internal female reproductive anatomy.

If a person does not become pregnant after ovulation, then the uterine lining, called the **endometrium**, is shed along with menstrual blood approximately every 28 to 32 days. The uterus is typically in alignment with the lower body region; however, it can also be angled forward or backward. A uterus angled toward the bladder is *anteverted* and one tilted toward the back, near the rectum, is *retroverted*. For most, these variations in uterine placement do not cause significant problems during sexual intercourse or pregnancy.

The **vagina** is a canal-like muscular organ that receives sperm during intercourse and serves as a passageway for menstrual blood leaving the body and for a baby during delivery. For this reason, it is also called the birth canal. The vagina is about 9 centimeters long and extends from the vaginal opening to the cervix, where the uterus attaches at approximately a 90-degree angle. The vaginal opening may be partially or completely obstructed by a thin membrane called the **hymen**. The hymen may vary in appearance—some are more intact, and others have small openings. The hymen can be ruptured during first sexual intercourse, and some people will notice a small amount of blood. It can also be torn as a result of activities not related to sexual intercourse, such as participating in recreational activities or sports. A torn or partially intact hymen does not mean a person is no longer a virgin. Some people have a hymen that is thick, obstructing menstrual blood; in this case, the hymen may need to be removed by a physician.

> Endometriosis occurs when segments of the uterine lining end up in the peritoneal cavity and cause pain. People who experience extreme pain and discomfort during their menstrual cycle need to consult with their physician or gynecologist.

Female External Genitalia

The external genitalia consist of the mons pubis, labia majora ("outer lips"), labia minora ("inner lips"), and clitoris. The **mons pubis** is the soft area made up of fatty tissue covering the pubis bone. Some people experience sexual pleasure when this region is touched. The vaginal vestibule is the region between the labia minora where the vagina, the urethra, and Bartholin's glands open. At the top of the vestibule is the **clitoris**, a small erectile organ that is the most sensitive area related to sexual pleasure for many. The **labia majora** and **labia minora** are elongated folds of skin that can vary in appearance (figure 12.4). They are composed of sensitive tissues that protect the internal organs and provide lubrication during sexual intercourse.

The **mammary glands** (or breasts) produce and store milk to provide nourishment for babies. Milk is produced when the glands are stimulated by hormones after birth. Each mammary gland has approximately 15 to 20 lobes that lead to the nipple. The nipple contains erectile tissue and is surrounded by the pigmented **areola**. During pregnancy, the areola becomes darker and enlarges. Breast milk is produced in the alveoli in the lobes when lactating, collected into tiny ducts, and then released from the nipple (figure 12.5).

Male Reproductive System

The primary role of the male reproductive system (figure 12.6) is to produce male sex hormones and to produce, store, and transport sperm and semen to aid in fertilization of the egg. The ability to produce sperm begins in puberty.

Preventing Pelvic Inflammatory Disease

The structure from the opening of the vagina to the peritoneal cavity creates the risk of pelvic inflammatory disease (PID). Bacterial infections, such as untreated sexually transmitted infections (STIs), in the Fallopian tubes can cause PID, leading to ectopic pregnancies and infertility.

PID can also be caused by infections that are not related to sexual activity or STIs. Water sports or recreational activities, like water skiing or sliding down a water slide, can also cause PID. When going against water at a high speed, people with vaginas should wear a wet suit or very tight bathing suit bottoms to prevent contaminated water from being propelled by pressure into their reproductive organs.

Protect your reproductive organs, both during sexual activity and recreational activities, in order to keep them free from PID.

Female Circumcision

Female genital mutilation (FGM), or female circumcision, is a nonmedical procedure in which the clitoris is partially or completely removed, or the labia are sewn shut. A small opening remains for menstrual blood to leave the body. Long-term health complications of this practice include severe bleeding, problems urinating, infections, cysts, complications during childbirth, and increased risk of newborns dying due to their mother's results of FGM. These procedures are mostly done to young females who live in certain countries in Africa, the Middle East, and Asia. Worldwide, approximately 4 million females are at risk of undergoing FGM each year—most of whom are under the age of 15 (UNICEF 2019). Many have fought to end this inhumane practice because it violates the rights of young children and women, causes lifelong health problems, and can be fatal (World Health Organization 2020).

Male Internal Organs

The two oval-shaped **testes,** or testicles, are housed in the external structure called the scrotum. The testes are where testosterone and sperm are produced. The **seminiferous tubules** are coiled tubes inside the testes, which produce sperm cells. The **epididymis** is another coiled tube (about 20 feet long when uncoiled!) that rests on the back of the testes and stores the sperm until maturation. Once the sperm are mature, the epididymis aids in transporting them out of the scrotum. During sexual arousal and eventually ejaculation, sperm are forced into the **vas deferens**, a muscular tube connecting the epididymis to the urethra, which is located just behind the bladder. The **urethra** is responsible for transporting urine out of the body; however, it also provides the means for the sperm and semen to leave the body during an ejaculation. One of the physiological responses during sexual

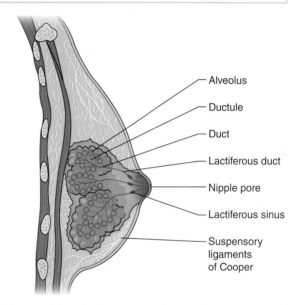

Figure 12.5   The breast is made up of mammary glands that, when stimulated by hormones, produce milk to feed a newborn baby.

intercourse is that urine flow to the urethra is blocked by a small valve, the **ejaculatory duct**, so that the semen can be expelled from the body.

The **seminal vesicles** are small pouches attached to the vas deferens. They produce a liquid high in fructose that gives sperm the energy necessary to be motile. The **prostate gland** is shaped like a walnut and located in close proximity to the rectum and bladder. It also provides fluids that nourish the sperm. The final internal reproductive organs are the pea-sized **bulbourethral glands** (or Cowper's glands), which excrete a fluid to help lubricate and neutralize the urethra just prior to ejaculation. An **ejaculation** is the propulsion of semen from the male reproductive system that is initiated by sexual response. **Semen** is composed of sperm and secretions from the internal glands that provide the nutrients necessary for sperm motility and energy.

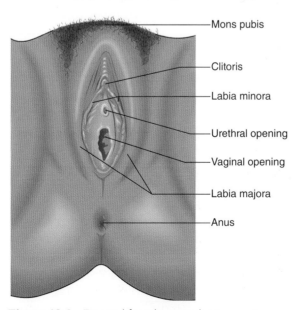

Figure 12.4   External female reproductive anatomy.

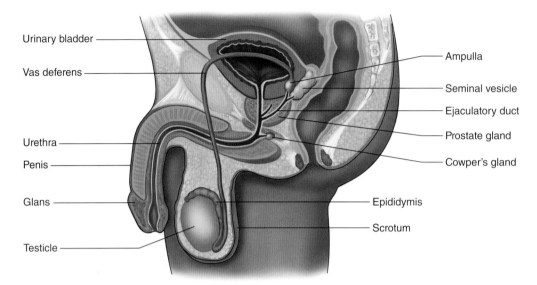

Figure 12.6   Male reproductive anatomy.

Male External Genitalia

The external organs of the male reproductive anatomy are the penis and the scrotum. The **penis** excretes urine out of the body. The shaft of the penis has a cylindrical shape and contains three cavities made of spongelike tissue. These tissues fill with blood to achieve an **erection**, which is necessary for sexual intercourse. The glans is the head of the penis and is shaped somewhat like a helmet. The foreskin is a layer of skin that, when the penis is not erect, covers the glans.

> Sperm production begins during puberty and continues throughout life. A single sperm cell can take between 72 and 74 days to mature (Rebar 2020). Each day, around 300 million sperm cells are produced.

The **scrotum** is an external part of the reproductive system that holds the testicles and provides a nurturing environment for optimal sperm production and maturation by keeping the testes at a slightly cooler temperature than the rest of the body.

Contraception and Birth Control Methods

What is the difference between contraception and birth control? Although both terms are related to family planning and preventing unwanted pregnancies, there are subtle differences between the two. **Contraception** is typically used to identify methods or devices to prevent conception (i.e., the meeting of sperm and ovum). These methods include gels such as spermicides, barrier methods such as condoms, and hormonal methods such as intrauterine devices (IUDs). **Birth control methods** is a broader term that typically include methods that prevent conception as well as the implantation of a fertilized egg into the uterine wall. Birth control methods help people plan when they want to have children and include practices (e.g., abstinence or natural family planning) and surgeries (e.g., vasectomy or tubal ligation). Many use these terms interchangeably, and while they have their own definitions and specifications, the results are the same: to prevent pregnancy and have more control when planning families.

According to data from the National Survey of Family Growth (Martinez and Abma 2020), 42 percent of never-married female and 38 percent of never-married male teenagers aged 15 to 19 have had sexual intercourse. In this study, 78 percent of females and 89 percent of males reported using some type of birth control the first time they had sexual intercourse. Table 12.1 shows the types of contraception that females use and how their choices change over time. College-aged females reported oral contraceptives as the most common form of birth control, followed by external (male) condoms and emergency contraception (Frederiksen et al. 2021). As teenagers got older (ages 18 to 19), they were much more likely to use birth control

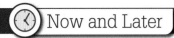
Now and Later

Male Circumcision

Now

Male babies are typically born with foreskin around the glans of the penis. The foreskin may be removed by a physician soon after birth or performed as a religious rite in a procedure called **circumcision**. Circumcision is a controversial topic for some parents because there is no medical evidence strong enough to mandate or prohibit the procedure. The American Academy of Pediatrics recommends supporting the wishes of new parents; however, they cite some potential benefits for circumcision, such as making it easier to wash the penis; a reduced risk of urinary tract infections, penile cancer, and transmission of some STIs and HIV; and possible reduced risk of cervical cancer for sexual partners (Mayo Clinic 2021a). Complications of this procedure, when performed by trained health care professionals, are rare. If circumcision is to be performed, it is recommended that it be done soon after the baby is born. If parents decide not to have their baby circumcised, they should wash beneath the foreskin to reduce the chance of infection. Parents need to consider their own medical, religious, ethical, and cultural beliefs along with the best interests of the child when deciding.

Later

Although you may not be planning to have a child soon, it's important to think about whether or not you would want your baby to be circumcised. What are your thoughts about circumcision? Would you have your baby circumcised? Why or why not?

Take Home

Research the facts on male circumcision now so that you and your partner are prepared to make decisions about this issue later.

with the first sexual encounter (figure 12.7). Among females using a contraceptive method during their reproductive years, they were most likely to have used external (male) condoms (39 percent), oral contraceptives (37 percent), and IUDs (23 percent) within the past 12 months (Frederiksen et al. 2021).

Birth control methods allow people the opportunity to plan when they want to have children. However, it can be challenging to avoid pregnancies, as well as plan the best time to have a child (or subsequent children). Those with the ability to become pregnant will be fertile for approximately three decades, a time during which birth control methods must be considered any time the person is sexually active. There are more than three million unintended pregnancies in the United States each year (Sonfield, Hasstedt, and Gold 2014), almost half of which are a result of inconsistent and incorrect use of birth control methods (Centers for Disease Control and Prevention 2021o).

The implant (Nexplanon), intrauterine device (IUD), and **sterilization** (tubal ligation or vasectomy) provide the lowest failure rates because they are long-term methods that do not require attention

to **perfect use**—that is, the user does not have to remember to take medication or correctly use a contraceptive during every sexual encounter. Couples rarely have perfect use of birth control methods that are not considered permanent or long term. Figure 12.8 shows the percentage rates of unintended pregnancy during the first year of birth control related to **typical use** (not perfect use). You can see that it is important to learn how to use these methods correctly to prevent pregnancy. It is also important to remember that some methods are highly reliable to prevent pregnancy but not infections, including HIV. Consider dual protection from pregnancy and STIs; correct and consistent use of the external (male) latex condom along with a contraception method can reduce the infection risks.

Learning how to properly use birth control can help you reduce the chances of pregnancy now and increase your chances of conception if you are ready to have a baby later. Most college students do not plan to have children while in school; therefore, it is important to consider when you want to begin having children and which birth control methods will help you and your partner meet this goal. If you

Table 12.1 Most Commonly Used Types of Contraception Among Females

Type of contraception used in past 12 months	ALL FEMALES	AGE GROUP		
	18-49	18-25	26-35	36-49
Oral contraceptives	37%	50%*	37%	28%
Injectables	4%	5%	5%	2%
Patch	2%	4%*	2%	0%
Ring	3%	3%	4%	2%
IUD	23%	13%	24%	28%*
Implants	7%	11%*	7%	2%
External (male condoms)	39%	47%*	36%	35%
Fertility awareness–based methods	8%	6%	11%*	7%
Emergency contraception	9%	15%*	11%	2%
Other	4%	6%	4%	3%

*Estimate is statistically different from estimate for all females ages 18 to 49 (*p* < 0.05). *Note:* Respondents were females ages 18 to 49 who have used contraception in the past 12 months; respondents could respond with more than one contraceptive method.

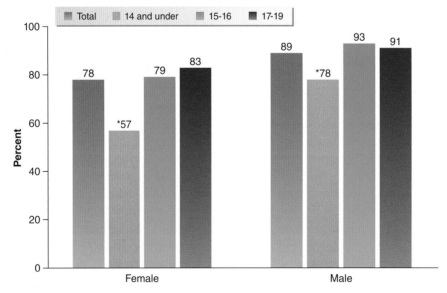

Figure 12.7 Use of contraception at first sexual intercourse among U.S. females and males, aged 15 to 24, who had sexual intercourse before age 20, 2015 to 2017.

*Significantly lower than the percentages for those ages 15 to 16 and 17 to 19 at first sexual intercourse (*p* < 0.05).

Most effective	Method	Unintended pregnancy with typical use (%)
		Most effective
Less than 1 per 100	Implant	.01%
	IUD	0.1-0.8%
	Vasectomy	0.15%
	Tubal ligation	0.5%
6-12 per 100	Shot (Depo-Provera)	4%
	Birth control pill	7%
	Patch	7%
	Vaginal contraceptive ring	7%
	Diaphragm	17%
18+ per 100	External condom	13%
	Internal condom	21%
	Withdrawal	22%
	Fertility awareness–based methods	23%
	Spermicide	21%
	No method	85%
		Least effective

Figure 12.8 If you use contraceptives, carefully evaluate which one to use, considering their failure rates.
The percentages indicate the number of every 100 people who experienced an unintended pregnancy during the first year of typical use.
Data from Trussell et al. (2018).

choose not to have children, which birth control methods would be the best options for you and your partner to consider for the long term?

Being aware of birth control methods and knowing how to use them consistently and correctly with every sexual encounter is being responsible to yourself and your partner. Consider these questions when choosing a birth control method:

1. What are your and your partner's values regarding conception? What are your opinions about the different types of birth control methods?

2. Do you both know the advantages and disadvantages of each method, including side effects?

3. What are the costs of different methods? Which ones are covered by insurance or government health care plans or are available at lower costs from community health clinics? Is cost a prohibiting factor when considering birth control?

4. Which methods will require the commitment of both partners? Which methods require that only one partner be responsible?

5. Do you need a method that also protects against STIs? Which methods can help prevent transmission of STIs?

6. Which methods require seeing a health care provider before use?

7. How long are you and your partner going to use this method?

8. Do you plan on having children? If so, when?

9. Which methods do you and your partner consider to be convenient?

10. Which methods do you and your partner consider to be too difficult or not worth using? What are the reasons?

Contraceptive Use by the Numbers

Check out these statistics on contraceptive use, compiled by the Guttmacher Institute (2021a).

- 85 percent: The chance of a sexually active heterosexual couple getting pregnant with no contraceptive use over the course of a year
- 2.7 children: The average desired family size in the United States
- 3 decades: The total time a female must use contraceptives, on average, to have 2.7 children
- 65 percent: Percentage of U.S. females of reproductive age using birth control
- >99 percent: Percentage of sexually experienced U.S. females aged 15 to 44 who have used at least one contraceptive method since 2008
- 4 out of 5: Number of sexually active females aged 15 to 44 who have used the birth control pill at some time

- 18 percent: Percentage of all contraceptive users between the ages of 15 and 44 who rely on long-acting reversible contraceptives such as the IUD or an implant (Guttmacher Institute 2021b)
- 2 primary reasons given for using emergency contraceptives: Fear that the regular birth control method would not work and having unprotected sex (Guttmacher Institute 2021c; Hussain and Kavanaugh 2021)

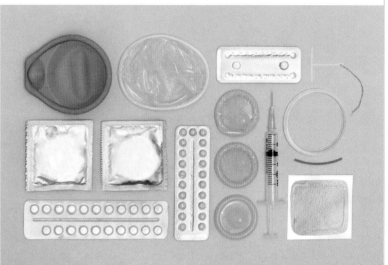

ABSTINENCE

Abstinence means choosing not to be sexually active until the time is right for you. For many, this means not engaging in sexual contact, sexual stimulation, kissing, oral sex, vaginal sex, or anal sex. Some people wait to engage in any or all these activities until marriage. No one can tell you when to become sexually active or which sexual activities you should engage in. Research shows that young people who delay sexual activity between the start of a relationship and the first sexual encounter with that partner are more likely to use birth control (Manlove, Ryan, and Franzetta 2003).

 Behavior Check

Abstinence

Why do people choose abstinence? What are the pros and cons? Can you still be a sexual person if you are not sexually active? What are the challenges of sticking to a decision to be abstinent?

Abstinence provides 100 percent protection from pregnancy and STIs. Abstinence means that no genital contact occurs. By not rushing into a relationship that includes sexual activities, partners can get to know each other better and build trust.

BARRIER BIRTH CONTROL METHODS

Barrier birth control methods provide a physical barrier that prevents the sperm and egg from meeting. External latex condoms (see figure 12.9), when used consistently and correctly with every sexual encounter, can provide an effective barrier and reduce the risk of acquiring STIs that are transmitted by genital fluids, including HIV, the virus that causes AIDS (Centers for Disease Control and Prevention 2021f).

Some of the terms for birth control products have changed to reflect gender-neutral language. For example, the male condom is now recognized as an "external condom" and the female condom is now referred to as the "internal condom" (Centers for Disease Control and Prevention 2021c). Using this language makes no specific gender or identity assumptions about the person using the birth control method.

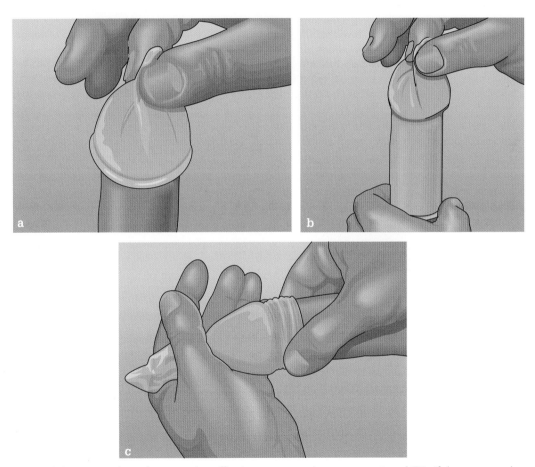

Figure 12.9   External condoms can be effective at preventing pregnancy and STIs if they are used consistently and correctly with every sexual encounter.

EXTERNAL CONDOM

Use. Read package instructions before using a condom. Check the expiration date and get a new one if the date has passed. Use external latex condoms to prevent pregnancy and transmission of STIs and HIV. Place the condom over an erect penis before intercourse and pinch the tip of the condom to prevent an air bubble from forming. It is important to leave a space at the tip of the condom to collect the semen. After ejaculation, remove the condom and dispose of it in the trash, making sure the semen remains in the condom (see figure 12.9).

Advantages. Many different types are available; partner can participate; no prescription needed. Most methods fall to the female for responsibility, but this method is one that does not.

Disadvantages. Cannot reuse condoms; need to use correctly and consistently every time; may cause irritation or allergic reactions; some people with a penis experience diminished sensation; must make sure condom is on correctly so it doesn't slip off during intercourse; can use only water-based lubricants; condoms made of animal skin (or natural condoms) do not prevent STIs or HIV.

INTERNAL CONDOM

Use. The internal condom is inserted into the vagina; the smaller circle covers the cervix, and the larger circle covers the vulva (see figure 12.10).

Advantages. Made of nitrile, not latex; can be inserted into the vagina up to eight hours before sexual intercourse.

Disadvantages. A new internal condom must be used with every sexual encounter; may cause irritation or allergic reaction; user must be comfortable inserting the end of the condom in the vagina, which takes practice; cannot be used with the external condom at the same time.

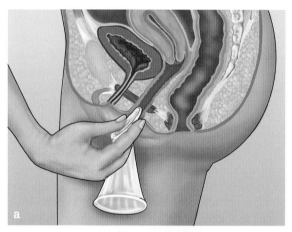

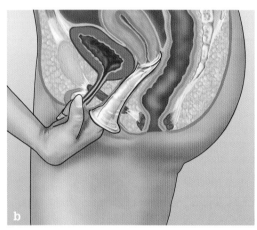
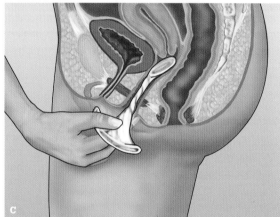

Figure 12.10   An internal condom can be inserted up to eight hours before intercourse.

DIAPHRAGM

Use. Fits over the cervix; must be inserted into the vagina and placed over the cervix before intercourse (see figure 12.11). A spermicide must be applied to the inside of the diaphragm before it is inserted; the diaphragm must remain over the cervix for six hours after the last sexual encounter and removed within 24 hours.

Advantages. Can be reused; inserted before sexual intercourse; can be used with external condom.

Disadvantages. Must be inserted before penile-vaginal intercourse and remain in place during intercourse; must be used with every sexual encounter; may cause irritation or allergic reaction; user must be comfortable inserting the diaphragm into the vagina, which takes practice; does not prevent HIV or STIs.

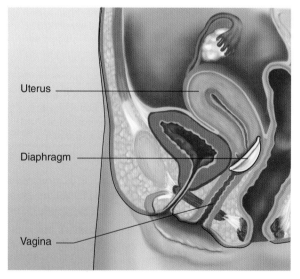

Figure 12.11   A diaphragm is a barrier method of birth control that prevents the sperm from fertilizing the egg.

CERVICAL CAP

Use. The cervical cap is smaller than the diaphragm; however, just like the diaphragm, it is used with spermicide and held in place over the cervix with suction. Must be inserted before penile-vaginal intercourse and used with a spermicide.

Advantages. Can be reused; inserted before sex; can be used with external condom.

Disadvantages. Must be inserted before penile-vaginal intercourse and remain in place during intercourse; must be used with every sexual encounter; may cause irritation or allergic reaction; user must be comfortable inserting cervical cap in the vagina, which takes practice; does not prevent HIV or STIs.

> If you are using the diaphragm or cervical cap and planning on having sex more than once in 24 hours, be sure to check the placement of these barrier methods and use more spermicide with each sexual encounter.

HORMONAL BIRTH CONTROL METHODS

Hormonal birth control methods contain estrogen and progestin to prevent pregnancy in those with female reproductive systems. They work through various mechanisms such as preventing ovulation; thickening the cervical mucus, which prevents sperm from entering the uterus; or causing the lining of the uterus to thin, which prevents implantation of the fertilized egg. Most hormonal methods must be prescribed by a health care provider. One exception is the emergency contraceptive pill, which is available over the counter.

> None of the hormonal birth control methods prevent sexually transmitted infections (Centers for Disease Control and Prevention 2019a).

BIRTH CONTROL PILL

Use. A pill that usually contains progestin and estrogen taken at the same time every day to prevent fertilization and inhibit ovulation. Some pills have only one hormone. Most packs have 21 days of pills with hormones and 7 days without hormones, the latter of which are taken when the period begins. Continuous birth control pills with low estrogen may stop bleeding during the menstrual cycle; absence of a period will not cause long-term health problems. Individuals interested in this method need to consult with their health care providers to determine which type of birth control pill is best for their overall health and quality of life.

Advantages. Does not interrupt penile-vaginal intercourse; user can stop taking the pill at any time; may help with acne or lead to shorter and lighter periods.

Disadvantages. Requires a prescription; user must take a pill every day; missing a pill decreases the effectiveness of the method and requires using another birth control method (e.g., external or internal condom) for at least seven days; increased risk of blood clots if user smokes cigarettes; may cause nausea, mood changes or depression, headaches, spotting in between periods, and breast tenderness; does not prevent HIV or STIs.

> Although the birth control pill has been used by millions of people since the 1960s and is considered very safe, be sure to contact your health care provider if you take the birth control pill and experience any of the following symptoms, or ACHES: abdominal pain, chest pain, headaches, eye problems, or severe leg pain.

IMPLANT (NEXPLANON)

Use. Progestin only; small flexible rod is surgically placed under the skin on the underside of the upper arm; suppresses ovulation and thickens cervical mucus.

Advantages. Lasts for three years; size of a small matchstick; fertility returns within days of removal.

Disadvantages. User must have new implant inserted every three years; side effects include irregular bleeding and spotting between periods, mood changes, weight gain, headaches, acne, depression, breast tenderness, painful periods, and nausea; does not prevent HIV or STIs.

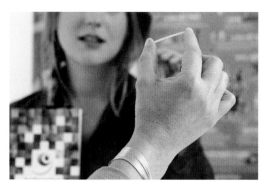

With the implant Nexplanon, the tiny rod is placed just under the skin and the body absorbs the progestin to prevent ovulation.

PATCH

Use. A small 1-1/2-inch patch containing estrogen and progestin is applied to the abdomen, shoulder, side of upper arm, or buttocks; prevents ovulation; thickens cervical mucus.

Advantages. Simple to use; adheres to body; user does not have to change daily.

Disadvantages. Requires a prescription; must be placed on body before intercourse and remain in place during penile-vaginal intercourse; user must change patch weekly on the same day for three weeks, then on fourth week wear no patch to begin the menstrual cycle; patch may become detached from skin or cause irritation; contains higher levels of estrogen than the birth control pill; may be less effective for individuals who weigh over 198 pounds (90 kg); does not prevent HIV or STIs.

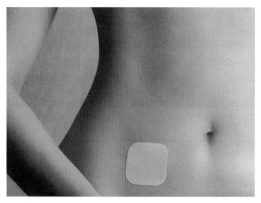

The birth control patch is worn on the skin and delivers hormones that prevent ovulation.

VAGINAL RING

Use. A flexible ring is inserted into the vagina. This method releases low doses of estrogen and progestin and stops ovulation. Unlike other hormonal birth control methods, this method requires the user to insert the ring into the vagina. If the user experiences some discomfort, then the ring is not in place. Most sexual partners have indicated that they cannot feel the ring during intercourse.

Advantages. Remains in place for three weeks and is removed during the menstrual cycle; user does not have to change daily.

Disadvantages. Must be inserted before penile-vaginal intercourse and remain in place during intercourse; user must be comfortable inserting and removing the ring; user must replace ring every month; possibility of irritation; does not prevent HIV or STIs.

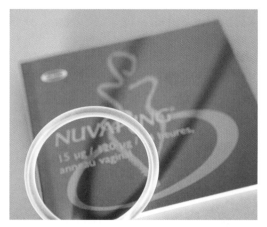

The vaginal ring is flexible so it can be inserted into the vagina and placed around the cervix.

SHOT (DEPO-PROVERA)

Use. A progestin-only shot given in the upper arm or buttocks every three months.

Advantages. No estrogen; begins providing protection against pregnancy within 24 hours of the first injection; no menstrual bleeding after one year of use.

Disadvantages. Requires injection every three months; must see a health care provider to get the injection; possible weight gain, hair loss, and mood changes; bone density decreases after long-term use; does not prevent HIV or STIs.

IUD (INTRAUTERINE DEVICE)

Use. A tiny, T-shaped device is inserted into the uterus by a health care provider; different types are available with and without hormones (copper T); works by thickening cervical mucus and inhibiting fertilization (see figure 12.12).

Advantages. Lighter periods; less cramping during periods; some can be in place for 3 to 12 years; user does not have to do anything once it is inserted; easily removed.

Disadvantages. Some IUDs may increase bleeding and cramps during period; may cause irregular menstrual cycle, pelvic discomfort, acne, headaches, nausea, and breast tenderness; does not prevent HIV or STIs.

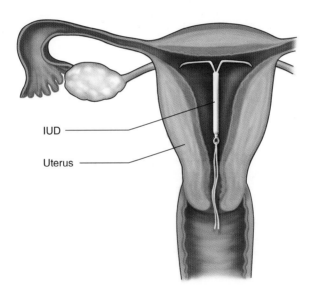

IUD

Uterus

Figure 12.12   The IUD is placed in the uterus by a health care provider to prevent pregnancy. Three different types are available that can stay in the uterus for 3, 5, or 10 years.

EMERGENCY CONTRACEPTION (MORNING-AFTER PILL)

Use. Taken after unprotected penile-vaginal intercourse to prevent pregnancy; should be taken within three days for optimal effectiveness; delays or prevents ovulation to prevent fertilization; inhibits the Fallopian tubes from drawing the egg toward the uterus.

Advantages. An option for individuals who have been sexually assaulted; helpful for when a birth control method was not used, the method failed to work as intended, or the method was used incorrectly; can be up to 95 percent effective in preventing pregnancy if taken within the first 24 hours after unprotected penile-vaginal intercourse.

Disadvantages. Loses effectiveness if taken more than three days after unprotected penile-vaginal intercourse; ineffective for users who weigh more than 165 pounds (75 kg); will not work if the user is already pregnant; cannot be taken before penile-vaginal intercourse as a birth control method; may cause nausea and vomiting; does not prevent HIV or STIs.

In 2014, the FDA removed the age requirements for the sale of Plan B and generic versions of this type of emergency contraception, and it can be obtained over the counter (Kaiser Family Foundation 2022).

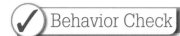

Behavior Check

Reasons for Not Using Birth Control

With all the reliable and affordable birth control methods available for preventing pregnancy, why do you think sexually active college students choose not to use them? Which of the following reasons have you heard from your friends?

- Lack of information and knowledge about methods and how to use them
- Too embarrassed to talk to their sexual partner or their health care provider
- Don't want others to know they are sexually active
- Afraid of the side effects like potential weight gain or mood swings
- Afraid that methods may reduce sexual desire, excitement, or pleasure
- Methods are too expensive
- Methods are too complicated and bothersome
- Drug or alcohol use prevents them from using birth control methods
- Religious or cultural reasons
- Not sure where to get them

Now that you know about the methods of birth control, what would you say to friends who gave these reasons for not using birth control?

OTHER METHODS

Other types of birth control do not require the use of a barrier method or hormones. These options are available for couples who want to use a method that is in alignment with their religious or personal values. They do not require getting a prescription or using a medication or products that may cause irritations or allergies. None of these methods protect against HIV or STIs.

FERTILITY AWARENESS–BASED METHODS, OR NATURAL FAMILY PLANNING

Use. Users recognize fertile days during the menstrual cycle by charting changes in cervical mucus and basal body temperature (which are slightly elevated during ovulation) and abstain from intercourse during those days. To use this method correctly, it's best to get training from a health care professional.

Advantages. Involves both partners; avoids the side effects of other methods; helps to plan a pregnancy; users and their partners learn to understand the menstrual cycle.

Disadvantages. Cannot have spontaneous penile-vaginal intercourse and must plan according to the menstrual cycle; need to keep track of ovulation; will have to use alternate birth control methods if choosing to have sex during ovulation days; hard to track ovulation with an irregular menstrual cycle; does not prevent HIV or STIs.

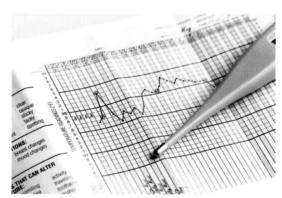

Fertility awareness requires the careful calculation and charting of ovulation during the menstrual cycle. Couples who do not want children abstain from sexual intercourse during these days.

WITHDRAWAL

Use. When using the **withdrawal** method, a person with a penis withdraws it from the person with a vagina before ejaculation; may prevent fertilization.

Advantage. No prescription or devices needed; may be better than no birth control method.

Disadvantages. Requires cooperation of both partners; may disrupt sexual pleasure; pre-ejaculatory fluid from previous ejaculations during this sexual intercourse encounter may contain sperm; does not prevent HIV or STIs.

SPERMICIDES

Use. **Spermicide** contains a chemical that kills sperm. It comes in the form of foam, jelly, cream, or film that is placed inside the vagina before sex. Some types must be put in place 30 minutes ahead of time but no more than 1 hour before intercourse. Spermicides are most often used along with other birth control methods such as the external condom, diaphragm, or cervical cap.

Advantages. Easy to use, inexpensive, available at most drug stores.

Disadvantages. May cause irritations; could increase risk of getting HIV or STIs.

STERILIZATION: VASECTOMY

Use. Permanent surgical procedure that severs the vas deferens; prevents sperm from leaving the testicles (see figure 12.13).

Advantages. Permanent procedure; highly effective; does not alter sexual pleasure or desire.

Disadvantages. Surgical procedure; user experiences soreness at incision site, some swelling in the testicles; does not provide immediate protection against pregnancy and can take somewhere between 15 and 20 ejaculations to clear sperm from semen; user must submit semen samples to health care provider to make sure semen no longer contains sperm; not intended to be a reversible procedure (Mayo Clinic 2021b); does not prevent HIV or STIs.

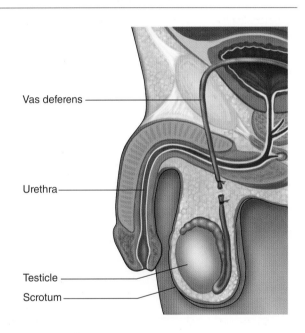

Figure 12.13 A vasectomy is a permanent surgical procedure in which the vas deferens is cut and sealed to prevent the sperm from leaving the testicles.

STERILIZATION: TUBAL LIGATION

Use. Permanent surgical procedure that severs the Fallopian tubes and prevents eggs from entering the uterus (see figure 12.14).

Advantages. Permanent procedure; quick recovery; highly effective; does not alter sexual pleasure or desire.

Disadvantages. Surgical procedure; user experiences soreness at incision site; not intended to be a reversible procedure (American College of Obstetricians and Gynecologists 2019); does not prevent HIV or STIs.

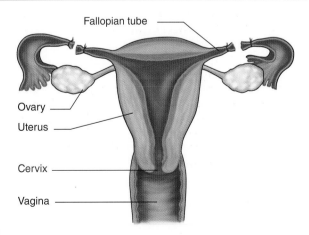

Figure 12.14 A tubal ligation is a permanent surgical procedure in which the Fallopian tubes are cut or sealed to prevent eggs from entering the uterus.

Sexually Transmitted Infections

Sexually transmitted infections (STIs) can cause a lifetime of health problems; therefore, you should have conversations about preventing these infections with all sexual partners. Talking to sexual partners about your sexual history can be uncomfortable, but it is necessary to make sure you are taking care of yourself and practicing responsible behaviors. Understanding more about your body, recognizing when something just isn't right, and knowing how to communicate about your sexual health can help you make responsible decisions. Knowing your STI status, as well as that of your partner, is important for remaining infection free throughout your life.

Sexually transmitted infections are common diseases caused by viruses, bacteria, or parasites that are transmitted through vaginal intercourse, anal intercourse, and oral sex. Most, if caught early, can be treated with antibiotics. However, viral STIs are with you for life. Some can lead to further complications, such as cancers, infertility, and problems during pregnancy and childbirth. Unfortunately, some infections do not lead to obvious symptoms, and symptoms do not have to be present for an infection to be transmitted to another person. People with female reproductive systems are more susceptible to acquiring STIs than those with male reproductive systems are.

On any given day in 2018 in the United States, approximately 1 in 5 people had an STI, equaling almost 68 million infections (National Academies of Sciences, Engineering, and Medicine 2021). Of these reported cases, they are diagnosed most often among teens and young adults between the ages of 15 and 25. The most diagnosed bacterial STIs are chlamydia, gonorrhea, and syphilis, and the most common viral STIs are genital herpes simplex virus (HSV), HIV/AIDS, and human papilloma virus (HPV). The Centers for Disease Control and Prevention (2021a) reported that from 2014 to 2019, STIs reached an all-time high for six years in a row (figure 12.15).

> Most STIs, if detected early, can be treated. However, some can lead to cancer, infertility, complications during pregnancy and childbirth, and death. Viral STIs are with you for life.

RECORD HIGH STDs THREATEN MILLIONS OF AMERICANS

2,554,908
COMBINED CASES REPORTED IN 2019

Chlamydia
1,808,703 cases
553 per 100,000 people

Gonorrhea
616,392 cases
188 per 100,000 people

Syphilis (all stages)
129,813 cases
40 per 100,000 people

Syphilis (primary and secondary)	Syphilis (congenital)
38,992 cases	1,870 cases
12 per 100,000 people	49 per 100,000 live births

Figure 12.15   Six consecutive years of record-breaking STI cases in the United States, 2014 to 2019.

Reprinted from Centers for Disease Control and Prevention (2021m).

- STIs continue to be a significant health challenge in our country today (figure 12.16). According to the CDC's report on STIs in the United States, data show the following (Centers for Disease Control and Prevention, 2021m):

- Because many cases of STIs are undiagnosed and not reported to the CDC or state health departments, the existing data is only a snapshot of the full STI epidemic in the United States.

STI Treatment for Partners

Did you know that if you are diagnosed with an STI, you may be able to get medication to give to your sexual partner? If you are diagnosed with gonorrhea, chlamydia, or trichomoniasis, ask your health care provider about expedited partner therapy. After you have taken the prescribed medication and no longer have symptoms, see your health care provider to make sure the infection is gone (Guttmacher Institute 2021d).

• There are effective treatments for some STIs, but when left untreated, some people can have severe lifelong health outcomes like chronic pain, neurological complications, and infertility, and without treatment, they are more likely to transmit infections to others.

• More than 20,000 females are infertile as a result of undiagnosed and untreated STIs every year.

• Almost half of gay and bisexual males who have been diagnosed with syphilis also have HIV.

The Centers for Disease Control and Prevention reports that STIs are increasing across many racial and ethnic minority groups (figure 12.17). Compared to non-Hispanic white people, STI rates were 1 to 2 times higher among Hispanic or Latino people, 3 to 5 times higher among American Indian or Alaska Native and Native Hawaiian or other Pacific Islander people, and 5 to 8 times higher among African American or Black people.

Reported new STD cases per year:

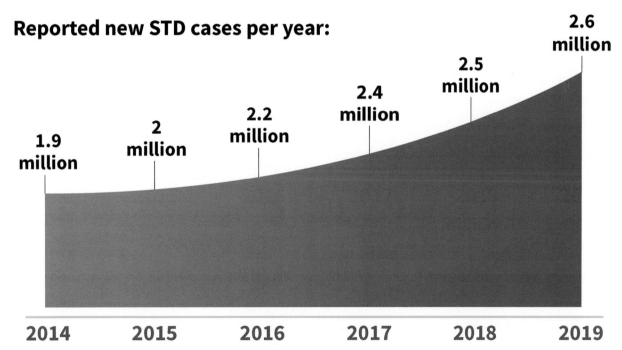

1.9 million — 2014
2 million — 2015
2.2 million — 2016
2.4 million — 2017
2.5 million — 2018
2.6 million — 2019

Figure 12.16   CDC fact sheet: Reported STIs in the United States, 2019.

Reprinted from Centers for Disease Control and Prevention (2021a).

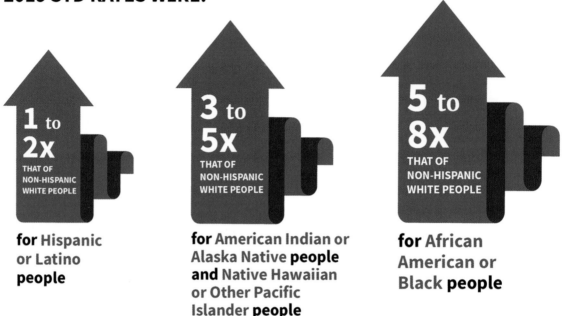

Disparities in STDs persist among racial & ethnic minority groups

While STDs are increasing across many groups, 2019 STD RATES WERE:

1 to 2x THAT OF NON-HISPANIC WHITE PEOPLE

for **Hispanic or Latino people**

3 to 5x THAT OF NON-HISPANIC WHITE PEOPLE

for **American Indian or Alaska Native people and Native Hawaiian or Other Pacific Islander people**

5 to 8x THAT OF NON-HISPANIC WHITE PEOPLE

for **African American or Black people**

Figure 12.17   Disparities in STIs among racial and ethnic minority groups in the United States, 2019.
Reprinted from Centers for Disease Control and Prevention (2021a).

MOST COMMON VIRAL STIs

Viral STIs enter the body through skin or body fluids. A virus can survive only by attaching to living cells in the body. Viral STIs can be treated but not cured. For example, herpes is a viral STI that can be successfully treated with medications prescribed by a physician to alleviate the symptoms (e.g., sores or blisters), which may include reducing the frequency of the outbreaks in addition to reducing their severity and duration. Hepatitis and human papilloma virus are the only viral STIs that can be prevented with a vaccine.

HIV/AIDS

Facts. The human immunodeficiency virus (HIV) causes acquired immunodeficiency syndrome (AIDS). The virus is transmitted through breast milk, vaginal secretions, semen, and blood. HIV attacks the body's immune system and affects its ability to fight infections. The body becomes susceptible to serious opportunistic infections that are typically rare in people without HIV. Examples of these unique infections are a skin cancer called Kaposi's sarcoma and pneumocystis pneumonia.

Prevalence. According to the Centers for Disease Control and Prevention (2021h), there were 36,801 new HIV diagnoses in 2019. Of these, 66 percent were related to male-to-male sexual contact, 23 percent were among heterosexuals, 7 percent were among people who used intravenous drugs, and 4 percent were related to both male-to-male sexual contact and injection drug use. Heterosexual women accounted for 16 percent of the new cases as compared to 7 percent of heterosexual men. With regard to race and ethnicity, Black or African American and Hispanic or Latino people are disproportionately affected; 42 percent of new HIV diagnoses were among Black or African American people and 29 percent were among Hispanic or Latino people. Figure 12.18 shows the number of new HIV diagnoses was highest among people aged 25 to 34 (Centers for Disease Control and Prevention 2021g).

Transmission. The primary modes of transmission are sharing needles and having anal intercourse, vaginal intercourse, or oral sex with an HIV-infected person where these body fluids come in contact with a mucosal lining or damaged tissues. These delicate membranes are in the rectum, vagina, penis, and mouth. Detectable amounts of the virus show up on blood or oral secretion tests between one week and three months after exposure. The virus can be transmitted to another person by someone who is HIV positive but does not show any specific symptoms of infection. Only 87 people out of 100 with HIV know their status.

Symptoms. When a person has been diagnosed with HIV, they may be symptom free for many years. As the infection progresses, symptoms may include fevers, weight loss, swollen lymph nodes, or oral yeast infections. A person is diagnosed with AIDS based on the progression of the disease and its toll on the immune system, causing opportunistic infections, increased levels of HIV in the body, and lower levels of infection-fighting antibodies.

Treatment. No cure or vaccine exists to prevent HIV; however, medications are available to reduce the amount of HIV in the body and can help HIV-positive individuals live a long and productive life. These medications are called antiretroviral therapy (ART) and are recommended for anyone with HIV; these should start as soon as possible after diagnosis by a health care professional (Centers for Disease Control and Prevention 2021i). These medications decrease the viral load (the amount of HIV in the blood) and can reduce the chances of transmitting the virus to others. At the time HIV/AIDS was first discovered in the early 1980s, many died within a few years of diagnosis. Today, with our better understanding of how the virus affects the immune system and access to medications, HIV is no longer the death sentence it once was.

New HIV Diagnoses in the US and Dependent Areas by Age, 2019

The number of new HIV diagnoses was highest among people aged 25 to 34.

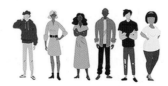

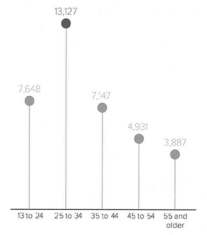

13 to 24	25 to 34	35 to 44	45 to 54	55 and older
7,648	13,127	7,147	4,931	3,887

Figure 12.18   HIV infections among youth in the United States, 2019.

Reprinted from Centers for Disease Control and Prevention (2019).

✓ Behavior Check

HIV Testing and Prevention

The Centers for Disease Control and Prevention's Get Tested program is focused on motivating people to learn their HIV status. Knowing your status enables you to get the medical care you need to treat these infections or prevent their progress, inform your sexual partners so they can be treated, and remain infection free. On the Centers for Disease Control and Prevention's website, you can locate a testing site in your community and learn the specific types of testing you need by answering a few questions related to your sex, age, and sexual behaviors and history. Behaviors that can put you at risk for HIV are having more than one sexual partner, engaging in sexual activities without knowing your partner's sexual health history, not using condoms, having been diagnosed with other STIs, and sharing needles or syringes. The Centers for Disease Control and Prevention recommends that everyone between the ages of 13 and 64 get tested for HIV as part of a routine health examination. For more information about getting tested, visit the Centers for Disease Control and Prevention's website at https://gettested.cdc.gov.

PrEP (pre-exposure prophylaxis) is a highly effective prevention method for people who are not HIV positive but engage in behaviors that may put them at risk of acquiring HIV. This medication works to prevent the virus from becoming a permanent infection in the body and can reduce the risk of HIV infection by up to 99 percent when taken as prescribed. Increased protection from acquiring HIV can be achieved by also using external and internal condoms consistently and correctly with all sexual partners, not sharing needles, and visiting a health care provider every three months (Centers for Disease Control and Prevention 2021k).

HUMAN PAPILLOMA VIRUS (HPV)

Facts. HPV is so common that most sexually active people will be diagnosed with the virus at some point (Centers for Disease Control and Prevention 2021j).

Prevalence. HPV is not a reportable STI to state health departments or the Centers for Disease Control and Prevention. It is estimated that 42.5 million Americans between the ages of 15 to 59 were infected with HPV in 2018. Approximately 13 million new infections are diagnosed annually (Kreisel et al. 2021).

Symptoms. Warts appear internally or externally in the genital area between six weeks and eight months after exposure, although some people never develop the warts.

Diagnosis. Visual examination or biopsy of the warts; people with a cervix may require a Pap smear or colposcopy (microscopic examination of cervix).

It's important to keep in mind that the HPV vaccination works to prevent new infections and does not treat or cure existing HPV infections, so be proactive and talk to your medical provider if you haven't received your HPV vaccinations yet.

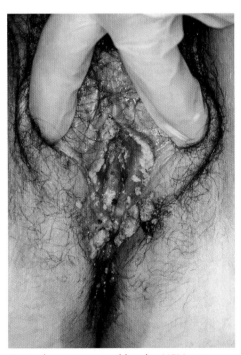

Genital warts, caused by the HPV, are typically flesh colored. They can be found in the genital (internal and external), anal, mouth, and throat regions.

Treatment. The warts can go away on their own without treatment, but the virus never goes away. A health care provider can remove the warts through cryotherapy (freezing with liquid nitrogen), burning them off with a topical solution like trichloroacetic acid, cauterization with electrical heat, or a laser treatment. A prescription topical cream can also be applied to the warts if they are external.

Complications. People with a cervix are at an increased risk of cervical cancer when exposed to certain HPV strains. People with a penis can develop anal and penile cancers. Pregnant people with the virus will have to deliver a baby by cesarean section if warts are present during delivery. All people exposed to HPV can develop throat cancers.

Vaccine. The HPV vaccine for young people, Gardasil 6, protects against six types of the virus that are linked to cancers. The vaccine is only two doses, with the second dose given 6 to 12 months after the first dose. If two doses of the vaccine are received less than the recommended five months apart, then a third dose will be required. The CDC recommends that young people be vaccinated between ages 11 and 12; however, people vaccinated as young adults can still benefit from the vaccine's protective factors if they have never been exposed to HPV or the specific types that can cause cancer (Centers for Disease Control and Prevention 2020).

HERPES SIMPLEX VIRUS (HSV)

Facts. Two different types of HSV exist—herpes simplex virus type 1 (HSV-1; oral) and herpes simplex virus type 2 (HSV-2; genital). HSV-1 can be transferred from the mouth to the genitals and HSV-2 can be transferred from the genitals to the mouth through oral sex or if an infected person touches the infected genitals and then touches the mouth (or vice versa). Most fever blisters or cold sores on the mouth are HSV-1 and tend to flare up during very stressful times. This virus can be transmitted when symptoms are not present.

Prevalence. HSV is not a reportable STI by law to state health departments or the Centers for Disease Control and Prevention. It is estimated that in 2018, there were 18.6 million people aged 15 to 49 with HSV-2 (Kreisel et al. 2021).

HSV type 1, a cold sore on the lip, tends to reoccur in the same place during each outbreak.

Symptoms. For people exposed to HSV, outbreaks of small sores or lesions appear around the mouth or genitals (depending on the type of contact) 2 to 12 days after exposure. Sores can last up to two weeks. When the sores are gone, the virus remains dormant until the next outbreak.

Diagnosis. It is recommended to be tested when people have symptoms or an outbreak of sores that look like blisters. Diagnosis involves examination and viral culture of the lesions, which involves taking a sample of the lesion tissue (Centers for Disease Control and Prevention 2017).

Treatment. Herpes cannot be cured because it is a virus; however, medications can reduce the intensity and frequency of the outbreaks and may reduce the chances of the virus being spread to a sexual partner (Centers for Disease Control and Prevention 2021d).

Complications. Pregnant people who have an active outbreak may not be able to deliver the baby vaginally.

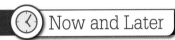 Now and Later

HPV Vaccine

The HPV vaccine is the best method for preventing many types of cancers, including cervical, penile, anal, and throat cancers. The vaccination is effective and the cervical cancer rates have dropped significantly. These are just a few reasons why parents need to talk to their health care providers about vaccinating their children (see figure 12.19).

Now

The HPV vaccine was approved by the FDA in June 2006. When it was first introduced as a safe and effective method of preventing cervical cancer caused by certain strains of the virus, many parents were concerned. Some of the controversial aspects of the vaccine included the mandate that all young people with a cervix must get the vaccine. Parents thought the age at which to give the vaccine, 11 to 12 years old, was premature because individuals are typically not sexually active at this age and felt that the primary message their young children would receive is that it is safe for them to become sexually active at an earlier age. Parents who are against the vaccine often express their concerns about their child's sexual development and do not feel ready to deal with such uncomfortable issues with their preteens.

Later

The vaccine is safe and effective for young females through age 26 and young males through age 21; however, the vaccine, which consists of two shots given 6 to 12 months apart, should be given at age 11 or 12 (Centers for Disease Control and Prevention 2020. You may be a parent in the future, so what are your thoughts about the HPV vaccine? How will you plan to protect your children from HPV in the future?

- Should the HPV vaccine be mandatory for all young people? Why or why not?
- Why should preteens get the HPV vaccine if they are not yet sexually active?

Take Home

Learn more about the HPV vaccine so that you and your future children can be protected from acquiring the virus.

ZIKA

Facts. Zika was first discovered in 1947, but very few cases were reported until recently. It is transmitted when an infected *Aedes* species mosquito bites a human. Once Zika infects a human, it can be passed from a pregnant person to the fetus, through sexual activity, and possibly through blood transfusions. Zika infections are primarily concentrated in certain areas of the world, specifically in tropical Africa, Southeast Asia, and the Pacific Islands (Centers for Disease Control and Prevention 2019b). Cases of Zika transmission were reported in in south Florida and Texas in 2015 and 2016; however, there have been no confirmed cases of transmission within the continental United States since 2018 and none in the U.S. territories since 2019 (Centers for Disease Control and Prevention 2021q).

Research studies are being conducted in the United States and other countries to determine how long Zika can remain in semen and vaginal fluids, how long Zika can be passed to sexual partners, and whether there is a difference in the risk for birth defects if the pregnant person acquires Zika during sex rather than directly from a mosquito bite (Centers for Disease Control and Prevention 2019b).

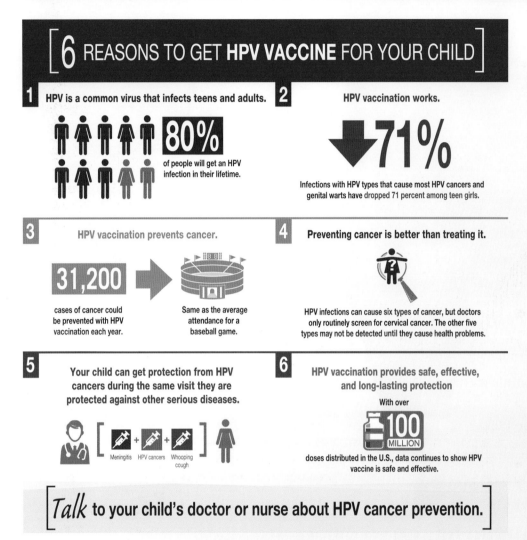

Figure 12.19   Six reasons to get the HPV vaccine for your child.
Reprinted from Centers for Disease Control and Prevention (2018).

Prevalence. Zika is a notifiable infection and is reported to state health departments and the Centers for Disease Control and Prevention. Since 2019, there have been only a few cases reported in the United States, and all of the cases were travelers returning from countries with high rates of infection (Centers for Disease Control and Prevention 2021p).

Symptoms. Most people infected with Zika have no symptoms. When experienced, symptoms are mild and last for several days to weeks. The most commonly reported symptoms are fever, rash, joint pain, red eyes, muscle pain, and headaches. Zika is not considered fatal.

Diagnosis. Zika is diagnosed through a comprehensive health and travel history, especially to countries with high rates such as tropical Africa, Southeast Asia, and the Pacific Islands. A blood or urine test will confirm the infection.

Treatment. Currently, no vaccine or medication is available to treat or cure Zika.

Complications. In pregnant people who are infected with Zika, the virus causes a birth defect called microcephaly (the baby's head and brain are smaller than they should be at birth), eye and hearing defects, and compromised growth.

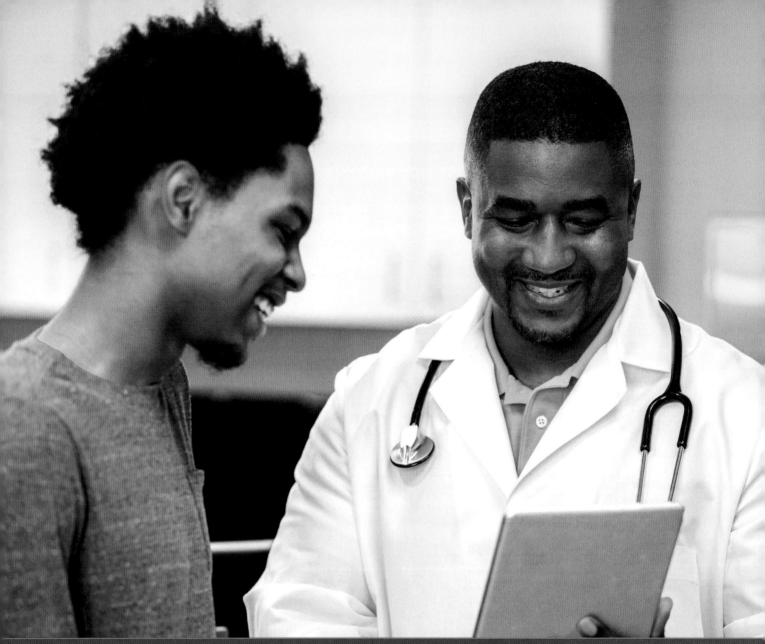

If you have not received the HPV vaccine, consider talking with your medical provider about it.

MOST COMMON BACTERIAL STIs

Bacterial STIs come from cells that cause infection and enter the body through the skin or body fluids (e.g., semen or vaginal fluids). If the bacterial infection is detected early, it can be successfully treated and often cured with antibiotics; however, if the infection is not treated, it could lead to long-term negative health consequences like sterility or death. Medications that treat the infection do not prevent recurrence if exposed to the bacteria in the future. Therefore, if you are sexually active, it is important to protect yourself by using condoms or other barrier methods that prevent the exchange of body fluids. See a health care provider if you are concerned about any abnormal symptoms such as discharge from the genitals or if a sexual partner has been diagnosed with a bacterial STI so that you can be diagnosed and treated in the early stages of the infection.

CHLAMYDIA

Facts. Most frequently reported bacterial STI in the United States (Centers for Disease Control and Prevention 2021b).

Prevalence. Reported cases are the highest among people aged 15 to 24. In 2019, this age group accounted for 61 percent of chlamydia cases (see figure 12.20).

Symptoms. Appear 7 to 30 days after exposure; many people do not experience symptoms.

- *Male reproductive organs:* Discharge from penis, pain in testicles, swollen testicles, painful urination
- *Female reproductive organs:* Odorous discharge from vagina, mid-cycle bleeding

Diagnosis. Everyone who is sexually active should be tested. Sexually active females age 25 and younger need to be tested annually. Testing methods involve urine analysis or testing of discharge for the bacteria.

Treatment. Can be easily cured with antibiotics if diagnosed in early stages.

Complications. If not detected and treated in the early stages of the infection, people with female reproductive organs can develop PID, which can lead to infertility. People with male reproductive organs can also develop infertility.

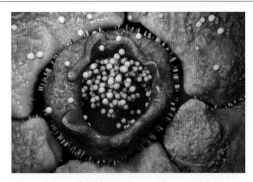

Illustration of *Chlamydia trachomatis* bacteria emerging from a cell. Not all people infected with chlamydia will have symptoms, but those who do may have an odorous or purulent discharge from the cervix (vagina) or penis.

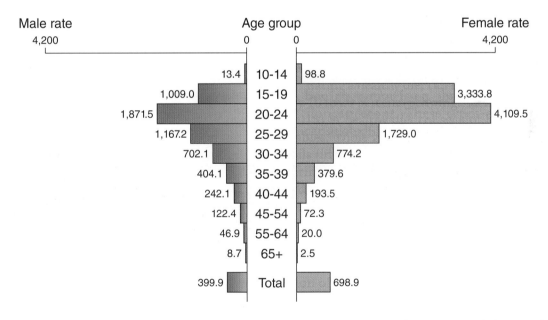

Age group	Male rate	Female rate
10-14	13.4	98.8
15-19	1,009.0	3,333.8
20-24	1,871.5	4,109.5
25-29	1,167.2	1,729.0
30-34	702.1	774.2
35-39	404.1	379.6
40-44	242.1	193.5
45-54	122.4	72.3
55-64	46.9	20.0
65+	8.7	2.5
Total	399.9	698.9

Figure 12.20 U.S. chlamydia rates per 100,000, 2019. Americans aged 15 to 24 account for 61 percent of all reported cases.

From: Centers for Disease Control and Prevention (2021j). Available: https://www.cdc.gov/std/statistics/2019/figures/F_CTSEXAGE-medium.png

GONORRHEA

Facts. Known as "the clap" or "the drip," gonorrhea is the second most commonly reported STI in the United States (Centers for Disease Control and Prevention 2021e). It can infect not only the genitals but also the rectum and throat.

Prevalence. Cases are up 56 percent from 2015 (Centers for Disease Control and Prevention 2021m); rates are high among teens and college-age individuals.

Symptoms. Appear two to seven days after exposure.

- *Male reproductive organs:* White or yellowish discharge from penis, pain when urinating, fever
- *Female reproductive organs:* White or yellowish vaginal discharge, mid-cycle bleeding, pain when urinating, fever, severe abdominal pain

Diagnosis. Urine analysis.

Treatment. Can be easily cured with antibiotics if diagnosed in early stages.

Complications.

- *Male reproductive organs:* Infertility, inflammation of the urinary tract and organs (prostate gland, seminal vesicles, bladder, and epididymis)
- *Female reproductive organs:* PID and infertility; infection can be transmitted to a baby during childbirth

PELVIC INFLAMMATORY DISEASE (PID)

Pelvic inflammatory disease is a serious, and sometimes fatal, complication that affects people with female reproductive organs. It is caused by untreated chlamydia or gonorrhea that has made its way to the female reproductive organs. Many individuals do not experience obvious signs of infection. The Fallopian tubes are the most vulnerable organs to these bacteria, which cause inflammation, severe abdominal pain, fever, and possible scarring of the tubes (see figure 12.21). Scarring of the Fallopian tubes leads to infertility by blocking the sperm from meeting the egg or causing a fertilized egg to get caught in the tubes, causing an ectopic pregnancy. Individuals who are diagnosed with PID may have to undergo a hysterectomy due to the irreversible damage to the reproductive organs.

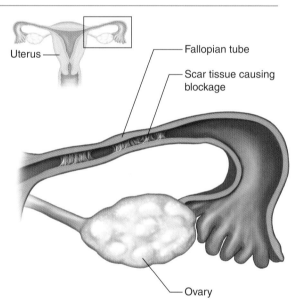

Figure 12.21   Scarring of the Fallopian tubes caused by PID. PID is a leading cause of infertility. It is typically caused by bacterial STIs that lead to scarring of the Fallopian tubes, preventing the sperm from fertilizing the egg.

SYPHILIS

Facts. The rate of syphilis increased more than 70 percent from 2015 to 2019. This increase was recorded among both sexes, among all racial/Hispanic ethnicity groups, and in all areas of the United States (U.S. Department of Health and Human Services 2021). This infection is transmitted by direct contact with the chancre lesion.

Prevalence. The occurrence of syphilis continues to increase annually at a high rate. Since 2000, the rates among men continue to increase, and men who have sex with men (MSM) account for most of the cases (56.7%). The rates for women are lower when compared to men, increasing 30 percent during 2018-2019 (U.S. Department of Health and Human Services 2021). Figure 12.22 shows the dis-

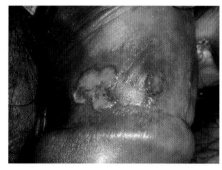

A chancre of primary syphilis.

tribution of cases by sex and sex of partners in 2019. These data indicate that heterosexual transmission of syphilis continues to be a major concern (U.S. Department of Health and Human Services 2021).

Symptoms. For individuals exposed to or diagnosed with syphilis, symptoms develop over time and in stages. Symptoms of primary syphilis include a painless chancre, or ulcer, at the site of the infection; examples are on the glans (head of the penis) and labia minora. In the secondary stages of syphilis, a distinctive rash may appear on the palms of the hands and soles of the feet.

- *Primary stage:* A painless lesion, called a chancre, appears at the site of sexual contact 10 to 90 days after exposure and goes away in approximately 3 weeks.
- *Secondary stage:* The bacteria spreads in the body and causes a painless rash on the body, swollen glands, fever, sore throat, weight loss, and low energy. Symptoms can last two to six weeks.
- *Tertiary stage:* The infection will continue to spread throughout the body and cause permanent organ damage.

Diagnosis. Blood test or culture from chancre sore.

Treatment. Can be cured with penicillin in the primary and secondary stages if the infection does not spread to other parts of the body and cause irreversible organ damage.

Complications. It can take years for the bacteria to reach the tertiary stage, leading to paralysis, strokes, blindness, and heart damage. A pregnant person with syphilis can transmit the bacterium to the fetus. As the rates continue to steadily increase in the general population, so have the rates of congenital syphilis. Syphilitic stillbirths are the devastating outcomes of congenital syphilis, primarily as a result of lack of treatment during pregnancy despite diagnosis of syphilis; the second most common contributing factor was lack of prenatal care and timely testing (U.S. Department of Health and Human Services 2021).

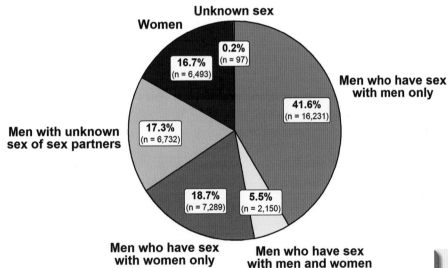

Figure 12.22   Distribution of cases of syphilis in the United States, 2019.

From: Centers for Disease Control and Prevention (2021). Available: https://www.cdc.gov/std/statistics/2019/figures/F_SYPH-SEXBEHAV.png

Reducing the Risks

Sexual activity can positively influence emotional and spiritual development and intimate relationships with others, but it brings the risk of STIs and other negative outcomes. Therefore, you need to make decisions now about how you plan to reduce your risks for STIs. Risk reduction methods include abstinence, mutual monogamy, using condoms, communicating, and having honest conversations with partners, and reducing or eliminating the use of alcohol and drugs.

Routine Testing

Getting tested is the only way you can know your STI status, so begin getting tested for HIV and STIs as part of your routine medical examinations. Knowing your status

STI symptoms include pain with urination, urethra or vaginal discharge that may have an odor, sores in the genital or mouth area, or pain in the pelvic region. Be sure to see a health care provider if you or a partner experience any of these symptoms.

can help you and your partners be safe and reduce the infection rates among young people.

Who should be tested? Recommendations from the Centers for Disease Control and Prevention (2021n) are as follows:

- All adolescents and adults aged 13 to 64 should be tested at least once for HIV.

- Annual chlamydia and gonorrhea screenings should be done for all sexually active females aged 25 and younger, as well as for older females who have new or multiple sex partners or a sex partner who has a sexually transmitted infection.

- People who are pregnant should be screened for syphilis, HIV, chlamydia, and hepatitis B and C early in the pregnancy. At-risk pregnant people should be screened for gonorrhea starting early in pregnancy, with repeat testing done as needed.

- All sexually active gay and bisexual males and any other individuals who have sex with people who have a penis should be screened at least once a year for syphilis, chlamydia, and gonorrhea. Individuals who have multiple or anonymous partners should be screened more frequently for STIs (e.g., at three- to six-month intervals), may benefit from frequent HIV testing (e.g., every three to six months), and tested annually for hepatitis C, if living with HIV.

- Anyone who has unsafe sex or shares intravenous drug equipment should get tested for HIV at least once a year.

- Individuals who have engaged in oral or anal sex should discuss throat and anal testing options with their health care provider.

- Individuals who have completed treatment for an STI should go back to their health care provider for another test to make sure that they are no longer infected.

✓ **Behavior Check**

Attitudes and Behaviors About STIs

Place a check mark next to all of the statements that apply to you:

- ▦ I have been or am currently sexually active.
- ▦ I have had multiple sexual partners.
- ▦ I do not use an internal or external condom for each and every sexual encounter.
- ▦ I use alcohol or drugs before I engage in sexual activities with a partner.
- ▦ I do not get routine checkups from my health care provider.
- ▦ I am uncomfortable talking to my sexual partners about sexual health issues, including sexual health history and STIs.
- ▦ I have used intravenous drugs and have shared the syringes with others.
- ▦ I am afraid to be tested for HIV and STIs.
- ▦ I am unsure of STI symptoms.

The more items you checked, the greater your risk of acquiring HIV or an STI. See your health care provider and discuss testing and ways to reduce your risks.

See your health care provider on a routine basis and get tested for HIV and STIs if you think you could be at risk of acquiring these infections due to risky sexual or drug behaviors.

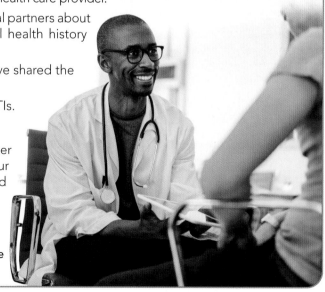

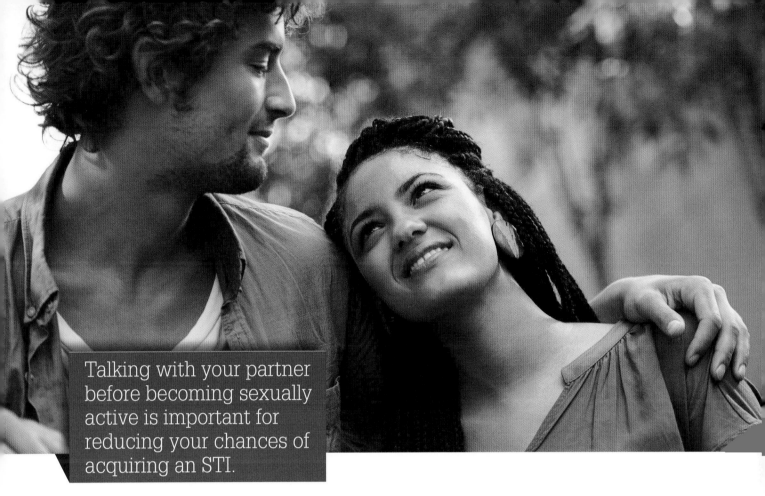

Talking with your partner before becoming sexually active is important for reducing your chances of acquiring an STI.

How to Talk With Partners About STI History

Communicating with current or potential sexual partners about sexual history can be uncomfortable and difficult. What are ways you can begin a conversation with a partner about behaviors that put them at risk for HIV and STIs? In addition to discussing higher-risk sexual behaviors, consider asking partners about their number of sexual partners, past diagnoses and treatments of STIs, and STI prevention methods.

It is a felony for someone with HIV to knowingly transmit the infection to a sexual partner without prior notification. Some infections do not have outward signs or symptoms and are spread unknowingly. What would you do if your sexual partner gave you HIV or another STI? How would you respond? When and how will you tell a future partner if you have been diagnosed with HIV or an STI? Think about the differences between viral and bacterial STIs and how that would affect the conversation.

Prevention of STIs

In short, follow these steps to prevent acquiring or spreading an STI (figure 12.23).

- Choose to be sexually abstinent.
- If you are sexually active, limit your number of sexual partners.
- Know your and your partners' STI status.
- Get routine medical exams that include STI screenings.

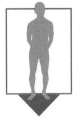
Choose abstinence

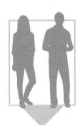
Limit number of sexual partners

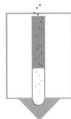
Get tested

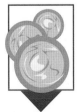
Use condoms

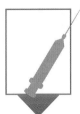
Get vaccinated

Figure 12.23 Following these steps will help you prevent an STI.

- Use condoms consistently and correctly with every sexual encounter.
- Get vaccinated against HPV.

Sexual Assault

Sexual assault is any type of sexual contact or behavior that happens without consent. Sexual assault includes rape and attempted rape, child molestation, sexual harassment or threats, and sexual coercion. Sexual coercion can include things that do not involve physical contact, such as forcing you to look at sexually explicit images, sending you a text with sexual photos or messages, or showing you their genitalia without your consent (i.e., "flashing" you). Sexual assault can happen to anyone of any age, race, ethnicity, religion, ability, appearance, sexual orientation, or gender identity (see figure 12.24). One in three females has experienced some type of sexual assault (Office on Women's Health 2019). In the United States, four out of five female rape victims report that the assault occurred before they

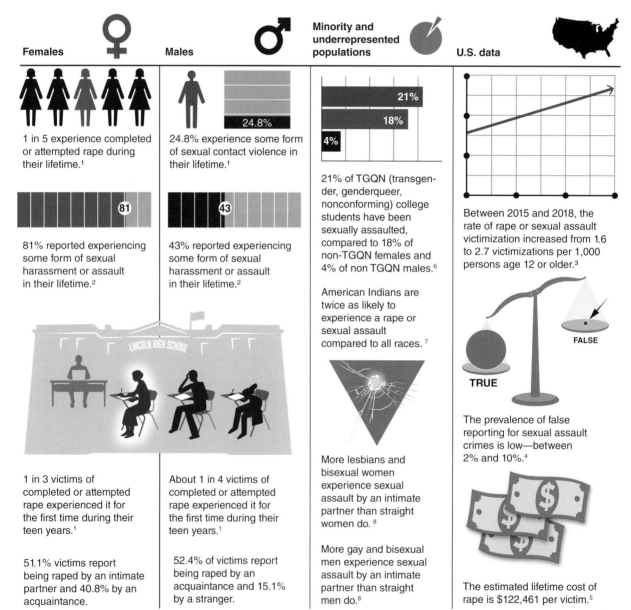

Females

1 in 5 experience completed or attempted rape during their lifetime.[1]

81% reported experiencing some form of sexual harassment or assault in their lifetime.[2]

1 in 3 victims of completed or attempted rape experienced it for the first time during their teen years.[1]

51.1% victims report being raped by an intimate partner and 40.8% by an acquaintance.

Males

24.8% experience some form of sexual contact violence in their lifetime.[1]

43% reported experiencing some form of sexual harassment or assault in their lifetime.[2]

About 1 in 4 victims of completed or attempted rape experienced it for the first time during their teen years.[1]

52.4% of victims report being raped by an acquaintance and 15.1% by a stranger.

Minority and underrepresented populations

21% of TGQN (transgender, genderqueer, nonconforming) college students have been sexually assaulted, compared to 18% of non-TGQN females and 4% of non TGQN males.[6]

American Indians are twice as likely to experience a rape or sexual assault compared to all races.[7]

More lesbians and bisexual women experience sexual assault by an intimate partner than straight women do.[8]

More gay and bisexual men experience sexual assault by an intimate partner than straight men do.[8]

U.S. data

Between 2015 and 2018, the rate of rape or sexual assault victimization increased from 1.6 to 2.7 victimizations per 1,000 persons age 12 or older.[3]

The prevalence of false reporting for sexual assault crimes is low—between 2% and 10%.[4]

The estimated lifetime cost of rape is $122,461 per victim.[5]

Figure 12.24 Who is sexually assaulted?

Data reported by the National Sexual Violence Resource Center (n.d.) from:

[1]Smith et al. (2018); [2]Kearl (2018); [3]Morgan and Oudekerk (2019); [4]Lisak et al. (2010); [5]Peterson et al. (2017); from RAINN (n.d.a); [6]Cantor et al. (2015); [7]Perry (2004); from the Human Rights Campaign (n.d.); [8]Black et al. (2011).

were 25 years old (Smith et al. 2017); 40 percent occurred before the age of 18 (Office on Women's Health 2019). Among high school students, 11 percent reported in 2021 being forced to do sexual activities when they did not want to, and American Indian or Alaska Native youth were more likely to experience forced sex (Centers for Disease Control and Prevention 2021l).

How to Recognize and Prevent Sexual Assault

All college students have a responsibility to recognize and prevent sexual assault on their campuses. This can begin by attending educational programs or joining organizations on your campus that focus on preventing sexual assault. So, what exactly is sexual assault? Sexual assault means that there was sexual contact or behavior that occurred without the explicit consent from the person who was sexually assaulted. It includes attempted rape; fondling or unwanted sexual touching; forcing the victim to perform sexual acts, such as oral sex or penetrating the perpetrator's body; and penetration of the victim's body, which is defined as rape (RAINN n.d.a). Rape is defined by the FBI as "the penetration, no matter how slight, of the vagina or anus with any body part or object, or oral pene-

tration by a sex organ of another person, without the consent of the victim" (U.S. Department of Justice 2017).

Force does not have to be physical; it can also be emotional and involve manipulating or intimidating the victim into sexual activity. Explicit, affirmative consent must be obtained before engaging in sexual activity. Silence is not consent. Finally, consent cannot be given when someone is mentally or physically helpless, is under the influence of drugs or alcohol, or is unconscious (RAINN n.d.c).

One example of an organization that helps men understand their role in the prevention of sexual assault is Male Athletes Against Violence. This is an initiative on many college campuses that is focused on educating and involving students in understanding how to recognize and prevent sexual assault. These students take a pledge to be a positive role model, educate others, have the courage to correct the violent behaviors of others, support all victims of sexual assault, and implement strategies to reduce and end sexual violence. In 2014, eight leading national fraternities also joined together to address sexual

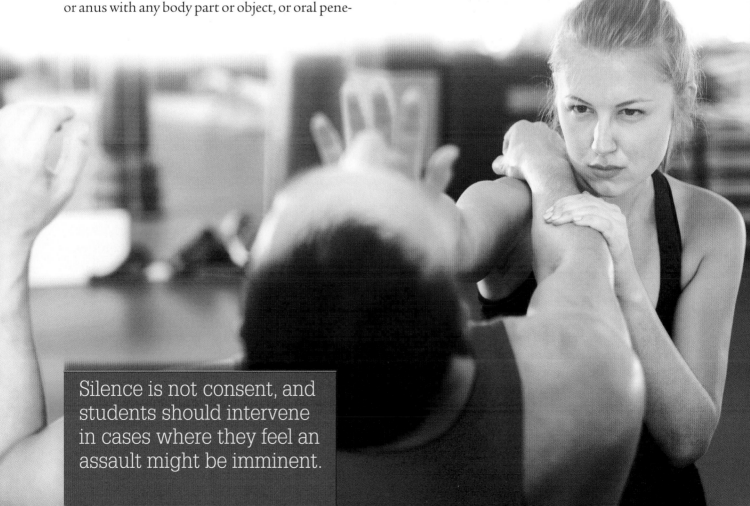

Silence is not consent, and students should intervene in cases where they feel an assault might be imminent.

✓ Behavior Check

Reduce Your Risk of Sexual Assault

Take an active role in reducing sexual assault by incorporating safety strategies. You cannot always prevent sexual assault. However, you can take the following steps to help stay safe in general:

- Go to parties or gatherings with friends. Arrive together, check in with each other, and leave together.

- Look out for your friends and ask them to look out for you. If a friend is acting out of character or seems too drunk to stay safe in general, get them to a safe place.

- Have a code word you can text to your family and friends that means, "Come get me, I need help" or "Call me with a fake emergency." You can also use a hand signal with friends or on a video call (see figure 12.25).

- Download a safety app on your phone. Some apps share your location with your friends or the police if you need help. You can also set up an app to send you texts throughout the night to make sure you're safe. If you don't respond, the app will notify police.

- Avoid drinks in punch bowls or other containers that can be easily spiked with alcohol or drugs. If you think that you or one of your friends has been drugged, call the police. Tell them what happened so that you can be tested for the right drugs.

- Know your limits when using alcohol or drugs. Don't let anyone pressure you into drinking or doing more than you want to.

- Trust your instincts. If you find yourself alone with someone you don't know or trust, leave. If you feel uncomfortable in any situation for any reason, leave.

- Be aware of your surroundings. Especially if you are walking alone, avoid talking on your phone or listening to music with headphones. Stay in busy, well-lit areas (Office on Women's Health 2018).

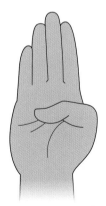 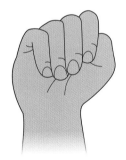

Turn your palm to the camera and tuck your thumb.　　Turn your palm to the camera and tuck your thumb.

Figure 12.25 Sometimes social media can be a positive influence: A hand gesture created and shared on social media by the Canadian Women's Foundation to signal for help without alerting an attacker went viral in 2021. A 16-year-old girl was rescued after she used the gesture to let others know she had been kidnapped (Edwards 2021).

misconduct, hazing, and binge drinking by forming the Fraternal Health and Safety Initiative (Market Wired 2014). The goal of this initiative is to educate fraternity members to make positive and healthy decisions, understand the risks and consequences of their actions, and recognize and intervene during potential harmful situations. It is important for members to participate in educational programs and initiatives on campus that emphasize their roles and responsibilities related to the prevention of sexual assault. Sexual assault is a campus-wide issue that can be solved only when everyone works together toward solutions.

Another campus initiative that may exist on your campus for all students is the It's On Us campaign (www.itsonus.org). The goals of this college-based campaign are to recognize that nonconsensual sex is sexual assault, identify situations in which sexual assault may occur, intervene in situations where consent has not been or cannot be given, and create an environment in which sexual assault is unacceptable and survivors are supported.

Consent

Consent is a clear yes to sexual activity. Just because someone has not said no does not mean they have given consent. Consent means the following:

- You know and understand what is going on (you are not unconscious, blacked out, or otherwise mentally or intellectually impaired).
- You know what you want to do.
- You are able to say what you want to do.
- You are sober (not under the influence of alcohol or drugs).

Sometimes you cannot give legal consent to sexual activity or contact. For example, you cannot consent in any of the following conditions:

- You are threatened, forced, or manipulated into agreeing.
- You are physically unable to (e.g., drunk, high, drugged, passed out, or asleep).
- You are mentally unable to as a result of illness or disability.
- You are under the age of consent (16 in most states, 17 or 18 in others).

Getting Help

If you are in danger or need medical care, call 911. If you can, get away from the person who assaulted you and go to a safe place as fast as you can. After a sexual assault, you may feel fear, shame, guilt, or shock. These feelings are normal. You might be afraid to talk about the assault, but it is important to get help. You can call these organizations at any time, day or night:

- National Sexual Assault Hotline, 800-656-HOPE (4673)
- National Domestic Violence Hotline, 800-799-SAFE (7233) or 800-787-3224 (TTY)

COVID and Sexual Health

The COVID-19 pandemic has affected every aspect of our lives in ways we could have never imagined, including our sexual and reproductive health. It was imperative to learn the ways the virus could be transmitted; because we know that some viruses such as

HIV can be transmitted through semen or vaginal fluids, one of the earliest research studies was to determine whether the COVID-19 virus could be transmitted this way. Although there is no evidence that it can be transmitted through semen or vaginal fluid, the virus was found in the semen of those who were recovering from COVID-19 (Marshall 2021).

Because the pandemic limited personal interactions, additional research was conducted to determine changes in sexual activity and behaviors early in the pandemic. The results of a survey among adults aged 18 to 94 indicated that almost half of the participants reported a decrease in sexual behaviors, mostly as a result of having young children at home, increased depression and loneliness, and not engaging in behaviors that would increase the risk of acquiring COVID-19 (Hensel et al. 2020). Although the results of this study are not surprising given the limitations the participants had in interacting with others, the researchers point out that because sexual health is an important component of overall well-being, public health resources to support this issue should still be made available during a pandemic. Providers who have expertise in sexual health should continue to support positive sexual behaviors and provide recommendations for balancing basic human needs for intimacy with personal safety and pandemic control measures (Turban, Keuroghlian, and Mayer 2021).

Summary

This chapter focuses on how college students can develop and sustain a sexually healthy lifestyle. In order to be sexually healthy, you must understand your own reproductive anatomy and physiology, as well as that of others. Knowing more about how your body works allows you to become aware of how your body matures, changes, and develops over your lifetime. This information can prepare you for preventing or planning to have a child. A variety of methods are available for sexually active people to reduce the chances of an unintended pregnancy and plan for the future. When used consistently and correctly, these methods are very reliable.

Being sexually healthy also means learning more about the risks associated with sexually transmitted infections. Keep in mind that some STIs cannot be cured and could be fatal. Knowing

⊕ Immunity Booster

How STIs Affect the Immune System

It is important to protect yourself from sexually transmitted infections, specifically HIV, which attacks the immune system and reduces the body's ability to defend itself against other illnesses. We are still learning more about the comorbidities that impact how COVID-19 reacts in the body, so do all you can to prevent exposure to all types of infections.

your partner's sexual health history and practicing safe sex (e.g., using an external or internal condom) can reduce your chances of acquiring a sexually transmitted infection. Before you become sexually active, take time to consider how you might sustain a healthy sexuality. If you are currently sexually active, think about how you can discuss sexual health issues with your partner, share how you plan to prevent STIs, and consider how you can plan for children in the future.

Finally, preventing sexual assault must be a collective effort among all college students. Make a commitment to learn how to prevent sexual assault, educate others, and stand up against these violent behaviors. Prioritizing your sexual health can help you develop positive and respectful relationships, reduce your chances of negative physical and emotional health outcomes, plan pregnancies, and enjoy sex.

ⓦⓦⓦ ONLINE LEARNING ACTIVITIES

Go to HK*Propel* and complete all of the online activities to further facilitate your learning:

Study Activities: Review the main concepts of the chapter.

Labs: Complete the labs your instructor assigns.

Videos: Look through the videos and choose which ones you want to try this week.

REVIEW QUESTIONS

1. How does conception happen?
2. What are examples of barrier birth control methods?
3. What are examples of hormonal birth control methods?
4. Which birth control methods have the highest rate of preventing pregnancy with typical use?
5. Which birth control methods also protect against STIs?
6. What are the symptoms of chlamydia, gonorrhea, and syphilis?
7. What are the symptoms of HPV and HSV?
8. Which STIs can be cured?
9. Which STIs can be treated but not cured?
10. What is PID?
11. What are some ways you can help prevent sexual assault?
12. What is consent?

Reducing the Risks for Metabolic Syndrome

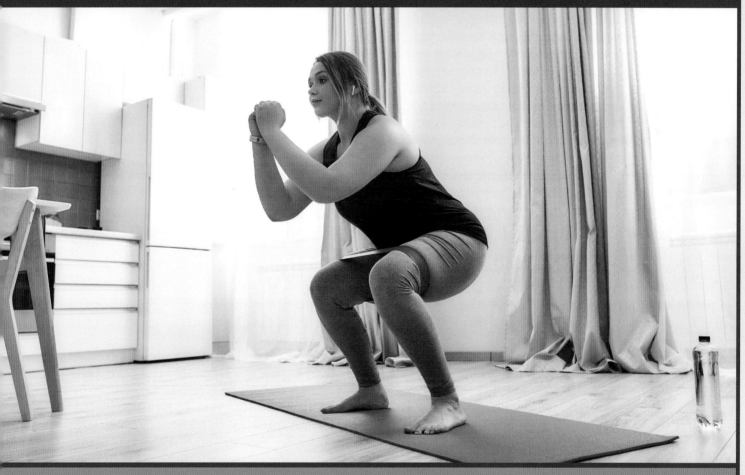

OBJECTIVES

- Define metabolic syndrome and understand the risk factors for it.
- Appreciate that metabolic syndrome increases the risk for other chronic diseases, including type 2 diabetes and cardiovascular disease.
- Understand that healthy dietary and physical activity habits can reduce the risk for type 2 diabetes.
- Know the main cardiovascular diseases, the risk factors for them, and strategies for protecting yourself from these diseases.
- Recognize that preventing metabolic syndrome early in life can decrease your risk of cardiovascular disease as you age.

KEY TERMS

angina

arrhythmias

arteriosclerosis

atherosclerosis

cardiovascular disease (CVD)

cholesterol

chronic diseases

chronic systemic inflammation

coronary heart disease (CHD)

C-reactive protein (CRP)

diabetes

endothelium

gestational diabetes

heart failure

hemorrhagic stroke

high-density lipoprotein cholesterol (HDL-C)

hypercholesterolemia

hyperglycemia

hyperlipidemia

hypertension

ischemic stroke

low-density lipoprotein cholesterol (LDL-C)

metabolic syndrome (MetS)

myocardial infarction (heart attack)

pathophysiology

peripheral arterial disease (PAD)

prediabetes

stroke

triglycerides

type 1 diabetes

type 2 diabetes (T2D)

Do you know someone who has diabetes or has suffered a heart attack? Although these health conditions typically occur in middle-aged or older adults, the disease process begins earlier in life than you may realize. Your genetics, weight status, and current health behaviors, especially your dietary and physical activity habits, can greatly influence your health later in life. This chapter introduces you to metabolic syndrome, and, relatedly, type 2 diabetes and cardiovascular disease, their risk factors, and how you can reduce your risk, especially with regular physical activity.

Are You at Risk for Metabolic Syndrome?

Many young adults are at risk for developing metabolic syndrome (MetS) because of overweight and obesity. If you have been or are one day diagnosed with MetS, think of it as a wake-up call to reassess your health status and behaviors. However, also be confident that you can get back on track.

Definition and Diagnosis

Metabolic syndrome (MetS) can be thought of as a clustering of biological factors that raise your risk for other chronic conditions, especially diabetes and cardiovascular disease. Recall that the term *metabolic* refers to your biochemical processes and energy production systems. A syndrome is a set of signs and symptoms related to each other or occurring simultaneously. A risk factor is a trait, condition, or habit that increases your risk of developing a disease.

Although the cause of MetS and its components are complex, it is well established that central obesity is a key factor (International Diabetes Federation 2006). To be diagnosed with MetS, a person must have central obesity (defined by a high waist circumference based on ethnicity-specific values) plus two of the four other factors, listed as follows:

High Waist Circumference

- Males: ≥94 centimeters (37 in.)
- Females: ≥80 centimeters (31.4 in.)

Other Factors (Any Two)

- Elevated triglycerides: ≥150 mg/dL or using medication for this condition
- Low HDL cholesterol: <40 mg/dL for females, <50 mg/dL for males, or using medication for this condition

- Elevated blood pressure: Systolic ≥130 mmHg, diastolic ≥85 mmHg, diagnosed with hypertension, or using medication to control it

- Elevated fasting blood glucose: ≥100 mg/dL, diagnosed with type 2 diabetes, or using medication to control it

Why Do We Care About MetS?

Being diagnosed with MetS is not the critical issue. We care about MetS because if you have several metabolic risk factors, your chances of developing one of the metabolic big three increases substantially. A person who has MetS has at least a fivefold greater risk of developing type 2 diabetes (T2D), one of the worldwide major causes of premature illness and death. Critically, T2D increases the risk of cardiovascular disease (CVD), which is responsible for over 80 percent of all deaths. Thus, MetS and T2D are currently driving the CVD epidemic (International Diabetes Federation 2006). Finally, much emerging research also supports a link between MetS and several types of cancer (Stocks et al. 2015). If you want to avoid the metabolic big three, you need to avoid MetS. This means that, first and foremost, you need to learn personal strategies for managing your waistline.

Your Traits, Conditions, and Habits = Risk of MetS

The risk for MetS involves a complex mix of genetic factors, certain conditions, and personal

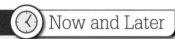
Now and Later

MetS Can Lead to the Metabolic Big Three

Now

Do you think that heart attacks, diabetes, and cancer happen only to older adults? Do you ever rationalize putting off exercise or eating foods that are not "heart smart" with the thought that you'll have more time to take care of your health later? In fact, the risk for these primary causes of death begins much earlier in life than is often recognized and is frequently linked to MetS. Due to our poor dietary behaviors and our physically inactive lifestyles, approximately 10 percent of young adults and over one-third of the adult population have MetS (Moore, Chaudhary, and Akinyemiju 2017). Do you know anyone your age who has been diagnosed with MetS? You or some of your friends may have it and not even know it.

Later

Body composition often changes (e.g., abdominal fat increases) and physical activity is typically reduced as part of the aging process. Therefore, the rates for MetS increase even more with age. For example, approximately 50 percent of middle-aged adults in the United States have MetS, and the rates climb to nearly 65 percent for U.S. adults over age 70 (Moore, Chaudhary, and Akinyemiju 2017). MetS rates are predicted to reach 25 percent of the world's population in future decades (International Diabetes Federation 2006). When people are lean and highly physically active, their chance of having MetS is drastically reduced to nearly zero. MetS is another example of how our genetics unfavorably interact with our environment.

Take Home

Take steps now to know your risk factors for MetS. Invest in your health, and make lifestyle changes to reduce your risk factors for MetS and other chronic conditions, especially the metabolic big three.

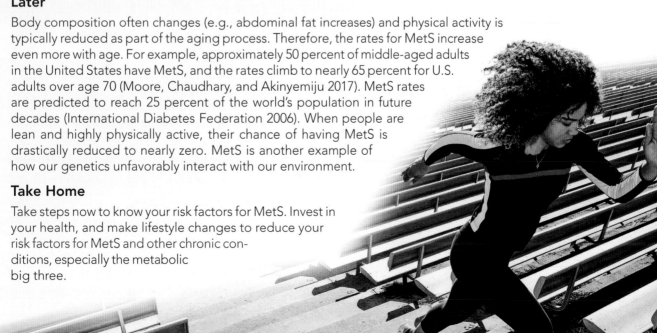

habits. For example, if your family tree includes many people with MetS, your risk increases. However, if you eat a relatively balanced diet, engage in regular physical activity and exercise, and manage your weight, you will go a long way toward preventing MetS. These key health choices also help you lower **chronic systemic inflammation**.

Chronic Inflammation: A Flame for Chronic Diseases

Chronic diseases such as T2D are designated as such because they are lifelong or recurrent, unlike communicable diseases such as the flu. Rather, chronic diseases are caused by the interaction between our genes, our environment, and our health behaviors. Nearly everyone who gets diagnosed with a chronic disease develops a subclinical version of the disease first. *Subclinical* means undetectable or not meeting the criteria. Thus, there may not be any signs and symptoms, but the **pathophysiology** associated with the disease is present, often many years prior to diagnosis. A low-level chronic systemic inflammation is often related to this subclinical disease state.

Cellular Inflammation Basics

If you have ever scraped your knee, sprained your ankle, or had strep throat, you have probably become aware of acute inflammation. White blood cells travel to the scene to destroy bacteria and the immune process repairs your tissues. This healing process is termed the *inflammatory response* and is one of the body's most basic survival mechanisms. Typically, this response stays local and then resolves after the injury or infection heals, which you recognize when the pain and swelling go away. However, sometimes the system does not shut off and inflammatory-promoting compounds spread throughout the body, damaging cells and tissues. In this case, our defense mechanisms have turned against us. This low-level systemic inflammation can simmer for years, contributing to a range of chronic conditions, including T2D, CVD, and some cancers (Libby, Ridker, and Hansson 2009). Understanding the role that inflammation plays in your risk for chronic disease is important. Even more critical is the need to recognize how your health behavior choices influence your levels of inflammation.

Detection of Chronic Inflammation

To detect this silent inflammation, physicians might measure levels of **C-reactive protein (CRP)** or other markers in the blood. If the levels are elevated, they will conduct additional testing to determine what is triggering the inflammation and then pursue treatment. Inflammation is a key factor in almost all chronic degenerative and lifestyle diseases, especially vascular diseases such as atherosclerosis (Roitman and LaFontaine 2012). Obesity (especially abdominal obesity), diet quality, physical activity or exercise, physical fitness, and smoking are key factors associated with this stealthy condition. See figure 13.1 and ask yourself if you might be igniting your inflammatory flame.

Evaluating Your Risk for Type 2 Diabetes

Diabetes is a chronic disease that occurs when the pancreas cannot make the hormone insulin or when the insulin the body produces does not work very well (American Diabetes Association n.d.a). All carbohydrate foods are broken down and released as glucose into the blood. Insulin helps glucose get into the cells and produce energy. When insulin is not available or cannot be used effectively, glucose cannot enter cells; thus, glucose begins to build up in the blood. This condition is called **hyperglycemia** (high blood sugar). If these high-glucose conditions continue for long periods of time, tissues and organs get damaged. The following is a list of primary conditions that often occur with long-term diabetes if it is not well controlled with diet, exercise, or medication:

> Keeping your blood sugar under control not only helps prevent diabetes but also reduces the risk for many other chronic health conditions.

- *Cardiovascular disease (CVD).* High blood glucose is linked to artery vessel damage, which accelerates risk for cardiovascular disease.
- *Eye complications.* Many eye conditions that increase in prevalence with age (such as glaucoma) are also increased in people with diabetes.

Inflammation Fuels Chronic Disease

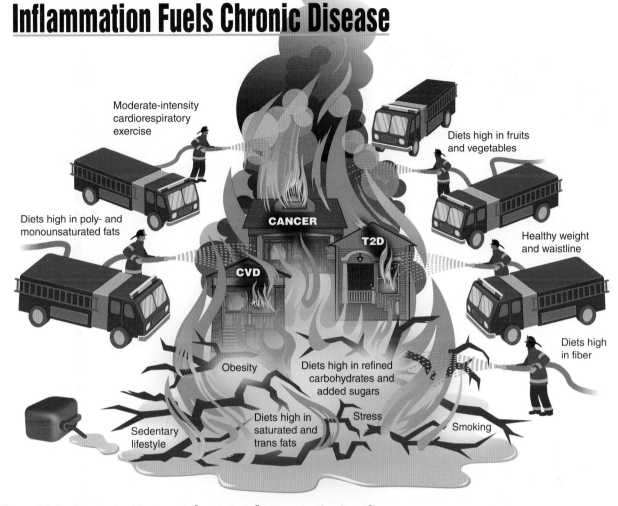

Figure 13.1   Are you igniting your inflammatory flame or putting it out?

- *Kidney disease.* Kidneys are large filters with millions of tiny blood vessels. Because small blood vessels are more likely to be damaged with high blood glucose, kidney failure is common in people with diabetes.
- *Neuropathy.* Nerves become damaged, resulting in loss of feeling and often pain.
- *Skin changes.* People with diabetes often have more bacterial and fungal infections and itchy skin.

If possible, it is best to avoid diabetes. But if you have diabetes, good blood sugar control is essential for preventing numerous other chronic conditions, many of which can be fatal, such as CVD.

Types and Definitions

Two main types of diabetes exist. First, **type 1 diabetes**, which affects only about 5 percent of people with diabetes, is caused by the body's inability to produce insulin. Your health behaviors are mainly linked to the most common type of diabetes, **type 2 diabetes (T2D)**, which is primarily caused by insulin resistance. A less common and very specific type of diabetes is **gestational diabetes**, which develops during pregnancy as a result of multiple factors, including pregnancy-related hormones and insulin resistance. Insulin resistance means that the body's tissues, especially the muscles, become less receptive to the action of insulin. In response, the pancreas must work harder and create more insulin to maintain blood glucose in the normal range. Over time, the pancreas becomes exhausted and is unable to manage blood sugar levels, so blood sugar begins to rise (Centers for Disease Control and Prevention 2022a).

Note that there is also a **prediabetes** category related to T2D, which is when a person has a level of elevated glucose that is above normal but has not yet reached the level clinically defined as diabetic. This is important because prediabetes almost always precedes T2D; relatedly, prediabetes starts with insulin resistance. In fact, more than one-third of the population has prediabetes, and most of those people have no idea they have it. Like MetS, prediabetes also increases your risk for T2D and CVD (Centers for Disease Control and Prevention 2022b). The good news is that prediabetes can be reversed!

Diagnosis

All types of diabetes are diagnosed with blood tests using several well-established clinical techniques (American Diabetes Association n.d.b). When reviewing table 13.1, notice how the normal, prediabetes, and diabetes categories are ranked in order of increasing A1C, or blood glucose levels.

Symptoms and Risk Factors for Prediabetes

Like MetS, prediabetes should be a wake-up call to make some changes in your lifestyle so you can prevent the progression to T2D. There are no symptoms of prediabetes or T2D until the disease becomes advanced. If you have several of the following risk factors, you are advised to consult your physician (Centers for Disease Control and Prevention 2022b).

- Age: Being age 45 or older
- Family history: Having a parent or sibling with T2D
- Race or ethnicity: Being African American, Hispanic or Latino American, American Indian, Pacific Islander, or Asian American
- Overweight: Having a high BMI and a high waist circumference
- Physical activity: Being physically active fewer than three times per week
- Gestational diabetes: Being diagnosed with gestational diabetes or having a baby who weighs more than nine pounds at birth

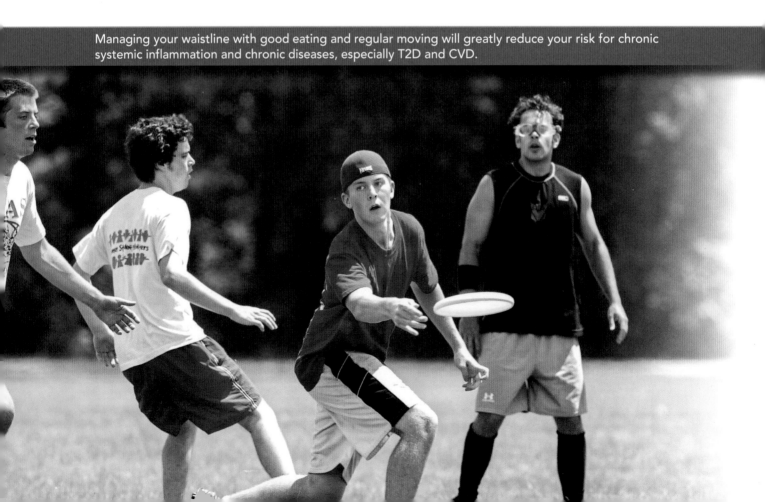

Managing your waistline with good eating and regular moving will greatly reduce your risk for chronic systemic inflammation and chronic diseases, especially T2D and CVD.

Table 13.1 Common Clinical Tests for Diabetes

Test	Description	Normal	Prediabetes	Diabetes
A1C	• A marker that measures your average blood glucose for the past two to three months • Does not require you to fast or drink anything	<5.7%	5.7%-6.5%	≥6.5%
Fasting plasma glucose (FPG)	• Tests your fasting glucose • Requires you to fast at least 8 hours (typically completed in the morning before breakfast)	<100 mg/dL	100-126 mg/dL	≥126 mg/dL
Oral glucose challenge test (OGTT)	• Tests how your body handles a glucose load • Requires you to fast, then drink a glucose beverage and have your blood retested two hours later	<140 mg/dL	140-200 mg/dL	≥200 mg/dL

- Polycystic ovary syndrome: Being diagnosed with this hormonal disorder characterized by higher-than-normal levels of androgens, which cause enlarged ovaries and lead to infertility and insulin resistance

Treatment Options

Treatment options for prediabetes and T2D center around lifestyle changes and medication.

- *Weight loss.* If a person has prediabetes and is overweight, losing a small amount of weight can greatly reduce the progression to T2D. This can be as little as 5 percent of body weight. For a 200-pound (91 kg) person, that means losing 10 to 14 pounds (4.5 to 6.4 kg) (Centers for Disease Control and Prevention 2022b).

- *Regular physical activity.* Meeting the HHS Physical Activity Guidelines can greatly reduce the risk of prediabetes in general and the progression to T2D, specifically. Repeated muscle contraction increases the action of insulin that helps move blood glucose into cells, thereby lowering blood glucose.

- *Diet quality.* In addition to reducing caloric intake to cause weight loss, improving diet quality can help manage blood glucose. Be sure to limit added sugars and refined carbohydrates.

- *Medications.* If a person does not adhere to lifestyle changes or if the condition has progressed too far, oral medications or injectable insulin may be needed to control blood sugar.

Prevent and Manage T2D With Quality Resources

You have likely heard that an ounce of prevention is worth a pound of cure. This is absolutely true for your blood glucose management and the prevention of MetS, prediabetes, and T2D (figure 13.3). Unfortunately, if you are genetically predisposed to be at high risk for hyperglycemia, you will need to be extra vigilant about your diet quality, physical activity, and waistline. Most adults diagnosed with T2D will have to manage this disease for the rest of their lives. If you are at high risk for diabetes, keeping your blood glucose in the healthy range is critical for preventing comorbidities later in life. An excellent resource for more information about T2D is the American Diabetes Association (www.diabetes.org).

✓ Behavior Check

Preventing Insulin Resistance Is the Key to Preventing T2D

You may recall the basics of how insulin works from other classes such as biology or physiology. Essentially, insulin works like a key to open the receptor lock on the cell. It unlocks the door to let glucose into cells, removing glucose from the blood and preventing high blood sugar (see figure 13.2). When the key does not fit well in the lock and work like it should (quickly and easily!), this is termed insulin resistance (i.e., the cells are resistant to the action of insulin). The pancreas then must work harder to produce more insulin to clear the glucose from the bloodstream, setting the course for prediabetes and T2D.

Recent data indicates that about 40 percent of adults aged 18 to 44 in the United States are insulin resistant (Parcha et al. 2022). In this nondiabetic population, being insulin resistant was associated with having high blood pressure and unhealthy cholesterol levels. Importantly, although also linked to obesity, nearly half of the young adults with insulin resistance *were not obese*. Behaviorally, poor physical activity levels were linked to insulin resistance.

The take-home point is that youth does not protect you from starting the disease process of T2D. It is important to fuel with quality foods and move often to prevent insulin resistance, prediabetes, and ultimately T2D. Are your eating and moving habits keeping your insulin-receptor "lock and key" combos working well?

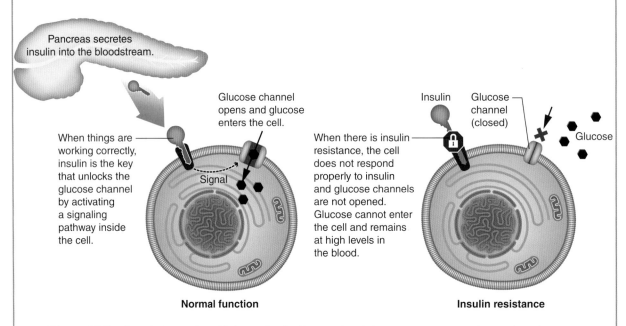

Figure 13.2   Regularly moving, high-quality fueling, and weight management are key to keeping your cell's lock-and-key combination in good working order, helping you avoid MetS.

Cardiovascular Disease: Our Number One Killer

Cardiovascular disease (CVD)—specifically **coronary heart disease (CHD)**, also known as coronary artery disease (CAD)—is the leading cause of death in the United States and has been for the past several decades (Centers for Disease Control and Prevention 2023a). Over 50 percent of young adults (18-24 years) have at least one risk factor for CHD and almost 25 percent have evidence of atherosclerosis (i.e., plaque buildup) in their arteries. Notably, the extent of the atherosclerosis is directly related with the number of risk factors (Arts, Fernandez, and Lofgren 2014). Therefore, to reduce your chances of developing CVD later in life, you should examine your lifestyle factors now, along with your genetics and family history.

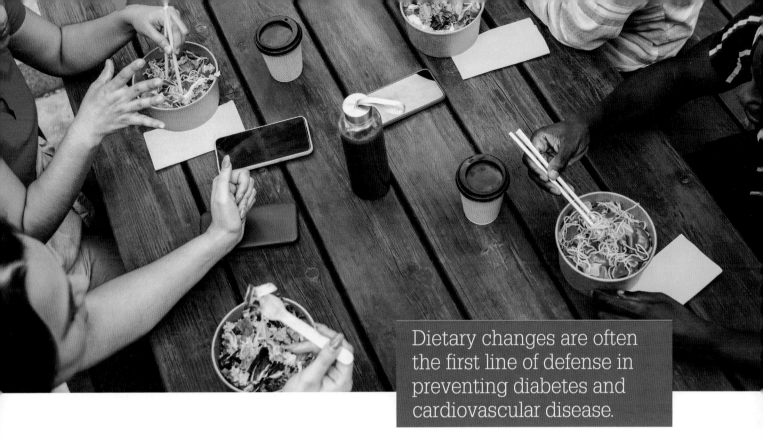

Dietary changes are often the first line of defense in preventing diabetes and cardiovascular disease.

Will You Get Type 2 Diabetes?

Weight and waist line

Exercise and physical activity

Genetics

Physical Activity: Being physically active less than 3 times per week.

Family history: Having a parent or sibling with T2D.

Age: Being 45 years or older.

Overweight: Having a high BMI (and also a high waist circumference).

Gestational diabetes: Being diagnosed with gestational diabetes or having a baby greater than 9 pounds.

?

Polycystic Ovary Syndrome: A hormonal disorder characterized by higher than normal levels of androgens, which causes enlarged ovaries and leads to infertility and insulin resistance.

Race/ethnicity: African Americans, Hispanic/Latino Americans, American Indians, Pacific Islanders, and some Asian Americans are at higher risk.

Figure 13.3 Progression from being metabolically healthy to MetS to prediabetes to T2D involves a complex mix of your genetics, physical activity habits, and how well you manage your waistline.

Evaluating your personal risk for CVD, including talking to your parents and family members about your family history, is a critical first step toward the prevention of CVD.

Major Forms of Cardiovascular Disease: Definitions and Diagnosis

Cardiovascular disease (CVD) is defined as a variety of conditions that can prevent the heart from circulating blood and oxygen throughout the body. Without blood flow, and hence oxygen delivery, cells and tissues die. Although most situations occur in the heart itself, which is why many people refer to CVD as *heart disease*, blood-flow problems can occur all over the body. Major sites of concern are the neck, brain, and large arteries in the arms, abdomen, and legs. Although blood flow can be reduced by **arrhythmias** (abnormal rhythms of the heart) or heart valve problems, the majority of CVD is caused by **atherosclerosis**, which is when plaque builds up on the walls of arteries, reducing blood flow (figure 13.4). The plaque causes the arteries to become narrower, preventing optimal blood flow to all tissues downstream. Most heart attacks and strokes are caused by a plaque rupture or a blood clot that gets caught in the narrowed artery, subsequently preventing blood from flowing.

Another factor that alters the work of the heart and cardiovascular system is **arteriosclerosis**, more commonly known as hardening of the arteries. Arteriosclerosis is a condition where the walls of the arteries are thickened and hardened, which reduces blood flow to organs and tissues. Arteriosclerosis is related to atherosclerosis and also typically occurs as part of the aging process.

Atherosclerotic Heart Disease: The Heart Attack

When the atherosclerosis process progresses in the arteries of the heart and the artery becomes very narrow, a ruptured plaque or a blood clot often completely blocks a heart artery and stops blood flow. This is called a **myocardial infarction**, more commonly known as a heart attack. A heart attack most often occurs when the heart tissue supplied by the blocked artery begins to die. Because various arteries deliver oxygen-rich blood to different parts of the heart, where the clot occurs has major implications for survival and recovery. Sometimes people will refer to a "mild" or "massive" heart attack to describe the extent of the damage based on the size of the vessel and the chamber of the heart it supplies. Know the common signs of a heart attack and act quickly.

CHD can be completely silent, with no symptoms, or it might present with **angina** (chest pain), especially under conditions of higher oxygen demand for the heart when heart rate and blood pressure increase, such as during exercise or emotional distress (e.g., anger or anxiety). Sometimes CHD is suspected when routine activities start to cause breathlessness and chest heaviness. A physician might have a person complete a graded exercise stress test by walking on a treadmill, which increases the speed and grade to increase demand on the heart. During this physical challenge, the patient is monitored for arrhythmias, heart rate, blood pressure, and any other signs and symptoms like chest pain. Medical imaging techniques are often used to determine if there are blood-flow issues caused by blocked arteries or value abnormalities.

Stroke

Stroke is the fifth leading cause of death in the United States (Centers for Disease Control and Prevention 2023a) and a leading cause of disability. Strokes can be caused by a blood vessel bursting (**hemorrhagic stroke**), but the great majority of strokes are caused by a clot (**ischemic stroke**). The latter type of stroke is very similar to a heart attack, but the clot occurs in the brain rather than the heart, depriving brain cells of blood and oxygen. If blood flow is restored quickly, some of the brain cells may only be injured and over time can repair in response to therapy, which allows speech, memory, and body movement and functioning to improve. Unfortunately, stroke is the leading cause of disability in middle-aged and older adults. The good news is that, like CHD, the great majority of strokes are preventable. The number one cause of stroke is high blood pressure, or hypertension (American Stroke Association 2021), which is a risk factor you can control.

Peripheral Artery Disease (PAD)

Peripheral arterial disease (PAD), sometimes referred to as *peripheral vascular disease*, is a lesser-known form of CVD. It is often caused by a process of atherosclerosis like CHD and stroke. PAD is the narrowing of the peripheral arteries, which reduces blood flow and oxygen delivery; it occurs mainly in major vessels of the legs where

Progression of Plaque Buildup

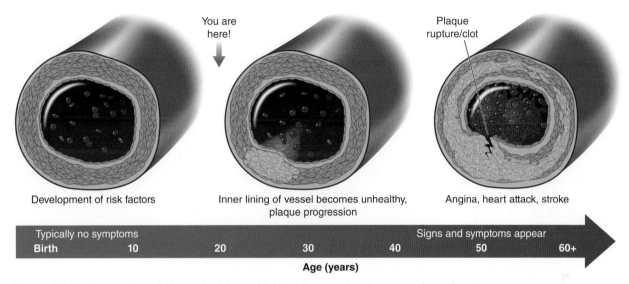

Figure 13.4 Progression of plaque buildup, which leads to angina, heart attack, and stroke.

symptoms are noticed. When we walk, our leg muscles have greater need for oxygen and hence blood flow. Classic symptoms of PAD include cramping, pain, or tiredness in the legs when walking that subsides with rest. Over and above the reduction in physical function and pain that occurs with this condition, the presence of PAD also increases the risk for CHD and stroke. Early detection is key to prevent leg or foot amputation, a heart attack, or a stroke (American Heart Association n.d.a).

Heart Failure

Heart failure occurs when the heart muscle has been permanently damaged, typically because of atherosclerosis, a heart attack, chronic uncontrolled high blood pressure, birth defects, or other less common factors. Heart failure does not mean that the heart stops beating; rather, pumping action is impaired and can greatly limit the amount of physical activity or exercise a person can perform, including basic activities around the house. When the heart rate and contraction force is compromised to a certain degree, fluids can start to back up in the lungs or in the lower legs, which can make breathing or walking very difficult. In addition to a heart-healthy lifestyle, this condition requires medications to help the heart pump effectively and control the fluid. Unfortu-

nately, people with heart failure have a high level of disability and a greatly shortened life span.

Address Risk Factors to Prevent Future Disease

Several factors can increase your risk for CVD in general and CHD and heart attack specifically. These can be categorized into major risk factors that you cannot change, behaviors that you can change, and conditions that are *related to your behaviors* that you can manage. Check out tables 13.2 and 13.3 to get an overview of these factors. Essentially, the more risk factors you have and the greater the level of each risk factor, the higher chance of a future heart attack. You will explore your personal risk factors for cardiometabolic diseases in the chapter 13 labs on HK*Propel*. Because the presence of a strong family history (a risk factor in itself) will mean you need to work harder to prevent these chronic diseases as you age, the labs will involve exploring your genetic family tree for risk factors and known diseases, including T2D and CVD.

> Preventing CVD begins with knowing your personal CVD risk factors, especially the ones that are under your control. Know your numbers!

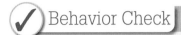 Behavior Check

Automatic External Defibrillator (AED)

Defibrillators can save lives by restoring a normal heart rhythm, especially after a heart attack. They are found in schools, airports, fitness centers, and public buildings. Do you see any AEDs on campus? The American Red Cross and the American Heart Association offer courses on how to use AEDs. We recommend becoming trained so you can save a life.

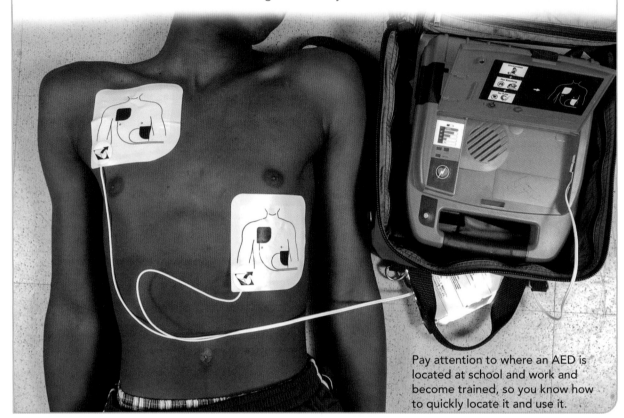

Pay attention to where an AED is located at school and work and become trained, so you know how to quickly locate it and use it.

Detecting Strokes

Strokes can be very evident or hard to detect (see figure 13.5). The American Stroke Association uses an acronym of FAST:

Face drooping. Does one side of the face droop or is it numb? Ask the person to smile and check to see if the face is uneven or lopsided.

Arm weakness. Is one arm weak or numb? Ask the person to raise both arms and check to see if one arm drifts downward.

Speech difficulty. Is speech slurred? Is the person unable to speak or hard to understand? Ask the person to repeat a simple sentence like "The sky is blue" and determine if the words are correctly repeated.

Time. If the preceding symptoms are present, even if they appear to be going away, call 911 to get help. Time is of the essence: The sooner the treatment can be started, the less permanent damage will occur to the brain cells. Also note the time you think the symptoms started so you can inform the emergency responders.

Warning Signs of Heart Attack and Stroke

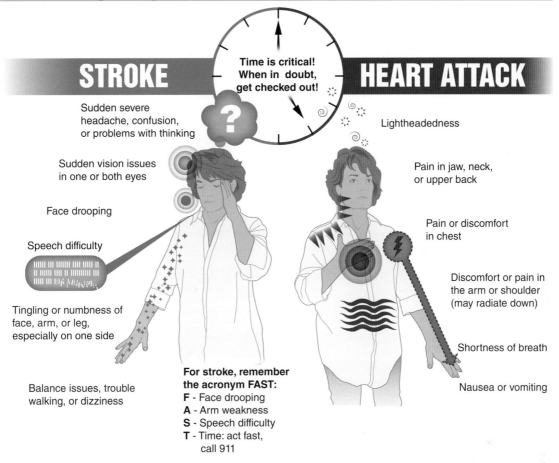

Figure 13.5   Know the warning signs of a heart attack and stroke. If you suspect someone is experiencing any of these symptoms, call 911 immediately. Minutes may prevent disability and save lives!

Additional clues might be remembered as STROKE:

Speech. Trouble speaking or understanding speech.

Tingling. Sudden numbness or weakness of face, arm, or leg, especially on one side.

Remember. Sudden confusion and problems with thinking.

Off balance. Trouble walking, dizziness, or loss of balance or coordination.

Killer headache. Sudden severe headache with no known cause.

Eyes. Sudden trouble seeing in one or both eyes.

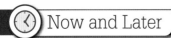 Now and Later

Heart-Healthy Behaviors

Now

The atherosclerosis process begins very early in life. By making good behavior choices now, you can prevent plaque buildup that might cause a heart attack or stroke later in your life. Understanding your risk factors related to your genetics is also important. Having candid conversations with parents and grandparents about their health can help you understand your personal risk of CVD. Finally, getting regular medical checkups is key. Most checkups provide a screening for CVD by assessing weight, blood pressure, and your blood lipid profile.

Later

Once you have graduated, try to keep a regular schedule for medical checkups. Adherence to a heart-healthy lifestyle can often become challenging as your life gets more complicated with employment, families, hobbies, and friends. Remember that healthy habits will make you feel great in the short term and can also increase your chances of having a long and disability-free life.

Take Home

Atherosclerosis, the major cause of CVD, begins early in life and is greatly influenced by your health behaviors. CVD can largely be prevented. If detected early, it can be treated to avoid a severe cardiovascular event such as a heart attack or stroke. Taking care of your arteries now can save your life later. Be heart smart!

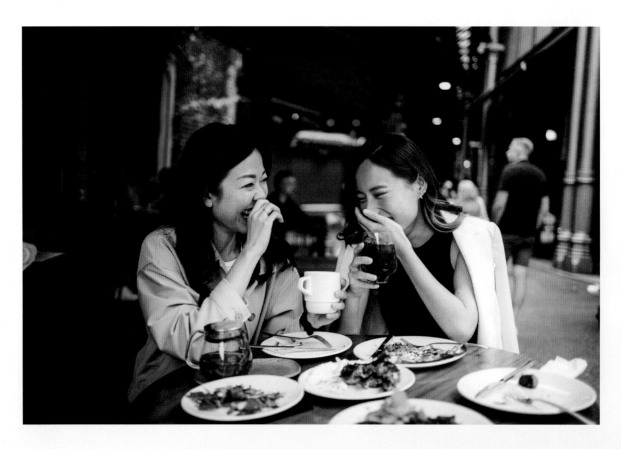

Table 13.2   Nonmodifiable Risk Factors for Coronary Heart Disease and Heart Attack

Factors you cannot change	
Age	Risk increases with age, with the majority of heart attacks occurring in older adults (over the age of 65).
Biological sex	Males have a greater risk of CVD and CHD compared to females, and they have heart attacks at an earlier age than females do.
Family history	Risk increases from genetic factors or shared environments and lifestyles if you have a parent or sibling who developed CVD or CHD.
Race or ethnicity	African Americans and non-Hispanic Blacks are at a greater risk than whites and non-Hispanic whites. Rates among Hispanics, American Indians, native Hawaiians, and some Asian Americans are also higher than among whites.

Adapted from "Heart Disease: Know Your Risk for Heart Disease," Centers for Disease Control and Prevention, last modified March 21, 2023, www.cdc.gov/heartdisease/risk_factors.htm.

Table 13.3   Modifiable Risk Factors for Coronary Heart Disease and Heart Attack

Factors you can manage over time (with behavior and medications)	Factors you can manage today (with lifestyle choices)
Overweight and obesity (see chapter 9)	Diet quality and alcohol (see chapter 8)
MetS, prediabetes, and type 2 diabetes (see previous text in this chapter)	Smoking (see chapters 11 and 14)
High blood pressure (see following section)	Stress (see chapter 10)
High cholesterol (see following section)	Exercise, physical activity, and fitness (see chapter 4)

Adapted from "Heart Disease: Know Your Risk for Heart Disease," Centers for Disease Control and Prevention, last modified March 21, 2023, www.cdc.gov/heartdisease/risk_factors.htm.

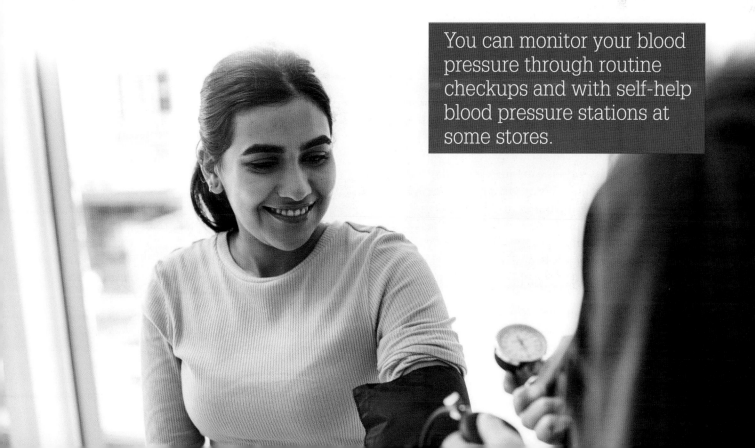

You can monitor your blood pressure through routine checkups and with self-help blood pressure stations at some stores.

Immunity Booster

The Impact of T2D and CVD on COVID-19

As described in chapter 9, being obese and physically inactive have negative implications for immune function. COVID-19, currently the greatest acute challenge to our collective immune function, serves as an important example. Baseline health status can influence a person's experience with COVID-19, including their likelihood of getting the virus, severity of illness, residual effects (e.g., long COVID), and effectiveness of the vaccine.

The Centers for Disease Control and Prevention (2023c) urges people with T2D, CVD, CHD, and especially heart failure to take extra precautions to prevent COVID-19. Although it currently appears that having T2D, CVD, or CHD (or other heart diseases plus high blood pressure) does not increase the likelihood of getting the virus, it does increase the risk that a person could get very sick from COVID-19. This is yet another reason to invest in your health behaviors now to prevent these common chronic diseases during your middle and older years. By fueling with high-quality food, maintaining a regular physical activity program, managing your weight and waistline, and not smoking, you are also reducing your risks of viruses, especially COVID-19.

Chronic Conditions to Be Managed

Several of the risk factors that you can manage with your daily lifestyle choices are discussed in other chapters (cardiorespiratory fitness, nutrition, weight management, stress, and smoking) or previously in this chapter (MetS, T2D). These factors often coexist with the other risk factors of high blood pressure and an unhealthy blood lipid profile. When high blood pressure or blood lipid profile cannot be managed with lifestyle changes alone, these conditions are often treated with prescription medications.

High Blood Pressure

Blood pressure (BP) is the pressure exerted against the arteries during heart contraction (systolic blood pressure; the first number) and relaxation (diastolic blood pressure; the second number). **Hypertension** is the medical term to describe chronically elevated resting blood pressure. Chronic high blood pressure increases the heart's workload with each beat and causes the heart muscle to adapt in an unhealthy manner, contributing to many forms of heart disease, including risk for a heart attack. Hypertension can also greatly increase the risk of a stroke. Hypertension can be completely silent, even if it is severe. Thus, it is important to monitor your resting blood pressure on at least an annual basis. Getting your blood pressure monitored is a quick, simple, painless procedure that is included in routine visits to the doctor as a vital sign. Blood pressure machines are also conveniently located in grocery stores with clinics, at pharmacies, and often at worksites. Remember that your target is to keep your resting blood pressure at or below normal range, which is below 120/80 mmHg (American Stroke Association 2021; Centers for Disease Control and Prevention 2021b):

- Normal: Systolic BP <120 mmHg *and* diastolic BP <80 mmHg
- Elevated: Systolic BP 120 to 129 mmHg *and* diastolic BP <80 mmHg
- Hypertension (or high blood pressure): Systolic BP ≥130 mmHg *or* diastolic ≥BP 80 mmHg

Hypertension can be caused by genetics, certain medications, or lifestyle behaviors. For most college students, the latter is generally the cause. You can help prevent hypertension by making healthy lifestyle choices in the following areas:

- *Physical activity and exercise.* Beyond weight management, regular activity is effective for reducing the risk for hypertension, especially moderate- to vigorous-intensity cardiorespiratory exercise. Adhering to the HHS Physical Activity Guidelines by obtaining at least 150 minutes of physical activity per week is very important.
- *Not smoking or vaping.* The chemicals in tobacco and vape nicotine increase blood pressure. If you smoke or vape, make every attempt to quit. If you don't smoke or vape, do not start.

- *Weight management.* Maintaining a healthy weight and keeping your waistline in check is very important for managing blood pressure.
- *Diet quality.* Over and above managing your diet to help manage your weight, high-quality dietary fuel reduces your risk for hypertension. This involves consuming a variety of fruits and vegetables, choosing low-fat dairy products, reducing the amount of sodium in your diet, and moderating your alcohol consumption. DASH (Dietary Approaches to Stop Hypertension) is a popular and well-researched diet that reinforces many of the healthy dietary strategies discussed in chapter 8 (see www.dashdiet.org).
- *Stress.* Chronic stress can increase risk for hypertension. Managing your stress, including getting high-quality sleep, is important for managing your blood pressure.

If you are diagnosed with hypertension, in addition to the lifestyle changes just described, your doctor will prescribe one or more medications to keep your blood pressure in the normal range.

High Cholesterol

Your body requires some blood **cholesterol** (a waxy, fatlike substance) in order to function. However, too much cholesterol in your blood, or **hypercholesterolemia**, can accelerate the atherosclerosis process. The importance of keeping your blood cholesterol levels in a healthy range cannot be understated. The challenge is that this risk factor for a heart attack or stroke is typically silent and requires a blood test to detect.

A simple way to think about blood lipids is that too many of them in the blood provide material for plaques to develop (i.e., they can clog your arteries). **Hyperlipidemia** occurs when there is too much lipid (fat) in your blood, including cholesterol and triglycerides. A blood test called a *lipid profile* provides measurements that help assess your risk for CVD. A conventional lipid profile includes total cholesterol, high-density lipoprotein cholesterol (HDL-C), low-density lipoprotein cholesterol (LDL-C), and triglycerides.

- **High-density lipoprotein cholesterol (HDL-C)** is a "good" cholesterol. It carries the LDL away from the arteries; therefore, higher levels are protective against CVD.
- **Low-density lipoprotein cholesterol (LDL-C)** is a "bad" cholesterol; it is the primary type of cholesterol that contributes to the buildup of plaque in the arteries that can cause a heart attack or stroke.
- **Triglycerides**, although needed for energy production, increase the risk of a heart attack or stroke if levels are too high.

The American Heart Association (n.d.b) and other health organizations such as the Centers for Disease Control and Prevention (2023b) provide information to raise awareness about blood cholesterol and encourage Americans to make healthier lifestyle choices. Although you should always check with your personal physician regarding your own health, these sources provide important information for you to consider for the prevention of CVD.

Blood cholesterol levels have traditionally been evaluated using specific ranges of values. However, recent scientific advances now use the various blood values in context with other risk factors (e.g., age, sex) to predict a 10-year risk for atherosclerotic CVD. The guidelines provide specific recommendations for primary prevention (i.e., person has not been diagnosed with CVD)

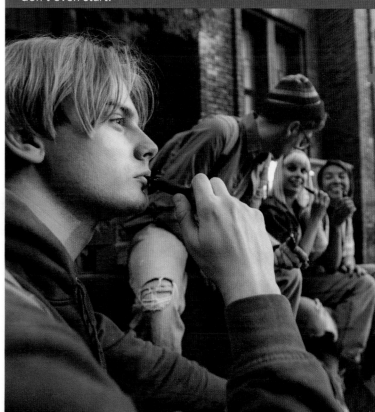

Smoking and vaping increase your risk for CVD. They also increase your risk for osteoporosis and cancer, especially lung cancer, and they even contribute to wrinkles as you age. Smoking and vaping are very hard habits to break. Just don't even start!

and secondary prevention (i.e., a person has already been diagnosed with CVD) and for treatment in people aged 20 to 79 (Stone et al. 2014). For young adults under the age of 20, specific blood lipid values are often evaluated (see table 13.4); however, clinical practice and guidelines are rapidly changing. Thus, the clinical significance of your personal blood lipid values, including the treatment plan, should be evaluated by a physician familiar with your health history, including your family history.

> High cholesterol is affected by more than weight management. You can also maintain healthy blood lipids by improving the quality of your diet, being physically active, and not smoking or vaping.

Hyperlipidemia can be genetic or caused by lifestyle behaviors. Like hypertension, lifestyle choices are the primary way you can change an unhealthy lipid profile, even if someday you must take medications to keep your blood lipids in the healthy range:

- **Weight management.** Being overweight or obese tends to raise LDL-C and lower HDL-C. Managing your weight and waistline is critical for preventing hyperlipidemia.
- **Diet quality.** From a dietary standpoint, the best strategy for lowering your cholesterol is to reduce the intake of your cholesterol, saturated fats, and trans fats. Another key is to have a diet high in fiber, which can lower cholesterol. Of course, other recommendations include following a healthy diet by eating fruits, vegetables, whole grains, poultry, fish, and nuts and limiting foods and beverages with added sugars. A diet high in refined carbohydrates and added sugars can elevate triglycerides. High levels of alcohol in the diet can also increase triglycerides. Your fuel quality greatly affects your blood lipids.
- **Regular physical activity and exercise.** A sedentary lifestyle is linked with lower HDL-C, which means there is less good cholesterol to combat the bad cholesterol. Regular physical activity also helps reduce triglycerides in the blood.
- **Smoking and vaping.** Smoking also lowers HDL-C, the good cholesterol. This is another important reason to never start.

If you are diagnosed with hyperlipidemia and you are unable to improve your blood values with lifestyle changes, you might be prescribed one or more medications, such as statin drugs, which are very effective in bringing your blood lipids closer to healthy values (Stone et al. 2014).

Exercise and Physical Activity as Key Prevention Behaviors

It should be clear that exercise, physical activity, and cardiorespiratory fitness are very important for preventing MetS, T2D, and CVD, especially CHD. People who have cardiorespiratory fitness greatly reduce their risk for obesity, hypertension, and hyperlipidemia and thus reduce risks for MetS, T2D, and CVD. Most of the beneficial effects of exercise and physical activity for preventing CHD can be explained indirectly through their positive influence on these traditional risk factors.

Cardiorespiratory exercise and fitness also directly reduce risk of CVD through their effects on the arteries and heart. The inner lining of the arteries, called the **endothelium**, controls physiological functions such as blood flow, which is linked to wear and tear on the lining of the vessel and risk for hypertension, and vessel permeability, which is important to the atherosclerotic process and plaque buildup. Moderate to vigorous exercise and physical activity

Table 13.4   Blood Cholesterol Levels for Young Adults (Under Age 20)

Type of cholesterol	Acceptable	Borderline risk	High
Total cholesterol	<170	170-199	≥200
LDL-C	<110	110-129	≥130
HDL-C	>45	40-45	<40
Triglycerides	<90	90-129	≥130

Data from U.S. Department of Health and Human Services (2012).

positively change the endothelium, making the vessels more flexible in response to physical demand and facilitating repair processes. The chambers of the heart are also favorably affected by movement, especially the left ventricle, which is responsible for pumping oxygenated blood to the body (Roitman and LaFontaine 2012). Thus, exercise and physical activity provide powerful indirect *and* direct benefits to prevent heart attack (see figure 13.6).

Prevention of CVD Starts Early in Life

Although it should be clear by now, the prevention of CVD and its risk factors, including MetS, prediabetes, and T2D, are key to cardiovascular health. Maintaining good cardiovascular health comes down to these top strategies:

1. Do not smoke or vape (not even a little bit!).
2. Eat a healthy and balanced diet (most of the time!).
3. Have a high level of physical activity (especially cardiorespiratory exercise of a moderate to vigorous intensity!).
4. Manage your waistline (which should happen naturally if you follow 2 and 3 on this list!).

Unless you happen to have genetics that are working against you, you can greatly reduce your chance of CVD if you invest in these strategies. It will also be very unlikely that you will develop high blood pressure, hyperlipidemia, or MetS (or prediabetes or T2D).

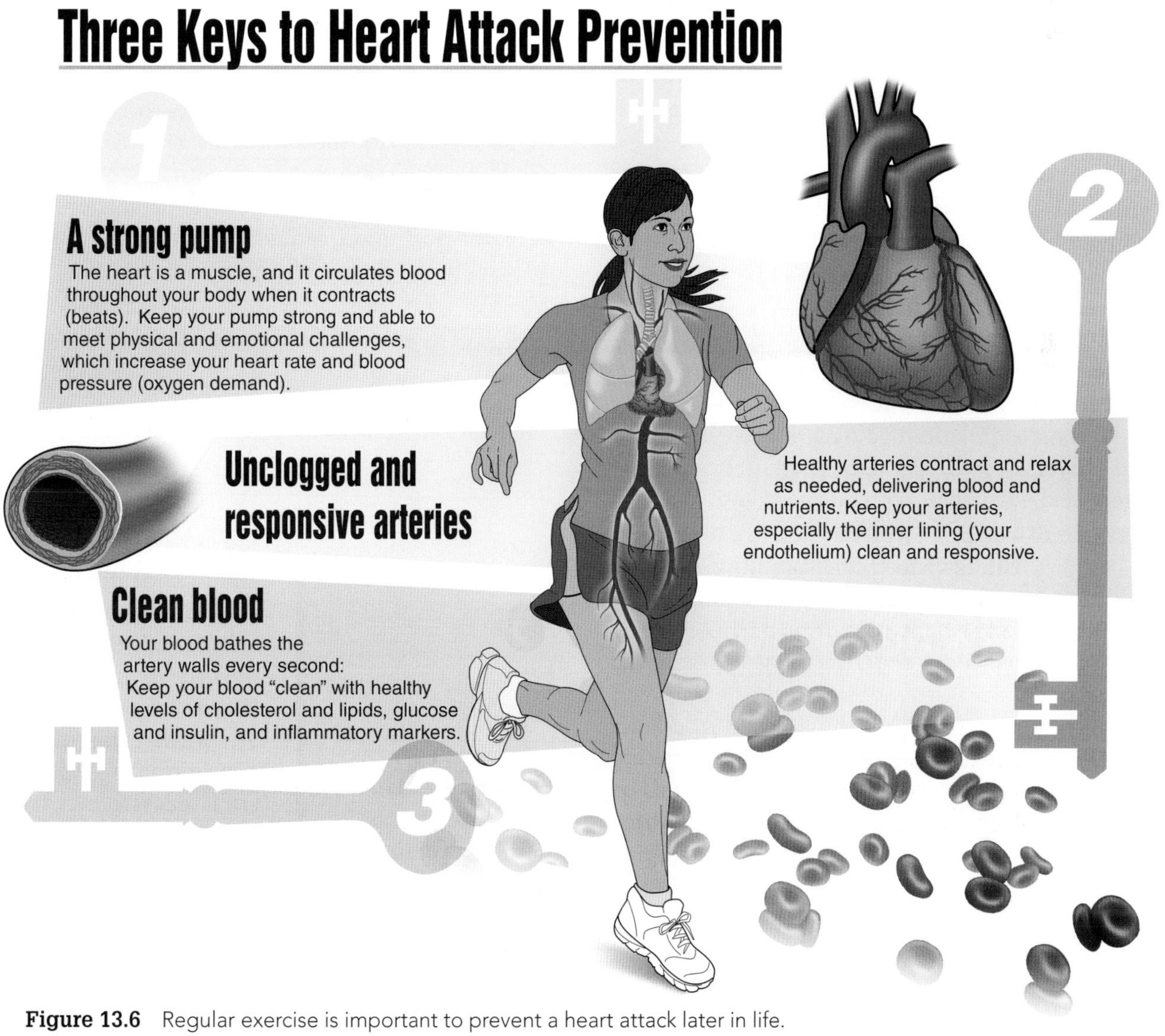

Three Keys to Heart Attack Prevention

A strong pump
The heart is a muscle, and it circulates blood throughout your body when it contracts (beats). Keep your pump strong and able to meet physical and emotional challenges, which increase your heart rate and blood pressure (oxygen demand).

Unclogged and responsive arteries

Healthy arteries contract and relax as needed, delivering blood and nutrients. Keep your arteries, especially the inner lining (your endothelium) clean and responsive.

Clean blood
Your blood bathes the artery walls every second: Keep your blood "clean" with healthy levels of cholesterol and lipids, glucose and insulin, and inflammatory markers.

Figure 13.6 Regular exercise is important to prevent a heart attack later in life.

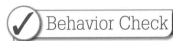

Behavior Check

Know Your Numbers

Many young adults think if their weight is reasonably managed, they must have good blood pressure and blood lipid numbers and are therefore protected from chronic diseases like CVD and CHD. To some degree this is true; however, some people can reasonably manage their weight without eating very well (i.e., they manage their calories, but their fuel quality is low). A diet high in saturated fats, refined carbohydrates and simple sugars, sodium, and alcohol can negatively affect your blood lipid profile and blood pressure even if you are not overweight or obese. If you also have chronically high stress and do not engage in regular cardiorespiratory exercise, your lipid profile and blood pressures might not be in the healthy range. Get tested and know your numbers, especially if you have a family history of hypertension or hyperlipidemia.

Summary

The cornerstone of prevention strategies for T2D and CVD are your lifestyle choices, including avoiding smoking, secondhand smoke, and vaping; limiting alcohol consumption; eating a balanced and healthy diet; engaging in regular moderate- to vigorous-intensity cardiorespiratory exercise; and managing your weight and waistline. T2D and CVD disease processes often start as a young adult with insulin resistance and MetS. As the decades progress, MetS becomes prediabetes, which becomes T2D, which leads to CVD in the following decade. Prevention starts today. Know the risk factors for these diseases, know your personal family history, and chart your risk numbers for life. Investing in heart-healthy behaviors will help you feel good today and prevent chronic diseases in the decades to come.

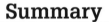

ONLINE LEARNING ACTIVITIES

Go to HK*Propel* and complete all of the online activities to further facilitate your learning:

Study Activities: Review the main concepts of the chapter.

Labs: Complete the labs your instructor assigns.

Videos: Look through the videos and choose which ones you want to try this week.

REVIEW QUESTIONS

1. How does MetS influence the risk for T2D and CVD?
2. List the risk factors for T2D and CVD. Which factors are the same and which are different?
3. What are the primary risk factors for T2D and CVD that you can change through your lifestyle choices?
4. Which type of exercise is most effective for enhancing your cardiovascular health? Describe the specifics of the exercise in terms of FITT (review chapter 4 as needed).
5. Which specific components of a healthy diet help reduce the risk of CVD?
6. When does the atherosclerotic process for CHD typically begin? Explain how early health choices can prevent subclinical disease with respect to this process.
7. How does regular cardiorespiratory exercise directly and indirectly reduce the risk for CHD?

14

Reducing the Risks for Cancer

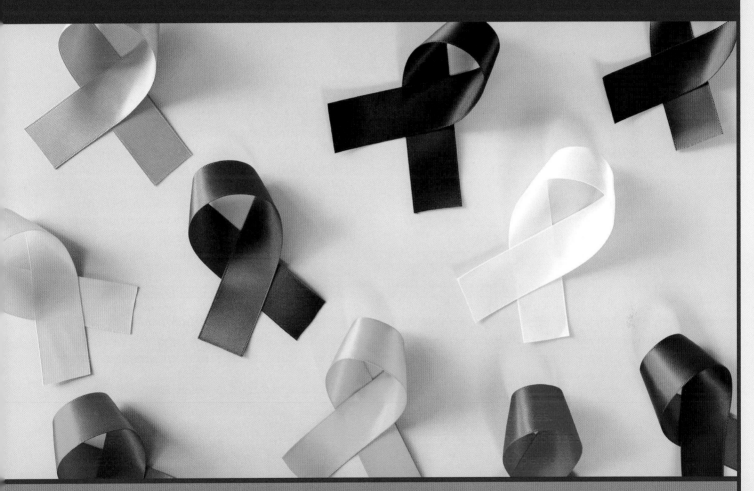

OBJECTIVES

- Define how cancer develops in the body.
- Identify the most commonly diagnosed cancers in the United States.
- Identify the cancers with the highest mortality rates in the United States.
- Explain how cancer develops related to genetics, lifestyle, and personal behaviors.
- Differentiate between the different types of cancer treatments.
- Develop a plan to prevent cancer.

KEY TERMS

benign

biopsy

cancer

carcinogen

carcinogenesis

carcinoma in situ

chemotherapy

endoscopy

malignant

melanoma

metastasis

mutation

polyp

prognosis

radiation therapy

TNM system

Cancer affects one in three people and is the second leading cause of death in the United States. This chapter provides a basic explanation of what cancer is, how it develops, how it is detected, and how it is treated. The chapter includes information about commonly diagnosed cancers and what you can do to prevent cancer. In addition, this chapter will cover the COVID-19 pandemic and the increased risks for those with specific health conditions such as cancer. It is estimated that cancer rates may increase in the years to come as a result of delays in diagnosis and treatment caused by the pandemic.

Cancer has been a medical mystery for centuries. Tumors were described in pictures and written records in many ancient civilizations in Asia, South America, and Egypt. In 400 BC, Hippocrates observed abnormal growths from breast tumors in his patients that looked like limbs of a crab. In 1700, Italian physician Bernardino Ramazzini speculated whether the increased incidence of breast cancer seen among Catholic nuns was related to their oath of celibacy, making him one of the first to propose a direct cause-and-effect relationship between lifestyle and cancer. Another such relationship was noted in 1775 by British physician Percivall Pott, who saw many patients in their 20s who worked as chimney sweepers. These young males were being diagnosed with cancers of the scrotum at a very high rate. Dr. Pott concluded that the chimney soot, or tar, was the causative agent and recommended that his patients wash their hands and body and change their clothes after cleaning chimneys to reduce their exposure to the tar. These simple recom-

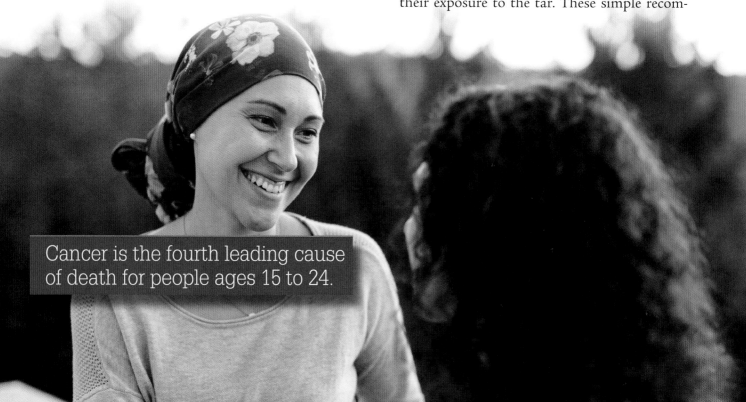

Cancer is the fourth leading cause of death for people ages 15 to 24.

mendations reduced the rates of cancer. In more recent history, in 1971, President Richard Nixon signed the National Cancer Act with the goal of eradicating cancer as a leading cause of death.

The Nature of Cancer

Cancer is not considered a single disease; well over 100 different types of cancer exist. The common factors in these diseases are the characteristics of the cells. **Cancer** is a malignant tumor that develops from an abnormal growth in healthy cells that the body is unable to stop from growing; the spread of the growth can become uncontrollable. Some of the distinct characteristics of these abnormal cells are large nuclei, larger than normal cell size, and variations in shape and size. Eventually, these cells invade the space in which the cancer began, and if the disease is not detected early, these cells often spread to other parts of the body.

Cancer is a significant leading cause of death and disability in the United States. Age happens to be one of the most significant risk factors, with more than 9 out of 10 cancers diagnosed among those aged 45 and older (Martin 2020); this is especially significant as our country's older population increases. Despite the current numbers, however, the overall number of cancer cases and deaths have followed a steady decline since peaking in 1991, with the death rate decreasing 31 percent. This

is partly a result of changes in lifestyle behaviors such as decreased tobacco use, as well as improved treatment options and advances in medical technology that detect cancer in the earlier stages and lead to longer survival rates.

Figure 14.1 shows the leading causes of death in the United States in 2019 (Kochanek, Xu, and Arias 2020). Cancer is the second leading cause of death overall and the fourth leading cause of death for young people ages 15 to 24. The relative survival rate for cancer gives an idea of life expectancy and is calculated based on the percentage of people who are still alive five years after their cancer diagnosis. Since the early 1960s, the five-year survival rate for all cancers has increased 31 percent among white people and 37 percent among Black people (70 percent and 64 percent, respectively; American Cancer Society 2021c). The cancers with the most significant survival rates over the past five decades are prostate, breast, colon, and rectum cancers, and leukemia. Certain cancers can be defined as curable if they are detected early and have not spread to other parts of the body and if the treatment options are successful.

Tumors: Benign Versus Malignant

A **benign** tumor is an abnormal growth that is noncancerous. These types of tumors are encapsulated, meaning that they have a defined

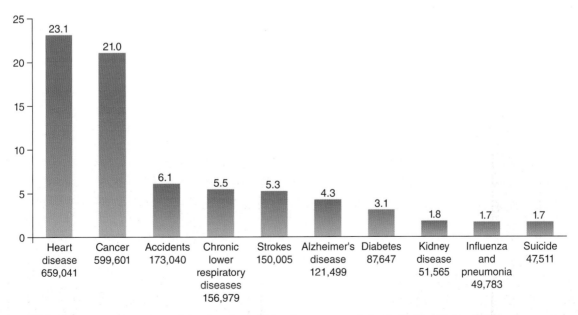

Figure 14.1   Percent and number of deaths of top 10 leading causes of death, United States, 2019.
Data from Heron et al. (2021).

border that does not allow the cells to break free and spread (figure 14.2). Although these types of tumors are not cancerous, they may still be fatal if left untreated or not removed from the site. For example, a benign tumor located in the lower abdominal cavity could fill that space as it becomes larger, which could affect the ability to urinate or have a bowel movement.

A **malignant** tumor is also a mass of abnormal cells; however, these cancerous cells look and act different than those of benign tumors (figure 14.3). Malignant tumors have the ability to grow in size and shape, and the cells can separate from

the primary tumor and spread to other parts of the body. These cells invade nearby tissue and then spread by way of the circulatory or lymphatic system. This is a multistage and multiyear process.

How Does Cancer Develop?

Chemicals, radiation, viruses, and heredity can all cause changes to the cell's genes that lead to cancer. Chemicals (such as those in cigarettes), radiation, and viruses invade normal cells and lead to a **mutation**, which is the alteration of the genetic makeup of a normal cell. Specific cancers have been identified as hereditary. The development of cancer, **carcinogenesis**, is a multistep process consisting of a series of mutations over many years.

A **carcinogen** is an agent that is capable of causing permanent damage to the molecular structure of the cell's DNA. This initiating agent is either inherited or acquired though carcinogenic chemicals, radiation, or viruses. Exposure is often repeated over time. Initiating agents include the chemicals in cigarettes, ultraviolet radiation from the sun, air pollution, or the human papilloma virus (which can cause cervical cancer).

Who Gets Cancer?

Information from the American Cancer Society (2023) gives us insight on who develops cancer. In

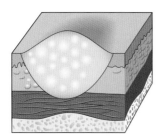

Type: Tumor
Description: A swelling or enlargement, any mass lesion; may be either malignant or benign
Examples: Lipoma, inflammatory reaction

Figure 14.2   Cross-section of a benign tumor.

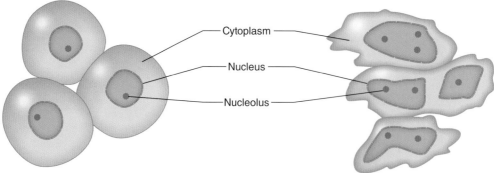

Figure 14.3   Comparison of normal cells and cancer cells.
Reprinted from National Cancer Institute (1990).

the United States in 2023, it is expected there will be 1.95 million new cancer cases and almost 609,820 deaths. This is equivalent to approximately 5,300 new cases and over 1,600 deaths every day. Figure 14.4 shows the leading sites of new cancer cases.

In the United States, it is estimated that 41 out of 100 males and 39 out of 100 females will be diagnosed with cancer at some point in their lifetime. Lifestyle and behaviors are the primary reasons why people develop cancer. Knowing which behaviors can lead to certain cancers will help you plan ways to reduce your chances of developing cancer.

Cancer: Race and Ethnicity

Cancer affects all populations and groups in the United States. However, specific groups have higher incidence rates, more cancer-related health complications, decreased survival rate and quality of life after treatment, more incidences of late-stage diagnosis, and higher mortality rates than others, which can be related to social, environmental, and economic disadvantages. Health inequities are evident in quality of life; life expectancy; incidence, prevalence, and severity of disease and disability; access to screenings and treatment; and mor-

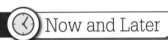

Should You Worry About Cancer?

Now

Should you worry about cancer? Let's put it in perspective. Are you more afraid of a shark attack, being in an airplane crash, contracting the West Nile virus, or being diagnosed with cancer, heart disease, or Alzheimer's disease? Many fears are rooted in emotions rather than facts. Cancer can be caused by genetics or lifestyle behaviors such as a poor diet or using tobacco products. Knowing the causes now can help you reduce the chances of developing cancer in the future. Let's add some perspective. Table 14.1 shows the odds over a lifetime that a U.S. citizen will die by certain causes.

Table 14.1 Odds of Dying

Common fears	Common causes of death
Shark attack: 1 in 3.7 million	Cancer: 1 in 5
Bear attack: 1 in 1.2 million	Heart disease: 1 in 6
Amusement park rides: 1 in 950,000	Stroke: 1 in 23
Anthrax: 1 in 730,000	Diabetes: 1 in 53
Fireworks: 1 in 340,733	Alzheimer's disease: 1 in 75
Lightning: 1 in 138,849	Intentional self-harm (suicide): 1 in 88
Commercial airplane: 1 in 40,000	Opioid overdose: 1 in 92
West Nile virus: 1 in 15,000	Motor vehicle accident: 1 in 107

Data from Ropeik and Gray (2002); American Cancer Society (2021d): National Safety Council (2021); National Geographic (2018).

Later

Cancer develops over time and is more likely to develop after repeated exposure to carcinogens, like radiation from the sun or the toxic chemicals in cigarettes. What can you do to reduce your odds of dying from cancer in the future?

Take Home

Although cancer can take years to develop and is typically thought of as a disease of older people, you can take steps now, as a college student, to prevent your chances of being diagnosed with cancer. Begin setting your cancer prevention goals now: It's never too early to use sunscreen, limit alcohol, quit smoking, and begin age-appropriate health screenings like breast self-exams. Do all you can to learn how to catch cancer early and prevent cancer from starting in the first place.

tality. Cancer disparities are evident when data show there have been an improvement overall, but when these data are broken down to specific categories or groups, these improvements are not evident. Although the information shown in

> Health equity is achieved when every person has the opportunity to attain their full health potential and no one is disadvantaged because of socially determined circumstances (Centers for Disease Control and Prevention 2020a).

this section focuses on race and ethnicity, disparities exist among other population groups, defined by disability, sexual orientation, gender identity, geographic location, income level, educational attainment, age, and national origin (National Cancer Institute 2020a). Figures 14.5 and 14.6 show that the incidence of cancer and the death rates are highest among Black males.

Cancer Disparities in the United States (National Cancer Institute 2020a)

- Black and African American people have higher death rates than all other racial and ethnic

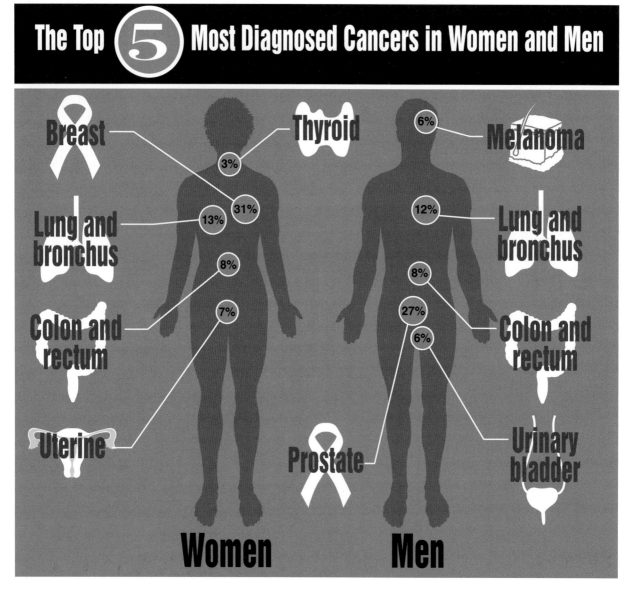

Figure 14.4 Leading types of cancer diagnosed in females and males, by percentage of new cancer cases, 2022.
Data from American Cancer Society (2022).

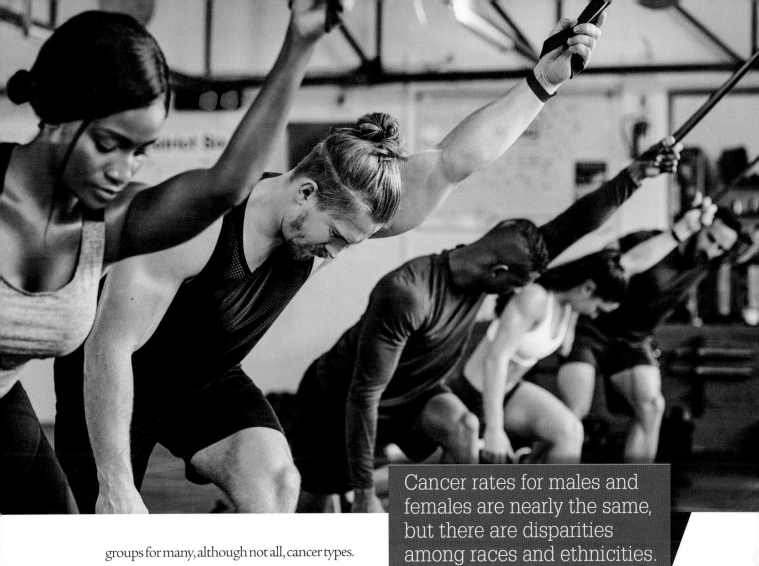

Cancer rates for males and females are nearly the same, but there are disparities among races and ethnicities.

groups for many, although not all, cancer types.

- Black and African American females are much more likely than white females to die of breast cancer even though the rates of breast cancer among the groups are similar.
- Rural Appalachia has higher rates of colorectal, lung, and cervical cancers than urban areas in the same region.
- Black and African American males are twice as likely as white males to die of prostate cancer.
- People with less education have a higher likelihood of dying prematurely from colorectal cancer regardless of race or ethnicity.
- Hispanic, Latina, and Black or African American females have higher rates of cervical cancer than females of other racial and ethnic groups.
- Black and African American females have the highest rates of death from cervical cancer.

- American Indian and Alaska Native people have higher death rates from kidney cancer than people of other racial and ethnic groups.
- Both the incidence of lung cancer and death rates from the disease are higher in Black males than in males of other racial and ethnic groups.
- Youth who identify as lesbian, gay, or bisexual have higher rates of smoking and drinking alcohol, which increases cancer risks, than heterosexual youth.
- Liver and intrahepatic bile duct cancer is highest among American Indian and Alaska Native people, which is linked to heavy alcohol use and cigarette smoking.

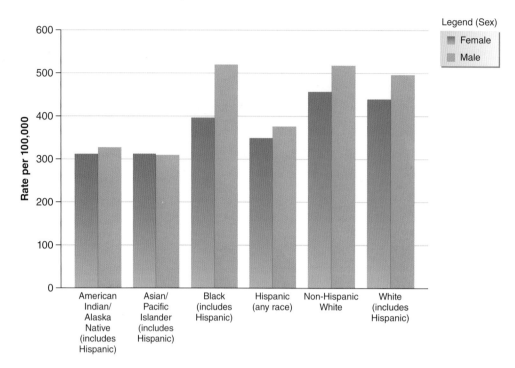

Figure 14.5   Combined incidence rates of all cancer sites by race and ethnicity, United States, 2014 to 2018.

Note. Created by https://seer.cancer.gov/explorer on Thu Sep 02 2021. SEER 21 areas [http//seer.cancer.gov/registries/terms.html]. Rates are per 100,000 and are age-adjusted to the 2000 US Std Population (19 age groups - Census P25-1130). See SEER Race Recode Documentation for Spanish-Hispanic-Latino Ethnicity [http://seer.cancer.gov/seerstat/variables/seer/race_ethnicity/#hispanic].

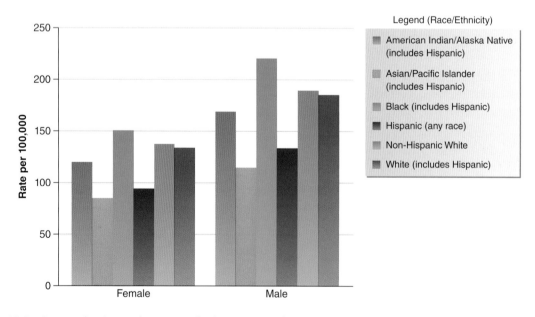

Figure 14.6   Cancer death rates by race and ethnicity, United States, 2014 to 2018.

Note. Created by https://seer.cancer.gov/explorer on Thu Sep 02 2021. US Mortality Files, National Center for Health Statistics, CDC. Rates are per 100,000 and are age-adjusted to the 2000 US Std Population (19 age groups - Census P25-1130).

Cancers by Age and Sex: The Risks Change Over Your Lifetime

Consider your risk of developing cancer as a young adult and then the risk over your lifetime, as shown in table 14.2. Then consider the differences between males and females in the same age categories. Females have a higher overall lifetime risk of developing cancer than males, and their risk is higher than males for some specific cancers as well. Why do you think males have a higher risk of developing lung cancer at a young age than females, but the overall lifetime risk is higher for females?

The incidence rates of lung cancer among females began to rise in the early 1980s because of an increased smoking rate among this population, but the incidence of cancer soon surpassed males at a rate not commensurate with the smoking prevalence among these populations. Studies have been conducted to determine why females are more susceptible to lung cancer and whether the differences are related to the changes in the composition of cigarettes or how female bodies respond to the carcinogenic agents in tobacco (Fidler-Benaoudia et al. 2020). Specifically, these two variables are worth further exploration (American Cancer Society 2020b):

Table 14.2   Probability of Developing Invasive Cancers by Age and Sex, United States, 2015 to 2017

Site	Sex	Birth to age 49	Birth to death
All sites1	M	1 in 29	1 in 2
	F	1 in 17	1 in 3
Breast	F	1 in 49	1 in 8
Prostate	M	1 in 451	1 in 8
Colon and rectum	M	1 in 254	1 in 23
	F	1 in 266	1 in 25
Lung	M	1 in 776	1 in 15
	F	1 in 679	1 in 17
Skin2	M	1 in 230	1 in 27
	F	1 in 156	1 in 40

[1]All sites exclude basal cell and squamous cell skin cancers and in situ cancers except urinary bladder.

[2]Statistic is for non-Hispanic whites.

Data from American Cancer Society (2021b).

- Filtered cigarettes increase the risk of adenocarcinoma lung cancer because the tobacco smoke is distributed to the outer parts of the lungs, and many females began smoking when filtered cigarettes were common.
- Females may have different genetic risk factors than males, such as an inability to repair damaged DNA or having abnormal genes related to cancer development.

Skin cancer shows a similar trend as lung cancer, except in reverse: Females are more likely to develop skin cancer at a young age than males, but the overall lifetime risk is higher for males than for females. What are your hypotheses related to these differences? This is most likely linked to higher rates of occupations and recreational activities where males are exposed to ultraviolet radiation over many years.

Why Do Specific Racial and Ethnic Groups Have Higher Incidence and Mortality Rates?

The most common reasons why other races and ethnic groups have higher cancer incidence and death rates than whites are related to social, environmental, and economic disadvantages (National Cancer Institute 2020a). Some examples include experiencing obstacles to getting necessary health care, including low income, no insurance, lack of transportation to a medical facility, or low health literacy. Limited opportunities for quality health care and inability to afford medical care makes people from disadvantaged racial and ethnic groups less likely to receive recommended screenings and more likely to be diagnosed with a late-stage cancer.

Understanding the role biological differences play among various populations can also help researchers develop early screening and interventions to prevent late-stage diagnosis and improve quantity and quality of life for diverse racial and ethnic groups. For example, one such difference is seen among African American males, who have approximately 60 percent higher rates of prostate cancer than white males do, as well as a mortality rate two to three times higher (National Cancer Institute 2015). Unfortunately, the continued lack of diversity in clinical research participation has led to little insight related to these racial and ethnic differences.

Approaches to Reducing Cancer Disparities:

- Provide health care to all regardless of one's ability to pay.
- Fund screening programs to be implemented in specific geographical locations where programs are scarce or do not exist.
- Implement educational programs in community-based organizations that increase knowledge and teach skills for changing behavioral and lifestyle factors that contribute to developing cancer.

- Allocate additional funding that supports understanding the role of biological differences across all racial and ethnic groups.

Detection, Staging, and Treatment of Cancer

Learning about health screenings and the early detection of cancer will increase your chances of surviving the disease, should you ever have it. Once a cancer has been detected, determining its size and location and whether it has spread to other locations in the body will help guide the treatment

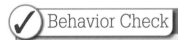 Behavior Check

Advocating for Yourself

Although health disparities are frequently related to economic disadvantages, people of color who have health insurance or a higher socioeconomic status (e.g., have more access to financial, educational, social, and health resources) may also experience disparities as a result of institutional racism and the resulting chronic stress. Conscious or unconscious bias from health care providers can lead individuals to develop mistrust of the health care system or adopt fatalistic attitudes about cancer (National Cancer Institute 2020a). Be sure to explore your options when it comes to a health care provider—consider making an interview appointment so you can decide if the provider is a good fit for you!

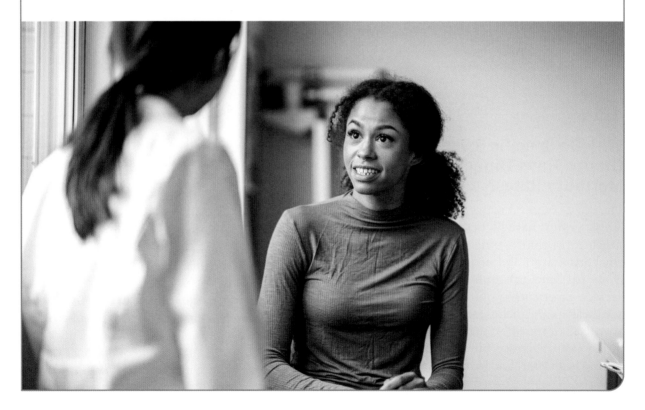

plan and prognosis. All of this information helps the cancer patient and the team of health care providers determine the appropriate treatment plan to support an optimal quality of life.

Early Detection of Cancer

Detecting the disease in its early stages leads to a better prognosis, better quality of life, and better chance of survival (figure 14.7). When early-detection techniques are implemented as part of routine medical care, you and your physician can note immediate changes. The cancer is most likely to be localized rather than distant. Cancer treatment involves removal of the tumors and use of medications or radiation to prevent the cancer cells from dividing and spreading; these are less invasive than later-stage treatments and do not greatly affect quality of life.

The most common types of early-detection techniques conducted by medical professionals are biopsies, X-rays, genetic testing, endoscopy,

and blood tests. However, you can do certain techniques yourself on a monthly basis. Talk with your doctor about the need for additional medical screenings.

Biopsy

A **biopsy** is when a physician or surgeon removes a sample of cells or tissues from the tumor site. A screening of the cells or tissue will allow the health care provider to determine whether the tumor is malignant or benign.

- *Fine-needle aspiration.* A small sample of cells is taken from the tumor with a syringe. This technique removes the least number of cells compared to the others. Typically, no scarring or damage occurs to the surrounding area.
- *Core needle biopsy.* A small core sample of cells is removed from the tumor. There may be a small scar and the potential need for stitches.

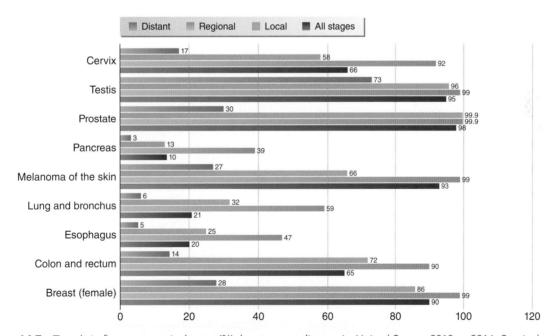

Figure 14.7   Trends in five-year survival rates (%), by stage at diagnosis, United States, 2010 to 2016. Survival rates for most cancers have increased due to earlier detection and advances in treatment.

Local: An invasive malignant cancer confined entirely to the organ of origin. *Regional:* A malignant cancer that 1) has extended beyond the limits of the organ of origin directly into surrounding organs or tissues; 2) involves regional lymph nodes; or 3) has both regional extension and involvement of regional lymph nodes.

Distant: A malignant cancer that has spread to parts of the body remote from the primary tumor either by direct extension or by discontinuous metastasis to distant organs, tissues, or via the lymphatic system to distant lymph nodes.

Reprinted by permission from N. Howlader, A.M. Noone, M. Krapcho M, et al., "SEER Cancer Statistics Review, 1975-2017," National Cancer Institute, last modified April 15, 2020, https://seer.cancer.gov/archive/csr/1975_2017/.

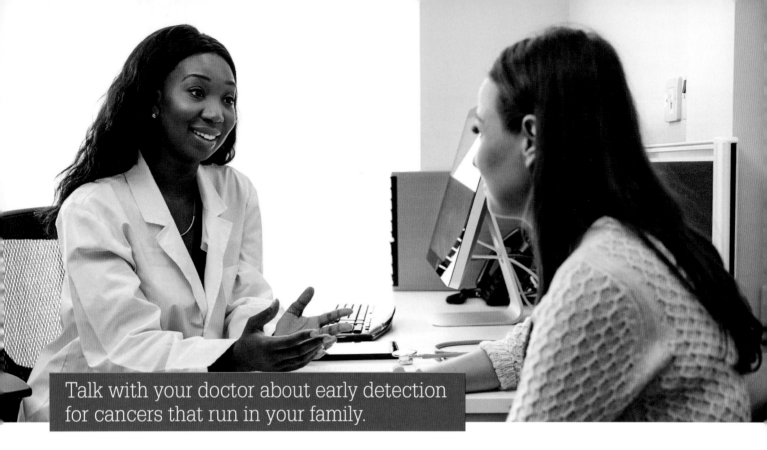

Talk with your doctor about early detection for cancers that run in your family.

- **Incisional.** A small wedge sample of cells is taken from the tumor. There may be a somewhat large scar and the need for stitches or other treatment to close the incision site.
- **Excisional.** The entire tumor area is extracted, and no surrounding tissue remains. There will be a noticeable scar and the need for stitches or another treatment to close the incision site.
- **Ductal lavage.** Cells are extracted from milk ducts in the breast with a syringe.

X-Rays

Table 14.3 shows the various types of imaging techniques that allow health care providers to determine the location and size of tumors in the body.

Genetic Testing

Hereditary cancers can be detected early through medical techniques such as chromosome analysis. Some of these tests are covered by insurance and others are not. It is important to discuss options with your health care and insurance providers. If you determine you have a predisposition to cancer based on your family history, share the results with your health care provider and discuss which tests may be able to help you detect cancers early. According to Simon (2019) from the American Cancer Society, you should consider genetic testing if you have any of the following:

- You have several first-degree relatives (parents, siblings, children) with cancer.
- Many relatives on one side of your family have had the same type of cancer.

Table 14.3 Types of Imaging Used to Detect Cancer

Type of imaging	Description
Ultrasound	A device called a transducer transmits high-frequency sound waves to examine the inside of the body
Mammogram	An X-ray is taken of the breast
Magnetic resonance imaging (MRI)	Magnet and radio waves examine the inside of the body
Computed tomography (CT)	A scanning X-ray technique takes cross-sectional photos of the body

- A cluster of cancers in your family have been linked to a single gene mutation (such as some types of breast, ovarian, colorectal, and pancreatic cancers).
- A family member has more than one type of cancer.
- Family members have had cancer at a younger age than normal for that type of cancer.
- Close relatives have cancers that are linked to hereditary cancer syndromes.
- A family member has a rare cancer, such as male breast cancer or retinoblastoma (a type of eye cancer).
- You are an ethnicity known to be at risk (for example, Ashkenazi Jewish ancestry is linked to ovarian and breast cancers).
- A physical finding is linked to an inherited cancer (such as having many colon polyps).
- One or more family members have already had genetic testing that found a mutation.

Endoscopy

Physicians may perform an **endoscopy** to check for cancer by inserting a thin, flexible illuminated tube (called an endoscope) into internal body cavities. Common sites for endoscopy are the throat, esophagus, bladder, colon, and rectum. Endoscopies allow physicians to detect and locate possible tumors, ulcers, **polyps**, and areas of inflammation or bleeding and to remove tissue samples or suspicious tumors during the procedure. Endoscopes are used for colon cancer screenings to detect cancers in the large intestine (figure 14.8).

Self-Detection Techniques

You can take an active part in early detection by performing personal cancer screenings monthly so that you are aware of what is normal and what is not. The American Cancer Society developed the acronym CAUTION to help people identify signs and symptoms of cancer (figure 14.9).

Both females and males can do monthly breast and skin self-examinations, and males can conduct a monthly testicular self-examination. See figures 14.10 and 14.11 for instructions on how to do these self-exams. If you have a vision impairment that makes it difficult for you to visually inspect your body, ask a trusted friend or a family member to help you.

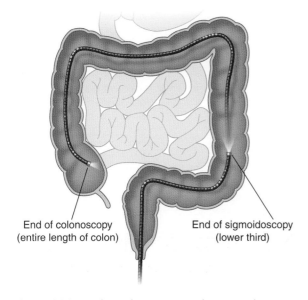

End of colonoscopy (entire length of colon)   End of sigmoidoscopy (lower third)

Figure 14.8 Both a colonoscopy and a sigmoidoscopy use a thin, flexible tube with a light and camera to examine the colon. A colonoscopy examines the entire length of the colon, whereas the sigmoidoscopy examines only the lower third of the colon (MedlinePlus 2021).

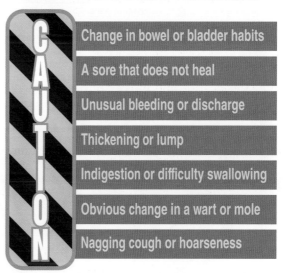

The CAUTION Acronym

- Change in bowel or bladder habits
- A sore that does not heal
- Unusual bleeding or discharge
- Thickening or lump
- Indigestion or difficulty swallowing
- Obvious change in a wart or mole
- Nagging cough or hoarseness

Figure 14.9 The acronym CAUTION can help you notice changes that you should report to your doctor.

Mirror exams

Step 1: While standing in front of a mirror, straighten your body, make sure your shoulders are not rounded, and put your hands on your hips. Look at both breasts, looking for any differences in the shape and size of both breasts: Do they look the same? Check for differences in the skin tone or color (e.g., redness), if the skin has the look of an orange peel, or if it has any puckering, dimpling, a rash, or inflammation. Pay attention to your nipples: Have they changed in position, or are they inverted, sore, or red?

Step 2: While still standing in front of the mirror, raise your arms over your head and do the same checks as you did in step 1.

1 Hands on hips

2 Arms raised

Nipple check **3**

Step 3: Focus on your nipples: Check for fluid discharge from the nipples and note if it is yellow, cloudy, or bloody.

| Retracted nipple | Nipple discharge | Lump or thickening | Change in color of skin | Change in breast size or shape |

Lying down **4**

Step 4: This step focuses on checking your breasts while lying down. Place a pillow under your right shoulder to flatten the breast, and put your right hand underneath your head. With your left hand, begin to check the right breast for any lumps or changes in the consistency of the breast by using the finger pads of your three middle fingers. Using your middle fingers, check the entire breast, from the collarbone to the top of the rib cage, and from your armpit to the sternum. Use three different patterns to check your breast: an up and down pattern, a circular pattern, and moving inward toward the nipple. Repeat this for the left breast.

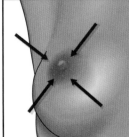

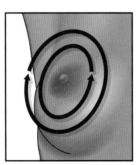

5 Shower

Step 5: Checking your breasts in the shower is recommended because some women find checking their breasts when they are warm, wet, and slippery makes it easier to detect abnormalities or changes. Implement the same three techniques in the shower as described in step 4.

Figure 14.10   Both males and females should follow these instructions to examine their breasts.
Based on Breastcancer.org (2017).

Testicular Self-Exam

1 **Step 1:** While standing, move your penis out of the way so you can see your scrotum. Examine the scrotum for any changes in skin color, swelling, soreness, or thickening. It is normal for one testicle to be slightly larger than the other and for one of the testicles to hang a bit lower than the other.

2 **Step 2:** Using both hands, specifically your thumbs and fingers, locate one of the testicles and begin to gently roll the testicle between your fingers and thumbs noticing any changes which may include hard lumps, painless lumps, smooth rounded bumps, swelling, shape, or consistency. Do this for both testicles.

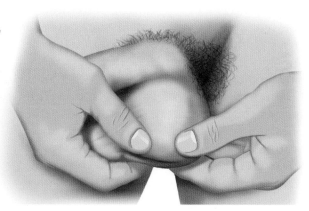

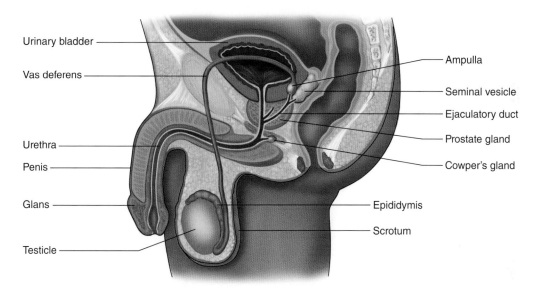

Urinary bladder — Vas deferens — Urethra — Penis — Glans — Testicle —
— Ampulla — Seminal vesicle — Ejaculatory duct — Prostate gland — Cowper's gland — Epididymis — Scrotum

Figure 14.11   Males should follow these instructions to examine their testicles.
Based on American Cancer Society (2018).

Staging of Cancer

Once someone is diagnosed with cancer, the physician or oncologist (a physician who specializes in cancer) will determine the stage, or seriousness, of the disease. This assists the physician in determining the types of treatments and the **prognosis**, which is the physician's best estimate of

Testicles can change for other reasons besides cancer. Fluid building around the testicle is called a hydrocele, and a varicocele is when veins dilate, causing enlargement or lumpiness (American Cancer Society 2018).

the time it will take to recover and how the cancer may affect the patient's quality of life.

The stage of the cancer is based on the size of the primary tumor, the extent to which it has invaded the space where it is located, and if it has spread to lymph nodes or other locations in the body. If the cancer cells have not spread or penetrated any layers of tissues, and are confined to the original cells, then this is known as **carcinoma in situ**. If the cells have gone beyond the original layer of cells, then the cancer is defined as invasive, or taking up more space or spreading to other parts of the body. The physician will need to determine if the cancer is localized, regional, or distant and will use different imaging techniques to determine the extent of the invasiveness. Some primary cancers have a distinctive path through which they have traditionally been known to spread to other parts of the body by invading the lymph or circulatory system. For example, metastatic lung cancer tends to spread to other lobes of the lung and the bones, adrenal gland, liver, or brain, and metastatic breast cancer spreads to the bones, lungs, liver, and brain (National Cancer Institute 2020b).

The **TNM system** is used to determine the extent or size of the primary tumor (T), whether or not the cancer cells have spread to lymph nodes (N), and if **metastasis** (M) has occurred—that is, the cells have traveled to other parts of the body. Based on the TNM findings, the patient will be given a diagnosis of stage 0, I, II, III, or IV cancer. Stage 0 is carcinoma in situ, meaning that the cancer has not spread and is not invasive. Stage I indicates the cancer is in the very early stages, and stage IV is the most advanced. For example, a diagnosis of stage IV breast cancer means that a malignant tumor (T) of any size has been diagnosed, the cancer has most likely spread to local or distant lymph nodes (N), and the cancer has metastasized (M) to distant sites in the body (American Cancer Society 2021b).

When cancer has spread to other sites, it is still considered the primary type of cancer. Thus, breast cancer that has spread to the lungs would be called metastatic breast cancer, not lung cancer, and the patient's health care team would treat this as stage IV breast cancer (American Cancer Society 2021a). There are many factors that oncologists consider before staging cancer; therefore, it is important to keep in mind that two patients with the same stage of cancer may have a different combination of factors (National Cancer Institute 2020b).

Common Treatments of Cancer

The most common treatments for most cancers are surgery, chemotherapy, and radiation. **Surgery** involves the removal of the malignant tumor. For more advanced cancers, it may also require the removal of surrounding tissues and lymph nodes. The goal of **chemotherapy** is to introduce powerful medications into the body that stop the cancer cells from reproducing and the tumor from growing larger, thus preventing the cancer from spreading to other sites in the body. Chemotherapy can be administered by pill, IV or infusion, or injections through the skin or in muscles. In many cases, oncologists use chemotherapy medications in conjunction with other treatments such as surgery or radiation. However, in some cases, chemotherapy alone can treat cancer; no other treatments are necessary. Additionally, chemotherapy may be prescribed on a long-term basis to prevent the recurrence of cancer. **Radiation therapy** involves the use of radioactive waves, such as X-rays, gamma rays, neutrons, and protons, to kill cancer cells or shrink the size of the tumor. The radioactive beams can target specific cancer cells from a machine that delivers the beam either externally (outside of the body) or internally in the form of a small pellet that is placed in the body near the cancer cells (National Cancer Institute 2021a).

World War II sailors were accidentally exposed to mustard gas, which resulted in low white blood cell counts. This led to the discovery of medications that slow down or stop the division of cancer cells (DeVita and Chu 2008).

Causes of Cancer

Approximately 5 percent of all cancers are clearly hereditary, but the majority of cancers—up to 95 percent—are a result of genetic mutations caused by exposure to environmental toxins and lifestyle factors such as tobacco use, sun exposure, alcohol, drugs, an unhealthy diet, and lack of physical activity (American Cancer Society 2021b). Figure 14.12 shows the extent to which each risk factor contributes to specific types of cancer. More than half of all cancer deaths in the United States are preventable—these risk factors can be reduced with lifestyle changes (American Association for Cancer Research 2014). Consider the importance of implementing preventive behaviors now to decrease your chance of developing cancer later in life.

Heredity

You have no control over your genetics, which include your eye color, hair color, body build, and

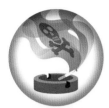

Smoking
81.7% of lung cancers
73.8% of laryngeal cancers
50% of esophageal cancers
46.9% of bladder cancers

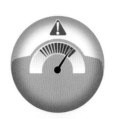

Excess body weight
60.3% of uterine cancers
33.9% of liver cancers
11.3% of breast cancers in females
5.2% of colorectal cancers

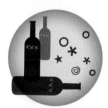

Alcohol
46.3% of oral cavity and
pharyngeal cancers in males,
27.4% in females
24.8% of liver cancers in males,
11.9% in females
17.1% of colorectal cancers in males,
8.1% in females
6.4% of breast cancers in females

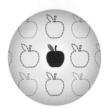

Few fruits and veggies
17.6% of oral cavity and
pharyngeal cancers
17.4% of laryngeal cancers
8.9% of lung cancers

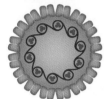

HPV infection
All cervical cancers
88.2% of anal cancers
64.6% of vaginal cancers
56.9% of penis cancers

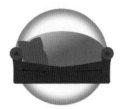

Physical inactivity
26.7% of uterine cancers
16.3% of colorectal cancers
3.9% of breast cancers in females

UV radiation
96.0% of melanomas of the
skin in males
93.7% of melanomas of the
skin in females

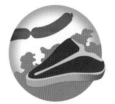

Red meat and processed meat
5.4% of colorectal cancers in males
8.2% of colorectal cancers in females

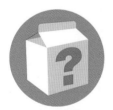

Low dietary calcium
4.9% of colorectal cancers

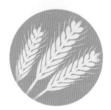

Low dietary fiber
10.3% of colorectal cancers

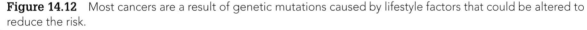

Figure 14.12 Most cancers are a result of genetic mutations caused by lifestyle factors that could be altered to reduce the risk.
Data from American Cancer Society (2017).

cancer genes. Overall, inherited cancers are rare, and many are diagnosed in childhood. An example of a childhood inherited cancer is retinoblastoma, an eye tumor. If detected early, it can be successfully treated. Adult inherited cancers include some types of breast and colon cancer. It is important to know your family medical history to understand your risks of developing cancer in your lifetime. The risks of developing some inherited cancers can be determined through screenings such as blood tests that can be discussed with your health care provider.

Lifestyles, Behaviors, and Cancer

Tobacco use and poor diet are the leading causes of cancer, and tobacco use is the leading cause of cancer deaths in the United States. An unhealthy diet, lack of physical activity, excessive sun exposure, and pollutions in the environment also contribute to cancer deaths. Learning more about your own lifestyle and behaviors can help you make choices to reduce your risks of developing cancer in the future.

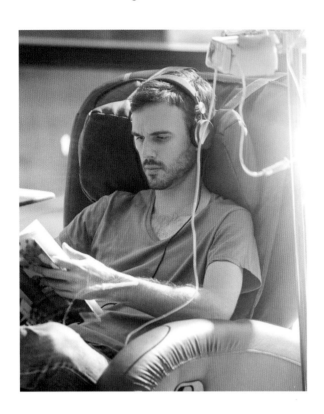

Tobacco Use

The first Surgeon General's report related to smoking and tobacco, *Smoking and Health: Report of the Advisory Committee of the Surgeon General of the Public Health Service*, was published in 1964 in response to increasing lung cancer rates in the United States (Centers for Disease Control and Prevention 2020b). Fortunately, these rates have since declined and tobacco use has significantly decreased in the United States since the early 2000s.

Despite this decline, however, smoking continues to be the leading cause of preventable disease and death in the United States (U.S. Department of Health and Human Services 2014). Tobacco use accounts for about one in five deaths each year, and lung cancer remains the leading cause of cancer deaths in the United States (American Cancer Society 2020a). Many chemicals found in cigarettes and other tobacco products are known carcinogens; smoking is linked to 13 different

✓ Behavior Check

Genetic Screening

Would you want to know if you are at an increased risk of developing cancer? If you were able to get genetic screening today to find out which diseases and conditions you are most likely to develop in the future, what would you do with this information? Would you change your lifestyle by eating healthier, using sunscreen, reducing your drinking habits, or abstaining from alcohol, not smoking, or becoming more physically active? Would you consider more aggressive approaches like getting a mastectomy if you tested positive for the BRCA gene? Or would you prefer not to know or make any changes in your life? What are the advantages and disadvantages to knowing your future when it comes to potentially fatal illnesses or diseases?

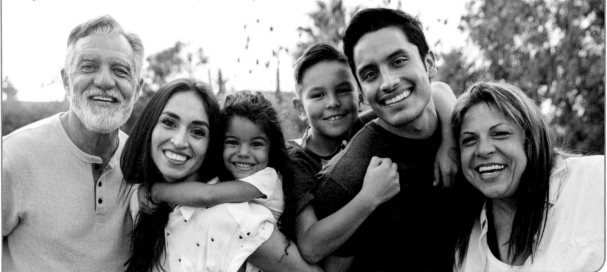

Behavior Check

Is Tobacco Harmless?

There are many myths that claim using tobacco is harmless. Be aware of these claims and don't start smoking; if you do smoke, quit now. Consider these myths (Centers for Disease Control and Prevention n.d.):

- **Myth: Filters make cigarettes safer.** The filters are designed to make the tobacco particles smaller, so the nicotine is more easily absorbed in the body, which increases the addiction.
- **Myth: An occasional cigarette is no big deal.** Tobacco smoke causes immediate harm and can trigger sudden heart attacks and death—and this can happen to nonsmokers, too.
- **Myth: Secondhand smoke isn't dangerous, just annoying to others.** Secondhand smoke is full of poisonous chemicals that can cause deadly clots and block arteries to the heart and brain.
- **Myth: Kids are not harmed by a little bit of secondhand smoke.** Kids exposed to cigarette smoke have increased risk of bronchitis, pneumonia, and ear infections.
- **Myth: It's too late, the damage is done.** As soon as you quit, your body begins to heal.

What steps do you want to take to reduce your risk?

types of cancers (U.S. Department of Health and Human Services 2014), including lung, upper respiratory tract, esophagus, oral, tongue, bladder, pancreas, stomach, liver, and kidney. It may also contribute to cancers of the colon and rectum. Nonsmokers live, on average, 10 years longer than smokers (Centers for Disease Control and Prevention 2021b).

It is never too late to quit smoking or using tobacco products! The body begins to heal within 20 minutes of that last cigarette, cigar, or pipe! Talk to your health care provider, call 800-QUIT-NOW, or go to www.smokefree.gov for help.

Diet and Physical Activity

Obesity has become a common, serious, and costly disease, and rates are only increasing: By 2018, the obesity prevalence in the United States was 42.4 percent (Centers for Disease Control and Prevention 2021a). Being overweight or obese is linked to an increased risk of certain types of cancers, shown in figure 14.13 (American Institute for Cancer Research 2020).

Eating a healthy diet can lower your cancer risk by 10 to 20 percent (Schwingshackl and Hoffman 2015). A healthy diet consists of fruits and vegetables, whole grains, lean proteins, healthy plant oils (in moderation), and limited alcohol, sugary drinks, and milk and dairy products (Harvard School of Public Health n.d.). According to Rock et al. (2020), dietary guidelines to reduce your chances of developing cancer include following the U.S. Dietary Guidelines to eat at least 2-1/2 to 3 cups of vegetables and 1-1/2 to 2 cups of fruits

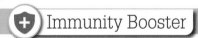

Immunity Booster

Serious Complications: COVID-19 and Cigarette Smoking

Research has shown that smokers who are diagnosed with COVID-19 have an increased risk of more severe illnesses that can lead to hospitalization, intensive care, or death. Why are smokers at a higher risk for severe illness? The chemicals and nicotine cause inflammation and cell damage throughout the body, which lead to a weakened immune system that is less able to fight infections (U.S. Food and Drug Administration 2021). Increasing your chances for a full recovery from a COVID-19 infection includes refraining from smoking and staying smoke-free. Although we are still learning about the long-term effects of COVID-19, we do know that nonsmokers are less likely to get very sick from COVID-19, the flu, and other infections that affect the lungs.

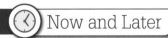
Now and Later

Smoking Sucks the Life Out of You

Now

Smoking can affect your health in more ways than just increasing your risk of cancer. If you currently smoke, you may find that you get winded easily, your hair and clothes smell, your breath smells bad, and your teeth are becoming more stained or yellowed. Smoking has immediate effects on your health and image, so choosing to quit now will save you time and money on breath mints, doing extra laundry, fewer dental visits, and having fun being active without having to stop and catch your breath.

Later

Think about how smoking and using tobacco products can affect many other aspects of your health throughout your life. All of the following are adverse health outcomes that you do not want to experience (American Cancer Society 2020a):

- Gum disease and tooth loss
- Lowered immune system function
- Increased risk of developing type 2 diabetes
- Decreased sense of taste and smell
- Premature aging of the skin
- Bad breath and stained teeth
- Delayed wound healing
- Eye problems (e.g., cataracts and macular degeneration)

Take Home

Smoking is a detriment to your health now and later. Honor your body and embrace your health—don't start smoking, and if you are already a smoker, please quit. Contact your local American Cancer Society (cancer.org) or your campus health center for resources and support to help you quit. Practice self-talk and have the words ready to refuse tobacco products when offered to you. Your current and future self will thank you.

per day based on your personal caloric needs. Eating a variety of fruits and vegetables may prevent cancers of the mouth and pharynx, esophagus, lungs, stomach, and colon and rectum. So, eat your fruits and veggies!

In order to get a head start on preventing cancer, try to be physically active most days for a weekly total of approximately 150 minutes. Maintaining a weight that is healthy for your body will decrease your risk. According to research, college students have an average of 20 hours a week that they can devote to leisure activities that include spending time with friends and extracurricular activities (Fosnacht, McCormick, and Lerma 2018). According to Yarnal and colleagues (2013), how college students should spend their leisure time (e.g., participation in physical activities, becoming involved in civic and academic programs) should be promoted as examples to avoid unhealthier alternatives because these types of activities can support improvements in their mood and coping skills.. You can increase your physical activity on campus by walking to class, riding your bike, taking advantage of campus recreational facilities, or joining an intramural sport.

Sun Exposure

Spring break is typically a time for college students to hit the road and head to sunny beaches. The majority of skin cancers are a result of spending too much time unprotected in the sun, especially between the hours of 10 a.m. to 2 p.m., when ultraviolet radiation exposure is highest and sunburns are most likely to occur. Sunburns, which increase the chance of developing skin cancer, occur after too much exposure to ultraviolet light, either from the sun or other sources such as sun lamps or tanning beds.

Skin cancer is the most commonly diagnosed cancer in the United States. Nonmelanoma skin cancer is defined based on where the cancer cells develop: in the basal, squamous, or Merkel cells of the skin. **Melanoma** is a cancer that develops in the skin's melanocytes, which are the cells that give

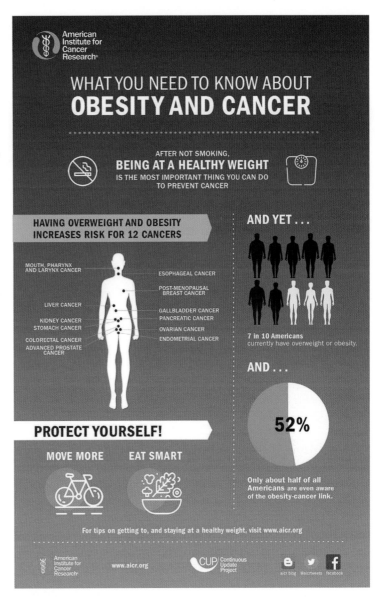

Figure 14.13   Being at a healthy weight can help prevent cancer.
Reprinted from American Institute for Cancer Research (2020). Available: www.aicr.org.

you your skin color. The American Cancer Society (2022) estimates that ultraviolet exposure is linked to over a million cases of basal and squamous cell skin cancers, which are classified as nonmelanoma skin cancers. It was estimated that there would be 99,780 new cases of malignant melanoma diagnosed in 2022. Malignant melanoma is the most dangerous type of skin cancer and the most likely to metastasize quickly if not detected early.

Melanoma can develop from existing moles or as a new mole. Conducting monthly skin self-examinations using the ABCDE method (figure 14.14) can help detect skin cancer in early stages. Treatment of skin cancer involves the removal by

Signs and Symptoms of Skin Cancer

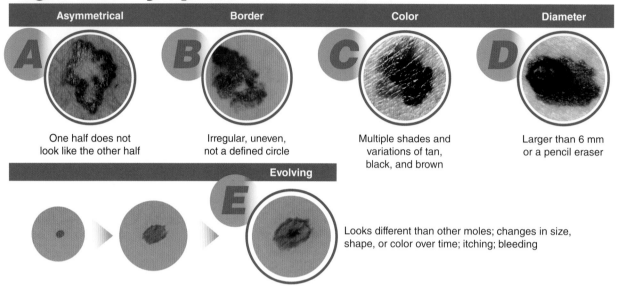

Figure 14.14   Use the ABCDE method to identify suspicious moles that need to be examined by a health care provider.

Reprinted from National Cancer Institute (1990).

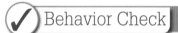 Behavior Check

Reduce Your Risk of Skin Cancer

Many college students and young adults spend a lot of time in the sun and at tanning salons. However, overexposure to ultraviolet radiation over many years causes not only skin cancer but also premature aging and wrinkles, damage to the eyes, and other types of infections. You are at an increased risk of developing skin cancer if you have any of the following traits or behaviors (Centers for Disease Control and Prevention 2021c):

- A lighter natural skin color
- A family history of skin cancer
- A personal history of skin cancer
- Exposure to the sun through work and play
- A history of sunburns, especially early in life
- A history of indoor tanning
- Skin that burns, freckles, reddens easily, or becomes painful in the sun
- Blue or green eyes
- Blond or red hair
- Certain types and a large number of moles

Think about your exposure to ultraviolet radiation and make a commitment to check your body every month for changes in moles or the development of new moles. Wear sunscreen, reapply it often, and try to stay out of the sun during the hottest times of the day, between 10 a.m. and 2 p.m.

electrocautery (burning), cryotherapy (freezing), or excision (cutting or shaving) of the suspicious lesion and perhaps an additional margin of skin and tissue around the mole.

Environment

Carcinogens in the environment that have been known to cause cancer include arsenic, asbestos, benzene, radon, soot, tar, vinyl chloride, and ultraviolet light. For example, radon is a naturally occurring odorless gas found underground that increases the risk of lung cancer. Because it can leak through the foundation in homes, many health departments in the United States offer home radon gas testing kits. Soot and tar, known to cause lung, skin, and liver cancers, can be found in many industrial settings. Environmental and occupational specialists work closely with businesses to make sure their employees are using protective gear, including masks, clothing, and sunscreen, to reduce their exposure to these chemicals and substances. Until the 20th century, asbestos was used as insulation in homes, schools, and other buildings, and many construction workers exposed to this substance developed lung cancer. The implementation of strict policies and laws preventing the use of this and certain other chemicals and substances has reduced the rates of some cancers associated with their use and long-term exposure.

> Females who have a first-degree relative (a mother, a sister, or daughter) with breast cancer are about twice as likely to develop breast cancer; females with two first-degree relatives with breast cancer are about five times more likely than average to be diagnosed with breast cancer (Breastcancer. org 2021).

Most Commonly Diagnosed Cancers

Tables 14.4 and 14.5 present the incidence, risk factors, warning signs, detection, treatment, and survival rates for the most commonly diagnosed cancers. You can discuss this information with your health care provider to decide when you should begin screenings based on your age, sex, lifestyle, and health behaviors.

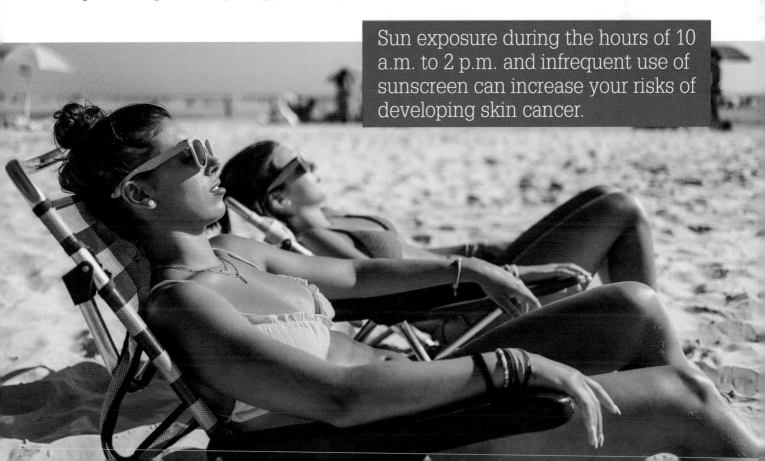

Sun exposure during the hours of 10 a.m. to 2 p.m. and infrequent use of sunscreen can increase your risks of developing skin cancer.

Table 14.4   Selected Cancers: Incidence, Risk Factors, and Warning Signs

Cancer site	Incidence trends	Risk factors	Warning signs
Lung Second most commonly diagnosed cancer and leading cause of cancer death	Rates declining annually by about 2% but decreasing faster among males than females	80% of lung cancer cases are caused by smoking. Other causes are exposure to radon gas, secondhand smoke, organic chemicals, air pollution, and diesel exhaust; occupational hazards such as paving, roofing, painting, and chimney sweeping; and genetic predisposition	Symptoms appear in late stages: persistent cough, blood in mucus, chest pain, voice changes, shortness of breath, and recurrent pneumonia or bronchitis
Breast Most frequently diagnosed cancer in females Second leading cause of death in females	Rates continue to increase by 0.5% per year	Overweight or obesity, postmenopausal hormone use (estrogen and progestin), physical inactivity, alcohol use, smoking, family history, genetic predisposition, high breast tissue density, type 2 diabetes, early onset of menstruation (before age 12) or late menopause (after age 55), use of oral contraceptives, never having had children or having a child after age 30	Lump or mass in breast; persistent changes in breast: thickening, swelling, distortion, tenderness, skin irritation, redness, scaliness, nipple abnormalities, nipple discharge
Colon/rectum Third most common cancer in males and females	Diagnosis rates have declined among older adults; however, there has been an increase among individuals younger than 50 years old	Obesity, physical inactivity, smoking, high consumption of red meats, low calcium intake, alcohol use, diet low of fruits and vegetables, family history, genetic predisposition, history of ulcerative colitis or Crohn's disease	Typically does not have early symptoms; symptoms include rectal bleeding, blood in stool, change in bowel habits or stool shape, cramping in lower abdomen, decreased appetite, weight loss
Prostate Most commonly diagnosed cancer and third leading cause of cancer deaths in males	Black males in the United States and Caribbean have the highest rates in the world	Increasing age, African heritage, family history, genetic predisposition, smoking	Early symptoms typically not present; advanced symptoms include weak or interrupted urine flow, urge to urinate more frequently, difficulty starting or stopping urine flow, blood in urine, pain or burning sensation when urinating, pain in hips, spine, or ribs
Cervix Increased risk of cervical cancer due to infection with human papilloma virus (HPV)	Rates have declined by more than half since 1975 due to HPV vaccine and Pap screening tests	HPV, sexual intercourse beginning at an early age, multiple sexual partners, suppressed immune system, multiple childbirths, smoking, long-term oral contraceptive use	Abnormal vaginal bleeding, mid-cycle bleeding, menstrual bleeding that is heavier and longer than normal, bleeding or vaginal discharge after menopause, bleeding after intercourse, douching, or a pelvic exam

Data from American Cancer Society (2021b).

Table 14.5   Selected Cancers: Recommendations for Screening, Treatment Options, and Survival Rates

Who should be screened	Test or procedure	Detection recommendation	Treatment options*	5-year survival rate
Lung Current or former smokers with a history of smoking 20+ packs per year	Low-dose helical CT	Annual lung cancer screenings for people with 20-pack per year smoking history starting at age 50 and continuing through age 80 if patient is in good health; current smokers or those who have quit within the last 15 years should be screened	Surgery, radiation, chemotherapy, immunotherapy, targeted therapy	17% for males, 24% for females 59% if localized
Breast Females age 40+	Mammography	Regular screening between ages 40 and 44; annually starting at age 45; biennially at age 55+	Surgical removal of tumor (lumpectomy), mastectomy (removal of breast), radiation post mastectomy, chemotherapy	90% 99% if localized
Colon/rectum Everyone age 50+	gFOBT (guaiac-based fecal occult blood test) or FIT (fecal immunochemical test) OR	Annual testing of stool	Surgery is most common; chemotherapy alone or in combination with radiation	65% 90% if localized
	Multi-target stool DNA test	Every 3 years		
	Flexible sigmoidoscopy OR	Every 5 years		
	Colonoscopy	Every 10 years		
	CT colonography	Every 5 years		
Prostate Males ages 50+; African American males ages 45+	Prostate-specific antigen (PSA) with or without digital rectal examination (DRE)	Negative result: Future screenings depend on a PSA of less than 2.5 ng/mL retested every 2 years Annual test if PSA level is 2.5 ng/mL or higher Prostate cancer advances slowly. Those without symptoms with a life expectancy of less than 10 years would not benefit from PSA screening. Health status is the primary consideration related to screenings.	Depends on age; younger males and early stages: observation over time instead of treatment; surgery; external beam radiation, radioactive seed implants (brachytherapy), hormonal therapy with surgery or radiation	98% >99% if localized

(continued)

Who should be screened	Test or procedure	Detection recommendation	Treatment options*	5-year survival rate
Cervix				
Females ages 25 to 65 Begin screening at age 25	HPV DNA test OR	Every 5 years	Loop electrosurgical excision procedure (LEEP) to remove abnormal tissue, cryotherapy (destroy cells with extreme cold), laser ablation, conization (cone-shaped removal of abnormal tissue); invasive treated with surgery or radiation with chemotherapy; targeted therapy	78% for white females younger than 50, 46% for Black females ages 50+ 92% if localized
	Pap test and HPV DNA test OR	Every 5 years		
	Pap test	Every 3 years		
Everyone age 65+		No screenings recommended if results from regular screenings were negative within the last 10 years and most recent test within the past 5 years		

*Treatment options are always dependent on the stage of the cancer.

Data from American Cancer Society (2021b).

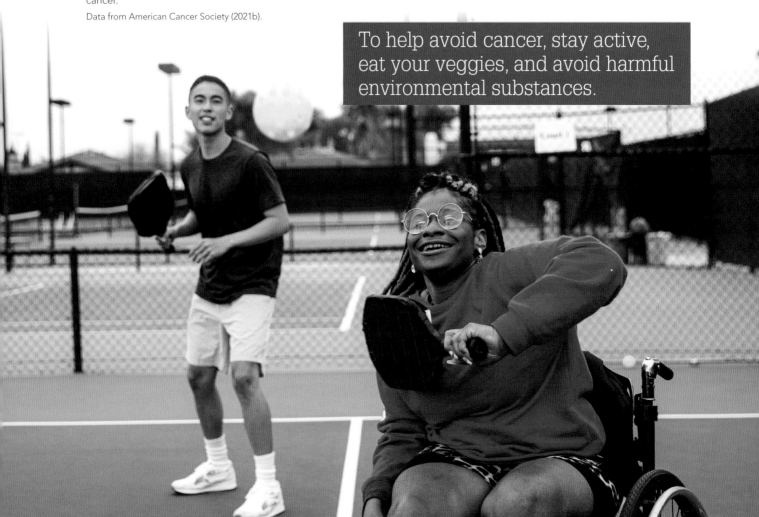

To help avoid cancer, stay active, eat your veggies, and avoid harmful environmental substances.

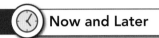 **Now and Later**

Cancer and COVID-19

Now

Certain groups who are more at risk of becoming infected with COVID-19 include older individuals and those who have comorbidities like high blood pressure, heart disease, and diabetes. What does this mean for people with cancer? Cancer and its treatments (e.g., radiation, surgery, chemotherapy) can impair the immune system, lowering the body's defenses against disease, including viruses like COVID-19. According to the American Cancer Society (2021b), initial studies about the risk of disability and death among cancer patients with COVID-19 showed an increased risk compared to those without cancer, especially those patients with lung and blood cancers or those who had had treatments within the past 30 days. However, more recent studies (Kuderer et al. 2020) indicate that there is no conclusive evidence that there was an increased risk of dying or that there was an increased death rate based on the timing of cancer treatment, and that risk factors such as smoking, older age, and obesity had similar outcomes that may have more of an influence on mortality and COVID-19 (American Cancer Society 2021b).

Later

We still have more to understand about the relationship of cancer on COVID-19 outcomes and the factors that influence serious illness and death. The National Cancer Institute (2020c) is studying cancer patients undergoing treatment while infected with COVID-19 to determine the effects of a compromised immune system and the body's ability to fight the virus; the American Cancer Society (2021b) is also conducting a cohort study about COVID-19 and effects on cancer outcomes.

Take Home

In order to keep your cancer risk low and avoid the possibility of complications from COVID-19, you need to practice positive health behaviors discussed in this book—eat well, move often, increase your strength, get plenty of sleep, and be proactive about early detection and screenings! Information about COVID-19 and its long-term effects is constantly evolving. Resources for current information include the following:

- American Cancer Society (cancer.org/coronavirus)
- National Cancer Institute (cancer.gov/about-cancer/coronavirus)
- Centers for Disease Control and Prevention (cdc.gov/coronavirus)
- Johns Hopkins University Coronavirus Resource Center (coronavirus.jhu.edu/map.html)

Summary

So, now what? The bad news is that not all cancers can be prevented or cured. Many research efforts are still focused on the prevention, detection, and treatment of cancers. The good news is that we know how to prevent many cancers, and there have been significant medical advancements in the early detection of cancer. More treatments exist that are specific to the type and stage of cancer, as well as new and improved medications and complementary therapies. Reducing your cancer risks means reducing your chances of getting cancer and having a great quality of life for decades to come.

www ONLINE LEARNING ACTIVITIES

Go to HK*Propel* and complete all of the online activities to further facilitate your learning:

Study Activities: Review the main concepts of the chapter.

Labs: Complete the labs your instructor assigns.

Videos: Look through the videos and choose which ones you want to try this week.

REVIEW QUESTIONS

1. What is the difference between benign and malignant tumors?
2. What does the acronym CAUTION mean?
3. List and describe the primary ways cancer can be treated.
4. What are the most diagnosed cancers among males and among females?
5. What are the reasons for health disparities related to cancer prevention and treatment?
6. List environmental chemicals and substances that are linked to cancer.
7. What are the primary causes of cancer?
8. How does smoking affect someone with COVID-19?

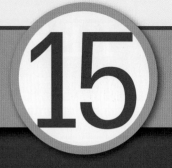

Fitness and Well-Being: Today and Beyond

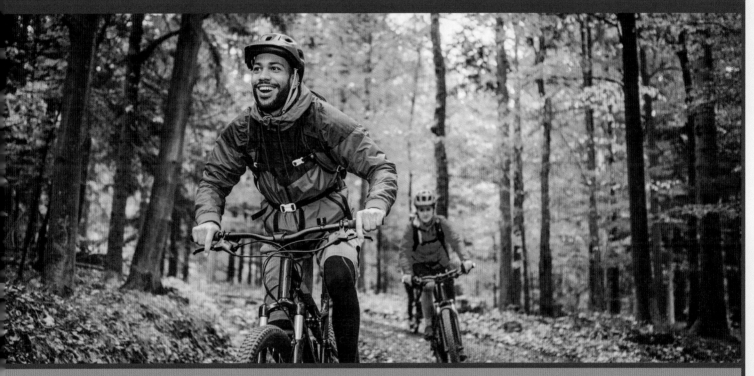

OBJECTIVES

- Gain an understanding of how our society is rapidly aging worldwide, and how health choices greatly influence a person's life span and health span.
- Understand the concept of intrinsic capacity and how it greatly influences functional fitness across the life span but especially in the last decades of life.
- Define and discuss differences between conventional medical practices and complementary and alternative medicine.
- Identify and discuss resources that will be needed to maintain health behaviors and ultimately fitness and well-being in our culture where the healthy choice is often not the easy choice.
- Discuss the benefits of wearable technologies to monitor and encourage adherence to one's movement program and to assess health parameters.
- Consider the similarities and differences between lifestyle coaching and personal fitness training and how they may assist a person with health behavior adherence.
- Revisit SMART goals and begin to consider how they will need to be adapted throughout the life span.

KEY TERMS

Well-Being Across the Decades

In the first few chapters, we discussed the importance of a positive outlook on well-being. We promised to minimize scare tactics, avoid prescriptive recommendations (e.g., you must do this or that!), and discourage quick fixes. Rather, we wanted to provide general guidelines for healthy moving, eating, and sleeping choices, and provide ideas so that you can make healthier choices. Finally, we wanted you to build your behavioral toolkit and motivational muscles. We hope we have broadened your outlook on the importance of integrating movement and well-being practices into your life—not just during your college years but for a lifetime.

We hope this culminating overview of fitness and wellness concepts will help you remember that life is precious, and that how you choose to live it will dictate your life span and, as importantly, your health span. Investing in these behaviors that enhance your

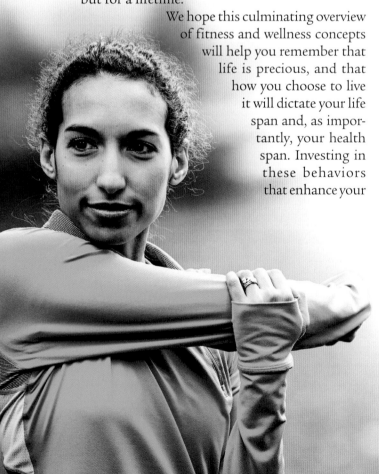

well-being will give you energy and vitality to not only do what you have to do but also what you want to do every day. And because we are social animals, it is imperative to surround yourself with people who also invest in healthy behaviors to maximize their well-being. This choice will ultimately make your own decisions to move more and sit less much easier. You will know when you have arrived at "living well" because you will not have to think about it—you will be too busy living it.

Putting positive well-being practices at the forefront of our daily lives can and will make a difference in your quality of living now and in your future decades. However, you will need to be very intentional about your well-being practices because our modern world makes the less healthy choice the easy choice at every turn. For example, as shown in figure 15.1, the U.S. workplace has become increasingly sedentary over the decades, and the trends continue—note the increase in sedentary and light work compared to the reduction in moderate work from 1960 to 2010 (Church et al. 2011). This means we are sitting more and moving less at work because our jobs require less daily physical activity. As discussed in previous chapters, the World Health Organization's guidelines on physical activity and sedentary living (Bull et al. 2020) recommend reducing sedentary behavior and increasing physical activity for better health—remember, some physical activity is better than none.

The majority of the research introduced in this book tells us that in order to be well, we need to move more, sit less, and sleep better. The integrated ebb and flow of the wellness continuum (chapter 1) reminds us that our relative efforts (i.e., how much and what we do) to improve the various areas of wellness differ across the life span. Concepts introduced in chapter 2 remind us that all movement counts, and some days you will engage in intentional exercise, whereas other days you will have lots of physical activity. Ideally, most

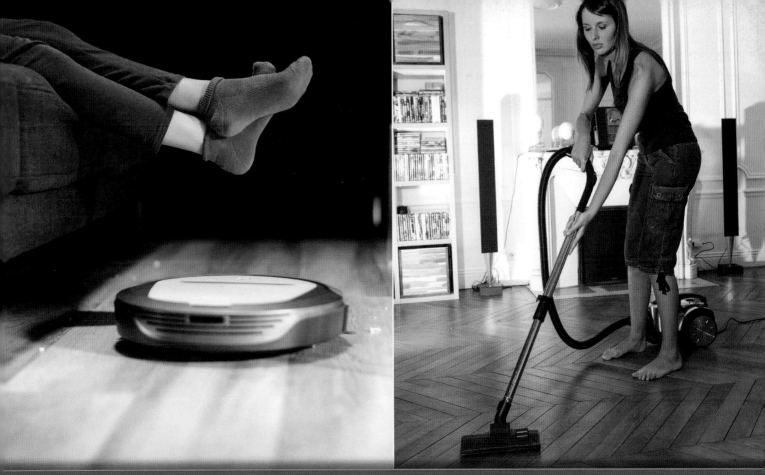

Has the robot vacuum cleaner taken away daily movement opportunities?

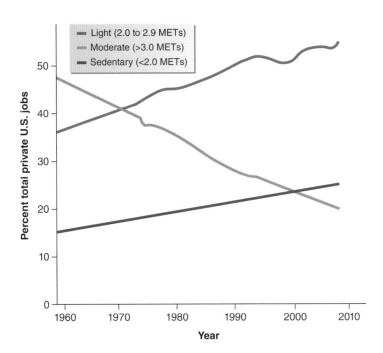

Figure 15.1 The reduction of activity levels in the workplace. Between 1960 and 2010, U.S. jobs required less physical work. Note the increase in light daily work versus the decrease in moderate daily work.

days you will have both types of movement. Reducing your sedentary behavior and your sitting time should also be a goal every single day. Remember the equation: human movement = exercise + physical activity – sedentary behavior. In addition, the importance of your movement pattern over a 24-hour period (an average day) is gaining more importance. The 24-hour activity cycle paradigm reminds us that time spent in sleep, sedentary behavior, light-intensity physical activity, and moderate-to vigorous-intensity physical activity interact and impact multiple domains of health in complicated and unknown ways.

However, adult physical inactivity rates are at an all-time high as a result of the continued decline in daily movement practices. According to the Centers for Disease Control and Prevention (2022), the highest prevalence of inactivity in the United States is in Puerto Rico (49.4 percent), compared to the lowest in Colorado (17.7 percent). Regionally, states in the South have the highest prevalence of physical inactivity (27.5 percent), followed by the Midwest (24.7 percent) and West (21.0 percent). On average, a quarter of the people

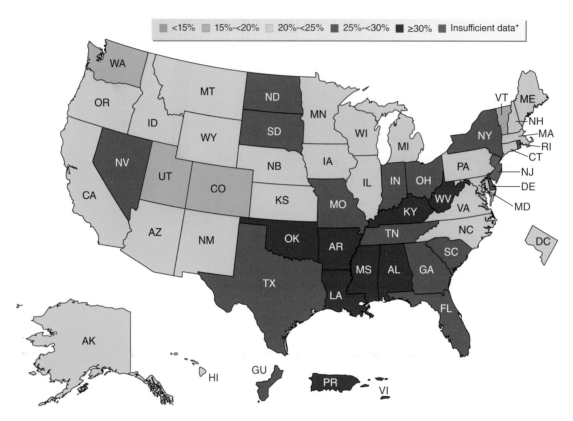

Figure 15.2   The prevalence of adult physical inactivity in the United States.

Reprinted from "Adult Physical Inactivity Prevalence Maps," Centers for Disease Control and Prevention, last modified February 17, 2022, www.cdc.gov/physicalactivity/data/inactivity-prevalence-maps/index.html#overall.

living in the United States are physically inactive (see figure 15.2).

Living Longer or Living Better?

The World Health Organization (2022) reports that by 2050, the world's population of people aged 60 and older will double to 2.1 billion, and the number of persons aged 80 and older is expected to triple to reach 426 million. By 2030 (just around the corner), 1 in 6 people in the world will be aged 60 years or over. The choices you make now will likely influence if you make it to 80 years of age and how well you live in these older years. A landmark study following Harvard alumni from ages 35 to 74 taught us that moving throughout the life span might add more years to your life (Paffenbarger et al. 1986). Although all your body systems decline with advancing age, starting a physical activity program early and keeping it up throughout your life will help "bend the aging curve" for key systems, helping you retain your functional fitness with age. For example, being a consistent mover will help delay muscle decline as you age, which will keep you active and independent in your older years (see

figure 15.3). There is much research supporting the importance of intentional exercise (especially resistance training), regular physical activity, and

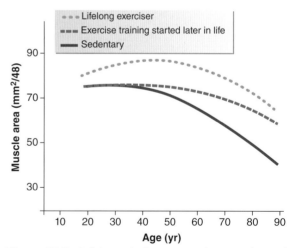

Figure 15.3   Lifelong decline in muscle area, depending on physical activity level. Starting and sticking with an active lifestyle will delay physical decline later in life and can give you more years of life.

Reprinted by permission from J.F. Signorile, *Bending the Aging Curve: The Complete Exercise Guide for Older Adults* (Champaign, IL: Human Kinetics, 2011), 13.

minimal sedentary behavior to preserve function for the heart, brain, and metabolic and immune systems, to name a few. This protection becomes obvious in midlife and beyond.

Another example of this current data is the 2018 Physical Activity Guidelines Advisory Scientific Report (Katzmarzyk et al. 2019) that described a strong link between sedentary behavior (mostly sitting time) and increased risk of cardiovascular disease (CVD) and type 2 diabetes (T2D). As these two diseases influence other chronic diseases and conditions (e.g., cancer), and with CVD being our top cause of mortality, it is not surprising that sedentary behavior is also linked to mortality. As an example, figure 15.4 shows the association between sitting time and moderate to vigorous physical activity with risk of all-cause mortality. Beyond life span and health span, most middle-age and older adults value living independently in their own homes, having autonomy, and making decisions about how and where they spend their time. Your well-being will directly influence your ability to go and do in your later stages of life. Invest in your future self now.

> It is up to you to move more so that you can overcome the trend of sedentary living and live a longer, more independent life.

Chronological Age and Functional Fitness

The definitions of various age dimensions have been proposed, changed, and of increasing interest in the past few decades. For example, according to Stanton (1996), there are differences between the following ages: chronological, biological, psychological, and functional. More contemporary thinking endorses the use of chronological age, biological age, and

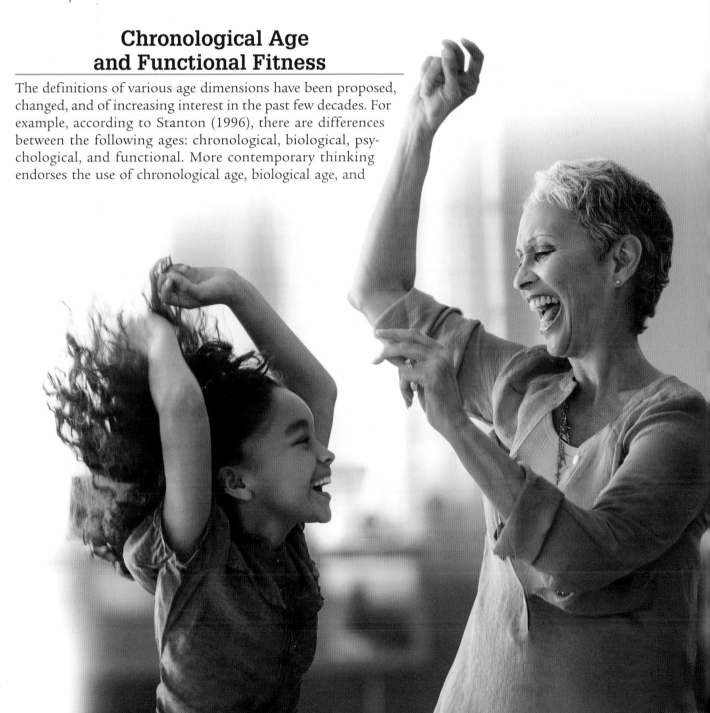

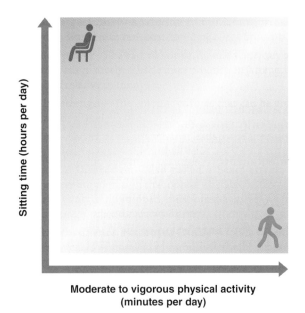

Figure 15.4 Sitting time and moderate to vigorous physical activity time interact to impact risk of all-cause mortality.

Adapted from *2018 Physical Activity Guidelines Advisory Committee Scientific Report.*

psychological age. However, world experts are also moving toward an integrated concept termed **intrinsic capacity**. As we unpack these various definitions of age (see figure 15.5), we encourage you to think about your own aging process and the aging process of your family members and close friends, especially those in late middle age (50s and 60s) and in their 70s and 80s. Does someone you know have great walking function and capacity for physical work or leisure activities but perhaps less robust cognitive function (i.e., memory and reasoning) or vice versa? Does someone you know have lots of energy and vitality? Which health behaviors did these people have that likely contributed to them aging well or poorly (e.g., daily movement, healthy eating, smoking, excessive alcohol intake, etc.)?

Intrinsic capacity is the term that the World Health Organization (2015) has developed to describe a public health model to support the idea that the older age stage of life is not merely progressive functional decline and diseases. The definition is the composite of all physical and mental capacities of a person within the five

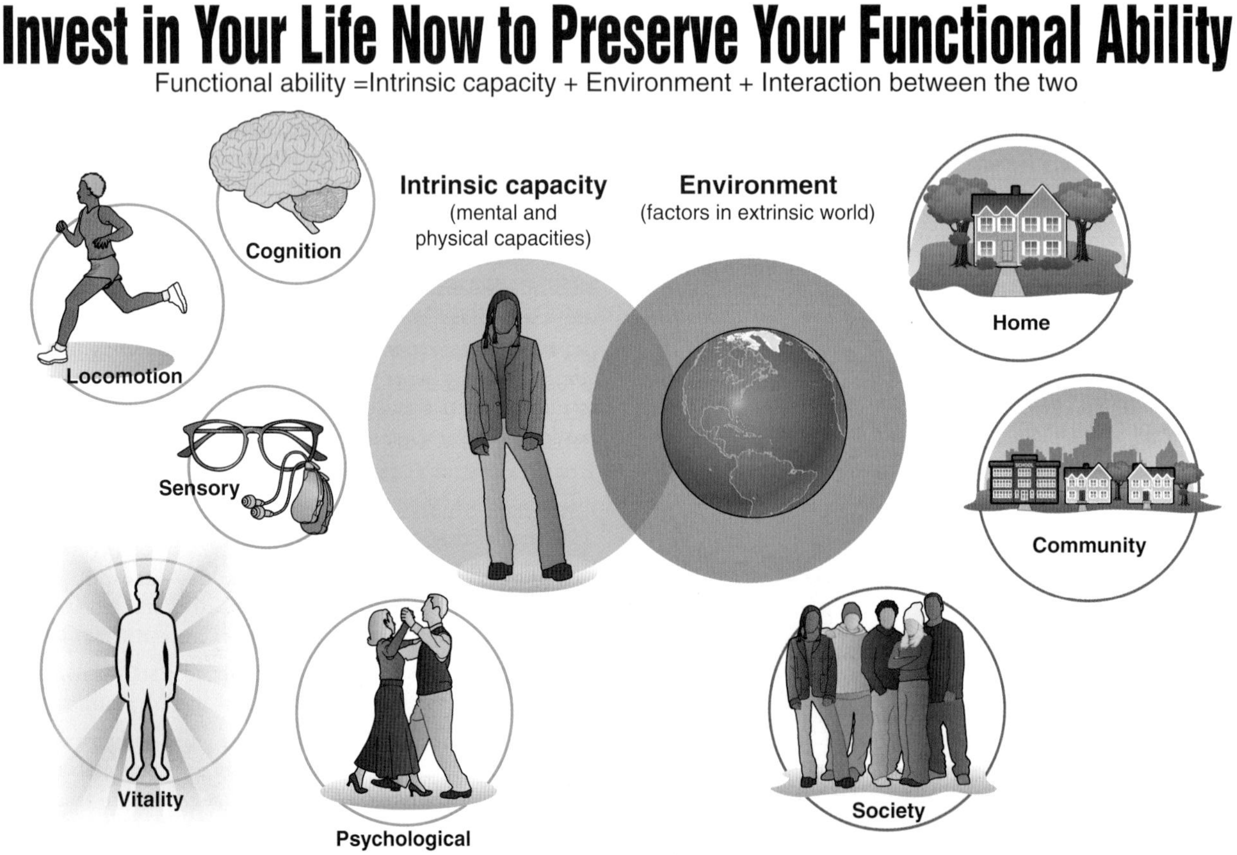

Invest in Your Life Now to Preserve Your Functional Ability

Functional ability =Intrinsic capacity + Environment + Interaction between the two

Locomotion

Cognition

Intrinsic capacity
(mental and physical capacities)

Environment
(factors in extrinsic world)

Home

Sensory

Community

Vitality

Psychological

Society

Figure 15.5 A key to your well-being, especially in middle age and older, is your functional ability determined by your intrinsic mental and physical capacities and how you interact with your environment.

subdomains of cognition, locomotion, sensory, vitality, and psychological. This current view is that older adults can maintain functioning and well-being and remain productive members of society. Simply, functional ability is determined by the intrinsic capacity of the individual, relevant environmental factors, and the interaction between the two. It is acknowledged that intrinsic capacity generally declines from adulthood to advanced age; however, less appreciated is how variable this decline can be, even among family members who share genetics and lifestyles. Functional ability can also be maintained with environmental support and compensation strategies. For example, an older person can maintain mobility by using a cane or walker. Another common example are eyeglasses or hearing aids to maintain sensory abilities (Koivunen et al, 2022).

With your current focus on personal fitness and well-being and plans for your future self, do you

✓ Behavior Check

The Dallas Bed-Rest Study

Over 50 years ago, a group of scientists (Saltin et al. 1968) did an experiment in which they paid five healthy 20-year-old men to lie in bed for three weeks to see what would happen to their health. The scientists then analyzed the subjects' $\dot{V}O_2$max, body composition, and other health parameters. In just three weeks, these 20-year-olds developed physiologic characteristics of men twice their age. The scientists then put the men on an eight-week exercise-training program following the three-week bed rest. Exercise did more than reverse the bed-rest deterioration: The subjects were healthier than before the study. This study was a demonstration of the dramatic effects of not moving followed by exercise training on fitness and health parameters.

An identical study was performed on these same five men 30 years later (McGuire et al. 2001). The scientists found that three weeks of bed rest for the subjects, now 50 years old, had a more profound effect on their physical work capacity than did 30 years of aging. Finally, McGavock and colleagues (2009) repeated this same experiment again 10 years later, when the men were 60 years old. The men's decline in cardiorespiratory fitness ($\dot{V}O_2$max) was comparable with what they experienced after three weeks of strict bed rest when they were 20. This unique set of studies shows the dramatic effects of not moving and the immediate response of the body to increased exercise.

These studies also remind us of the importance of human movement over the life span. If you have done the lab activities with this textbook, you have acquired personal information about your physical abilities at a young age. Consider retesting yourself yearly. Perform a well-check and keep the information in a personal health folder on your computer. Keep track of your own changes throughout your life span. Be your own well-being champion for life!

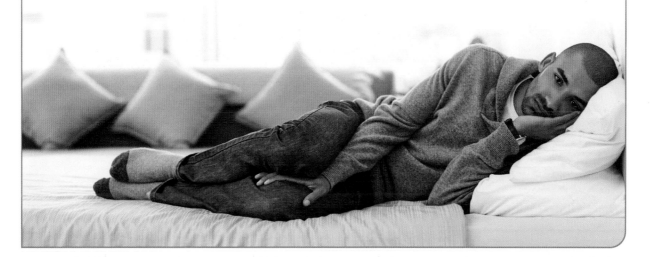

think you will age well and travel through your older ages with a high level of intrinsic capacity? You might know older adults who are not thriving well and have greatly compromised well-being. We might say to ourselves, "I'm not going to be like that when I am older." Yet if you do not take care of yourself now, that may be who you become. What investments do you want to make in your moving, eating, sleeping, connecting, and stress management behaviors? Consider and enact the steps you want to take so that you do not become any "older" than your actual chronological age.

Behavioral Systems Approach to Healthy Living

There is no question COVID-19 impacted population health and well-being globally. Improving healthy living choices (e.g., regularly moving, making healthy nutritional choices, getting adequate rest) are important to reduce negative outcomes of future pandemics or other disease outbreaks (Pronk and Faghy 2022). For decades our healthy living focus has been on changing individuals as opposed to looking at complex causes and factors that prevent people from making the healthy choice the easy choice. These models are not new, but they are complex because they involve a multidisciplinary approach.

As a society we are living longer, but we must ask ourselves: Are we living better? And how does society support our healthy choices? According to the National Association of Chronic Disease Directors (2022), 16 states receive funding to support physical activity and healthy eating through state-based public health programs. Public health programming per-capita expenditure is approximately $0.25, far below the estimated $1,429 per-capita cost of obesity-related medical care. For years we have been discussing community prevention, but we continue to kick the can down the road, and it is clearly catching up to us. The "right to move" (Antonucci et al. 2012) predicted problems that society will face by 2030 if we do not become more proactive in combating our decline in levels of physical activity and increasing obesity. COVID-19 ought to be a wake-up call that we need to not only take individual action, but also community action. Be the functional fitness change agent for the healthy behaviors you want to see in your community.

Approaches to Medicine

Conventional Western medicine is a system in which medical doctors and other health care professionals (such as nurses, pharmacists, physician's assistants, and therapists) treat symp-

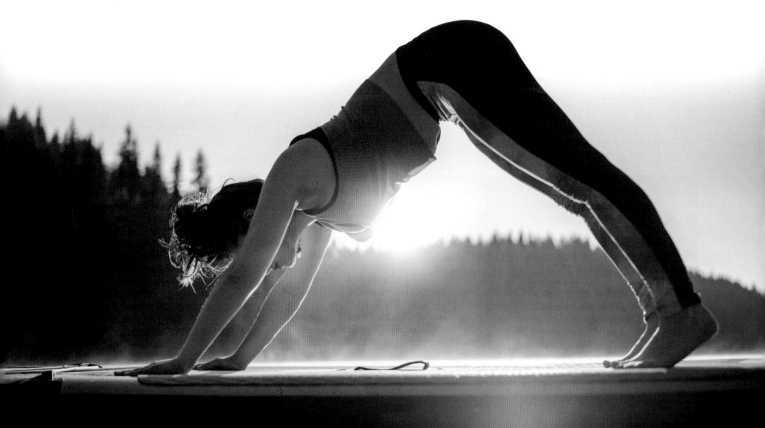

toms and diseases. For example, if you need a knee replacement, the painful knee is thought to be fixed once it has been replaced and you have completed physical therapy. These types of **conventional medical practices** are also called allopathic medicine, biomedicine, or just plain mainstream medicine. Medical doctors, doctors of osteopathy, and allied health professionals practice standard care.

Complementary and alternative medicine (CAM) is another approach that honors your body as a system and works with it to heal you. A few examples of alternative practices include yoga, meditation, and chiropractic medicine. According to the National Center for Complementary and Integrative Health (Clarke et al. 2018), yoga was the most used complementary health approach among U.S. adults in 2017 (14.3 percent). The use of meditation increased more than threefold, from 4.1 percent in 2012 to 14.2 percent. In terms of who uses CAM, those who identify as females are more likely to use yoga (19.8 percent versus 8.6 percent), meditation (16.3 percent versus 11.8 percent), and see a chiropractor (11.1 percent versus 9.4 percent, see figure 15.6) than individuals who identify as males.

CAM approaches have usually not gone through the same research rigor as double-blind clinical research trials of conventional medical practices. However, the standards of lab research may not fully apply to CAM because its benefits involve not only physical health but also mental and psychological health, which are difficult to quantitatively evaluate through rigorous studies. CAM approaches tend to be more individual in their outcomes; many people who feel better after CAM treatments cannot explain why. You may want to consider these less-invasive options for well-being. Given the lack of research on the benefits, however, this is a choice best left up to the individual.

Finding Resources to Enhance Your Fitness and Well-Being

One traditional way to improve your fitness and well-being is to hire a personal fitness trainer or a lifestyle coach to help you learn how to exercise and make other healthy choices. Fitness facilities and businesses across the nation offer personal training, and many are also beginning to offer lifestyle coaching. Personal trainers might speak with you about sedentary living and physical activity, but remember that if they are employed by exercise facilities, they often focus on exercise routines using the facility's equipment. Lifestyle coaches, on the other hand, are typically required to be knowledgeable about a variety of topics and may work in places such as schools, hospitals, private practice, long-term care centers, government agencies, and even some large companies. You might also be surprised to see what health and wellness options

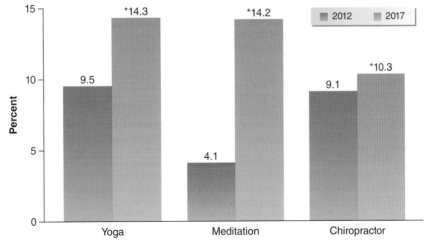

Figure 15.6 Increases in yoga, meditation, and chiropractor care from 2012 to 2017.

*Significantly different from 2012 (*p* < 0.05).

Notes: Estimates are age adjusted using the projected 2000 U.S. population as the standard population and three age groups: 18 to 44, 45 to 64, and 65 and over. Estimates are based on household interviews of a sample of the civilian noninstitutionalized population. Access data table for figure 15.6 at https://www.cdc.gov/nchs/data/databriefs/db325_table-508.pdf#1.

Reprinted from National Center for Health Statistics (2012 and 2017).

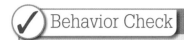

Behavior Check

How to Evaluate Complementary and Alternative Medicine

When evaluating CAM options, consider the following:

1. Check out the online resources located on the National Center for Complementary and Integrative Health: https://nccih.nih.gov. Look at the Health Info page or consult a specialist through the NCCIH Clearinghouse.
2. Talk to your health care provider about safety and effectiveness of the treatment and potential interactions with any medications and vitamins you are taking.
3. Take precautions. Don't just try a treatment—do some research, read peer-reviewed research studies, listen to your body, and make sure CAM is a safe and effective approach for you.

your local pharmacy offers. Finally, if you want to go it alone, consider purchasing an activity tracker to monitor your daily movement habits. Recall that the human movement paradigm discussed in chapter 2 includes getting enough physical activity and exercise as well as minimizing sedentary living.

Wearable Technology

In 2022, ACSM named wearable technology the number one trend in their worldwide fitness trends survey; this is its fifth time at the top spot since it was first included in the survey in 2016 (Thompson 2022). Wearable technology, which includes **activity trackers** such as smart watches, heart rate monitors, and GPS trackers, can be used for a variety of purposes. These can track step count, heart rate, body temperature, calories used, and sitting time. Newer innovations of wearable technology include reliable and valid measures of blood pressure, oxygen saturation, respiratory rate, and even an electrocardiogram. Wearable technology can also be multimodal, monitoring other aspects of health and well-being beyond movement to include, as an example, sleep.

A systematic review of the literature (Laranjo et al. 2021) reveals that activity trackers in combination with apps are effective at increasing daily physical activity. However, wearable activity tracker technology is changing constantly, making it challenging to find up-to-date evidence-based research. The accuracy of these devices may also vary widely. Despite these issues, wearable technology is estimated to be a $100 billion industry.

Activity Trackers as an Alternative to Fitness Centers

In her book *The Joy Choice* (2022), Michelle Segar describes numerous accounts of clients who did not know that moving throughout the day counted toward health and fitness, believing the only way to get fit was to join a fitness facility. The obvious barriers to using a formal fitness program or facility—cost, discomfort using equipment, or difficulty attending classes at a specific time or day—are reduced or overcome by activity trackers. Many people also find using an activity tracker less intimidating than joining a fitness facility. These devices can offer objective accountability as well as social connection with apps; they may be a game changer for a population-based explosion of movement.

The COVID-19 pandemic has also provided many individuals the incentive and opportunity to consider using activity trackers as an alternative to their fitness routine in a facility. The International Health and Racquet Sports Association (2021) reported that the U.S. fitness facility industry lost $20.4 billion in 2020 after a previous record year of sales. The pandemic resulted in over 17 percent of fitness facilities in the United States closing—and as high as 40 to 50 percent in other countries. Many people turned to activity trackers for an alternative for accountability and connection.

Activity Trackers in Combination With Coaching

Activity trackers can assist you in behavior change by helping you set more realistic movement goals that are specific to the demands of your own life. They can also prompt you to move more and sit less, hold you accountable for your goals, and record your movement in an easy and convenient manner. Research suggests that using a wearable activity tracker as either the primary component of an intervention or as part of a broader physical activity intervention has the potential to increase physical activity participation (Brickwood et al. 2019). Coaches have also been found to have more success working with clients who had activity trackers after both parties had acquired personal experience using the devices (Kiessling and Kennedy-Armbruster 2016). Because physical activity interventions are often short term, the inclusion of an activity tracker may provide an effective tool to assist health professionals to provide ongoing monitoring and support.

Personal Training and Lifestyle Coaching

If you are already physically active and want to enhance your exercise options, working with a personal trainer or lifestyle coach may be effective for you. Working with a personal trainer can be especially helpful if you join a fitness facility and want to learn how to use equipment.

Which One Is Right for You?

Once you have decided that you would like to work with a professional, the next step is to determine whether you need a **personal trainer**, a **lifestyle coach**, or someone who practices a blend of these approaches. Personal trainers will help you learn how to use equipment correctly, teach you how to do movements in a strength and conditioning area, and help design or adapt a fitness program to meet your needs. Certified lifestyle coaches, on the other hand, will work on the behavioral aspects of changing your perspective and setting realistic goals. Make sure you know the ultimate goal and training background of the coach you select. This will help you find out if you are getting the coaching you need to continue on your path for consistent movement and lifestyle improvements.

If you prefer instruction and motivation, check out a facility that offers small group training. It helps to be trained in a small group so you can eventually venture out on your own. Once you know what to do, motivation and commit-

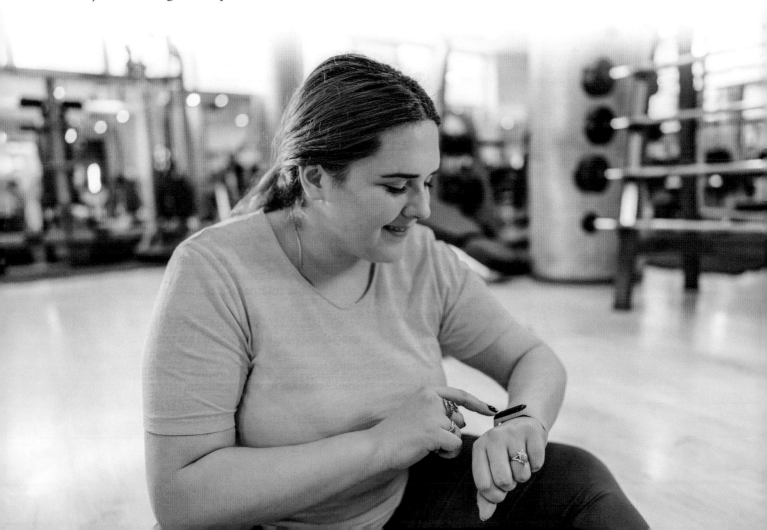

ment become the key drivers of success. You can stay motivated and committed, and perhaps meet others on the well-being path, by working with a coach who checks in on your goals and holds you accountable to them in these small groups. Ultimately, remember: The movement program that will give you the most benefit is the one that you will sustain over time.

> Personal training is about transferring knowledge and skills related to fitness instruction and goal setting, whereas lifestyle coaching is about behavioral skill development where you are encouraged to set your own personal goals.

Credentialing Process

Before you hire a personal trainer or lifestyle coach, be sure that they have a professional fitness certification approved by the National Commission for Certifying Agencies (NCCA). Local or in-house certifications or training programs may not be rigorous enough to meet clinical practice standards. NCCA-accredited certification tests are developed by exercise and fitness professionals based on specific knowledge, skills, and attributes necessary to enhance healthy movement practices and prevent injury. Many national certifications include both written and practical examinations for which a fitness professional must demonstrate basic skills in exercise leadership and knowledge of its related components (e.g., anatomy and physiology, intensity monitoring, injury prevention). All NCCA-accredited fitness certifications also involve cardiopulmonary resuscitation (CPR) and automated external defibrillator (AED) training.

The United States Registry of Exercise Professionals (USREPS) is a nonprofit corporation composed of organizations that offer NCCA-accredited exercise certifications. The mission of USREPS is to secure recognition of registered exercise

> One of the best ways to know if an exercise professional has an NCCA-accredited certification is to check the United States Registry of Exercise Professionals at www.usreps.org.

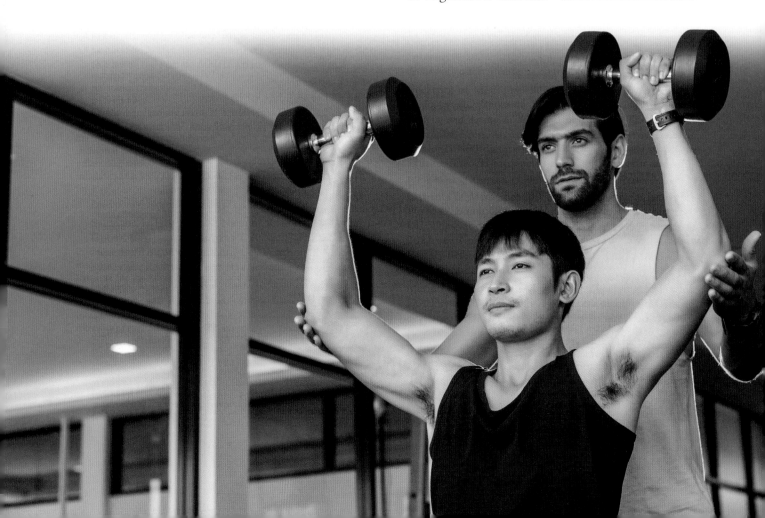

professionals for their distinct roles in medical, health, fitness, and sports performance fields. Use both the NCCA accreditation and www.usreps.org websites when looking for fitness professionals. If you already have a personal trainer, you can find out if they have an NCCA-accredited certification by viewing the registry at www.usreps.org.

SMART Goals Are Smart for Life

Let's take a moment to rethink the SMART goals you established earlier in chapters 2 and 3. How did you do? Did you meet your goals? What worked and what did not work? How will you continue to work toward wellness goals in the future? Most of us start our fitness and well-being journeys with physical fitness goals because they seem to be the easiest and are the priority. Now that you have learned more about broader wellness concepts such as nutrition, stress, addiction, and sexual health, your next steps might be integrating a well-being goal across multiple domains. Do you want to reduce stress, improve your nutrition practices, sleep better, or improve your relationships with others? To truly function and feel well, most people are meeting their wellness goals in many dimensions at the same time. Start slow, gain some wins, add more goals, and continue to spiral up!

As you know by now, wellness is more than looking good and being physically fit. It is also about pondering your dreams, living your best present while mapping your awesome future. Setting specific SMART goals, working toward them, and meeting most of them for all your well-being categories will greatly enhance the chance that you will live a long, productive, and fulfilling life. This life well lived will also be aligned with your values, giving you peace of mind. Circling back to the World Health Organization's definition of intrinsic capacity for the aging process, you will notice that it mirrors the notion of functional fitness described throughout this textbook. Intrinsic capacity is reflected by observations of vitality, including energy and metabolism, neuromuscular function,

and immune and stress response functions of the body (Bautmans et al. 2022). If you use your favorite browser to search a definition of vitality, you will see phrases like "exuberant physical strength or mental vigor," "capacity for the continuation of a meaningful or purposeful existence," or "the power to live or grow." We all know people who have a lot of vitality and those who do not, and this is typically obvious when you interact with them. We all admire others with a high level of vitality, especially those who maintain vitality as they get older. Your decisions about health behavior and lifestyle, especially physical activity and exercise, have major implications for your vitality, and therefore your intrinsic capacity, as you age. How might you embrace life's opportuni-

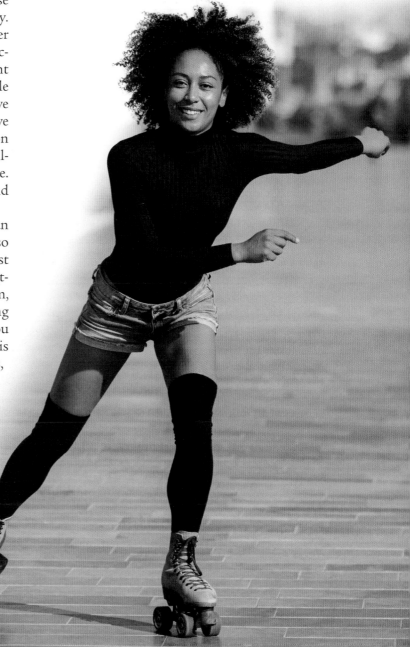

ties and overcome life's challenges in decades to come to maintain your well-being and keep your vitality?

Procrastination: Just Do It!

Now that we have reviewed some of the larger wellness concepts related to living well throughout the life span, let's focus on a specific trait that commonly sabotages us: **procrastination**. You may be thinking, "It's all fine and good that we've learned about wellness, but I think I'll start working on it tomorrow."

It is generally quite easy to work on wellness concepts when you are with a group or enrolled

> Every day spent procrastinating is another day spent worrying about that thing. Do it *now* and move on with your life.

in a class; goal setting on your own can be a bigger challenge. Think about one or two specific things related to your own personal well-being that you often procrastinate. If you are not a procrastinator, think of a time in the past when this was a problem for you. Do you know why you procrastinate? For some people, lack of motivation is a key factor in procrastination. For many others, it a puzzle. You may tell yourself that you really want to do something, but for some mysterious reason, you just cannot seem to get around to it. We all have our own reasons why we tend to forget about our functional fitness and wellness goals. If this is something you feel you need to consider, search online for procrastination tests, and see how you fare on this issue. Your favorite browser can also provide many tips and strategies to overcome this sabotaging and stress-producing habit.

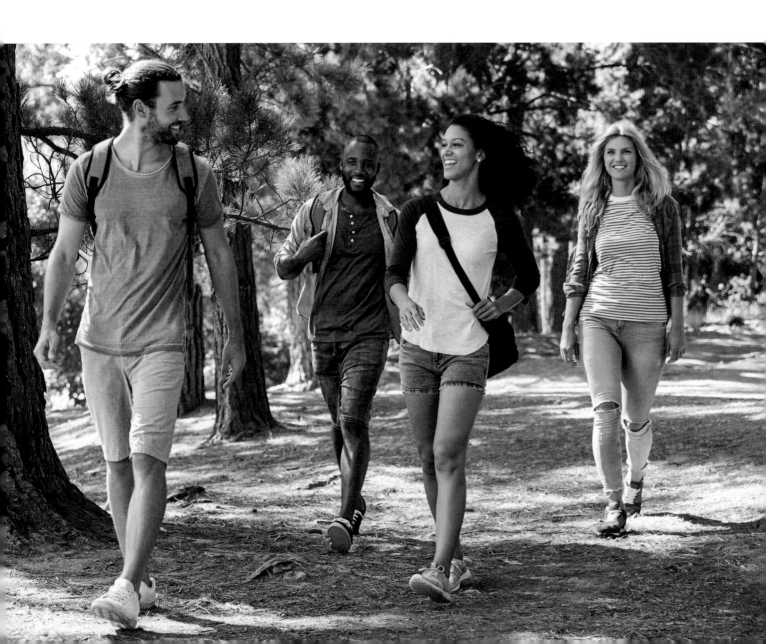

Fitness and Well-Being: Choosing Your Way of Life

The goal of this book is to provide you with information to help you set your own goals and priorities related to fitness and wellness practices. If you have implemented any of the information from this book, you are on your way to attaining a higher quality of life.

We hope as you chart your life path, you will also integrate your fitness and wellness plan. Fitting your personal fitness and wellness goals into your life plan will help you bridge the gap between college and career. Keep in mind that fitness and well-being best practices are processes. We are all a work in progress. If you continue to put your best foot forward and work to improve the various dimensions of well-being (which ultimately may improve your life span and health span), you will reap the benefits of a life well lived. Remember to think globally but work locally: What each person contributes is what makes us better as a society. We wish you well as you continue to make forward-thinking choices toward your own fitness and wellness way of life.

ONLINE LEARNING ACTIVITIES

Go to HK*Propel* and complete all of the online activities to further facilitate your learning:

Study Activities: Review the main concepts of the chapter.

Labs: Complete the labs your instructor assigns.

Videos: Look through the videos and choose which ones you want to try this week.

REVIEW QUESTIONS

1. How are social demographics changing in the United States and worldwide that will greatly impact every aspect of society?
2. How did the U.S. workplace change between 1960 and 2010, and what effect did this have on the physical activity patterns of individuals?
3. Define intrinsic capacity and list and describe the five main subcategories.
4. Describe how a healthier physical fitness can influence the intrinsic capacity and functional fitness of a typical older adult (around 70 years old).
5. Describe how wearable technology can monitor health outcomes and influence health behavior adherence with respect to one of your current SMART goals.
6. How is a personal trainer different from a lifestyle coach?
7. Revisit your personal movement SMART goal from an earlier chapter and anticipate how you might change it when you are 50 years of age and then again at 80 years of age.

GLOSSARY

24-hour activity cycle (24-HAC) paradigm—Represents the physiological mechanisms by which sleep, sedentary behavior, light-intensity physical activity, and moderate-to-vigorous physical activity (MVPA) affect health collectively.

abstinence—The choice not to engage in any type of sexual activity, which may include oral sex, anal intercourse, or vaginal intercourse.

ACSM exercise guidelines—The American College of Sports Medicine (ACSM)'s evidence-based recommendations to help the general public approach intentional exercise practices, which are categorized into cardiorespiratory exercise, resistance exercise, flexibility exercise, and neuromotor exercise.

activity trackers—A device or application for monitoring and tracking fitness-related data such as distance walked or run, nutritional information, and in some cases heartbeat and quality of sleep.

addiction—When someone becomes dependent on a drug, alcohol, or a behavior (e.g., exercising) and cannot stop despite the negative effects.

adenosine triphosphate (ATP)—The energy source for cellular processes.

adenosine triphosphate–phosphocreatine (ATP-PC) system—The energy system that supplies immediate but limited energy to muscle cells through the breakdown of cellular stores of ATP and creatine phosphate (CP).

adiposity—An expression of how much stored energy, or fat, the body contains, similar to the term *body fat*.

adrenal glands—Endocrine glands located near the kidneys that produce several hormones important for the stress response, including adrenaline and cortisol.

adrenocorticotropic hormone (ACTH)—In the stress cascade, ACTH stimulates the release of cortisol from the cortex of the adrenal gland.

air displacement plethysmography—A technique for measuring body density that uses air displacement rather than water.

allostasis—An organism's process of achieving stability, or homeostasis, through physiological or behavioral change.

allostatic load—The wear and tear on the body that results from chronic stress; the physiological consequences of chronic exposure to changing or elevated neuroendocrine response.

anabolic-androgenic steroids (AAS)—Synthetic variations of the male hormone testosterone that both build muscle and produce male sexual characteristics.

angina—A condition caused by a reduced blood supply to the heart muscle; typically characterized as severe pain or pressure in the chest that often spreads to the shoulders, arms, and neck.

anorexia nervosa—An eating disorder characterized by low weight, fear of gaining weight, and a strong desire to be thin that results in food restriction.

antioxidants—Substance found in food that can block the formation and action of free radicals and repair damage that they cause.

areola—Darker skin around the nipple of the breast.

arrhythmia—A condition in which the heartbeats with an irregular or abnormal rhythm.

arteriosclerosis—A condition whereby the walls of the arteries are thickened and hardened; typically occurs with advanced age.

atherosclerosis—A disease of the arteries that can occur anywhere in the body; characterized by the deposition of plaques of fatty material on the inner walls of the vessels that, when advanced, reduces blood flow.

autonomic nervous system (ANS)—The main branch of the nervous system that is responsible for control of bodily functions not under direct conscious control, such as breathing, heartbeat, and digestion.

barrier birth control methods—Pregnancy prevention methods that use a barrier to inhibit sperm from fertilizing the egg (e.g., male or female condom).

behavioral addiction—Certain behaviors, like gambling or compulsive shopping, that become chronic and out of control; can cause the same euphoric feelings as abusing drugs or other substances.

benign—A tumor, or lump, or swelling in the body that is not cancerous.

binge drinking—Consuming large quantities of alcohol over a short period of time with the intention of getting drunk.

binge-eating disorder—An eating disorder characterized by frequent and recurrent episodes of eating much faster and in greater quantities than normal until uncomfortably full, and sometimes with subjective loss of control.

bioelectrical impedance analysis (BIA)—A technique that measures body composition by sending a small electrical current through the body and measuring the resistance to the current, which relates to water content of the body.

biopsy—The surgical removal of a benign (noncancerous) or malignant (cancerous) tumor.

birth control methods—Methods that prevent a fertilized egg from implanting into the uterine wall.

blood alcohol concentration (BAC)—The level of alcohol that can be detected in the blood after drinking.

body composition—The makeup of the body tissues; often expressed in percentages of fat, muscle, and bone.

body dysmorphic disorder—A mental disorder characterized by the obsessive idea that some aspect of one's own appearance, either imagined or severely exaggerated, is severely flawed and requires exceptional measures to hide or fix it.

body image—How you see yourself in the mirror or picture yourself in your mind; encompasses your beliefs about your appearance, how you evaluate yourself, and how you sense and control your body.

body mass index (BMI)—A weight-to-height ratio calculated by dividing weight in kilograms by height in meters squared; used to assess weight status.

bone density T-score—The number of standard deviations that your bone density is above or below what is normal for someone of your age and biological sex (i.e., someone with peak bone mass); a proxy for bone strength.

bulbourethral glands—Also called *Cowper's glands*; small glands in men that contribute to the fluid in semen.

bulimia nervosa—An eating disorder characterized by binge eating followed by purging, either by vomiting or laxatives.

calorie—A simplified or abbreviated term commonly used to represent a kilocalorie; there are 1,000 calories in a kilocalorie.

cancer—A mass of cells that have characteristics of uncontrolled growth and large nuclei, varying in shape and size, that develop into a malignant tumor.

carbohydrates—An essential nutrient typically found in sugar, starch, or dietary fiber; provides 4 kilocalories per gram.

carcinogen—An agent that is capable of causing permanent damage to the molecular structure of the cell's DNA, causing cancer.

carcinogenesis—The process in which healthy cells become cancerous cells.

carcinoma in situ—Cancerous cells that have not penetrated any layers of tissues and are confined to the area of the originating cells.

cardiorespiratory endurance—The ability of the circulatory and respiratory systems to supply oxygen during sustained physical activity.

cardiorespiratory fitness—The ability to perform large muscle movements during exercise or physical activity for a sustained period of time.

cardiovascular disease (CVD)—Most often refers to conditions that involve narrowed or blocked blood vessels that lead to a reduction in blood flow.

chemotherapy—Powerful medications that are introduced into the body in the form of pills or liquids administered through an IV, infusion, or injection; designed to stop cancer cells from reproducing and spreading to other sites in the body.

cholesterol—A waxy, fatlike substance that is found in cells of the body and acts as precursor of steroid compounds; an important part of cell membranes.

chronic disease—A disease that lasts greater than three months, cannot be prevented with vaccines or cured by medication, and does not go away on its own.

chronic systemic inflammation—A condition caused by the release of proinflammatory cytokines from immune system cells and the chronic elevation of the innate immune system that can contribute to the development or progression of chronic diseases, including heart disease.

circumcision—Surgical removal of the foreskin around the glans (head) of the penis.

clitoris—Small organ made of erectile tissue located at the top of the vulva that develops from the same embryonic tissue as the penis. Its only function is sensitivity to sexual stimulation.

club drugs—Psychoactive drugs that cause hallucinogenic effects and lowered inhibitions; examples include MDMA and Rohypnol.

cocaine—A highly addictive psychoactive drug derived from coca leaves.

complementary and alternative medicine (CAM)—Medical products and practices that are not part of standard medical care.

complex carbohydrates—Carbohydrates comprising sugar molecules connected together in long, complex chains.

connective tissue—The parts of the body (such as ligaments, tendons, and cartilage) that support and hold together the other parts of the body (such as muscles, organs, and bones).

contraception—Devices and techniques used to prevent pregnancy, specifically preventing the sperm and egg from uniting.

conventional medical practices—The form of medical treatment, focused on treating illnesses, that is currently in wide use by health care professionals.

coronary heart disease (CHD)—Also called coronary artery disease (CAD); the blockage of arteries that supply blood to the heart muscle as a result of atherosclerosis.

corticotropin-releasing hormone (CRH)—A hormone released from the hypothalamus in response to stress; it binds to corticotropic-releasing hormone receptors and stimulates the release of adrenocorticotropic hormone from the pituitary gland.

cortisol—In the glucocorticoid class of hormones; primarily released from the adrenal glands during the stress response and often called the stress hormone.

COVID-19—An acute infectious disease caused by the SARS-CoV-2 virus; also called coronavirus disease.

C-reactive protein (CRP)—A common marker of chronic systemic inflammation; located in the blood.

dependence—When someone who uses addictive substances cannot stop using them, is unable to complete daily tasks, and has mental health problems as a result of substance use.

depressants—Drugs that lower or depress normal functioning in the body along the central nervous system of the brain and spinal cord.

depression—A common but serious mood disorder with symptoms presenting for at least two weeks that affects how a person feels, thinks, or handles daily activities such as sleeping, eating, or working.

diabetes—A chronic disease that occurs when the pancreas cannot make insulin or when the insulin the body produces does not work very well, resulting in high blood sugar.

diastole—Relaxation or filling phase of the heart.

dietary fats—Also commonly called dietary lipids, a nutrient that typically comes from tropical oils and animal and plant sources in our contemporary diets; provides 9 kilocalories per gram.

distress—A type of stress that is considered negative and is characterized by anxiety and emotional pain; it is perceived as not manageable, and it is not beneficial.

dose–response association—Concept related to physical activity and exercise whereby a greater volume or intensity of training causes greater health and fitness benefits.

drug abuse—When an individual takes a drug not as prescribed or intended consistently and over a long period of time.

drug misuse—When a drug is taken for reasons other than intended by the prescriber.

dual-energy X-ray absorptiometry (DEXA)—A technique that measures body composition (fat, lean soft tissue, and bone mass) and density using a small dose of radiation to produce an image of the body.

dynamic stretching—A type of movement routine in which momentum and active muscular effort are used to stretch a muscle and the end position is not held (e.g., walking lunges).

ectopic fat—Fat depots in the body that are not primary and are located in an abnormal place, such as in the liver or around the heart.

ectopic pregnancy—When a fertilized egg settles in the Fallopian tube or the peritoneal cavity instead of the uterus.

ejaculation—The ejection of semen from a man's body through the penis.

ejaculatory duct—Small vessels that transport the sperm out of a man's body through the prostate and the urethra.

embryo—The beginning stage of cells that represent an undeveloped fetus that has implanted into the uterine wall.

endocrine system—The glands in the body that secrete hormones directly into the circulatory system to be carried to target organs.

endometrium—The lining of the uterus where an embryo implants for nourishment and grows; a blood lining that is released during a woman's period if no embryo is present.

endoscopy—A procedure in which a physician inserts a thin, lighted, flexible tube, called an endoscope, into internal body cavities to check for cancer.

endothelium—A thin layer of cells that lines the interior surface of the blood vessels and lymphatic vessels, forming an interface between circulating blood and the rest of the vessel wall.

energy balance—The relationship between calories taken in through foods and drinks and energy expended, typically expressed as calories per day.

energy density—The number of calories per gram of food.

epididymis—System of small ducts that is the site of sperm maturation in the testes.

epinephrine—Sometimes called adrenalin; a hormone secreted by the medulla of the adrenal glands that is responsible for increased heart rate and blood pressure and other responses that prepare the body for fight or flight.

erection—When the cavernous tissue in the penis becomes dilated with blood and the penis becomes hard.

ergogenic—In the context of exercise or sport, a technique or substance that enhances performance.

essential fat—Minimally required fat for health, especially reproductive function in biological women.

eustress—A type of stress that is considered positive and is perceived as manageable and motivating, because it leads to a beneficial response.

exercise—Bodily exertion for the sake of developing and maintaining physical fitness. Specific guidelines have been established by the ACSM and U.S. Department of Health and Human Services.

exercise addiction—A state characterized by a compulsive engagement in any form of physical exercise to burn energy, despite having negative consequences that could include physical injuries or problems in one's professional life or personal relationships.

Fallopian tubes—Pair of tubes along which eggs travel from the ovaries to the uterus.

fast-twitch fiber—White muscle fibers that have a faster contraction speed but fatigue more easily.

female athlete triad—A syndrome of three interrelated conditions, including energy deficiency with or without disordered eating, menstrual disturbances, and bone loss or osteoporosis.

fertility awareness–based contraception methods (natural family planning)—The identification of the fertile days during the menstrual cycle through the observation of changes in cervical secretions, the basal body temperature, and monitoring the days of the menstrual cycle when ovulation is most likely to occur.

fertilization—The process of combining sperm and egg.

fetus—Term used to describe a baby in utero during the gestational period spanning from two months after conception to birth.

fight-or-flight response—Also termed the acute stress response; a physiological reaction coordinated by the neurological and endocrine systems that occurs in response to an actual or perceived harmful event or threat to survival.

flexibility—The range of motion in a joint or group of joints or the ability to move joints effectively through a complete range of motion.

free radicals—Chemically unstable molecules produced

from natural metabolic processes of various fats and proteins that, once formed, can react with other fats, proteins, and DNA, damaging cell membranes and mutating genes; have been implicated in aging, cancer, and other degenerative diseases.

functional fitness—Possessing the necessary fitness to optimally perform daily functional tasks, especially physical activities, throughout life.

functional fitness training—Deliberate and intentional training to improve functional fitness, usually using resistance training and stretching and often simulating functional movements.

generalized anxiety disorder—A disorder that causes uncontrollable anxiety and reduces focus on daily tasks even when there is little reason to worry.

gestational diabetes—A specific type of diabetes that occurs during pregnancy as a result of pregnancy hormones and other lifestyle behaviors that contribute to insulin resistance.

glucose—A simple sugar within the bloodstream that is broken down to produce ATP.

glycemic index—A relative ranking of carbohydrate in foods based on how slowly or quickly the foods cause increases in blood glucose levels. A value of 100 represents the standard, an equivalent of pure glucose.

glycogen—The form of glucose stored in the liver and skeletal muscles for rapid delivery to muscles; it is broken down to produce ATP.

gonads—Biological sex organs (testes and ovaries).

health span—The length of time that a person is not only alive but also healthy.

Healthy People 2030—A plan that identifies public health priorities to help individuals, organizations, and communities across the United States improve health and well-being; the initiative's fifth iteration builds on knowledge gained over the first four decades.

heart failure—Sometimes referred to as chronic or congestive heart failure; an impairment in the pumping ability of the heart caused by structural or functional abnormalities that compromises blood circulation to the rest of the body and causes abnormal fluid levels within various tissues, including in the lower legs and lungs.

heart rate reserve (HRR) method—The difference between maximal heart rate and resting heart rate; often used to determine exercise intensity.

hemorrhagic stroke—Occurs when a blood vessel in the brain breaks or ruptures, causing damage to brain cells; most commonly caused by high blood pressure and a weakness in the artery wall.

heroin—A highly addictive white powder derived from morphine that has a sedative effect on the body but causes a euphoric feeling.

HHS Physical Activity Guidelines—Recommendations to perform 150 minutes of cumulative movement per week in any sequence of bouts, focusing on moving more throughout the day.

high-density lipoprotein cholesterol (HDL-C)—A subtype of cholesterol in the blood known to act as a scavenger to remove LDL-C.

high-intensity interval training (HIIT)—Form of cardiorespiratory training that alternates high-intensity activities of a short duration with longer lower-intensity activities in a repetitive sequence.

hormonal birth control methods—Pregnancy prevention methods that require the use of hormones (e.g., birth control pill or patch).

hydrodensitometry—A technique for measuring body density (the mass per unit of a living human being) that is a direct application of Archimedes' principle that an object displaces its own volume of water.

hydrogenated oils—Created by a chemical process whereby hydrogen is added to liquid oils to create a solid form; partially hydrogenated oils contain trans fats.

hymen—A thin membrane that surrounds the opening to the vagina.

hypercholesterolemia—An excess of cholesterol in the bloodstream.

hyperglycemia—High blood sugar.

hyperlipidemia—An abnormally high concentration of fats or lipids in the blood.

hypertension—Abnormally high blood pressure.

hypothalamus—A region of the forebrain that coordinates the autonomic nervous system and the activity of the pituitary gland, controlling body temperature, thirst, hunger, and other homeostatic systems; also involved in the control of sleep and emotional activity.

hypothalamus-pituitary-adrenal axis (HPA axis)—A major neuroendocrine system that controls reactions to stress and many other body processes, using a complex set of direct influences and negative feedback control mechanisms among the hypothalamus, the pituitary glands, and adrenal cortex.

illegal drugs—Drugs that are regulated and considered forbidden by law; examples include cocaine, LSD, and heroin.

illicit drugs—Drugs that are considered socially forbidden or improper when not used as intended; they may or may not be illegal but go against social norms or values based on the manner in which they are used (e.g., prescription opioids are legal, but when they are not acquired from a prescription and a pharmacy, this would be considered an illicit use of a drug).

intention—An idea that you plan (or intend) to carry out. It is something you mean to do, whether you do it or not.

intermuscular adipose tissue—A type of fat located underneath the deep fascia and between adjacent muscle groups that is linked to metabolic diseases including type 2 diabetes mellitus.

intrinsic capacity—The combination of all physical and mental capacities of a person within the subcategories of cognition, locomotion, sensory, vitality, and psychological.

ischemic stroke—A stroke caused by a clot in a blood vessel in the brain; is the most common type of stroke and is similar to a heart attack.

isometric—A type of muscle contraction where the muscle lengthens or the joint angle does not change.

isotonic concentric—A type of muscle contraction where the muscle shortens and the joint angle decreases.

isotonic eccentric—A type of muscle contraction where the muscle lengthens and the joint angle increases.

kilocalorie—Commonly abbreviated as calorie; a unit of food energy of 1,000 calories. 1 kilocalorie is the amount of heat needed to raise the temperature of 1 liter of water 1 degree Celsius.

labia majora—The outer skin folds of the vulva that are composed of fatty tissue and covered with pubic hair.

labia minora—The inner skin folds of the vulva; are not covered with pubic hair.

licensed dietitian (LD)—In addition to the RDN credentialing, many states have regulatory laws for dietitians and nutrition practitioners.

life expectancy—The average number of years that a person is expected to live, based on demographic factors such as biological sex, age, country, and geographic area.

life span—The length of time a person lives.

lifestyle coach—A professional, different from a counselor, who addresses specific personal conditions and encourages personal discovery in order to make the individual's life what he or she wants it to be.

low back pain (LBP)—A common disorder involving the muscles, nerves, and bones of the back; pain can vary from a dull constant ache to a sudden sharp feeling.

low-density lipoprotein cholesterol (LDL-C)—A subtype of cholesterol in the blood known to accelerate the atherosclerotic process.

macronutrients—Chemical compounds found in food, primarily carbohydrate, protein, and fat; provide humans with the majority of their energy.

magnetic resonance imaging (MRI)—A noninvasive medical test that that uses a magnetic field and pulses of radio-wave energy to map structures inside the body, including the location and amount of adipose, muscle, and bone tissues.

malignant—A tumor, lump, or swelling in the body that is diagnosed as cancer based on an abnormal mass of cells that have the ability to grow in size and shape and separate from the primary tumor and spread to other parts of the body. These cells invade nearby tissue and then spread by way of the circulatory (blood) and lymphatic systems.

mammary glands—Also called breasts; located on the chest, when stimulated by pregnancy hormones, these organs secrete milk to provide nourishment for a baby.

mantra—A word or phrase that is repeated, often during meditation, that enables the mind and body to get to a calm state.

marijuana—A drug made from dried leaves of the hemp or cannabis plant that is illegal in many U.S. states; typically smoked to get a euphoric feeling.

maximal oxygen consumption ($\dot{V}O_2$max)—The maximal amount of oxygen the body can take in and use during maximal physical effort; provides the best objective measure of cardiorespiratory fitness.

medical model—A health model used by trained medical experts that focuses on prescribing drugs and procedures to combat illness.

melanoma—A type of dangerous skin cancer; the most commonly diagnosed cancer in the United States.

metabolic equivalents (METs)—A measure of exercise intensity based on the assumption that a single MET is equal to the amount of oxygen a person consumes (i.e., energy expended) per unit of body weight while at rest.

metabolic syndrome (MetS)—A clustering of biological factors that raises your risk for other chronic conditions, especially diabetes and cardiovascular disease.

metabolism—The breakdown of food and its transformation into energy.

metastasis—When cancer cells have left the original site and traveled to other parts of the body through the circulatory or lymphatic system.

methamphetamine—a white odorless crystalline powder that is a highly addictive stimulant that affects the central nervous system.

micronutrients—Chemical elements or substances required in very small amounts for healthy growth, development, and physiological function.

mindfulness meditation—A meditation technique that focuses on reducing psychological stress through being mindful of the present moment rather than thinking about the past or future.

minerals—An inorganic compound required by living organisms that must be obtained through the diet.

mons pubis—Soft area covering the pubis bone that is composed of fatty tissue.

muscle dysmorphia disorder—Sometimes called body dysmorphic disorder, a subtype of body dysmorphic disorder where a person obsesses about being small and undeveloped or frail.

muscle fiber—An individual muscle cell.

muscular endurance—The ability of the muscle to hold or repeat a contraction without fatigue.

muscular fitness—A term that collectively refers to the ability of muscles to generate movement at various speeds and typically includes strength, hypertrophy, power, and endurance.

muscular hypertrophy—An increase in muscle size generally gained in response to resistance training.

muscular power—The rate at which muscle force can be executed; alternatively, muscle force production (strength) expressed relative to time.

muscular strength—The amount of force that can be produced with a single maximum effort.

mutation—Abnormal cell growth that leads to the alteration of the genetic makeup of a normal cell.

myocardial infarction—Also called a heart attack; a life-threatening condition that occurs when blood flow to the heart is abruptly stopped, most often as a result of a clot that has blocked a narrowed artery.

neonatal abstinence syndrome (NAS)—Occurs when a baby experiences withdrawal symptoms after being exposed to certain types of drugs during pregnancy. NAS is most often caused by using opioids during pregnancy, but can also happen when taking antidepressants, barbiturates, or benzodiazepines.

neuromuscular fitness—Involves motor skills such as balance, agility, coordination, gait, and proprioceptive training. Also called neuromotor fitness, with the exercises called ceuromotor exercises or neuromotor training.

nicotine—A substance derived from a tobacco plant that causes smokers to become addicted to cigarettes.

nonoxidative (anaerobic) energy system—The energy system that supplies rapid but also limited energy to muscle cells through the breakdown of glucose and glycogen; does not need oxygen to function; also produces lactic acid.

norepinephrine—Sometimes called noradrenaline; a neurotransmitter that is released primarily from the sympathetic nerve fibers and secondarily from the adrenal glands during the fight-or-flight response, increasing arousal, reaction time, heart rate, and blood glucose levels.

obesity—Being above a weight that is considered healthy or desirable for a given height, typically defined as a body mass index of greater than 30 kilograms per square meter for adults. Also indicates having too much stored fat mass.

obesogenic environment—A term used to describe how our genetics have not evolved with our socially and physically built environment, which predisposes a large portion of the population to store too much energy or become obese.

oocytes—Immature eggs in the ovary.

opioids—Highly addictive drug derived from opium, sometimes prescribed to treat and manage pain.

osteoporosis—A bone disease whereby bone mass and density loss results in an increased risk of fracture from everyday activities and nontraumatic injuries such as falling.

ovaries—The reproductive organ in biological females that produces the egg (oocytes) and hormones.

overweight—Being above a weight that is considered healthy or desirable for a given height, typically defined as a body mass index of greater than 25 kilograms per square meter for adults.

ovulation—When a mature egg (ovum) is expelled from the ovaries.

ovum—Another term for the mature egg produced by the ovaries.

oxidative (aerobic) system—The energy system that supplies energy more slowly but for a longer duration to working muscles through the breakdown of glucose or glycogen and fats; this system requires oxygen.

panic disorder—An anxiety disorder characterized by unexpected and repeated episodes of intense fear accompanied by physical symptoms that may include chest pain, heart palpitations, shortness of breath, dizziness, or abdominal distress.

parasympathetic nervous system—The division of the ANS that slows the heart rate, increases intestinal and glandular activity, and relaxes sphincter muscles; responsible for the rest and digestion functions of the body.

PAR-Q+—A self-administered questionnaire that assesses your readiness to perform physical activity.

pathophysiology—Disordered physiological processes associated with disease or injury.

pelvic inflammatory disease—Infection of the uterus, fallopian tubes, or ovaries caused by untreated chlamydia or gonorrhea; can lead to sterility.

penis—The erectile organ in biological males; urine and semen are expelled from the body through the penis.

percent body fat—The relative amount of fat contained in the body; calculated as fat mass divided by body mass.

perfect use—When a contraception method is used correctly during every sexual encounter.

peripheral arterial disease (PAD)—Sometimes referred to as peripheral vascular disease; occurs with narrowing or occlusion of arteries outside the heart or brain due to atherosclerotic plaques; typically most evident in the legs.

personal trainer—An individual certified in general fitness who provides an exercise prescription through one-on-one exercise instruction.

personality—Individual differences in patterns of thinking, feeling, and behaving.

physical activity—Any bodily movement produced by skeletal muscles that requires energy expenditure.

phytochemicals—Substances that are found in plant foods that may help prevent chronic diseases; include antioxidants.

pituitary gland—Sometimes called the master gland; endocrine gland located at the base of the brain and controls other hormone glands, including the adrenals, thyroid, and ovaries and testes.

polyp—Areas of inflammation or bleeding in certain body cavities that could become cancerous tumors.

posture—The position in which someone holds his or her body when standing or sitting.

prediabetes—A condition when blood glucose levels are not normal but not quite high enough to be diagnosed as diabetes.

Prochaska's transtheoretical model (TTM)—An integrative theory of behavior change that assesses your readiness to act on a new, healthier behavior and provides strategies to guide your change process.

procrastination—The act of delaying or postponing something.

prognosis—A physician's best estimate of the time it can take to recover from a diagnosis (e.g., cancer, heart disease) and how having this diagnosis may affect the patient's quality of life.

proprioceptors—A sensory receptor located in subcutaneous tissues capable of detecting movement and position of the body through a stimulus produced within the body.

prostate gland—The organ that provides the majority of the fluid in semen.

protein—An essential nutrient composed of amino acids that are literally the building blocks of our body, forming muscles, bones, and cell membranes; 4 kilocalories per gram.

psychoactive drugs—Drugs that alter consciousness, moods, and thoughts; examples include alcohol, cocaine, tobacco, and cannabis.

radiation therapy—The use of radioactive waves (such as X-rays, gamma rays, neutrons, or protons) to kill cancer cells or shrink the size of the tumor by targeting specific cancer cells; treatment comes either from a machine that delivers the beam externally or in the form of a small pellet that is placed in the body near the cancer cells.

rating of perceived exertion (RPE)—A scale that allows a numerical estimation of the feelings of exertion during physical activity or exercise.

refined carbohydrates—Grain products that have been processed by a food manufacturer so that the whole grain is no longer intact and is missing the bran and germ.

registered dietitian nutritionist (RDN)—Food and nutrition experts who have met the rigorous criteria to earn the RDN credential, including a bachelor's degree, a supervised practice program, a national examination, and continuing professional educational requirements.

resting metabolic rate (RMR)—The minimal amount of energy needed to support basic physiological processes when the body is completely at rest.

RICE principle—An acronym for rest, ice, compression, elevation; a way to think about first aid for musculoskeletal injuries.

sarcopenia—Loss of mass, quality, and strength of skeletal muscle; associated with the normal aging process.

satiety—The feeling of fullness that is related to the suppression of hunger for a period of time after a meal.

saturated fatty acids—A type of fat in which the fatty acid chains have all or predominantly single bonds; are typically solid at room temperature.

scrotum—Sac that holds the testes; located behind the penis.

sedentary behavior—Habits and routines associated with relatively low levels of activity and movement, which could lead to health-related problems.

self-confidence—Belief in your ability to succeed at what you put your mind to; a combination of self-esteem and general self-efficacy.

self-determination theory (SDT)—A macro theory of human motivation and personality that concerns people's growth tendencies and psychological needs; it includes the motivation behind people's choices in the absence of external influences and distractions.

self-efficacy—Belief in your ability to perform specific behaviors in order to produce the outcomes you desire.

self-efficacy theory—Belief in your ability to succeed in specific situations or accomplish a task, which can play a large role in how you approach goals, tasks, and challenges.

semen—A whitish fluid that contains sperm; primarily produced by the prostate gland and seminal vesicles.

seminal vesicles—Vesicles that provide the sugar and protein fluid that contribute to the components of semen.

seminiferous tubules—Coiled tubules where sperm are produced.

simple carbohydrates—Sugars made of just one or two sugar molecules.

skinfold thickness—A measurement taken with a caliper that corresponds to the amount of subcutaneous fat a person has at a given region of the body.

slow-twitch fiber—Red muscle fibers that are fatigue resistant but have a slower contraction speed.

SMART goals—A process used for accountability in goal setting; SMART stands for specific, measurable, attainable, realistic, and time bound.

social anxiety disorder—Sometimes referred to as social phobia; characterized by a persistent, intense, and chronic fear of being watched and judged by others and feeling embarrassed or humiliated to the degree that it interferes with work, school, and other activities and may negatively affect the person's ability to form relationships.

social ecological model—Focuses on both population-level and individual-level determinants of health and interventions, including public policy, community, institutional, interpersonal, and intrapersonal factors.

social psychology—The study of how individual or group behavior is influenced by the presence and behavior of others.

specificity of training—Training principle that developing a particular fitness component requires performing exercises or activities specifically designed for that component in terms of muscle groups, muscle actions, and energy systems.

sperm—A cell in biological males that contributes to reproduction.

spermicide—A substance (e.g., foams, creams, gels) that contains chemicals that can kill sperm to prevent pregnancy.

static stretching—A stretch that is held in a challenging but comfortable position for a period of time, usually somewhere between 10 and 30 seconds.

sterilization—A surgical procedure that prevents the sperm from leaving the testicles (vasectomy) or the egg from leaving the ovaries (tubal ligation).

stimulants—Drugs that cause an increase to physiological responses in the body, which may include a rapid heart rate and increases in blood pressure, breathing, alertness and attention, and energy.

stress—A condition or feeling experienced when we perceive that demands in a physical, mental, or emotional domain exceed our personal or social resources to meet them.

stressor—An event or situation that potentially triggers the stress response.

stretch reflex—Sometimes called the myotatic stretch reflex; a muscle contraction in response to stretching within the muscle that provides automatic regulation of skeletal muscle length.

stroke—A condition in which atherosclerosis or a clot blocks blood flow to the brain, causing brain cells to die.

subcutaneous fat—A primary fat depot located just under the skin.

substance addiction—Dependence on a substance that, when stopped or reduced, leads to psychological and physiological tolerance and withdrawal symptoms.

sympathetic nervous system—The division of the ANS that speeds up the heart rate, depresses secretion, and reduces tone and contractility of smooth muscle; responsible for the fight-or-flight response.

systole—Contraction or ejection phase of the heart.

talk test—Another valid method for assessing exercise intensity that involves monitoring the difficulty of talking while exercising.

testes—Also called testicles; reproductive organs that produce and hold sperm.

theory of planned behavior (TPB)—Theory that links one's beliefs and behavior; states that attitude toward behavior, subjective norms, and perceived behavioral control in combination shape your behavioral intentions and behaviors.

thermic effect of activity (TEA)—Energy expended above RMR due to skeletal muscle contraction.

thermic effect of meals (TEM)—Energy expended associated with digestion, absorption, transport, metabolism, and storage of digested food.

time management—The ability to efficiently prioritize and schedule one's time to maintain productivity toward goals.

TNM system—A diagnostic system used to determine the extent or size of the primary tumor (T), whether the cancer cells have spread to lymph nodes (N), and if the cells have metastasized (M), or traveled to other parts of the body.

trans fatty acids—An unsaturated fatty acid found in margarines and manufactured cooking oils that occurs as a result of the hydrogenation process; the FDA banned their use in the food supply in 2018.

Transcendental Meditation—A meditation technique that involves repetition of a word or phrase while sitting with the eyes closed to quiet the mind.

triglycerides—Formed from glycerol and three fatty acid groups; high concentrations in the blood elevates risk for CVD.

type 1 diabetes—A metabolic disorder that is characterized by high blood sugar caused by lack of insulin; occurs most commonly as a result of beta-cell destruction in the pancreas.

type 2 diabetes (T2D)—A metabolic disorder characterized by high blood sugar, insulin resistance, and a relative lack of insulin.

typical use—Average, real-life use of birth control methods; accounts for human error (as opposed to correct, exact use with every sexual encounter, as occurs during clinical trials).

unsaturated fatty acids—A type of fat in which there is at least one double bond; typically liquid at room temperature.

urethra—Tubular structure through which urine exits the body.

uterus—Muscular organ in the lower abdominal cavity in which an embryo develops into a fetus.

vagina—A cylindrical space that begins at the opening of the vulva and ends at the opening of the cervix; the space for the penis during intercourse.

vaping—The act of inhaling and exhaling the water vapor produced by an electronic cigarette.

vas deferens—Tubular structure in men that transports semen out of the body.

visceral fat—A primary fat depot located deep within the abdominal cavity beneath the muscle wall.

vitamins—An organic compound that is an essential nutrient and is required in limited amounts; must be obtained through the diet.

well-being—The state of being comfortable, healthy, and happy.

well-being model—A health model that focuses on living well and encourages personal lifestyle choices and the use of self-management skills for preventing disease.

whole grains—A grain that is intact and contains the endosperm, germ, and bran.

withdrawal—A birth control method in which the penis is removed from the vagina before ejaculation.

zygote—The organism that develops after the blending of an egg and sperm.

REFERENCES

Chapter 1

Arloski, M. 2021. *Masterful Health and Wellness Coaching.* Duluth, MN: Real Balance Global Services.

Åstrand, P. 1992. "Why Exercise?" *Medicine & Science in Sports & Exercise* 24 (2): 153-62.

Baer, D. 2014. "Harvard Psychologist Says These 8 Principles Will Bring You the Most Happiness for Your Money." *Business Insider.* www.businessinsider.com/harvard-dan-gilbert-money-happiness-principles-2014-10.

Blair, S., H. Kohl III, and N. Gordon. 1992. "Physical Activity and Health: A Lifestyle Approach." *Medicine, Exercise, Nutrition, and Health* 1 (1): 54-56.

Buettner, D. 2020. *The Blue Zones of Happiness.* Washington, DC: National Geographic Society.

Bull, F.C., S.S. Al-Ansari, S. Biddle, K. Borodulin, M.P. Buman, G. Cardon, C. Carty, et al. 2020. "World Health Organization (WHO) 2020 Guidelines on Physical Activity and Sedentary Behaviour." *British Journal of Sports Medicine* 54: 1451-1462.

Centers for Disease Control and Prevention. 2020. "Age-Adjusted Death Rates for the 10 Leading Causes of Death in 2020: United States, 2019 and 2020. www.cdc.gov/nchs/images/databriefs/401-450/db427-fig4.png.

da Silveira, M.P., K.K da Silva Fagundes, M.R. Bizuti, É. Starck, R.C. Rossi, and D.T. de Resende E Silva. 2021. "Physical Exercise as a Tool to Help the Immune System Against COVID-19: An Integrative Review of the Current Literature." *Clinical and Experimental Medicine* 21 (1): 15-28. https://doi.org/10.1007/s10238-020-00650-3.

Helliwell J.F., Layard R., Sachs, J.D., De Neve J.E., Aknin, L.B., and Wang S. Sustainable Development Solutions Network. The World Happiness Report. https://worldhappiness.report/ed/2023/ and https://happiness-report.s3.amazonaws.com/2023/WHR+23.pdf. ISBN 978-1-7348080-5-6. Accessed May 26, 2023.

Jay, M. 2012. *The Defining Decade: Why Your Twenties Matter and How to Make the Most of Them Now.* New York: Hachette Book Group.

Kaur, H., T. Singh, Y.K. Arya, and S. Mittal. 2020. "Physical Fitness and Exercise During the COVID-19 Pandemic: A Qualitative Enquiry." Frontiers in Psychology 11: 590172. https://doi.org/10.3389/fpsyg.2020.590172.

McCoy, K. 2009. "Burning Calories With Everyday Activities." *Everyday Health.* www.everydayhealth.com/weight/everyday-activities-that-burn-calories.aspx.

Muldoon, C. 2021. "Our Well-Being Predictions for 2022." Accessed December 7, 2021. www.webmdhealthservices.com/2021/12/07/our-2022-well-being-predictions.

Office of Disease Prevention and Health Promotion (OODPHP). 2022. "Healthy People 2030." https://health.gov/healthypeople.

Peddie, M.C., C. Kessell, T. Bergen, T.D. Gibbons, H.A. Campbell, J.D. Cotter, N.J. Rehrer, and K.N. Thomas. 2021. "The Effects of Prolonged Sitting, Prolonged Standing, and Activity Breaks on Vascular Function, and Postprandial Glucose and Insulin Responses: A Randomised Crossover Trial." *PLoS ONE* 16 (1): e0244841. https://doi.org/10.1371/journal.pone.0244841.

Perkins, D. 2009. *Making Learning Whole: How Seven Principles of Teaching Can Transform Education.* San Francisco: Jossey-Bass.

Rakshit, S., M. McGough, K. Amin, and C. Cox. 2021. "Peterson KFF Health System Tracker: How Does U.S. Life Expectancy Compare to Other Countries?" Accessed January 8, 2022. www.healthsystemtracker.org/chart-collection/u-s-life-expectancy-compare-countries.

Segar, M. 2022. *The Joy Choice: How to Finally Achieve Lasting Changes in Eating and Exercise.* New York: Hachette Book Group.

Segar, M.L., M.M. Marques, A.L. Palmeira, and A.D. Okely. 2020. "Everything Counts in Sending the Right Message: Science-Based Messaging Implications From the 2020 WHO Guidelines on Physical Activity and Sedentary Behaviour." *International Journal of Behavioral Nutrition and Physical Activity* 17: 135.

Sharecare. 2020. "Community Well-Being Index: United States." Accessed January 23, 2022. https://wellbeingindex.sharecare.com/interactive-map.

Sharecare. 2022. "How Does the Gallup Sharecare Well-Being Index Work?" www.gallup.com/175196/gallup-healthways-index-methodology.aspx.

Well People. 2011. "A New Vision of Wellness." www.wellpeople.com/What_Is_Wellness.aspx.

Chapter 2

2018 Physical Activity Guidelines Advisory Committee. 2018. *2018 Physical Activity Guidelines Advisory Committee Scientific Report.* Washington, DC: U.S. Department of Health and Human Services.

American College of Sports Medicine. 1978. "American College of Sports Medicine Position Statement: The Recommended Quantity and Quality of Exercise for Developing and Maintaining Fitness in Healthy Adults." *Medicine & Science in Sports & Exercise* 10: vii-x.

American College of Sports Medicine. 1990. "American College of Sports Medicine Position Stand: The Recommended Quantity and Quality of Exercise for Developing and Maintaining Cardiorespiratory and Muscular Fitness in Healthy Adults." *Medicine & Science in Sports & Exercise* 43 (7): 1334-1359.

American College of Sports Medicine. 1998. "American College of Sports Medicine Position Stand: The Recommended Quantity and Quality of Exercise for Developing and Maintaining Cardiorespiratory and Muscular Fitness, and Flexibility in Healthy Adults." *Medicine & Science in Sports & Exercise* 30 (6): 975-991.

American College of Sports Medicine. 2006. *ACSM's Guidelines for Exercise Testing and Prescription.* 7th ed. Baltimore: Lippincott Williams & Wilkins.

American College of Sports Medicine. 2018. *ACSM's Guidelines for Exercise Testing and Prescription.* 10th ed. Philadelphia: Wolters Kluwer.

American College of Sports Medicine. 2022. *ACSM's Guidelines for Exercise Testing and Prescription.* 11th ed. Philadelphia: Wolters Kluwer.

Canadian Society for Exercise Physiology. 2020. "Canadian 24-Hour Movement Guidelines: An Integration of Physical Activity, Sedentary Behaviour, and Sleep." https://csepguidelines.ca. Accessed May 26, 2023.

Frederick, G., J. O'Connor, M. Schmidt, and E. Evans. 2021. "Relationships Between Components of the 24-Hour Activity Cycle and Feelings of Energy and Fatigue in College Students: A Systematic Review." *Mental Health and Physical Activity* 21: 100409. https://doi.org/10.1016/j.mhpa.2021.100409.

Levine, J. 2014. *Get Up: Why Your Desk Chair Is Killing You and What You Can Do About It.* New York: Palgrave Macmillan.

Nguyen, P., L.K.-D. Le, D. Nguyen, L. Gao, D.W. Dunstan, and M. Moodie. 2020. "The Effectiveness of Sedentary Behaviour Interventions on Sitting Time and Screen Time in Children and Adults: An Umbrella Review of Systematic Reviews." *International Journal of Behavioral Nutrition and Physical Activity* 17: 117. https://doi.org/10.1186/s12966-020-01009-3.

Pate, R., M. Pratt, and S. Blair. 1995. "Physical Activity and Public Health: A Recommendation From the Centers for Disease Control and Prevention and the American College of Sports Medicine." *Journal of the American Medical Association* 273 (5): 402-407.

Rosenberger, M.E., J.E. Fulton, M.P. Buman, R.P. Troiano, M.A. Grandner, D.M. Buchner, and W.L. Haskell. 2019. "The 24-Hour Activity Cycle: A New Paradigm for Physical Activity." *Medicine & Science in Sports & Exercise* 51 (3): 454-464. https://doi.org/10.1249/MSS.0000000000001811.

U.S. Department of Health and Human Services. 1996. *Physical Activity and Health: A Report of the Surgeon General.* Atlanta: Author.

U.S. Department of Health and Human Services. 2008. *2008 Physical Activity Guidelines for Americans.* ODPHP Publication No. U0036. Washington, DC: U.S. Department of Health and Human Services.

U.S. Department of Health and Human Services. 2018. *Physical Activity Guidelines for Americans.* 2nd ed. Washington, DC: Author.

Ussery, E.N., J.E. Fulton, D.A. Galuska, P.T. Katzmarzyk, and S.A. Carlson. 2018. "Joint Prevalence of Sitting Time and Leisure-Time Physical Activity Among U.S. Adults, 2015-2016." *JAMA* 320 (19): 2036-2038. doi:10.1001/jama.2018.17797.

Warburton, D., V. Jamnik, S. Bredin, and N. Gledhill. 2011. "The Physical Activity Readiness Questionnaire for Everyone (PAR-Q+) and Electronic Physical Activity Readiness Medical Examination (ePARmed-X+)." *The Health & Fitness Journal of Canada* 4 (2): 3-23.

World Health Organization. 2020. "WHO Guidelines on Physical Activity and Sedentary Behavior." Accessed May 26, 2023. 2020. https://www.who.int/publications/i/item/9789240015128.

Yang, L., C. Cao, E.D. Kantor, L.H. Nguyen, X. Zheng, Y. Park, E.L. Giovannucci, et al. 2019. "Trends in Sedentary Behavior Among the US Population, 2001-2016." *JAMA* 321 (16): 1587-1597. https://doi.org/10.1001/jama.2019.3636.

Young, D., M-F. Hivert, S. Alhassan, S.M. Camhi, J.F. Ferguson, P.T. Katmarzyk, C.E. Lewis, et al. 2016. "Sedentary Behavior and Cardiovascular Morbidity and Mortality: A Science Advisory from the American Heart Association." *Circulation* 134 (13): e262-e279. https://doi.org/10/1161/CIR.0000000000000440.

Chapter 3

2018 Physical Activity Guidelines Advisory Committee. 2018. *2018 Physical Activity Guidelines Advisory Committee Scientific Report.* Washington, DC: U.S. Department of Health and Human Services.

Ajzen, I., and B. Driver. 1992. "Application of the Theory of Planned Behavior to Leisure Choice." *Journal of Leisure Research* 24: 207-224.

American College of Sports Medicine. 2018. *ACSM's Guidelines for Exercise Testing and Prescription.* 10th ed. Philadelphia: Wolters Kluwer.

American College of Sports Medicine. 2022. *ACSM's Guidelines for Exercise Testing and Prescription.* 11th ed. Philadelphia: Wolters Kluwer.

Bandura A. 1977. "Self-Efficacy: Toward a Unifying Theory of Behavioral Change." *Psychological Review* 84: 191-215.

Bauman, A., R. Reis, J. Sallis, J. Wells, R. Loos, and B. Martin. 2012. "Correlates of Physical Activity: Why Are Some People Physically Active and Others Not?" *The Lancet* 380 (9838): 258-271.

Centers for Disease Control and Prevention. 2023. "Benefits of Physical Activity." Accessed October 28, 2023. https://www.cdc.gov/physicalactivity/basics/pa-health/index.htm

Deci, E.L., and R.M. Ryan. 1985. *Intrinsic Motivation and Self-Determination in Human Behavior.* New York: Plenum.

Downs, D.S., and H.A. Hausenblas. 2005. "The Theories of Reasoned Action and Planned Behavior Applied to Exercise: A Meta-Analytic Update." *Journal of Physical Activity and Health* 2: 76-97.

Duhigg, C. 2014. *The Power of Habit: Why We Do What We Do in Life and Business.* New York: Random House.

Fortier, M.S., J.L. Duda, E. Guerin, and P.J. Teixeira. 2012. "Promoting Physical Activity: Development and Testing of Self-Determination Theory-Based Interventions." *International Journal of Behavioral Nutrition and Physical Activity* 9-20.

Gaesser, G.A., and S.S. Angadi. 2021. "Obesity Treatment: Weight Loss Versus Increasing Fitness and Physical Activity for Reducing Health Risks." *iScience* 24 (September): 102995. https://doi.org/10.1016/j.isci.2021.102995.

McAuley, E. 1994. "Enhancing Psychological Health Through Physical Activity." In *Toward Active Living: Proceedings of the International Conference on Physical Activity, Fitness and Health,* edited by H. Quinney, L. Gauvin, and A. Wall, 83-90. Champaign, IL: Human Kinetics.

Nigg, C. 2014. *ACSM's Behavioral Aspects of Physical Activity and Exercise.* Philadelphia: Wolters Kluwer/Lippincott Williams and Wilkins.

Prochaska, J.O., and C.C. DiClemente. 1984. *The Transtheoretical Approach: Towards a Systematic Eclectic Framework.* Homewood, IL: Dow Jones Irwin.

Sallis, J., M. Floyd, D. Rodriguez, and B. Saelens. 2012. "Role of Built Environments in Physical Activity, Obesity, and Cardiovascular Disease." *Circulation* 125: 729-737.

Sallis, J., N. Owen, and E. Fisher. 2015. *Health Behavior: Theory, Research and Practice.* 5th ed. San Francisco: Jossey-Bass.

Sallis, J.F., and Spoon, C. 2015. "Making the Case for Designing Active Cities." Accessed August 17, 2021. https://activelivingresearch.org/sites/activelivingresearch.org/files/MakingTheCaseReport.pdf.

Segar, M. 2022. *The Joy Choice: How to Finally Achieve Lasting Changes in Eating and Exercise.* New York: Hachette Book Group.

Teixeira, P.J., E.V. Carraca, D. Markland, M.N. Silva, and R.M. Ryan. 2012. "Exercise, Physical Activity, and Self-Determination Theory: A Systematic Review." *International Journal of Behavioral Nutrition and Physical Activity* 9: 78.

Tudor-Locke, C., C. Leonardi, W.D. Johnson, P.T. Katzmarzyk, and T.S. Church. 2011. "Accelerometer Steps/Day Translation of Moderate-to-Vigorous Activity." *Preventive Medicine* 53: 31-33. https://doi.org/10.1016/j.ypmed.2011.01.014.

Vaillant, G. 2002. *Aging Well: Surprising Guideposts to a Happier Life From the Landmark Harvard Study of Adult Development.* New York: Hachette Book Group.

Van Cappellen, P., E.L. Rice, L.I. Catalino, and B.L. Fredrickson. 2017. "Positive Affective Processes Underlie Positive Health Behaviour Change." *Psychology & Health* 33 (1): 1-21. https://doi.org/10.1080/08870446.2017.1320798.

Yobbi, D. 2020. "Pandemic Boosts Share Bike and Scooter Business." *Bicycle Retailer Industry News.* Accessed August 16, 2021. www.bicycleretailer.com/industry-news/2020/08/10/pandemic-boosts-share-bike-and-scooter-business#.YRrVI-4hKiUk.

Zenko, Z., P. Ekkekakis, and G. Kavetsos. 2016. "Changing Minds: Bounded Rationality and Heuristic Processes in Exercise-Related Judgments and Choices." *Sport, Exercise, and Performance Psychology* 5 (4): 337-351.

Chapter 4

2018 Physical Activity Guidelines Advisory Committee. 2018. *2018 Physical Activity Guidelines Advisory Committee Scientific Report.* Washington, DC: U.S. Department of Health and Human Services.

American College of Sports Medicine. 2022. *ACSM's Guidelines for Exercise Testing and Prescription.* 11th ed. Philadelphia: Wolters Kluwer Health.

Martin, S.A., B.D. Pence, and J.A. Woods. 2009. "Exercise and Respiratory Tract Viral Infections." *Exercise and Sport Sciences Reviews* 37 (4): 157-164.

Milanovic, Z., G. Sporis, and M. Weston. 2015. "Effectiveness of High-Intensity Interval Training (HIT) and Continuous Endurance Training for $\dot{V}O_2$max Improvements: A Systematic Review and Meta-Analysis of Controlled Trials." *Sports Medicine* 45 (10): 1469-1481.

Nieman, D.C. 2021. "Exercise Is Medicine for Immune Function: Implication for COVID-19." *Current Sports Medicine Reports* 20 (8): 395-401.

U.S. Department of Health and Human Services. 2018. *Physical Activity Guidelines for Americans.* 2nd ed. Washington, DC: Author.

Chapter 5

American College of Sports Medicine. 2022. *ACSM's Guidelines for Exercise Testing and Prescription.* 11th ed. Philadelphia: Wolters Kluwer Health.

Clark, B.C. 2009. "In Vivo Alternations in Skeletal Muscle Form and Function after Disuse Atrophy." *Medicine & Science and Sports & Exercise* 41 (10): 1869-1875.

Kersey, R.D., D.L. Elliot, L. Goldberg, G. Kanayama, J.E. Leone, M. Pavlovich, and H.G. Pope Jr. 2012. "National Athletic Trainers' Association Position Statement: Anabolic-Androgenic Steroids." *Journal of Athletic Training* 47 (5): 567-588.

Roberts, B.M., G. Nuckols, and J.W. Krieger. 2020. "Sex Differences in Resistance Training: A Systematic Review and Meta-Analysis." *Journal of Strength and Conditioning Research* 34 (5): 1488-1460.

U.S. Department of Health and Human Services. 2018. *Physical Activity Guidelines for Americans.* 2nd ed. Washington, DC: Author.

Yoke, M., and C. Armbruster. 2020. *Methods of Group Exercise Instruction.* 4th ed. Champaign, IL: Human Kinetics.

Chapter 6

American College of Sports Medicine. 2022. *ACSM's Guidelines for Exercise Testing and Prescription.* 11th ed. Philadelphia: Wolters-Kluwer.

Centers for Disease Control and Prevention. 2020a. "QuickStats: Percentage of Adults Aged ≥ 18 Years Who Had Lower Back Pain in the Past 3 Months, by Sex and Age Group — National Health Interview Survey, United States, 2018." *Morbidity and Mortality Weekly Report* 68: 1196. Accessed January 3, 2022. https://stacks.cdc.gov/view/cdc/84421.

Centers for Disease Control and Prevention. 2020b. "Disability Impacts All of Us." Accessed January 4, 2022. www.cdc.gov/ncbddd/disabilityandhealth/infographic-disability-impacts-all.html.

National Institute of Neurological Disorders and Stroke. 2020. "Low Back Pain Fact Sheet." Accessed January 3, 2022. www.ninds.nih.gov/Disorders/Patient-Caregiver-Education/Fact-Sheets/Low-Back-Pain-Fact-Sheet.

U.S. Department of Health and Human Services. 2018. *Physical Activity Guidelines for Americans.* 2nd ed. Washington, DC: Author.

Yoke, M., and C. Kennedy. 2004. *Functional Exercise Progressions.* Monterey, CA: Healthy Learning.

Chapter 7

Addison, O., R.L. Marcus, P.C. Lastayo, and A.S. Ryan. 2014. "Intermuscular Fat: A Review of the Consequences and Causes." *International Journal of Endocrinology* 2014: 309570.

American College of Sports Medicine. 2022. *ACSM's Guidelines for Exercise Testing and Prescription.* 11th ed. Philadelphia: Wolters Kluwer Health.

Bone Health and Osteoporosis Foundation. 2022. "General Facts – Bone Health Basics: Get the Facts." Accessed January 6, 2022. www.bonehealthandosteoporosis.org/preventing-fractures/general-facts.

Bouchard, C., and L. Perusse. 1988. "Heredity and Body Fat." *Annual Review of Nutrition* 8: 259-277.

Centers for Disease Control and Prevention. 2022a. "About Adult BMI." Accessed August 12, 2022. https://www.cdc.gov/healthyweight/assessing/bmi/adult_bmi/index.html.

Centers for Disease Control and Prevention. 2022b. "Assessing Your Weight." Accessed August 12, 2022. https://www.cdc.gov/healthyweight/assessing/.

Centers for Disease Control and Prevention. 2022c. "Defining Adult Overweight & Obesity." Accessed August 12, 2022. https://www.cdc.gov/obesity/basics/adult-defining.html.

Gallagher, D., S.B. Heymsfield, M. Heo, S.A. Jebb, P.R. Murgatroyd, and Y. Sakamoto. 2000. "Healthy Percentage Body Fat Ranges: An Approach for Developing Guidelines Based on Body Mass Index." *The American Journal of Clinical Nutrition* 72 (3): 694-701.

Heymsfield, S.B., T.G. Lohman, Z. Wang, and S.B. Going. 2005. *Human Body Composition.* Champaign IL: Human Kinetics.

Joy, E., M.J. De Souza, A. Nattiv, M. Misra, N.I. Williams, R.J. Mallinson, J.C. Gibbs, et al. 2014. "2014 Female Athlete Triad Coalition Consensus Statement on Treatment and Return to Play of the Female Athlete Triad." *Current Sports Medicine Reports* 13 (4): 219-232.

Kohrt, W. 2010. "Physical Activity and Risk of Obesity in Older Adults." In *Physical Activity and Obesity*, edited by C. Bouchard and P.T. Katzmarzyk, 117-120. Champaign IL: Human Kinetics.

Looker, A.C., L.J. Melton III, T. Harris, L. Borrud, J. Shepherd, and J. McGowan. 2009. "Age, Gender, and Race/Ethnic Differences in Total Body and Subregional Bone Density." *Osteoporosis International* 20 (7): 1141-1149.

Salimans, L., Liberman, K., Njemini, R., Kortekaas Krohn, I., Gutermuth, J., and Bautmans, I. 2022. "The Effect of Resistance Exercise on the Immune Cell Function in Humans: A Systematic Review." *Experimental Gerontology* 164: 1118-1122.

Shapses, S.A., and D. Sukumar. 2012. "Bone Metabolism in Obesity and Weight Loss." *Annual Review of Nutrition* 32: 287-309.

Slaughter, M.H., and T.G. Lohman. 1976. "Relationship of Body Composition to Somatotype." *American Journal of Physical Anthropology* 44 (2): 237-244.

Weaver, C.M., C.M. Gordon, K.F. Janz, H.J. Kalkwarf, J.M. Lappe, R. Lewis, M. O'Karma, T.C. Wallace, and B.S. Zemel. 2016. "The National Osteoporosis Foundation's Position Statement on Peak Bone Mass Development and Lifestyle Factors: A Systematic Review and Implementation Recommendations." *Osteoporosis International* 27: 1281-1386.

Xiao, J., S.A. Purcell, C.M. Prado, and M.C. Gonzalez. 2017. "Fat Mass to Fat-Free Mass Ratio Reference Values From NHANES III Using Bioelectrical Impedance Analysis." *Clinical Nutrition* 37 (6 Pt A): 2284-2287.

Chapter 8

Academy of Nutrition and Dietetics. 2022. "How Much Protein Should I Eat?" Accessed January 16, 2023. www.eatright.org/food/nutrition/dietary-guidelines-and-myplate/how-much-protein-should-i-eat.

Academy of Nutrition and Dietetics. 2020a. "Benefits of Coffee." Accessed February 4, 2022. www.eatright.org/health/wellness/preventing-illness/benefits-of-coffee.

Academy of Nutrition and Dietetics. 2020b. "Food Allergies and Intolerances." Accessed February 4, 2022. www.eatright.org/health/allergies-and-intolerances/food-allergies/food-allergies-and-intolerances.

Aljada, B., A. Zohni, and W. El-Matary. 2021. "The Gluten-Free Diet for Celiac Disease and Beyond." *Nutrients* 13 (11): 3993. https://doi.org/10.3390/nu13113993.

American College of Sports Medicine. 2007. "Position Stand: Exercise and Fluid Replacement." *Medicine & Science in Sports & Exercise* 39 (2): 377-390. https://doi.org/10.1249/mss.0b013e31802ca597.

Casas, R., E. Sacanella, and R. Estruch. 2014. "The Immune Protective Effect of the Mediterranean Diet Against Chronic Low-Grade Inflammatory Diseases." *Endocrine, Metabolic & Immune Disorders – Drug Targets* 14 (4): 245-254.

Center for Science in the Public Interest. 2021. Accessed February 4, 2022. https://cspinet.org/eating-healthy/ingredients-of-concern/caffeine-chart.

Institute of Medicine. 2005a. *Dietary Reference Intakes for Energy, Carbohydrate, Fiber, Fat, Fatty Acids, Cholesterol, Protein, and Amino Acids.* Washington, DC: The National Academies Press. Accessed February 4, 2022. www.nap.edu/catalog/10490/dietary-reference-intakes-for-energy-carbohydrate-fiber-fat-fatty-acids-cholesterol-protein-and-amino-acids.

Institute of Medicine. 2005b. *Dietary Reference Intakes for Water, Potassium, Sodium, Chloride and Sulfate.* Washington, DC: The National Academies Press. Accessed February 4, 2022. www.nationalacademies.org/hmd/Reports/2004/Dietary-Reference-Intakes-Water-Potassium-Sodium-Chloride-and-Sulfate.aspx.

Merino, J., A.D. Joshi, L.H. Nguyen, E.R. Leeming, M. Mazidi, D.A. Drew, R. Gibson, et al. 2021. "Diet Quality and Risk and Severity of COVID-19: A Prospective Cohort Study." *Gut* 70 (11): 2096-2104.

Phillips, S.M., S. Chevalier, and H.J. Leidy. 2016. "Protein 'Requirements' Beyond the RDA: Implications for Optimizing Health." *Applied Physiology, Nutrition, and Metabolism* 41 (5): 565-572.

U.S. Department of Agriculture and U.S. Department of

Health and Human Services. 2020. *Dietary Guidelines for Americans, 2020-2025*. 9th ed. Accessed February 4, 2022. DietaryGuidelines.gov.

U.S. Food and Drug Administration. 2014. "Nutrition Labeling and Education Act (NLEA) Requirements—Attachment 1." Accessed February 4, 2022. www.fda.gov/nutrition-labeling-and-education-act-nlea-requirements-attachment-1.

U.S. Food and Drug Administration. 2018. "Final Determination Regarding Partially Hydrogenated Oils (Removing Trans Fat)." Accessed February 4, 2022. www.fda.gov/Food/IngredientsPackagingLabeling/FoodAdditivesIngredients/ucm449162.h.

U.S. Food and Drug Administration. 2019. "Information for Consumers on Using Dietary Supplements." Accessed February 4, 2022. www.fda.gov/Food/DietarySupplements/UsingDietarySupplements/default.htm.

U.S. Food and Drug Administration. 2020. "How to Understand and Use the Nutrition Facts Label." Accessed February 4, 2022. www.fda.gov/food/new-nutrition-facts-label/how-understand-and-use-the-nutrition-facts-label.

Whole Grains Council. n.d. "Whole Grains 101." Accessed February 4, 2022. https://wholegrainscouncil.org/whole-grains-101.

Chapter 9

American College of Sports Medicine. 2022. *ACSM's Guidelines for Exercise Testing and Prescription*. 11th ed. Philadelphia: Wolters Kluwer Health.

Bouchard, C., and P.T. Katzmarzyk. 2010. *Physical Activity and Obesity*. Champaign, IL: Human Kinetics.

Bray, M.S., R.J.F. Loos, J.M. McCaffery, C. Ling, P.W. Franks, G.M. Weinstock, M.P. Snyder, J.L. Vassy, and T. Agurs-Collins. 2016. "NIH Working Group Report—Using Genomic Information to Guide Weight Management: From Universal to Precision Treatment." *Obesity (Silver Spring)* 24 (1): 14-22.

Centers for Disease Control and Prevention. 2021. "Adult Obesity Causes and Consequences." Accessed February 20, 2022. www.cdc.gov/obesity/adult/causes.html.

Centers for Disease Control and Prevention. 2022. "COVID-19: People with Certain Medical Conditions." Accessed February 26, 2022. www.cdc.gov/coronavirus/2019-ncov/need-extra-precautions/people-with-medical-conditions.html.

Hales C.M., M.D. Carroll, C.D. Fryar, and C.L. Ogden. Prevalence of Obesity and Severe Obesity Among Adults: United States, 2017–2018. *NCHS Data Brief*, 360, 2020.

Hill, J.O., and H.R. Wyatt. 2013. *State of Slim: Fix Your Metabolism and Drop 20 Pounds in 8 Weeks on the Colorado Diet*. New York: Rodale.

Jensen, M.D., D.H. Ryan, C.M. Apovian, J.D. Ard, A.G. Comuzzie, K.A. Donato, F.B. Hu, et al. 2014. "2013 AHA/ACC/TOS Guideline for the Management of Overweight and Obesity in Adults: A Report of the American College of Cardiology/American Heart Association Task Force on Practice Guidelines and The Obesity Society." *Journal of the American College of Cardiology* 63 (25 Pt B): 2985-3023.

Malhotra, R., T. Ostbye, C.M. Riley, and E.A. Finkelstein. 2013. "Young Adult Weight Trajectories Through Midlife By Body Mass Category." *Obesity (Silver Spring)* 21 (9): 1923-1934.

Popkin, B.M., S. Du, W.D. Green, M.A. Beck, T. Algaith, C.H. Herbst, R.F. Alsukait, M. Alluhidan, N. Alazemi, and M. Shekar. 2020. "Individuals with Obesity and COVID-19: A Global Perspective on the Epidemiology and Biological Relationships. *Obesity Reviews* 21 (11): e13128. https://doi.org/10.1111/obr.13128.

Reinehr, T. 2018. "Long-Term Effects of Adolescent Obesity: Time to Act." *Nature Reviews Endocrinology* 14(3): 183-188.

Rubino R., R.M. Puhl, D.E. Cummings, R.H. Eckel, D.H. Ryan, J.I. Mechanick, J. Nadglowski, et al. 2020. "Joint International Consensus Statement for Ending Stigma of Obesity." *Nature Medicine* 26: 485-497. www.nature.com/articles/s41591-020-0803-x.pdf.

Tremblay, A., and F. Bellisle. 2015. "Nutrients, Satiety, and Control of Energy Intake." *Applied Physiology, Nutrition, and Metabolism* 40 (10): 971-979.

Chapter 10

American College Health Association. 2021. "National College Health Assessment Spring 2021 Reference Group Data Report." Accessed March 1, 2022. www.acha.org/documents/ncha/NCHA-III_FALL_2021_REFERENCE_GROUP_EXECUTIVE_SUMMARY.pdf.

American Academy of Sleep Medicine. 2020. "Healthy Sleep Habits." Accessed May 28, 2023. https://sleepeducation.org/healthy-sleep/healthy-sleep-habits.

American Sleep Association. n.d. "What Is Sleep?" Accessed January 22, 2018. www.sleepassociation.org/patients-general-public/what-is-sleep.

Bureau of Labor Statistics. 2016. "American Time Use Survey." Accessed December 20, 2016. www.bls.gov/tus/charts/students.htm.

Centers for Disease Control and Prevention. 2020. "Sleep and Sleep Disorders." Accessed March 1, 2022. www.cdc.gov/Sleep/index.html.

Centers for Disease Control and Prevention. 2023. "Coping With Stress." Accessed March 1, 2022. www.cdc.gov/mental-health/stress-coping/cope-with-stress.

Goyal, M., S. Singh, E.M. Sibinga, N.F. Gould, A. Rowland-Seymour, R. Sharma, Z. Berger, et al. 2014. "Meditation Programs for Psychological Stress and Well-Being: A Systematic Review and Meta-Analysis." *JAMA Internal Medicine* 174 (3): 357-368.

Lazarus. R.S., and S. Folkman. 1984. *Stress, Appraisal and Coping*. New York: Springer.

Morales, J.S., P.L. Valenzuela, A. Castillo-García, J. Butragueño, D. Jiménez-Pavón, P. Carrera-Bastos, and A. Lucia. 2021. "The Exposome and Immune Health in Times of the COVID-19 Pandemic." *Nutrients* 14 (1): 24. https://doi.org/10.3390/nu14010024.

National Institutes of Health. 2022. "Stress." Last modified April 2022. Accessed May 28, 2023. https://nccih.nih.gov/health/stress.

National Institutes of Mental Health. 2023a. "Anxiety Disorders." Accessed May 28, 2023. www.nimh.nih.gov/health/topics/anxiety-disorders.

National Institutes of Mental Health. 2023b. "Depression." Last modified April 2023. Accessed May 28, 2023. www.nimh.nih.gov/health/topics/depression.

Puetz, T.W., P.J. O'Connor, and R.K. Dishman. 2006. "Effects of Chronic Exercise on Feelings of Energy and Fatigue: A Quantitative Synthesis." *Psychological Bulletin* 132 (6): 866-876.

Sapolsky, R.M. 2004. *Why Zebras Don't Get Ulcers*. New York: St. Martin's Press.

U.S. Department of Health and Human Services. 2018. *Physical Activity Guidelines for Americans*. 2nd ed. Washington, DC: Author.

Watson, N.F., M.S. Badr, G. Belenky, D.L. Bliwise, O.M. Buxton, D. Buysse, D.F. Dinges, et al. 2015. "Recommended Amount of Sleep for a Healthy Adult: A Joint Consensus Statement of the American Academy of Sleep Medicine and Sleep Research Society." *Sleep* 38 (6): 843-844.

Chapter 11

Addiction Hope. 2017. "Sexual Addiction Causes, Statistics, Addiction Signs, Symptoms & Side Effects." www.addictionhope.com/sexual-addiction.

Addiction Policy Forum. 2022. "DSM-5 Criteria for Addiction Simplified." Accessed March 25, 2023. https://www.addictionpolicy.org/post/dsm-5-facts-and-figures.

American College Health Association. 2019. "American College Health Association-National College Health Assessment II: Reference Group Executive Summary Spring 2019." Silver Spring, MD. www.acha.org/documents/ncha/NCHA-II_SPRING_2019_US_REFERENCE_GROUP_EXECUTIVE_SUMMARY.pdf.

American Lung Association. 2016. "E-cigarettes and Lung Health." Last modified December 8, 2016. www.lung.org/stop-smoking/smoking-facts/e-cigarettes-and-lung-health.html.

American Lung Association. 2017a. "Nicotine." www.lung.org/stop-smoking/smoking-facts/nicotine.html.

American Lung Association. 2017b. "What's in a Cigarette?" www.lung.org/stop-smoking/smoking-facts/whats-in-a-cigarette.html.

American Lung Association. N.d. "I Want to Quit." www.lung.org/quit-smoking/i-want-to-quit.

American Psychiatric Association. 2022. Substance-related and Addictive Disorders. In *Diagnostic and statistical manual of mental disorders* (5th ed., text rev.). https://doi.org/10.1176/appi.books.9780890425787.x16_Substance_Related_Disorders.

Arria, A.M., K.M. Caldeira, B.A. Bugbee, K.B. Vincent, and K.E. O'Grady. 2015. "The Academic Consequences of Marijuana Use During College." *Psychology of Addictive Behaviors: Journal of the Society of Psychologists in Addictive Behaviors* 293: 564-575. doi:10.1037/adb0000108.

Ataei, M., F.M. Shirazi, R.J. Lamarine, S. Nakhaee, and O. Mehrpour. 2020. "A Double-Edged Sword of Using Opioids and COVID-19: A Toxicological View." *Substance Abuse Treatment and Prevention Policy* 15 (91). https://doi.org/10.1186/s13011-020-00333-y.

BBC News. 2014. "Many Young People Addicted to Net, Survey Suggests." www.bbc.com/news/technology-29627896.

Bragg, J. 2009. "Digging Out From $80,000 in Debt." www.cnn.com/2009/LIVING/worklife/09/21/mainstreet.digging.out.of.debt/index.html?_s=PM:LIVING.

Centers for Disease Control and Prevention. 1988. *Program Evaluation Handbook: Drug Abuse Education*. Office of Disease Prevention and Promotion, U.S. Department of Health and Human Services.

Centers for Disease Control and Prevention. 2011. "Drinking and Driving." Last modified October 3, 2011. www.cdc.gov/vitalsigns/drinkinganddriving.

Centers for Disease Control and Prevention. 2023. National Center for Health Statistics. Mortality Data on CDC WONDER.

Centers for Disease Control and Prevention. 2019. HIV Surveillance Report, vol. 32. www.cdc.gov/hiv/library/reports/hiv-surveillance.html.

Centers for Disease Control and Prevention. 2021a. "Alcohol and Public Health: Deaths From Excessive Alcohol Use in the United States." Last Modified January 14, 2021. www.cdc.gov/alcohol/features/excessive-alcohol-deaths.html.

Centers for Disease Control and Prevention. 2021b. "Alcohol and Substance Abuse." Last modified March 19, 2021. www.cdc.gov/coronavirus/2019-ncov/daily-life-coping/stress-coping/alcohol-use.html.

Centers for Disease Control and Prevention. 2021c. "Cigarette Smoking Is Down, but About 34 Million American Adults Still Smoke." Last modified June 21, 2021. www.cdc.gov/tobacco/infographics/adult/index.htm#down.

Centers for Disease Control and Prevention. 2021d. "Health Effects of Cigarette Smoking." Last modified October 29, 2021. www.cdc.gov/tobacco/data_statistics/fact_sheets/health_effects/effects_cig_smoking/index.htm.

Centers for Disease Control and Prevention. 2021e. "Hookas." Last modified April 22, 2021. www.cdc.gov/tobacco/data_statistics/fact_sheets/tobacco_industry/hookahs.

Cornelius M.E, C.G. Loretan, T.W. Wang, A. Jamal, and D.M. Homa. 2022. "Tobacco Product Use Among Adults—United States, 2020." *Morbidity Mortality Weekly Report*; 71:397–405. https://www.cdc.gov/tobacco/data_statistics/fact_sheets/adult_data/cig_smoking/index.htm.

Cranford, J.A. 2014. "DSM-IV Alcohol Dependence and Marital Dissolution: Evidence from the National Epidemiologic Survey on Alcohol and Related Conditions." *Journal of Studies on Alcohol and Drugs* 75 (3): 520-529. https://doi.org/10.15288/jsad.2014.75.520.

Dong, C., J. Chen, A. Harrington, K. Yaragudri Vinod, M.L. Hegde, and V.L. Hegde. 2019. "Cannabinoid Exposure During Pregnancy and Its Impact on Immune Function." *Cellular and Molecular Life Science* 76: 729-743. https://doi.org/10.1007/s00018-018-2955-0.

Drug Enforcement Administration. 2020. "Amphetamines." Last modified April 2020. www.dea.gov/factsheets/amphetamines.

Drug Enforcement Administration. 2021. "2020 National Drug Threat Assessment (NDTA)." U.S. Department of Justice. www.dea.gov/sites/default/files/2021-02/DIR-008-21%202020%20National%20Drug%20Threat%20Assessment_WEB.pdf.

Eating Disorder Hope. 2021. "Eating Disorder Statistics & Research." www.eatingdisorderhope.com/information/statistics-studies.

Esser, M.B., A. Sherk, Y. Liu, T. Stockwell, M. Stahre, D. Kanny, M. Landen, et al. 2020. "Deaths and Years of Potential Life Lost From Excessive Alcohol Use—United States, 2011-2015." *Morbidity Mortality Weekly Report* 69: 1428-1433. https://doi.org/10.15585/mmwr.mm6930a1.

Fifield, J. 2021. "Types of Therapy Used in Addiction Treatment and Recovery." American Addiction Centers. Last modified December 2, 2021. https://drugabuse.com/treatment/therapy/.

Foundation for a Drug-Free World. n.d. "The Truth About Crystal Meth and Methamphetamine." Accessed December 10, 2021. www.drugfreeworld.org/drugfacts/crystalmeth.html.

Grant J.E. and S.R. Chamberlain. 2016. "Expanding the Definition of Addiction: DSM-5 vs. ICD-11." *CNS Spectrums* (4):300-303. doi: 10.1017/S1092852916000183.

Grant, J., M. Potenza, A. Weinstein, and D. Gorelick. 2010. "Introduction to Behavioral Addictions." *American Journal of Drug and Alcohol Abuse* 35 (5): 233-241.https://doi.org/10.3109/00952990.2010.491884.

Han, B., N.D. Volkow, W.M. Compton, and E.F. McCance-Katz. 2020. "Reported Heroin Use, Use Disorder, and Injection Among Adults in the United States, 2002-2018." *Journal of the American Medical Association* 323 (6): 568-571. https://doi.org/10.1001/jama.2019.20844.

Hirai, A.H., J.Y. Ko, P.L. Owens, C. Stocks, and S.W. Patrick. 2021. "Neonatal Abstinence Syndrome and Maternal Opioid-Related Diagnoses in the US, 2010-2017." *Journal of the American Medical Association* 325 (2): 146-155. https://doi.org/10.1001/jama.2020.24991.

Institute for the Advancement of Food and Nutrition Science. 2021. "How Safe Is Caffeine in Coffee, Tea, and Other Drinks?" https://iafns.org/caffeine.

Jilani, S.M., M.T. Frey, D. Pepin, T. Jewell, M. Jordan, A.M. Miller, M. Robinson, et al. 2019. "Evaluation of State-Mandated Reporting of Neonatal Abstinence Syndrome—Six States, 2013–2017." *Morbidity Mortality Weekly Report* 68: 6-10. https://doi.org/10.15585/mmwr.mm6801a2.

Jones, C.M., W.M. Compton, and D. Mustaquim. 2020. "Patterns and Characteristics of Methamphetamine Use Among Adults—United States, 2015–2018." *Morbidity Mortality Weekly Report* 69: 317-323. https://doi.org/10.15585/mmwr.mm6912a1.

Kennedy, S. 2018. "Raising Awareness About Prescription and Stimulant Abuse in College Students Through On-Campus Community Involvement Projects." *Journal of Undergraduate Neuroscience Education* 17 (1): A50-A53.

Kilpatrick, S. 2016. "How to Help Prevent Students from Abusing Drug and Alcohol." www.campusanswers.com/prevent-student-drug-alcohol-abuse.

Koob, G.F., and N.D. Volkow. 2016. "Neurobiology of Addiction: A Neurocircuitry Analysis. *Lancet Psychiatry* 3(8):760-773.

Koran, L.M., R.J. Faber, E. Aboujaoude, M.D. Large, and R.T. Serpe. 2006. "Estimated Prevalence of Compulsive Buying Behavior in the United States." *American Journal of Psychiatry* 163 (10): 1806-1812.

Marczinski, C.A., and M.T. Fillmore. 2014. "Energy Drinks Mixed With Alcohol: What Are the Risks?" *Nutrition Reviews* 72 (Suppl. 1): 98-107. https://doi.org/10.1111/nure.12127.

Mayo Clinic. 2020. "Caffeine: How Much Is Too Much?" Last modified March 6, 2020. www.mayoclinic.org/healthy-life-style/nutrition-and-healthy-eating/in-depth/caffeine/art-20045678.

McCance-Katz, E.F. 2019. "The National Survey on Drug Use and Health: 2017." Substance Abuse and Mental Health Services Administration. www.samhsa.gov/data/sites/default/files/nsduh-ppt-09-2018.pdf.

Mumford, S.L., K.S. Flannagan, J.G. Radoc, L.A. Sjaarda, J.R. Zolton, T.D. Metz, T.C. Plowden, et al. 2021. "Cannabis Use While Trying to Conceive: A Prospective Cohort Study Evaluating Associations with Fecundability, Live Birth and Pregnancy Loss." *Human Reproduction* 6 (5): 1405-1415. https://doi.org/10.1093/humrep/deaa355.

National Center for Drug Abuse Statistics. 2021. "Drug Use Among Youth: Facts & Statistics." https://drugabusestatistics.org/teen-drug-use.

National Conference of State Legislatures. 2022. "State Medical Cannabis Laws." Last modified September 12, 2022. https://www.ncsl.org/health/state-medical-cannabis-laws#:~:text=As%20of%20Feb.,medical%20use%20of%20cannabis%20products.

National Council on Alcoholism and Drug Dependence. 2015. "Drugs and Alcohol in the Workplace." www.ncadd.org/about-addiction/addiction-update/drugs-and-alcohol-in-the-workplace.

National Council on Problem Gambling. 2014. "What Is Problem Gambling?" www.ncpgambling.org/help-treatment/faq.

National Eating Disorder Association. 2016. "Compulsive Exercise." www.nationaleatingdisorders.org/compulsive-exercise.

National Institute on Alcohol Abuse and Alcoholism. n.d.a. "Alcohol Myths." Accessed December 14, 2021. www.collegedrinkingprevention.gov/specialfeatures/alcoholmyths.aspx.

National Institute on Alcohol Abuse and Alcoholism. n.d.b.

"Alcohol's Effects on the Body." Accessed December 14, 2021. www.niaaa.nih.gov/alcohols-effects-health/alcohols-effects-body.

National Institute on Alcohol Abuse and Alcoholism. 2012. U.S. Department of Health and Human Services, National Institutes of Health. "A Family History of Alcoholism: Are You at Risk?" NIH Publication No. 03-5340. https://pubs.niaaa.nih.gov/publications/familyhistory/famhist.htm.

National Institute on Alcohol Abuse and Alcoholism. 2020. "Understanding Alcohol Use Disorder." Last modified April 2021. www.niaaa.nih.gov/publications/brochures-and-fact-sheets/understanding-alcohol-use-disorder.

National Institute on Alcohol Abuse and Alcoholism. 2021. "Understanding Binge Drinking." Last modified December 2021. www.niaaa.nih.gov/publications/brochures-and-fact-sheets/binge-drinking.

National Institute on Drug Abuse. 2017. "Over-the-Counter Medicines DrugFacts." Last modified December 17, 2017. www.drugabuse.gov/publications/drugfacts/over-counter-medicines.

National Institute on Drug Abuse. 2018. "Prescription Stimulants DrugFacts." Last modified June 6, 2018. www.drugabuse.gov/publications/drugfacts/prescription-stimulants.

National Institute on Drug Abuse. 2019a. "Hallucinogens DrugFacts." Last modified April 22, 2019. www.drugabuse.gov/publications/drugfacts/hallucinogens.

National Institute on Drug Abuse. 2019b. National Institutes of Health; U.S. Department of Health and Human Services. "Drug Use Trends Among College-Age Adults (19-22). From the 2018 Monitoring the Future College Students and Young Adults Survey Results." Last modified September 13, 2019. www.drugabuse.gov/drug-topics/trends-statistics/infographics/drug-alcohol-use-in-college-age-adults-in-2018.

National Institute on Drug Abuse. 2020a. "Drug Misuse and Addiction." Last modified September 13, 2020. www.drugabuse.gov/publications/drugs-brains-behavior-science-addiction/drug-misuse-addiction.

National Institute on Drug Abuse. 2020b. "Letter from the Director." Last modified May 28, 2020. www.drugabuse.gov/publications/research-reports/inhalants/letter-director.

National Institute on Drug Abuse. 2020c. "Most Commonly Used Addictive Drugs." Last modified June 25, 2020. www.drugabuse.gov/publications/media-guide/most-commonly-used-addictive-drugs.

National Institute on Drug Abuse. 2020d. "Vaping, Marijuana Use in 2019 Rose in College-Age Adults." Last modified September 15, 2020. www.drugabuse.gov/news-events/news-releases/2020/09/vaping-marijuana-use-in-2019-rose-in-college-age-adults.

National Institute on Drug Abuse. 2020e. "What Are the Risk Factors and Protective Factors?" Last modified May 25, 2020. www.drugabuse.gov/publications/preventing-drug-use-among-children-adolescents/chapter-1-risk-factors-protective-factors/what-are-risk-factors.

National Institute on Drug Abuse. 2021a. "Cocaine." Last modified December 12, 2021. https://teens.drugabuse.gov/drug-facts/cocaine.

National Institute on Drug Abuse. 2021b. "Inhalants." Last modified December 9, 2021. https://teens.drugabuse.gov/drug-facts/inhalants.

National Institute on Drug Abuse. 2021c. "Is Marijuana Addictive?" Last modified April 13, 2021. www.drugabuse.gov/publications/research-reports/marijuana/marijuana-addictive.

National Institute on Drug Abuse. 2021d. "Is There a Link Between Marijuana Use and Psychiatric Disorders?" Last modified April 13, 2021. www.drugabuse.gov/publications/research-reports/marijuana/there-link-between-marijuana-use-psychiatric-disorders.

National Institute on Drug Abuse. 2021e. "Marijuana." Last modified December 9, 2021. https://teens.drugabuse.gov/drug-facts/marijuana.

National Institute on Drug Abuse. 2021f. "Methamphetamine (Meth)." Last modified December 9, 2021. https://teens.drugabuse.gov/drug-facts/methamphetamine-meth.

National Institute on Drug Abuse. 2021g. "Naloxone DrugFacts." Last modified November 1, 2021. www.drugabuse.gov/publications/drugfacts/naloxone.

National Institute on Drug Abuse. 2021h. "Overdose Death Rates." Last modified January 29, 2021. www.drugabuse.gov/drug-topics/trends-statistics/overdose-death-rates.

National Institute on Drug Abuse. 2021i. "Prescription Opioids DrugFacts." Last modified June 1, 2021. www.drugabuse.gov/publications/drugfacts/prescription-opioids.

National Institute on Drug Abuse. 2021j. "Syringe Services Programs." Last modified June 7, 2021. www.drugabuse.gov/drug-topics/syringe-services-programs.

National Institute on Drug Abuse. 2021k. "What Is the Scope of Heroin Use in the United States?" Last modified April 13, 2021. www.drugabuse.gov/publications/research-reports/heroin/scope-heroin-use-in-united-states.

National Institute on Drug Abuse. 2021l. "What Are the Long-Term Effects of Heroin Use?" Accessed April 2, 2023. https://nida.nih.gov/publications/research-reports/heroin/what-are-long-term-effects-heroin-use.

National Institute on Drug Abuse. 2023. "Drug Overdose Death Rates." Accessed April 2, 2023. https://nida.nih.gov/research-topics/trends-statistics/overdose-death-rates.

PEW Trusts. 2020. "African Americans Often Face Challenges Accessing Substance Use Treatment." Last modified March 26, 2020. www.pewtrusts.org/en/research-and-analysis/articles/2020/03/26/african-americans-often-face-challenges-accessing-substance-use-treatment.

Schulenberg, J.E., L.D. Johnston, P.M. O'Malley, J.G. Bachman, R.A. Miech, and M.E. Patrick. 2019. "Monitoring the Future National Survey Results on Drug Use, 1975-2018: Volume II, College Students and Adults Ages 19-60." Ann Arbor: Institute for Social Research, University of Michigan. https://files.eric.ed.gov/fulltext/ED608266.pdf.

Schulenberg, J.E., L.D. Johnston, P.M. O'Malley, J.G. Bachman, R.A. Miech, and M.E. Patrick. 2020. "Monitoring the Future National Survey Results on Drug Use, 1975-2019: Volume II, College Students and Adults Ages 19-60." Ann

Arbor: Institute for Social Research, University of Michigan. http://monitoringthefuture.org/pubs/monographs/mtf-vol2_2019.pdf.

Sherburne, M. 2019. "Marijuana Use Among College Students Reaches New 25-Year High: National Study of College Students Also Shows Dramatic Increase in Vaping of Marijuana and Nicotine." *Michigan News*, University of Michigan. https://news.umich.edu/marijuana-use-among-us-college-students-reaches-new-35-year-high.

Sightes, E., B. Ray, D. Watson, P. Huynh, and C. Lawrence. 2018. "The Implementation of Syringe Services Programs (SSPs) in Indiana: Benefits, Barriers, and Best Practices." https://fsph.iupui.edu/doc/research-centers/SSP_Report_20180516.pdf.

Strain, E., A. Saxon, A., and M. Friedman, M. 2021. "Opioid Use Disorder: Epidemiology, Pharmacology, Clinical Manifestations, Course, Screening, Assessment, and Diagnosis." Last modified July 28, 2021. www.uptodate.com/contents/opioid-use-disorder-epidemiology-pharmacology-clinical-manifestations-course-screening-assessment-and-diagnosis.

Stop Medicine Abuse. 2021a. "The Size of the Problem." https://stopmedicineabuse.org/what-does-abuse-look-like/the-size-of-the-problem.

Stop Medicine Abuse. 2021b. "Slang Terms." http://stopmedicineabuse.org/what-does-abuse-look-like/slang-terms.

Substance Abuse and Mental Health Services Administration. 2014. "Results From the 2013 National Survey on Drug Use and Health: Summary of National Findings." NSDUH Series H-48, HHS Publication No. (SMA) 14-4863. Rockville, MD: Substance Abuse and Mental Health Services Administration. www.samhsa.gov/data/sites/default/files/NSDUHresultsPDFWHTML2013/Web/NSDUHresults2013.htm.

Substance Abuse and Mental Health Services Administration. Center for Behavioral Health Statistics and Quality. 2015. "Behavioral Health Trends in the United States: Results From the 2014 National Survey on Drug Use and Health." NSDUH Series H-50, HHS Publication No. (SMA) 15-4927. www.samhsa.gov/data.

Substance Abuse and Mental Health Services Administration. 2019. "National Survey on Drug Use and Health: Detailed Tables." Rockville, MD: Department of Health and Human Services. www.samhsa.gov/data/release/2019-national-survey-drug-use-and-health-nsduh-releases.

Substance Abuse and Mental Health Services Administration. 2020. "Key Substance Use and Mental Health Indicators in the United States: Results from the 2019 National Survey on Drug Use and Health." NSDUH Series H-55, HHS Publication No. (PEP) 20-07-01-001. Rockville, MD: Center for Behavioral Health Statistics and Quality, Substance Abuse and Mental Health Services Administration. www.samhsa.gov/data/sites/default/files/reports/rpt29393/2019NSDUHFFRPDFWHTML/2019NSDUHFFR090120.htm.

Substance Abuse and Mental Health Services Administration. 2022. "Key Substance Use and Mental Health Indicators in the United States: Results from the 2021 National Survey on Drug Use and Health (HHS Publication No. PEP22-07-01-005, NSDUH Series H-57)." Center for Behavioral Health Statistics and Quality, Substance Abuse and Mental Health Services Administration. https://www.samhsa.gov/data/report/2021-nsduh-annual-national-report.

U.S. Department of Health and Human Services. 2012. "Preventing Tobacco Use Among Youth and Young Adults: A Report of the Surgeon General." www.surgeongeneral.gov/library/reports/preventing-youth-tobacco-use/full-report.pdf.

U.S. Department of Health and Human Services. 2014. "The Health Consequences of Smoking—50 Years of Progress: A Report of the Surgeon General." www.cdc.gov/tobacco/data_statistics/sgr/50th-anniversary/index.htm.

U.S. Department of Health and Human Services. 2015. *2015-2020 Dietary Guidelines for Americans*, 8th ed. http://health.gov/dietaryguidelines/2015/guidelines.

U.S. Department of Health and Human Services. 2016. "E-Cigarette Use Among Youth and Young Adults: A Report of the Surgeon General." https://e-cigarettes.surgeongeneral.gov/documents/2016_SGR_Exec_Summ_508.pdf.

Chapter 12

American College of Obstetricians and Gynecologists' Committee on Practice Bulletins—Gynecology. 2019. "ACOG Practice Bulletin No. 208: Benefits and Risks of Sterilization." *Obstetrics and Gynecology* 133 (3): e194-e207. https://doi.org/10.1097/AOG.0000000000003111.

Black, M.C., K.C. Basile, M.J. Breiding, S.G. Smith, M.L. Walters, M.T. Merrick, J. Chen, and M.R. Stevens. 2011. "The National Intimate Partner and Sexual Violence Survey (NISVS): 2010 Summary Report." Atlanta: National Center for Injury Prevention and Control, Centers for Disease Control and Prevention. www.cdc.gov/violenceprevention/pdf/NISVS_Report2010-a.pdf.

Cantor, D., B. Fisher, S. Chibnall, R. Townsend, H. Lee, C. Bruce, and G. Thomas. 2015. "Report on the AAU Campus Climate Survey on Sexual Assault and Sexual Misconduct." Rockville, MD: Westat. www.aau.edu/sites/default/files/%40%20Files/Climate%20Survey/AAU_Campus_Climate_Survey_12_14_15.pdf.

Centers for Disease Control and Prevention. 2017. "Genital Herpes: Screening FAQ." Last modified February 9, 2017. www.cdc.gov/std/herpes/screening.htm.

Centers for Disease Control and Prevention. 2018. "6 Reasons to Get HPV Vaccine for Your Child." Last modified August 2018. www.cdc.gov/hpv/infographics/vacc-six-reasons.pdf.

Centers for Disease Control and Prevention. 2019a. "Know the Facts." Last modified February 26, 2019. www.cdc.gov/std/sam/gyt/knowthefacts.htm.

Centers for Disease Control and Prevention. 2019b. "Zika Virus: Overview." Last modified October 7, 2019. www.cdc.gov/zika/about/overview.html.

Centers for Disease Control and Prevention. 2020. "HPV Vaccine Recommendations." Last modified March 17, 2020. www.cdc.gov/vaccines/vpd/hpv/hcp/recommendations.html.

Centers for Disease Control and Prevention. 2021a. "CDC Fact Sheet: Reported STDs in the United States, 2019." www.cdc.gov/nchhstp/newsroom/docs/factsheets/STD-Trends-508.pdf.

Centers for Disease Control and Prevention. 2021b. "Chlamydia: Statistics." Last modified April 5, 2021. www.cdc.gov/std/chlamydia/stats.htm.

Centers for Disease Control and Prevention. 2021c. "Condom Effectiveness." Last modified June 2, 2021. www.cdc.gov/condomeffectiveness/index.html.

Centers for Disease Control and Prevention. 2021d. "Genital Herpes: Treatment and Care." Last modified July 22, 2021. www.cdc.gov/std/herpes/treatment.htm.

Centers for Disease Control and Prevention. 2021e. "Gonorrhea: Detailed Fact Sheet." Last modified July 22, 2021. www.cdc.gov/std/gonorrhea/stdfact-gonorrhea-detailed.htm.

Centers for Disease Control and Prevention. 2021f. "HIV and Youth: HIV Incidence." Last modified September 21, 2021. www.cdc.gov/hiv/group/age/youth/incidence.html.

Centers for Disease Control and Prevention. 2021g. "HIV in the United States and Dependent Areas." Last modified August 9, 2021. www.cdc.gov/hiv/statistics/overview/ata-glance.html.

Centers for Disease Control and Prevention. 2021h. HIV Surveillance Report, 2019; vol. 32. Published May 2021. Accessed December 16, 2021.www.cdc.gov/hiv/library/reports/hiv-surveillance.html.

Centers for Disease Control and Prevention. 2021i. "HIV Treatment." Last modified May 20, 2021. www.cdc.gov/hiv/basics/livingwithhiv/treatment.html.

Centers for Disease Control and Prevention. 2021j. "Human Papillomavirus (HPV) Statistics." Last modified April 5, 2021. www.cdc.gov/std/hpv/stats.htm.

Centers for Disease Control and Prevention. 2021k. "PrEP Effectiveness." Last modified May 13, 2021. www.cdc.gov/hiv/basics/prep/prep-effectiveness.html.

Centers for Disease Control and Prevention. 2021l. "The Youth Risk Behavior Survey Data Summary & Trends Report: 2011–2021." Accessed April 3, 2023. https://www.cdc.gov/healthyyouth/data/yrbs/pdf/YRBS_Data-Summary-Trends_Report2023_508.pdf.

Centers for Disease Control and Prevention. 2021m. *Sexually Transmitted Disease Surveillance 2019*. Atlanta: U.S. Department of Health and Human Services. Last modified July 29, 2021. www.cdc.gov/std/statistics/2019/std-surveillance-2019.pdf.

Centers for Disease Control and Prevention. 2021n. "Sexually Transmitted Diseases: Which STD Tests Should I get?" Last modified July 22, 2021. www.cdc.gov/std/prevention/screeningreccs.htm.

Centers for Disease Control and Prevention. 2021o. "Unintended Pregnancy Prevention." Last modified June 28, 2021. www.cdc.gov/reproductivehealth/unintendedpregnancy.

Centers for Disease Control and Prevention. 2021p. "Zika Virus: 2021 Case Counts." Last modified November 16, 2021. www.cdc.gov/zika/reporting/2021-case-counts.html.

Centers for Disease Control and Prevention. 2021q. "Zika Virus: Statistics and Maps." Last modified September 20, 2021. www.cdc.gov/zika/reporting/index.html.

Edwards, Jonathan. 2021. "A 16-Year-Old Girl Learned a Hand Gesture on TikTok to Signal for Help. Law Enforcement Says It Saved Her." *The Washington Post*. Last modified November 8, 2021. www.washingtonpost.com/nation/2021/11/08/tik-tok-hand-sign-kidnapper/.

Frederiksen, B., U. Ranji, A. Salganicoff, and M. Long. 2021. "Women's Sexual and Reproductive Health Services: Key Findings from the 2020 KFF Women's Health Survey." www.kff.org/womens-health-policy/issue-brief/womens-sexual-and-reproductive-health-services-key-findings-from-the-2020-kff-womens-health-survey.

Guttmacher Institute. 2021a. "Contraceptive Use in the United States by Demographics." Last modified May 2021. www.guttmacher.org/fact-sheet/contraceptive-use-united-states.

Guttmacher Institute. 2021b. "Contraceptive Use in the United States by Method." Last modified May 2021. www.guttmacher.ogr/fact-sheet/contraceptive-method-use-united-states.

Guttmacher Institute. 2021c. "Use of Emergency Contraception in the United States." Last modified September 2021. www.guttmacher.ogr/fact-sheet/use-emergency-contraceptive-united-states.

Guttmacher Institute. 2021d. "Partner Treatment for STIs." Last modified November 1, 2021. www.guttmacher.org/state-policy/explore/partner-treatment-stis.

Hensel, D., M. Rosenberg, M. Luetke, T. Fu, and D. Herbenick. 2020. "Changes in Solo and Partnered Sexual Behaviors During the COVID-19 Pandemic: Findings From a U.S. Probability Survey." https://doi.org/10.1101/2020.06.09.20125609.

Hussain, R. and M. Kavanaugh, 2021. "Changes in Use of Emergency Contraceptive Pills in the United States from 2008–2015." *Contraception: X*, 3:100065,. https://www.sciencedirect.com/science/article/pii/S2590151621000125.

Human Rights Campaign. n.d. "Sexual Assault and the LGBTQ Community." Accessed December 9, 2021. www.hrc.org/resources/sexual-assault-and-the-lgbt-community.

Kaiser Family Foundation. 2022. "Emergency Contraception." Accessed March 30, 2023. https://www.kff.org/womens-health-policy/fact-sheet/emergency-contraception/.

Kearl, H. 2018. "The Facts Behind the #MeToo Movement: A National Study on Sexual Harassment and Assault." www.stopstreetharassment.org/wp-content/uploads/2018/01/Full-Report-2018-National-Study-on-Sexual-Harassment-and-Assault.pdf.

Kreisel, K.M., I.H. Spicknall, J.W. Gargano, F.M. Lewis, R.M. Lewis, L.E. Markowitz, H. Roberts, et al. 2021. "Sexually Transmitted Infections Among U.S. Women and Men: Prevalence and Incidence Estimates." *Sexually Transmitted Diseases* 48 (4): 208-214. https://doi.org/10.1097/OLQ.0000000000001355.

Lisak, D., L. Gardinier, S.C. Nicksa, and A.M. Cote. 2010. "False Allegations of Sexual Assault: An Analysis of Ten Years of Reported Cases." *Violence Against Women* 16 (12): 1318-1334.

Manlove, J.S., S. Ryan, and K. Franzetta. 2003. "Patterns of Contraceptive Use Within Teenagers' First Sexual Relationships." *Perspectives on Sexual and Reproductive Health* 36 (6):

246-255. https://doi.org/10.1363/3524603.

Market Wired. 2014. "Eight Leading National Fraternities Form a Historic Consortium to Address Important Issues of Sexual Misconduct, Hazing and Binge Drinking Head On." Accessed July 11, 2017. https://finance.yahoo.com/news/eight-leading-national-fraternities-form-133500836.html.

Marshall, W. 2021. "Sex and Coronavirus: Can You Get COVID-19 From Sexual Activity?" Last modified May 18, 2021. www.mayoclinic.org/diseases-conditions/coronavirus/expert-answers/sex-and-coronavirus/faq-20486572.

Martinez, G.M., and J.C. Abma. 2020. "Sexual Activity and Contraceptive Use Among Teenagers Aged 15-19 in the United States, 2015-2017." NCHS Data Brief, no. 366. Hyattsville, MD: National Center for Health Statistics.

Mayo Clinic. 2021a. "Male Circumcision." Last modified September 21, 2021. www.mayoclinic.org/tests-procedures/circumcision/about/pac-20393550.

Mayo Clinic. 2021b. "Vasectomy." Last modified August 21, 2021. www.mayoclinic.org/tests-procedures/vasectomy/about/pac-20384580.

Morgan, R., and B. Oudekerk. 2019. *Criminal Victimization, 2018* (NCJ 253043). U.S. Department of Justice, Bureau of Justice Statistics. https://www.nsvrc.org/sites/default/files/2021-04/cv18.pdf.

National Academies of Sciences, Engineering, and Medicine. 2021. *Sexually Transmitted Infections: Adopting a Sexual Health Paradigm.* Washington, DC: The National Academies Press. https://doi.org/10.17226/25955.

National Sexual Violence Resource Center. n.d. "Statistics." Accessed December 9, 2021. www.nsvrc.org/statistics.

Office on Women's Health. 2018. "Sexual Assault on College Campuses." Last modified September 13, 2021. www.womenshealth.gov/relationships-and-safety/sexual-assault-and-rape/college-sexual-assault.

Office on Women's Health. 2019. "Sexual Assault." Last modified March 14, 2019. www.womenshealth.gov/relationships-and-safety/sexual-assault-and-rape/sexual-assault.

Pan American Health Organization. 2016. "What Is Zika?" Last modified October 24, 2016. www.paho.org/en/documents/infographic-what-zika-2016-png-version.

Perry, S. 2004. "A BJS Statistical Profile, 1992-2002: American Indians and Crime." U.S. Department of Justice, Office of Justice Programs, Bureau of Justice Statistics. https://bjs.ojp.gov/content/pub/pdf/aic02.pdf.

Peterson, C., S. DeGue, C. Florence, and C.N. Lokey. 2017. "Lifetime Economic Burden of Rape Among U.S. Adults." *American Journal of Preventive Medicine* 52 (6): 691-701.

RAINN. n.d.a. "Sexual Assault: What Is Sexual Assault?" Accessed December 9, 2021. www.rainn.org/articles/sexual-assault.

RAINN. n.d.b. "Victims of Sexual Violence: Statistics." Accessed December 9, 2021. www.rainn.org/statistics/victims-sexual-violence.

RAINN. n.d.c. "What Consent Looks Like." Accessed December 9, 2021. www.rainn.org/articles/what-is-consent.

Rebar, R. 2020. "Sperm Disorders." Last modified September 2020. www.merckmanuals.com/professional/gynecology-and-obstetrics/infertility/sperm-disorders.

Smith, S.G., J. Chen, K.C. Basile, L.K. Gilbert, M.T. Merrick, N. Patel, M. Walling, and A. Jain. 2017. *The National Intimate Partner and Sexual Violence Survey: 2010-2012 State Report.* Atlanta: National Center for Injury Prevention and Control, Centers for Disease Control and Prevention.

Smith, S.G., X. Zhang, K.C. Basile, M.T. Merrick, J. Wang, M. Kresnow, and J. Chen. 2018. *The National Intimate Partner and Sexual Violence Survey: 2015 Data Brief—Updated Release.* Atlanta: Centers for Disease Control and Prevention.

Sonfield, A., K. Hasstedt, and R.B. Gold. 2014. "Moving Forward: Family Planning in the Era of Health Reform." www.guttmacher.org/report/moving-forward-family-planning-era-health-reform#.

Trussell, J., A.R.A. Aiken, E. Micks, and K.A. Guthrie. 2018. "Efficacy, Safety, and Personal Considerations." In *Contraceptive Technology,* edited by R.A. Hatcher, A.L. Nelson, J. Trussell, C. Cwiak, P. Cason, M.S. Policar, A. Edelman, A.R.A. Aiken, J. Marrazzo, and D. Kowal, 21st ed. New York: Ayer Company Publishers, Inc.

Turban, J., A. Keurighlian, and K. Mayer. 2021. "Sexual Health in the SARS-CoV-2 Era." *Annals of Internal Medicine* 173: 387-389. https://doi.org/10.7326/M20-2004.

UNICEF. 2019. "What You Need to Know About Female Genital Mutilation: 7 Questions Answered." Last modified March 4, 2019. www.unicef.org/stories/what-you-need-know-about-female-genital-mutilation.

U.S. Department of Health and Human Services, Centers for Disease Control and Prevention, National Center for HIV, Viral Hepatitis, STD, and TB Prevention, Division of STD Prevention. 2021. "Sexually Transmitted Disease Surveillance 2019: Division of STD Prevention." Accessed March 31, 2023. https://www.cdc.gov/std/statistics/2019/std-surveillance-2019.pdf.

U.S. Department of Justice. 2017. "An Updated Definition of Rape." Last modified April 7, 2017. www.justice.gov/archives/opa/blog/updated-definition-rape.

World Health Organization. 2020. "Female Genital Mutilation." Last modified February 3, 2020. www.who.int/news-room/fact-sheets/detail/female-genital-mutilation.

Chapter 13

American Diabetes Association. n.d.a. "Diabetes Overview." Accessed May 28, 2023. www.diabetes.org/diabetes.

American Diabetes Association. n.d.b. "Diagnosis." Accessed May 28, 2023. www.diabetes.org/diabetes/a1c/diagnosis.

American Heart Association. n.d.a. "Peripheral Artery Disease (PAD)." Accessed May 28, 2023. www.heart.org/en/health-topics/peripheral-artery-disease.

American Heart Association. n.d.b. "Cholesterol" Accessed May 28, 2023. https://www.heart.org/en/health-topics/cholesterol.

American Stroke Association. 2021. "Risk Factors Under Your Control." Accessed May 28, 2023. www.stroke.org/en/about-stroke/stroke-risk-factors/risk-factors-under-your-control.

Arts, J., M.L. Fernandez, and I.E. Lofgren. 2014. "Coronary Heart Disease Risk Factors in College Students." *Advances in Nutrition* 5 (2): 177-187.

Centers for Disease Control and Prevention. 2021. "High Blood Pressure Symptoms and Causes." Accessed May 28, 2023. www.cdc.gov/bloodpressure/about.htm.

Centers for Disease Control and Prevention. 2022a. "Diabetes Basics." Accessed May 28, 2023. www.cdc.gov/diabetes/basics/index.html.

Centers for Disease Control and Prevention. 2022b. "Prediabetes—Your Chance to Prevent Type 2 Diabetes." Accessed May 28, 2023. www.cdc.gov/diabetes/basics/prediabetes.html.

Centers for Disease Control and Prevention. 2023a. "Leading Causes of Death." Accessed May 28, 2023. www.cdc.gov/nchs/fastats/leading-causes-of-death.htm.

Centers for Disease Control and Prevention. 2023b. "Heart Disease—Know Your Risk for Heart Disease." Accessed May 28, 2023. www.cdc.gov/heartdisease/risk_factors.htm.

Centers for Disease Control and Prevention. 2023c. "People with Certain Medical Conditions." Accessed February 26, 2022. www.cdc.gov/coronavirus/2019-ncov/need-extra-precautions/people-with-medical-conditions.html.

International Diabetes Federation. 2006. *The IDF Consensus Worldwide Definition of the Metabolic Syndrome.* Brussels: IDF Communications. Accessed February 26, 2022. www.idf.org/e-library/consensus-statements/60-idfconsensus-worldwide-definitionof-the-metabolic-syndrome.html.

Libby, P., P.M. Ridker, and G.K. Hansson. 2009. "Inflammation in Atherosclerosis: From Pathophysiology to Practice." *Journal of the American College of Cardiology* 54 (23): 2129-2138.

Moore, J.X., N. Chaudhary, and T. Akinyemiju. 2017. "Metabolic Syndrome Prevalence by Race/Ethnicity and Sex in the United States, National Health and Nutrition Examination Survey, 1988-2012." *Preventing Chronic Disease* 14: E24.

National Heart, Lung, and Blood Institute. 2012. *Expert Panel on Guidelines for Cardiovascular Health and Risk Reduction in Children and Adolescents.* NIH Publication No. 12-7486. Bethesda, MD: Author. www.nhlbi.nih.gov/files/docs/guidelines/peds_guidelines_full.pdf.

Parcha, V., B. Heindl, R. Kalra, P. Li, B. Gower, G. Arora, and P. Arora. 2022. "Insulin Resistance and Cardiometabolic Risk Profile Among Nondiabetic American Young Adults: Insights From NHANES." *Journal of Clinical Endocrinology and Metabolism* 107 (1): e25-e37. https://doi.org/10.1210/clinem/dgab645.

Roitman, J.L., and T. LaFontaine. 2012. *The Exercise Professional's Guide to Optimizing Health.* Baltimore: Lippincott Williams & Wilkins.

Stocks, T., T. Bjorge, H. Ulmer, J. Manjer, C. Haggstrom, G. Nagel, A. Engeland, et al. 2015. "Metabolic Risk Score and Cancer Risk: Pooled Analysis of Seven Cohorts." *International Journal of Epidemiology* 44 (4): 1353-1363.

Stone, N.J., J.G. Robinson, A.H. Lichtenstein, C.N. Bairey Merz, C.B. Blum, R.H. Eckel, A.C. Goldberg, et al. 2014. "2013 ACC/AHA Guideline on the Treatment of Blood Cholesterol to Reduce Atherosclerotic Cardiovascular Risk in Adults: A Report of the American College Of Cardiology/American Heart Association Task Force on Practice Guidelines." *Circulation* 129 (25 Suppl 2): S1-45.

Chapter 14

American Association for Cancer Research. 2014. "AACR Cancer Progress Report 2014." *Clinical Cancer Research* 20 (Suppl. 1): SI-S124.

American Cancer Society. 2018. "Can Testicular Cancer Be Found Early?" Last modified May 17, 2018. www.cancer.org/cancer/testicular-cancer/detection-diagnosis-staging/detection.html.

American Cancer Society. 2020a. "Health Risks of Smoking." Last modified October 28, 2020. www.cancer.org/healthy/stay-away-from-tobacco/health-risks-of-tobacco/health-risks-of-smoking-tobacco.html.

American Cancer Society. 2020b. "Study: Young Women Now Have Higher Rates for Lung Cancer Than Men Worldwide." Last modified February 14, 2020. www.canccr.org/latest-news/study-young-women-now-have-higher-rate-for-lung-cancer-than-men-worldwide.html.

American Cancer Society. 2021a. "Breast Cancer Stages." Last modified June 28, 2021. www.cancer.org/cancer/breast-cancer/understanding-a-breast-cancer-diagnosis/stages-of-breast-cancer.html.

American Cancer Society. 2021b. "Cancer Facts and Figures 2021. Special Section: COVID-19 and Cancer." www.cancer.org/content/dam/cancer-org/research/cancer-facts-and-statistics/annual-cancer-facts-and-figures/2021/special-section-covid19-and-cancer-2021.pdf.

American Cancer Society. 2021c. "Lifetime Risk of Developing or Dying From Cancer." Last modified January 13, 2021. www.cancer.org/cancer/cancer-basics/lifetime-probability-of-developing-or-dying-from-cancer.html.

American Cancer Society. 2022. "Cancer Facts & Figures 2022." Accessed April 1, 2023.

American Cancer Society. 2023. "Cancer Statistics Center." Accessed April 1, 2023. https://www.cancer.org/content/dam/cancer-org/research/cancer-facts-and-statistics/annual-cancer-facts-and-figures/2022/2022-cancer-facts-and-figures.pdf. https://cancerstatisticscenter.cancer.org/?_ga=2.170511715.238505627.1680361173-5820588.1676058690#!/.

American Institute for Cancer Research. 2020. "What You Need to Know About Obesity and Cancer." Last modified January 19, 2020. www.aicr.org/resources/media-library/what-you-need-to-know-about-obesity-and-cancer.

Breastcancer.org. 2019. "How to Do a Breast Self-Exam: The Five Steps." Last modified October 24, 2019. www.breastcancer.org/symptoms/testing/types/self_exam.

Breastcancer.org. 2021. "Family History." Last modified April 21, 2021. www.breastcancer.org/risk/factors/family_history.

Centers for Disease Control and Prevention. n.d. "Tobacco Myths." Accessed September 16, 2021. www.cdc.gov/tobacco/data_statistics/sgr/2010/myths/pdfs/myths.pdf.

Centers for Disease Control and Prevention. 2020a. "Health

Equity." Last modified March 11, 2020. www.cdc.gov/chronicdisease/healthequity/index.htm.

Centers for Disease Control and Prevention. 2020b. "Surgeon General's Reports on Smoking and Tobacco Use." Last modified January 23, 2020. www.cdc.gov/tobacco/data_statistics/sgr.

Centers for Disease Control and Prevention. 2021a. "Overweight & Obesity: Adult Obesity Facts." Last modified June 7, 2021. www.cdc.gov/obesity/data/adult.html.

Centers for Disease Control and Prevention. 2021b. "Smoking and Tobacco Use." Last modified June 2, 2021. www.cdc.gov/tobacco/data_statistics/fact_sheets/fast_facts/index.htm.

Centers for Disease Control and Prevention. 2021c. "What Are the Risk Factors for Skin Cancer?" Last modified April 28, 2021. www.cdc.gov/cancer/skin/basic_info/risk_factors.htm.

DeVita Jr., V.T., and E. Chu. 2008. "A History of Cancer Chemotherapy." *Cancer Research* 68 (21): 8643-8653. https://doi.org/10.1158/0008-5472.CAN-07-6611.

Fidler-Benaoudia, M.M., L.A. Torre, F. Bray, J. Ferlay, and A. Jemal. 2020. "Lung Cancer Incidence in Young Women vs. Young Men: A Systematic Analysis in 40 Countries." *International Journal of Cancer* 147 (3): 811-819. https://doi.org/10.1002/ijc.32809.

Fosnacht, K., A.C. McCormick, and R. Lerma. 2018. "First-Year Students' Time Use in College: A Latent Profile Analysis." *Research in Higher Education* 59(7): 958-978. https://doi.org/10.1007/ s11162-018-9497-z.

Harvard School of Public Health. n.d. "Healthy Eating Plate." Accessed September 23, 2021. www.hsph.harvard.edu/nutritionsource/healthy-eating-plate.

Heron, M. 2021. "Deaths: Leading Causes for 2019." *National Vital Statistics Reports* 70 (9). Hyattsville, MD: National Center for Health Statistics. doi: 10.15620/cdc:107021.

Kochanek, K.D., J.Q. Xu, and E. Arias. 2020. "Mortality in the United States, 2019." NCHS Data Brief, no 395. Hyattsville, MD: National Center for Health Statistics. www.cdc.gov/nchs/data/databriefs/db395-H.pdf.

Kuderer, N.M., T.K. Choueiri, D.P. Shah, et al. 2020. "Clinical Impact of COVID-19 on Patients With Cancer (CCC19): A Cohort Study." *Lancet* 395 (10241): 1907-1918. https://doi.org/10.1016/S0140-6736(20)31187-9.

Martin, L. 2020. "Cancer Incidence Rates by Age." WebMD. www.webmd.com/cancer/guide/cancer-incidence-age.

Medline Plus. 2021. "Colon Cancer Screening." Last modified September 1, 2021. https://medlineplus.gov/ency/article/002071.htm.

Mendes, E. 2017. "More Than 4 in 10 Cancers and Cancer Deaths Linked to Modifiable Risk Factors." www.cancer.org/latest-news/more-than-4-in-10-cancers-and-cancer-deaths-linked-to-modifiable-risk-factors.html.

National Cancer Institute. 1990. "Normal and Cancer Cell Structure." Last modified January 1, 2001. https://visualsonline.cancer.gov/details.cfm?imageid=2512.

National Cancer Institute. 2015. "The Biology of Cancer Health Disparities." Last modified September 11, 2015. www.cancer.gov/research/progress/discovery/biology-cancer-health-disparities#3.

National Cancer Institute. 2020a. "Cancer Disparities." Last modified November 17, 2020. www.cancer.gov/about-cancer/understanding/disparities.

National Cancer Institute. 2020b. "Metastatic Cancer: When Cancer Spreads." Last modified November 10, 2020. www.cancer.gov/types/metastatic-cancer.

National Cancer Institute. 2020c. "NCI COVID-19 in Cancer Patients Study (NCCAPS)." Last modified November 9, 2020. www.cancer.gov/research/key-initiatives/covid-19/coronavirus-research-initiatives/nccaps.

National Cancer Institute. 2021a. "NCI Dictionary of Cancer Terms." www.cancer.gov/publications/dictionaries/cancer-terms.

National Cancer Institute. 2021b. "Surveillance, Epidemiology, and End Results Program Explorer: An Interactive Website for SEER Cancer Statistics." Last modified April 15, 2021. https://seer.cancer.gov/explorer/.

National Geographic. 2018. "Shark Attack Facts." www.natgeotv.com/ca/human-shark-bait/facts.

National Safety Council. 2021. "Odds of Dying." https://injuryfacts.nsc.org/all-injuries/preventable-death-overview/odds-of-dying/.

Rock, C.L., C. Thomson, T. Gansler, S.M. Gapstur, M.L. McCullough, A.V. Patel, K.S. Andrews, et al. 2020. "American Cancer Society Guideline for Diet and Physical Activity for Cancer Prevention." *CA: A Cancer Journal for Clinicians* 70: 245-271. https://doi.org/10.3322/caac.21591.

Ropeik, D., and G. Gray. 2002. *Risk: A Practical Guide for Deciding What's Really Safe and What's Really Dangerous in the World Around You.* New York: Houghton Mifflin Company.

Schwingshackl, L., and G. Hoffmann. 2015. "Diet Quality as Assessed by the Healthy Eating Index, the Alternate Healthy Eating Index, the Dietary Approaches to Stop Hypertension Score, and Health Outcomes: A Systematic Review and Meta-Analysis of Cohort Studies." *Journal of the Academy of Nutrition and Dietetics* 115 (5): 780-800.e5. https://doi.org/10.1016/j.jand.2014.12.009.

Simon, S. 2019. "Should You Get Genetic Testing for Cancer Risk?" Last modified September 18, 2019. www.cancer.org/latest-news/should-you-get-genetic-testing-for-cancer-risk.html.

U.S. Department of Health and Human Services. 2014. "The Health Consequences of Smoking: 50 Years of Progress. A Report of the Surgeon General." Last modified January 16, 2014. www.hhs.gov/surgeongeneral/reports-and-publications/tobacco/consequences-smoking-factsheet/index.html.

U.S. Food and Drug Administration. 2021. "COVID-19 Frequently Asked Questions." Last modified December 15, 2021. www.fda.gov/emergency-preparedness-and-response/coronavirus-disease-2019-covid-19/covid-19-frequently-asked-questions#:~:text=Yes.%20Data%20shows%20that,%2C%20or%20even%20death.

Yarnal C., X. Qian, J. Hustad, and D. Sims. 2013. "Intervention for Positive Use of Leisure Time Among College Students." *Journal of College and Character* 14 (2). https://doi.org/10.1515/jcc-2013-0022.

Chapter 15

Antonucci, T.C., J.A. Ashton-Miller, J. Brant, E.B. Falk, J.B. Halter, L. Hamdemir, S.H. Konrath, et al. 2012. "The Right to Move: A Multidisciplinary Lifespan Conceptual Framework." *Current Gerontology and Geriatrics Research* 2012: 873937. https://doi.org/10.1155/2012/873937.

Brickwood, K.J., G. Watson, J. O'Brien, and A.D. Williams. 2019. "Consumer-Based Wearable Activity Trackers Increase Physical Activity Participation: Systematic Review and Meta-Analysis." *JMIR mHealth and uHealth* 7 (4): e11819. https://doi.org/10.2196/11819.

Bautmans, I., V. Knoop, J. Amuthavalli Thiyagarajan, A.B. Maier, J.R. Beard, E. Freiberger, D. Belsky, et al. 2022. "WHO Working Definition of Vitality Capacity for Healthy Longevity Monitoring." *The Lancet* 3 (11): e789-e796.

https://doi.org/10.1016/S2666-7568(22)00200-8.

Bull, F.C., S.S. Al-Ansari, S. Biddle, K. Borodulin, M.P. Buman, G. Cardon, C. Carty, et al. 2020. "World Health Organization (WHO) 2020 Guidelines on Physical Activity and Sedentary Behaviour." *British Journal of Sports Medicine* 54: 1451-1462.

Centers for Disease Control and Prevention. 2022. "Adult Physical Inactivity Prevalence Maps." Accessed June 8, 2022. www.cdc.gov/physicalactivity/data/inactivity-prevalence-maps/index.html#overall.

Church, T.S., D.M. Thomas, C. Tudor-Locke, P.T. Katzmarzyk, C.P. Earnest, R.Q. Rodarte, C.K. Martin, S.N. Blair, and C. Bouchard. 2011. "Trends Over 5 Decades in U.S. Occupation-Related Physical Activity and Their Associations With Obesity." *PLoS ONE* 6 (5): e19657. https://doi.org/10.1371/journal.pone.0019657.

Clarke, T.C., P.M. Barnes, L.I. Black, B.J. Stussman, and R.L. Nahin. 2018. "Use of Yoga, Meditation, and Chiropractors Among U.S. Adults Aged 18 and Older." NCHS Data Brief, no 325. Hyattsville, MD: National Center for Health Statistics.

Ekelund, U., J. Steene-Johannessen, W.J. Brown, M. Wang Fagerland, N. Owen, K.E. Powell, A. Bauman, et al. 2016. "Does Physical Activity Attenuate, or Even Eliminate, the Detrimental Association of Sitting Time With Mortality? A Harmonised Meta-Analysis of Data From More Than 1 Million Men and Women." *Lancet* 388 (10051): 1302-1310.

International Health and Racquet Sports Association. 2021. "Global Report." Accessed February 11, 2022. www.ihrsa.org/publications/the-2021-ihrsa-global-report.

Katzmarzyk, P., K.E. Powell, J.M Jakicic, R.P. Troiano, K. Piercy, and B. Tennant. 2019. "Sedentary Behavior and Health: Update from the 2018 Physical Activity Guidelines Advisory Committee." *Medicine & Science in Sports & Exercise* 51 (6): 1227-1241. https://doi.org/10.1249/MSS.0000000000001935.

Kiessling, P., and Kennedy-Armbruster, C. 2016. "Move More, Sit Less, Be Well. Behavioral Aspects of Activity Trackers." *ACSM Health and Fitness Journal* 20 (6): 26-31.

Koivunen, K., L.A. Schaap, E.O. Hoogendijk, L.J. Schoonmade, M. Huisman, N.M. an Schoor. 2022. "Exploring the Conceptual Framework and Measurement Model of Intrinsic Capacity Defined by the World Health Organization: A Scoping Review." *Ageing Research Review*, 80, 101685.

Laranjo, L., Ding, D., Heleno, B., B. Kocaballi, J.C. Quiroz, H.L. Tong, B. Chahwan, et al. 2021. "Do Smartphone Applications and Activity Trackers Increase Physical Activity in Adults? Systematic Review, Meta-Analysis and Metaregression." *British Journal of Sports Medicine* 55: 422-432.

McGavock, J., J. Hastings, P. Snell, D. McGuire, E. Pacini, B. Levine, and J. Mitchell. 2009. "A Forty-Year Follow-Up of the Dallas Bed Rest and Training Study: The Effect of Age on the Cardiovascular Response to Exercise in Men." *The Journals of Gerontology: Series A* 64A (2): 293-299. https://doi.org/10.1093/gerona/gln025.

McGuire, D.K., B.D. Levine, J.W. Williamson, P.G. Snell, C.G. Blomqvist, B. Saltin, and J.H. Mitchell. 2001. "A 30-Year Follow Up of the Dallas Bedrest and Training Study: II. Effect of Age on Cardiovascular Adaptation to Exercise Training." *Circulation* 104 (12): 1358-1366.

National Association of Chronic Disease Directors. 2022. "Nutrition, Physical Activity and Obesity FY 2022 Appropriations Fact Sheet." https://chronicdisease.org/wp-content/uploads/2021/06/NACDD-Fact-Sheet-2022_DNPAOFI-NALv3.pdf.

Paffenbarger, R., M.A. Hyde, A. Wing, and C. Hsieh. 1986. "Physical Activity, All-Cause Mortality, and Longevity of College Alumni." *New England Journal of Medicine* 314 (10): 605-613. https://doi.org/10.1056/NEJM198603063141003.

Pronk, N.P., and M.A. Fagh. 2022. "Causal Systems Mapping to Promote Healthy Living for Pandemic Preparedness: A Call to Action for Global Public Health." *International Journal of Behavioral Nutrition and Physical Activity* 19 (1): 13. https://doi.org/10.1186/s12966-022-01255-7.

Saltin, B., G. Blomqvist, J.H. Mitchell, R.L. Johnson Jr., K. Wildenthal, and C.B. Chapman. 1968. "Response to Exercise After Bed Rest and After Training." *Circulation* 38 (Suppl. 5): VII1-78.

Segar, M. 2022. *The Joy Choice: How to Finally Achieve Lasting Changes in Eating and Exercise.* New York: Hachette Book Group.

Signorile, J.F. 2011. *Bending the Aging Curve: The Complete Exercise Guide for Older Adults.* Champaign, IL: Human Kinetics.

Stanton, W.R. 1996. *From Child to Adult: The Dunedin Multidisciplinary Health and Development Study.* Oxford: Oxford University Press.

Thompson, W.R. 2022. "Worldwide Survey of Fitness Trends for 2022." *ACSM's Health & Fitness Journal* 26 (1): 1-20.

World Health Organization. 2022. "Ageing and Health." Accessed June 6, 2023. https://www.who.int/news-room/fact-sheets/detail/ageing-and-health.

World Health Organization. 2015. "World Report on Ageing and Health." Accessed June 6, 2023. https://apps.who.int/iris/bitstream/handle/10665/186463/9789240694811_eng.pdf?sequence=1&isAllowed=y.

INDEX

Note: The italicized *f* and *t* following page numbers refer to figures and tables, respectively.

A

AAS (anabolic-androgenic steroids) 107-108
abdominals 136-137
abstinence 290
academic performance 76, 78, 234, 236
Academy of Nutrition and Dietetics 184
acceptable macronutrient distribution range (AMDR) 191
ACSM. *See* American College of Sports Medicine
action stage of change 45, 47*f*, 48, 48*f*
active transportation 27, 31-32, 81, 84, 105, 214, 217, 220
activity. *See* exercise; movement; physical activity
activity trackers 82, 374-375
added sugars 178, 192, 218*t*
Adderall 264
addiction 247-277. *See also* behavioral addiction; substance addiction
adductor muscles 142-143
adenosine triphosphate (ATP) 70, 70*f*, 72-73, 90
adenosine triphosphate–phosphocreatine (ATP-PC) system 71*t*, 72
adequate intake (AI) 191
adipocytes 157
adiposity 157, 160, 166, 167
adolescents. *See* children and adolescents
adrenalin 228
AEDs (automated external defibrillators) 328, 376
aerobic fitness. *See* cardiorespiratory fitness
aerobic (oxidative) system 71*t*, 72, 73, 90
aerobic training. *See* cardiorespiratory training
aerosols, inhalation of 260
age. *See also specific age groups*
 biological 369, 370*f*
 body composition and 158, 167
 cancer and 339, 345, 345*t*
 chronic disease onset and 6, 6*f*
 chronological 369, 370*f*, 372
 flexibility and 110, 111
 low back pain and 122
 muscle decline and 368, 368*f*
 obesity rates and 204, 205*f*
 osteoporosis and 169
 percent body fat and 166, 167*t*
 prediabetes and 322
 psychological 370, 370*f*
 resting metabolic rate and 214
 weight changes and 209, 209*f*
 wellness priorities based on 9, 11
Aging Well (Vaillant) 53
AI (adequate intake) 191
AIDS. *See* HIV/AIDS
air displacement plethysmography 160
air quality 86

alcoholism, symptoms of 271
alcohol use. *See also* substance addiction
 binge drinking 267, 268*f*, 270
 blood alcohol concentration 268-270, 269*f*
 calories from 176, 177*f*, 188, 212
 by college students 254, 267-268, 268*f*
 energy drinks and 270, 271
 fatty liver disease and 167
 health risks and 267-268
 intake recommendations 188, 193
 myths vs. facts 270
 one drink by type 269*f*
 osteoporosis and 170
 prevalence of 249, 249*f*, 266
 treatment for 249-250
 weight management and 220
allocation of effort 231
all-or-none principle 90
allostasis 230
allostatic balance 230-232, 232*f*
allostatic load 230-232, 232*f*, 241
alpha linoleic acid 180
alternative medicine 373, 373*f*, 374
AMDR (acceptable macronutrient distribution range) 191
American Academy of Pediatrics 287
American Academy of Sleep Medicine 242
American Cancer Society 340, 348, 349, 357, 363
American College of Sports Medicine (ACSM)
 on cardiorespiratory training 28-29, 30*f*, 77-80, 82
 exercise guidelines 26, 28-33, 35, 45, 110
 on fitness categories 166
 on flexibility training 29, 30*f*, 110, 113
 on muscular fitness 88, 98
 on neuromuscular fitness 117
 on resistance training 29, 30*f*, 99-101, 104
 on wearable technologies 374
 on weight management 221
American Diabetes Association 323
American Heart Association 328, 333
American Medical Association 206
American Red Cross 328
American Sleep Association 241
American Stroke Association 328
amino acids 69, 182, 197
amphetamines 255, 255*f*
anabolic-androgenic steroids (AAS) 107-108
anaerobic (nonoxidative) system 71*t*, 72, 73, 90-92
android fat pattern 159, 159*f*
angina 326, 327*f*
anorexia nervosa 222, 251*f*
ANS (autonomic nervous system) 228
anterior deltoid muscles 144-145
antioxidants 185
anxiety

 binge-eating disorder and 223
 caffeine and 189, 190
 cardiorespiratory fitness and 75, 78
 generalized anxiety disorder 243
 HPA axis and 228
 lower back pain and 123
 management of 238
 panic disorder 243
 personality and 230
 sleep quality and 241
 social anxiety disorder 245
anxiolytics 252
apple body shape 159, 159*f*
areola 284
arm muscles 150-153
arrhythmias 326
arteries 64, 64*f*, 65
arteriosclerosis 326
arthritis 122
assault, sexual 312-315, 312*f*
asthma 38, 86
Åstrand, Per-Olof 18
atherosclerosis 324, 326, 330
ATP (adenosine triphosphate) 70, 70*f*, 72-73, 90
ATP-PC (adenosine triphosphate–phosphocreatine) system 71*t*, 72
atrophy 92-93
attitude, behavioral 51, 53
automated external defibrillators (AEDs) 328, 376
autonomic nervous system (ANS) 228
autonomy, in self-determination theory 51, 51*f*, 52

B

baby boomers, fitness practices of 29-30
BAC (blood alcohol concentration) 268-270, 269*f*
back muscles 138-139, 146-149
back pain. *See* low back pain
bacterial STIs 298, 298*f*, 306-309
balance training
 abdominals 137
 benefits of 119
 biceps 151
 calves 131
 chest and front shoulder 145
 gluteus maximus 135
 hamstrings 135
 hip abductors 141
 hip adductors 143
 latissimus dorsi 149
 lower back 139
 quadriceps 133
 triceps 153
 upper back and shoulders 147
ballistic stretching 115-116
bariatric surgery 219

ABOUT THE AUTHORS

Carol K. Armbruster, PhD, is the first teaching professor emeritus in the department of kinesiology in the School of Public Health at Indiana University (IU) at Bloomington. She previously served as a program director of fitness and wellness for the IU Division of Recreational Sports, where she managed a program that offered more than 100 group exercise sessions per week.

During her more than 35 years of teaching college students and training fitness leaders, she has served on the American College of Sports Medicine (ACSM) board of trustees and the American Council on Exercise (ACE) credentialing committees, and she is a fellow of ACSM. She is also an ACSM-certified exercise physiologist, holds the level 2 Exercise Is Medicine credential, and has enjoyed her work as a "pracademic" translating research to practice.

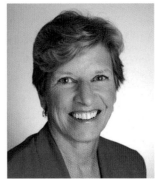

Courtesy of Indiana University School of Public Health-Bloomington.

Ellen M. Evans, PhD, is a department chair and professor at Indiana University. Previously, she was the associate dean for research and graduate education at University of Georgia (UGA) and director of the Center for Physical Activity and Health in the UGA College of Education. Prior to joining the faculty at UGA, she was a postdoctoral research fellow in geriatrics and gerontology and applied physiology at Washington University School of Medicine and was on the faculty of the University of Illinois at Urbana-Champaign.

Evans has been named a fellow of the American College of Sports Medicine (ACSM) and the National Academy of Kinesiology (NAK).

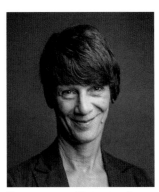

Photo courtesy of University of Georgia.

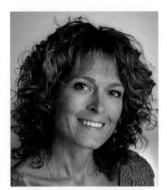

Catherine M. Laughlin, HSD, MPH, is a clinical professor and assistant department chair of the department of applied health science in the School of Public Health at Indiana University (IU) at Bloomington. Her research interests include sexual health education, cancer prevention and education, program planning, and implementation and evaluation in community-based organizations. She is regularly interviewed by media outlets as a human sexuality and sexual health education expert.

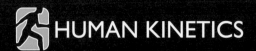
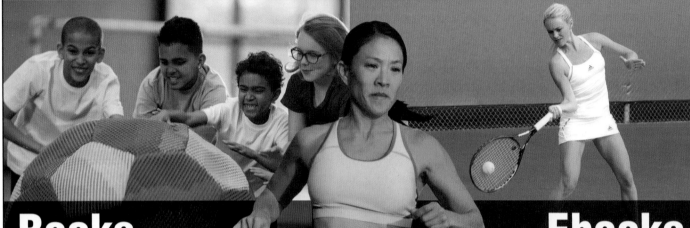
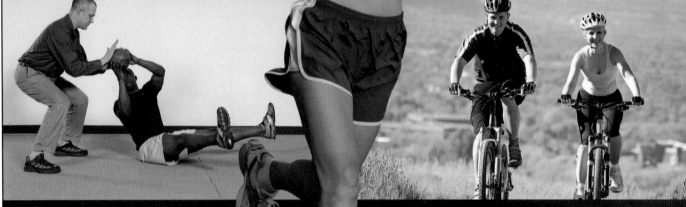